Inflammation: The Cause of All Diseases

Inflammation: The Cause of All Diseases

Editors

Vasso Apostolopoulos
Jack Feehan
Vivek P. Chavda

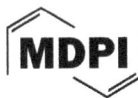

Basel • Beijing • Wuhan • Barcelona • Belgrade • Novi Sad • Cluj • Manchester

Editors

Vasso Apostolopoulos	Jack Feehan	Vivek P. Chavda
Victoria University	Victoria University	L M College of Pharmacy
Melbourne	Melbourne	Ahmedabad
Australia	Australia	India

Editorial Office
MDPI
St. Alban-Anlage 66
4052 Basel, Switzerland

This is a reprint of articles from the Topic published online in the open access journals *Biologics* (ISSN), *Cells* (ISSN 2079-9721), *Diseases* (ISSN 2076-328X), *International Journal of Molecular Sciences* (ISSN 1422-0067), and *Vaccines* (ISSN 2076-393X) (available at: https://www.mdpi.com/topics/inflammation).

For citation purposes, cite each article independently as indicated on the article page online and as indicated below:

Lastname, A.A.; Lastname, B.B. Article Title. *Journal Name* **Year**, *Volume Number*, Page Range.

ISBN 978-3-0365-8822-3 (Hbk)
ISBN 978-3-0365-8823-0 (PDF)
doi.org/10.3390/books978-3-0365-8823-0

© 2023 by the authors. Articles in this book are Open Access and distributed under the Creative Commons Attribution (CC BY) license. The book as a whole is distributed by MDPI under the terms and conditions of the Creative Commons Attribution-NonCommercial-NoDerivs (CC BY-NC-ND) license.

Contents

About the Editors ix

Preface xi

Hao Zhou and Qing Ye
Clinical Features of COVID-19 Vaccine-Associated Autoimmune Hepatitis:
A Systematic Review
Reprinted from: *Diseases* **2023**, *11*, 80, doi:10.3390/diseases11020080 1

Hayoung Choi, Jin Young Lee, Hongseok Yoo and Kyeongman Jeon
Bioinformatics Analysis of Gene Expression Profiles for Diagnosing Sepsis and Risk Prediction
in Patients with Sepsis
Reprinted from: *Int. J. Mol. Sci.* **2023**, *24*, 9362, doi:10.3390/ijms24119362 13

Mustafa Gandhi, Omar Elfeky, Hamza Ertugrul, Harleen Kaur Chela and Ebubekir Daglilar
Scurvy: Rediscovering a Forgotten Disease
Reprinted from: *Diseases* **2023**, *11*, 78, doi:10.3390/diseases11020078 27

Joanne M. Tang, Andrew McClennan, Linshan Liu, Jennifer Hadway, John A. Ronald, Justin W. Hicks, et al.
A Protocol for Simultaneous In Vivo Imaging of Cardiac and Neuroinflammation in
Dystrophin-Deficient MDX Mice Using [^{18}F]FEPPA PET
Reprinted from: *Int. J. Mol. Sci.* **2023**, *24*, 7522, doi:10.3390/ijms24087522 39

Luís Arpa, Carlos Batlle, Peijin Jiang, Carme Caelles, Jorge Lloberas and Antonio Celada
Distinct Responses to IL4 in Macrophages Mediated by JNK
Reprinted from: *Cells* **2023**, *12*, 1127, doi:10.3390/cells12081127 59

William Danilo Fernandes de Souza, Sofia Fernanda Gonçalves Zorzella-Pezavento, Marina Caçador Ayupe, Caio Loureiro Salgado, Bernardo de Castro Oliveira, Francielly Moreira, et al.
Lung Inflammation Induced by Inactivated SARS-CoV-2 in C57BL/6 Female Mice Is Controlled
by Intranasal Instillation of Vitamin D
Reprinted from: *Cells* **2023**, *12*, 1092, doi:10.3390/cells12071092 77

Yo Shimizu, Hiromi Sakata-Haga, Yutaka Saikawa and Toshihisa Hatta
Influence of Immune System Abnormalities Caused by Maternal Immune Activation in the
Postnatal Period
Reprinted from: *Cells* **2023**, *12*, 741, doi:10.3390/cells12050741 101

Marie-Claude Lampron, Isabelle Paré, Mohamed Al-Zahrani, Abdelhabib Semlali and Lionel Loubaki
annabinoid Mixture Affects the Fate and Functions of B Cells through the Modulation of the
Caspase and MAP Kinase Pathways
Reprinted from: *Cells* **2023**, *12*, 588, doi:10.3390/cells12040588 119

Xiyan Wang, Ruirui Ren, Bo Ma, Jing Xie, Yan Ma, Hong Luo, et al.
Comparative Study on MNVT of OPV Type I and III Reference Products in Different Periods
Reprinted from: *Diseases* **2023**, *11*, 28, doi:10.3390/diseases11010028 135

Puneetpal Singh, Nitin Kumar, Monica Singh, Manminder Kaur, Gurjinderpal Singh,
Amit Narang, et al.
Neutrophil Extracellular Traps and NLRP3 Inflammasome: A Disturbing Duo in
Atherosclerosis, Inflammation and Atherothrombosis
Reprinted from: *Vaccines* 2023, *11*, 261, doi:10.3390/vaccines11020261 145

Rose Calixte, Zachary Ye, Raisa Haq, Salwa Aladhamy and Marlene Camacho-Rivera
Demographic and Social Patterns of the Mean Values of Inflammatory Markers in U.S. Adults:
A 2009–2016 NHANES Analysis
Reprinted from: *Diseases* 2023, *11*, 14, doi:10.3390/diseases11010014 161

Zahid Ijaz Tarar, Umer Farooq, Mustafa Gandhi, Faisal Kamal, Moosa Feroze Tarar,
Veysel Tahan, et al.
Are Drugs Associated with Microscopic Colitis? A Systematic Review and Meta-Analysis
Reprinted from: *Diseases* 2023, *11*, 6, doi:10.3390/diseases11010006 177

Jolien Vandewalle, Bruno Garcia, Steven Timmermans, Tineke Vanderhaeghen,
Lise Van Wyngene, Melanie Eggermont, et al.
Hepatic Peroxisome Proliferator-Activated Receptor Alpha Dysfunction in Porcine Septic Shock
Reprinted from: *Cells* 2022, *11*, 4080, doi:10.3390/cells11244080 189

Yana Yang, Wenhui Qi, Yanyan Zhang, Ruining Wang, Mingyue Bao, Mengyuan Tian, et al.
Natural Compound 2,2′,4′-Trihydroxychalcone Suppresses T Helper 17 Cell Differentiation and
Disease Progression by Inhibiting Retinoid-Related Orphan Receptor Gamma T
Reprinted from: *Int. J. Mol. Sci.* 2022, *23*, 14547, doi:10.3390/ijms232314547 201

Zhijie Zheng, Yonghui Zheng, Xiaoben Liang, Guanhong Xue and Haichong Wu
Sanguinarine Enhances the Integrity of the Blood–Milk Barrier and Inhibits Oxidative Stress in
Lipopolysaccharide-Stimulated Mastitis
Reprinted from: *Cells* 2022, *11*, 3658, doi:10.3390/cells11223658 217

Yicheng Zhou, Zhangwang Li, Minxuan Xu, Deju Zhang, Jitao Ling, Peng Yu
and Yunfeng Shen
O-GlycNacylation Remission Retards the Progression of Non-Alcoholic Fatty Liver Disease
Reprinted from: *Cells* 2022, *11*, 3637, doi:10.3390/cells11223637 231

Gabriel Borges-Vélez, Juan A. Arroyo, Yadira M. Cantres-Rosario, Ana Rodriguez de Jesus,
Abiel Roche-Lima, Julio Rosado-Philippi, et al.
Decreased CSTB, RAGE, and Axl Receptor Are Associated with Zika Infection in the
Human Placenta
Reprinted from: *Cells* 2022, *11*, 3627, doi:10.3390/cells11223627 251

Yan Liu, Xuehua Kong, Yan You, Linwei Xiang, Yan Zhang, Rui Wu, et al.
S100A8-Mediated NLRP3 Inflammasome-Dependent Pyroptosis in Macrophages Facilitates
Liver Fibrosis Progression
Reprinted from: *Cells* 2022, *11*, 3579, doi:10.3390/cells11223579 269

Chenping Du, Rani O. Whiddett, Irina Buckle, Chen Chen, Josephine M. Forbes
and Amelia K. Fotheringham
Advanced Glycation End Products and Inflammation in Type 1 Diabetes Development
Reprinted from: *Cells* 2022, *11*, 3503, doi:10.3390/cells11213503 289

Avinash Khadela, Vivek P. Chavda, Humzah Postwala, Yesha Shah, Priya Mistry
and Vasso Apostolopoulos
Epigenetics in Tuberculosis: Immunomodulation of Host Immune Response
Reprinted from: *Vaccines* 2022, *10*, 1740, doi:10.3390/vaccines10101740 307

Amir Selimagic, Ada Dozic and Azra Husic-Selimovic
The Role of Novel Motorized Spiral Enteroscopy in the Diagnosis of Cecal Tumors
Reprinted from: *Diseases* **2022**, *10*, 79, doi:10.3390/diseases10040079 327

Tino Emanuele Poloni, Matteo Moretti, Valentina Medici, Elvira Turturici, Giacomo Belli, Elena Cavriani, et al.
COVID-19 Pathology in the Lung, Kidney, Heart and Brain: The Different Roles of T-Cells, Macrophages, and Microthrombosis
Reprinted from: *Cells* **2022**, *11*, 3124, doi:10.3390/cells11193124 335

Dhir Gala, Taylor Newsome, Nicole Roberson, Soo Min Lee, Marvel Thekkanal, Mili Shah, et al.
Thromboembolic Events in Patients with Inflammatory Bowel Disease: A Comprehensive Overview
Reprinted from: *Diseases* **2022**, *10*, 73, doi:10.3390/diseases10040073 359

He Li, Ya Meng, Shuwang He, Xiaochuan Tan, Yujia Zhang, Xiuli Zhang, et al.
Macrophages, Chronic Inflammation, and Insulin Resistance
Reprinted from: *Cells* **2022**, *11*, 3001, doi:10.3390/cells11193001 379

Asami Nishikori, Midori Filiz Nishimura, Yoshito Nishimura, Fumio Otsuka, Kanna Maehama, Kumiko Ohsawa, et al.
Idiopathic Plasmacytic Lymphadenopathy Forms an Independent Subtype of Idiopathic Multicentric Castleman Disease
Reprinted from: *Int. J. Mol. Sci.* **2022**, *23*, 10301, doi:10.3390/ijms231810301 403

Tor Persson Skare, Hiroshi Kaito, Claudia Durall, Teodor Aastrup and Lena Claesson-Welsh
Quartz Crystal Microbalance Measurement of Histidine-Rich Glycoprotein and Stanniocalcin-2 Binding to Each Other and to Inflammatory Cells
Reprinted from: *Cells* **2022**, *11*, 2684, doi:10.3390/cells11172684 413

Janice García-Quiroz, Bismarck Vázquez-Almazán, Rocío García-Becerra, Lorenza Díaz and Euclides Avila
The Interaction of Human Papillomavirus Infection and Prostaglandin E_2 Signaling in Carcinogenesis: A Focus on Cervical Cancer Therapeutics
Reprinted from: *Cells* **2022**, *11*, 2528, doi:10.3390/cells11162528 425

About the Editors

Vasso Apostolopoulos

Vasso Apostolopoulos is currently the Vice-Chancellor Distinguished Professorial Fellow (Distinguished Professor), Director of Immunology and Translational Research Group at Victoria University, Australia and Immunology Program Director at the Australian Institute for Musculoskeletal Science Australia. Previously, she has held several executive leadership roles including Pro Vice-Chancellor, Research Partnerships, Associate Provost. She received her PhD majoring in immunology from the University of Melbourne, and the Advanced Certificate in Protein Crystallography from Birkbeck College, University of London. Professor Vasso Apostolopoulos is a world-renowned researcher who has been recognized with over 100 awards for the outstanding results of her research. She has more than 510 research publications and 22 patents to her credit. Her interests include vaccine and drug development for cancer, chronic, infectious and autoimmune diseases. She is also interested in understanding inflammation and how to manipulate the immune system to treat diseases.

Jack Feehan

Jack Feehan is a Senior Research Fellow at the Institute for Health and Sport, Victoria University, with significant clinical and research expertise in the management of chronic diseases, particularly in older adults. Jack is a registered osteopath and gained a Ph.D. from the University of Melbourne in geriatric immunology, and now works on nutritional, exercise and pharmacological interventions in chronic cardiometabolic and musculoskeletal diseases. He also has a keen interest in inflammation and resulting diseases, such as type 2 diabetes and dementias. He has published over 70 papers, is an active supervisor of several PhD students and is an active presenter on the topics of inflammation and chronic diseases.

Vivek P. Chavda

Vivek P. Chavda is Assistant Professor (Selection Grade), Department of Pharmaceutics and Pharmaceutical Technology, L M College of Pharmacy, Ahmedabad, Gujarat, India. He is B Pharm and M Pharm Gold Medalist at Gujarat Technological University. Before joining academia, he served the biologics industry for almost 8 years in the Research and Development of Biologics with many successful regulatory filings. He has more than 170 peer-reviewed national and international publications, 18 book chapters, 10 book chapters under communication, 1 patent in pipeline and numerous newsletter articles to his credit. His research interests include the development of biologics process and formulations, medical device development, nano-diagnostics, and non-carrier formulations, long-acting parenteral formulations and nano-vaccines.

Preface

While inflammation is the body's natural response to stimuli and involved in healing following injury, if a stimulus persists over a long time, it can contribute to the development and progression of several diseases. Such diseases range from metabolic disorders, cancer, autoimmunity, to cardiovascular ailments and neurodegenerative syndromes. Herein, an array of topics are presented from an inflammation perspective on the diseases of COVID-19, zika infections, sepsis, tuberculosis, scurvy, polio, neuroinflammation, papilloma virus infections, Duchenne muscular dystrophy, atherosclerosis, colitis, inflammatory bowel disease, cancer, mastitis, non-alcoholic fatty liver disease, liver fibrosis, diabetes, insulin resistance, Castleman disease and the role of immune cells in inflammation, immune modulation and immune system abnormalities. We thank all authors who have contributed papers to make this Special Issue possible.

Vasso Apostolopoulos, Jack Feehan, and Vivek P. Chavda
Editors

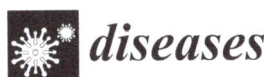

Systematic Review

Clinical Features of COVID-19 Vaccine-Associated Autoimmune Hepatitis: A Systematic Review

Hao Zhou and Qing Ye *

Department of Laboratory Medicine, Children's Hospital, Zhejiang University School of Medicine, National Clinical Research Center for Child Health, National Children's Regional Medical Center, Hangzhou 310000, China
* Correspondence: qingye@zju.edu.cn

Abstract: Autoimmune hepatitis (AIH) is an inflammatory liver disease wherein the body's immune system instigates an attack on the liver, causing inflammation and hepatic impairment. This disease usually manifests in genetically predisposed individuals and is triggered by stimuli or environments such as viral infections, environmental toxins, and drugs. The causal role of COVID-19 vaccination in AIH remains uncertain. This review of 39 cases of vaccine-related AIH indicates that female patients above the age of 50 years or those with potential AIH risk factors may be susceptible to vaccine-related AIH, and the clinical features of vaccine-associated AIH are similar to those of idiopathic AIH. These features commonly manifest in patients after the first dose of vaccination, with symptom onset typically delayed by 10–14 days. The incidence of underlying liver disease in patients with potential health conditions associated to liver disease is similar to that of patients without preexisting illnesses. Steroid administration is effective in treating vaccine-related AIH-susceptible patients, with most patients experiencing improvement in their clinical symptoms. However, care should be taken to prevent bacterial infections during drug administration. Furthermore, the possible pathogenic mechanisms of vaccine-associated AIH are discussed to offer potential ideas for vaccine development and enhancement. Although the incidence of vaccine-related AIH is rare, individuals should not be deterred from receiving the COVID-19 vaccine, as the benefits of vaccination significantly outweigh the risks.

Keywords: autoimmune hepatitis; COVID-19 vaccination; liver

Citation: Zhou, H.; Ye, Q. Clinical Features of COVID-19 Vaccine-Associated Autoimmune Hepatitis: A Systematic Review. *Diseases* **2023**, *11*, 80. https://doi.org/10.3390/diseases11020080

Academic Editors: Vasso Apostolopoulos, Jack Feehan and Vivek P. Chavda

Received: 30 March 2023
Revised: 17 May 2023
Accepted: 24 May 2023
Published: 30 May 2023

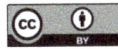

Copyright: © 2023 by the authors. Licensee MDPI, Basel, Switzerland. This article is an open access article distributed under the terms and conditions of the Creative Commons Attribution (CC BY) license (https://creativecommons.org/licenses/by/4.0/).

1. Introduction

Coronavirus disease 2019 (COVID-19), caused by severe acute respiratory syndrome coronavirus-2 (SARS-CoV-2) infection, quickly spread worldwide in December 2019. COVID-19 poses a significant threat to our lives and health and extensively damages society and the economy. There is an urgent need to treat and prevent COVID-19 in response to the fast-growing infection rate and escalating mortality toll, leading to COVID-19 vaccines being created and deployed at an unprecedented pace [1–3]. The United States Food and Drug Administration (FDA) granted an emergency use license for the Pfizer–BioNTech COVID-19 vaccine on 11 December 2020, and the Moderna vaccine on 18 December 2020. On 30 December 2020, the UK's Medicines and Healthcare Products Regulatory Agency (MHRA) authorized the Oxford–AstraZeneca vaccine [4].

A COVID-19 vaccination was administered to at least 68% of the world's population during the course of the following two years [5]. In phase III vaccine trials, the Pfizer–BioNTech and Moderna vaccine efficacies against COVID-19 were 91.3% and 93.2% in immunocompetent adults, respectively [6,7]. Solicited adverse events from BNT162b2 and the Moderna vaccine both involved fatigue, myalgia, arthralgia, and headache with moderate-to-severe systemic side effects. However, these effects resolved in most participants within two days and without sequelae [6,7]. Autoimmune conditions such as myocarditis and immunological thrombocytopenic purpura (ITP) are a noteworthy class of side effects associated with COVID-19 vaccinations [8,9]. There is no evidence of a causal relationship between the vaccine and autoimmune diseases due to a lack of data to investigate causality. Nevertheless, the occurrence of autoimmune diseases following COVID-19 vaccination should raise global public health concerns.

Case reports started to appear in 2021, and 39 patients with AIH-like syndromes have been reported thus far [10–34] (see Supplementary Materials). Autoimmune hepatitis, described by Waldenström in 1951, is a progressive inflammatory liver disease that may lead to cirrhosis, hepatocellular carcinoma, liver transplantation, and even death [35]. AIH is distinguished serologically by high alanine aminotransferase (ALT), aspartate aminotransferase (AST), immunoglobulin G (IgG), and autoantibody positivity, as well as histologically by interface hepatitis and lymphocytic infiltration of the liver [36,37]. AIH is not limited to any one racial or ethnic group, has a female-to-male ratio of 3.6:1, and affects both children and adults of all ages [38]. In this review, we describe the populations that may be susceptible to COVID-19 vaccine-associated AIH, the clinical features of vaccine-associated AIHs and the timing of the onset of symptoms and suggest how to administer treatment for vaccine-associated AIH and precautions to take. It provides reference for clinical diagnosis and treatment of vaccine-associated AIH.

2. Methods

A study of AIH syndrome after coronavirus disease 2019 (COVID-19) vaccination was performed. First, on 1 October 2022, we carried out a comprehensive search of the literature in the PubMed, Embase, and Web of Science databases. The search medical subjects heading (MeSH) terms included "COVID-19", "SARS-CoV-2", "autoimmune", and "hepatitis", along with "vaccine," "vaccination," and "mRNA." Second, to comprehensively collect relevant articles and cases, we eliminated all duplicate reports. Then, we screened the remaining articles based on their titles and abstracts and removed any reports that did not contain case studies, were irrelevant, or were missing critical clinical information. The filtering process is shown in Figure 1. This review was not registered in any registry and has no registration number.

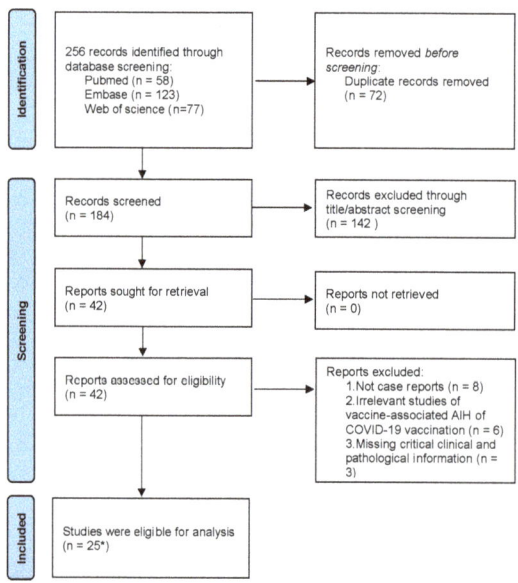

Figure 1. PRISMA flowchart describing the process of selecting eligible studies. * of the 25 articles included in the review, two contained three cases, two contained two cases, one was a series of case reports with nine cases, and the rest consisted of a single case. AIH, autoimmune hepatitis.

The patient's baseline characteristics were collected, such as age, sex, medication, and medical history, and clinical symptoms following the COVID-19 vaccine injection. We also gathered information on the COVID-19 vaccine, such as the type of vaccine, the timing of the first vaccination for patients, and the symptoms that appeared after the vaccine injection. Regarding AIH, we collected transaminase laboratory peak values, liver biopsies, and autoimmune antibodies. In addition, these patients' therapeutic drugs and clinical outcomes were documented.

3. Characteristics of Patients with Vaccine-Associated AIH before Vaccination

A total of 39 cases of COVID-19 vaccine-associated AIH syndromes were collected from databases [10–34]. The median age of diagnosis was 59.0 years, with 24 (61.5%) patients over 50 years old. The oldest and youngest ages were 80 and 23, respectively, and 30 (76.9%) patients were female (Figure 2A,B). In our study, except for five patients who were not recorded clearly, nine patients had a history of liver disease, eight patients had a history of autoimmune disease, four patients had a history of medication that induced AIH, and one patient had a history of both medication and autoimmune disease (Figure 2C). This generated 22 (64.7%) patients with a history of autoimmune disease, liver disease, or medications.

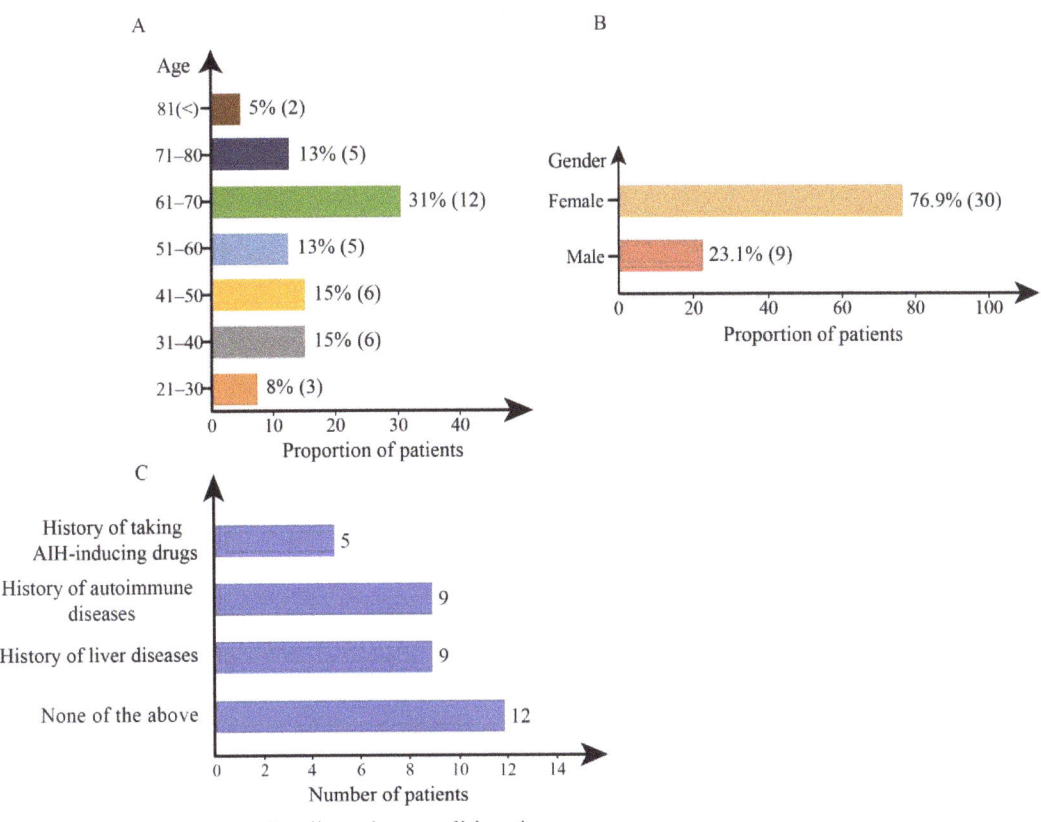

Figure 2. Pre-vaccination characteristics of patients with vaccine-associated AIH. Patient age (**A**), sex (**B**), and predisposing conditions (**C**). * one patient had a history of both taking AIH-inducing drugs and autoimmune diseases.

Twelve patients had no history of autoimmune or hepatic disease (Figure 2C). One patient was diagnosed with gestational hypertension during pregnancy and started on labetalol 100 mg bid. Three months postpartum, she developed AIH after COVID-19 vaccination [12]. One patient had a history of hypertension treated with olmesartan and laser eye surgery two weeks prior that required topical fluoroquinolone eye drops, 1 g acetaminophen TDS, and 400 mg ibuprofen TDS for one week total [16]. One patient was on a long-term course of omeprazole, losartan, and bromazepam treatment [27]. One patient had no side effects during replacement hormone therapy after a history of early ovarian failure [29]. One patient with sarcoidosis had not received treatment [32]. Another patient received ceftriaxone due to a urinary tract infection [33]. Two patients had taken Tylenol [33]. The remaining four patients had no medication or medical history [23,26,30,31].

Upon analyzing these 39 cases, the data suggest that a majority of the vaccinated patients who experienced onset symptoms were female, constituting 30 (76.9%) of the total cases. Furthermore, the age range for a significant portion of these patients was over 50 years, representing 24 (61.5%) of the observed cases. Additionally, an intriguing observation that emerged from the analysis was that 22 (64.7%) of the patients exhibited autoimmune disorders, had a history of liver disease, or had been administered medications that have the potential to induce AIH. Thus, it can be inferred that individuals belonging to this subset of the vaccinated population should be subjected to more vigilant monitoring.

4. Characteristics of Patients with Vaccine-Associated AIH after Vaccination

4.1. Time of Onset of Symptoms

AIH was documented following the Pfizer–BioNTech, Moderna, and Oxford–AstraZeneca vaccines in 18, 15, and 6 cases, respectively. Twenty-nine patients had clinical symptoms after receiving the initial vaccination, seven patients after receiving the second vaccination, three patients after receiving both the initial and second vaccination, and one patient had no record (Table 1). This suggests that most patients develop symptoms after receiving the first dose of the vaccine. After receiving the COVID-19 vaccine, the cohort included 39 cases from our collection, and the median time to symptom onset in patients was 14.0 days. This delay period ranged from 1 to 53 days. The presentation occurred 2–53 days after vaccination against SARS-CoV-2 with Pfizer–BioNTech, with a median of 10 days. The median time from the Moderna vaccine to presentation was 12.5 days, and patients presented between 3 and 46 days. In the reported case of vaccination AstraZeneca, the onset symptom occurred at median of 18.0 days with a range of 12 to 26 days. Next, we analyzed the time of onset of the first symptoms in patients with underlying health or medication conditions and patients without preexisting conditions. The median time for the onset of symptoms after vaccination was 13 days for patients with poor health or medication status related to liver disease and the median 10 days for patients without preexisting conditions. Overall, the data suggest a 10–14-day delay in the onset of symptoms after vaccination, which is similar between the patients with underlying health related to liver diseases and the cohort with no preexisting conditions.

Table 1. Clinical presentation of vaccine-associated AIH.

Type of Vaccines [a]	No. of Patients (%)	Autoantibodies [d]	No. of Patients (%)
Pfizer–BioNTech	18 (46.2%)	ANA	25 (78.1%)
Moderna	15 (38.4%)	ASMA	12 (37.5%)
Oxford–AstraZeneca	6 (15.4%)	ds-DNA	2 (6.3%)
Time of onset of symptoms [b]	No. of Patients (%)	Anti-SLA	1 (3.1%)
First vaccination	31 (81.6%)	Anti-LC1	1 (3.1%)
Second vaccination	7 (18.4%)	ANCA	1 (3.1%)
Symptoms [c]	No. of Patients (%)	None	4 (12.5%)
Jaundice	21 (75.0%)	Serum biochemical parameters [e]	Median (Range)

Table 1. Cont.

Type of Vaccines [a]	No. of Patients (%)	Autoantibodies [d]	No. of Patients (%)
Fatigue	7 (25.0%)	ALT (U/L)	1038 (171–2664)
Anorexia	5 (17.9%)	AST (U/L)	862 (111–2314)
Choluria	5 (17.9%)	ALP (U/L)	186 (24–2252)
Anorexia	5 (17.9%)	Tbil (U/L)	3.84 (0.33–45)
Pruritus	5 (17.9%)	GGT (U/L)	345 (98–810)
Abdominal pain	5 (17.9%)	Total IgG(mg/dL)	1998 (1081–4260)
Fever	5 (17.9%)	Liver biopsy [a]	No. of Patients (%)
Diarrhea	1 (3.6%)	Interface hepatitis	23 (59.0%)
Asymptomatic	1 (3.6%)	pycnotic necrosis	14 (35.9%)
		Lymphocyte/plasma cells infiltration	35 (89.7%)
		Eosinophils	11 (30.8%)

[a]: Thirty-nine patients had recorded the type of vaccine and liver biopsy. [b]: One out of 39 patients had no record of the type of vaccine. [c]: Eleven out of 39 patients had no documentation of symptoms. [d]: Seven out of 39 patients had no record of autoantibodies. [e]: The result of ALT, AST, ALP, Tbil, GGT, and total IgG were recorded for 39, 28, 28, 35, 13, and 26 patients, respectively. ALT, alanine aminotransferase; AST, aspartate aminotransferase; ALP, alkaline phosphatase; TBL, total bilirubin; GGT, gamma glutamyl transferase; IgG, immunoglobulin G; ANA, anti-nuclear antibodies; ASMA, anti-smooth muscle antibodies; ds-DNA; anti-double stranded DNA; anti-SLA, antibodies against soluble liver antigen; anti-LC1, anti-liver cytosol type 1.

4.2. Clinical Presentation of Patients with Vaccine-Associated AIH

Twenty-eight patients clinical symptoms were documented, and 11 patients were not recorded. The most common symptoms were jaundice in 21 (75.0%) patients and fatigue in 7 (25.0%). Choluria, anorexia, pruritus, abdominal pain, and fever each accounted for five (17.9%) patients. Diarrhea and asymptomatic symptoms were observed in only one (3.6%) patient (Table 1). Idiopathic AIH may present with one or more nonspecific symptoms, and fatigue is a more common presentation [36]. However, the primary clinical manifestation of vaccine-associated AIH is jaundice and multiple nonspecific symptoms, suggesting the need for concern about liver function in people who develop jaundice from vaccination.

Interestingly, three patients among all cases experienced a recurrence of symptoms after each of the vaccinations. The first patient exhibited malaise and jaundice after receiving the first vaccine. However, as his jaundice faded and liver function tests improved, these symptoms returned shortly after the second dose [17]. One day after receiving the first vaccination dosage, the second patient initially developed nausea, vomiting, and abdominal pain. Her symptoms resolved without a therapeutic record. After receiving her boost dose of vaccine, her symptoms—choluria and jaundice—returned with greater intensity [23]. Similarly, another patient who received the first and second doses of the vaccine presented pruritus and jaundice, respectively [29]. These data suggest that this may be the onset of vaccine-induced AIH.

4.3. Serological Profile of Patients with Vaccine-Associated AIH

The typical biochemical features of idiopathic AIH are aspartate aminotransferase (AST) and alanine aminotransferase (ALT), ranging from slightly above the upper limit of normal to more than 50-fold, and gamma-glutamyl transferase (GGT) and alkaline phosphatase (ALP), which are usually normal or only moderately elevated [39,40]. Hepatocellular liver damage was the most prevalent pattern in our data, with transaminase levels noticeably increasing to levels close to thousands. The median ALT level was 1043.0 U/L, the median AST was 854.6 U/L, the median ALP was 193.0 U/L, the median total bilirubin level was 3.9 mg/dl, and the GGT level was 361.0 U/L (Table 1). In addition, total immunoglobulin G (IgG) levels were recorded in 24 individuals, among whom 19 (79.2%) had elevated levels. Previous work has revealed that approximately 85% of individuals with idiopathic AIH have high IgG levels [40]. These results suggest that vaccine-associated AIH may be consistent with the biochemical profile of idiopathic AIH.

Autoantibodies are a defining feature of AIH and play a significant role in the diagnostic process. Of the data collected, autoantibodies were recorded in 32 cases and were undocumented in 7. Twenty-eight patients (87.5%) tested positive for at least one of the autoantibodies. Antinuclear antibody (ANA) and anti-smooth muscle (ASMA) were positive in 25 (78.1%) and 12 (37.5%) patients, respectively, and anti-double-stranded DNA (ds-DNA) antibodies were found in 2 (6.3%) patients. Furthermore, antibodies against soluble liver antigens (anti-SLA), anti-liver cytosol type 1 (anti-LC1), and anti-neutrophil cytoplasmic antibodies (ANCAs) were detected in only one (3.1%) patient each. In contrast, autoantibody screening yielded entirely negative results in four (12.5%) patients (Table 1). In a study of idiopathic AIH, 1152 patients (88%) were positive for ANA, and 1089 patients (83%) were positive for SMA at the time of diagnosis [41]. This result is higher than the autoantibodies expressed by vaccine-associated AIH. However, some patients with vaccine-associated AIH without elevated IgG or negative autoantibodies have also been observed. Such patients should not be ignored, as elevated serum IgG and antinuclear antibody levels are not observed in some patients with acute AIH [42]. It is essential to keep in mind the possibility of acute AIH, as a delay in diagnosis and initiation of treatment can lead to a poor prognosis of AIH.

4.4. Liver Histology with Vaccine-Associated AIH

Histological features of liver biopsy are considered a prerequisite for diagnosing AIH [43]. The typical hallmarks of AIH are interface hepatitis with dense plasma cell-rich lymphoplasmacytic infiltrates, hepatocellular rosette formation, emperipolesis, hepatocyte swelling, and/or pyknotic necrosis [43,44]. Typically, plasma cells are plentiful at the interface and throughout the lobule, but in 34% of instances, the lack of plasma cells in the inflammatory infiltrate does not rule out the diagnosis [45].

In the cohort, liver biopsy of all patients was performed. Twenty-three (59.0%) patients showed interface hepatitis. Fourteen (35.9%) patients had centrilobular necrosis. Thirty-five (89.7%) patients showed lymphocyte or plasma cell infiltration. Another two patients were compatible with AIH but did not describe the details of live biopsy (Table 1). Twenty patients were diagnosed with AIH using the Simplified AIH score [46] or the revised original score [47]. In 19 cases, clinical symptoms, laboratory data, and liver biopsy histology supported the probable diagnosis of AIH. Moreover, eosinophils were also found in liver biopsies of 11 patients (30.8%), suggesting that liver injury may be due to drugs or toxic substances.

5. Treatment and Outcomes in Patients with Vaccine-Associated AIH

The aim of treatment in idiopathic AIH is to obtain complete histological and biochemical remission [48,49]. Prednisolone, prednisone coupled with or without azathioprine, or budesonide and azathioprine alternately are therapeutic medicines with a high incidence of remission and a favorable prognosis [49,50]. In all cases, steroids were used as a first-line agent in 35 (89.7%) patients (Figure 3A). One patient's liver function test did not improve after receiving N-acetyl cysteine as a first-line therapy, and methylprednisolone had to be administered as a second medication [23]. Thirteen patients received prednisone, 14 received prednisolone, 4 received nonspecific steroids, and 1 received budesonide from the patients who received steroids as first-line therapy. Each of the remaining patients received ursodeoxycholic acid, endoscopic biliary dilation, or no treatment. All patients showed improved liver function except four who died (Figure 3B).

Four deaths in patients aged over 60 years were observed in this study. The first patient without autoimmune diseases was a 68-year-old woman who developed severe AIH after the AstraZeneca vaccination. After treatment with steroids for four weeks (1 mg/kg), the patient did not improve and developed hepatic encephalopathy and liver failure. After three days, the patient died of hepatic failure and sepsis [22]. In the second case, a 72-year-old woman was initially immunized with two doses of the AstraZeneca vaccine without incident. She was not known to have any medical conditions or be taking any medications.

She was diagnosed with AIH and initiated prednisolone 40 mg once daily for two weeks, with tapering doses subsequently. Although liver function improved initially, the patient died of severe sepsis two weeks later [23]. A 77-year-old woman without autoimmune disorders presented symptoms two days after receiving the second dose of the Pfizer–BioNTech vaccine and was hospitalized the following day. After three weeks on prednisone 60 mg/day, liver tests improved significantly. Two months later, azathioprine was added but discontinued due to rash, followed by budesonide 9 mg/day instead of prednisone. Five months later, the liver enzymes were in the normal range. Unfortunately, the patient developed a possible infectious brain injury and died one month later [27]. Another patient, a 62-year-old diabetic male, had been vaccinated with AstraZeneca and, after 13 days, developed symptoms lasting three days. After treatment with 30 mg/day prednisolone, a transient improvement in liver enzymes was observed. Due to cholestasis, he also had five rounds of therapeutic plasma exchange; however, his condition did not improve. Based on the clinical presentation, the patient required liver transplantation, and due to financial constraints, the patient eventually died [31].

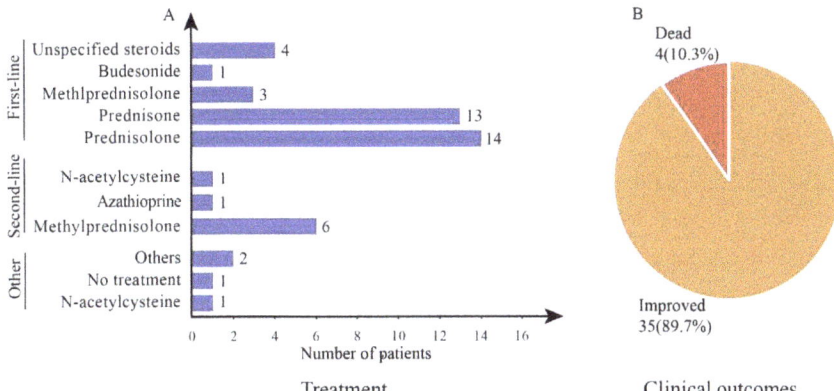

Figure 3. Treatment and outcomes of patients with vaccine-associated AIH. Patient medication (**A**) and clinical outcomes (**B**).

Among the cases in our collection, one case report demonstrated remission in a patient with vaccine-associated AIH without any treatment [33], and this phenomenon does not seem to be coincidental. A study on uncontrolled idiopathic AIH revealed that untreated asymptomatic patients had similar survival rates compared to patients undergoing immunosuppressive therapy with glucocorticoids or azathioprine [51], and spontaneous improvement of AIH may occur [52]. Therefore, this phenomenon may be justified. Should patients like this be ignored? The answer should be no. Studies indicate that a proportion of asymptomatic patients who exhibit symptoms during disease follow-up are at risk of developing end-stage liver disease with liver failure and developing hepatocellular carcinoma (HCC) [51,53]. In addition, since nearly half of all instances of idiopathic AIH have an asymptomatic subclinical course [41], it is unclear whether the cases reported thus far are the full scope of vaccine-associated AIH. However, there are no data on the overall recurrence rates and long-term outcomes for vaccine-related AIH. Therefore, we must remain vigilant and require regular follow-up and liver function testing after vaccination in patients with risk factors.

By assessing the clinical prognosis of patients diagnosed with vaccine-induced AIH, we found that treatment with steroids for vaccine-associated AIH proved effective, leading to a favorable prognosis in 35 (89.7%) patients. Regrettably, four patients were unable to recover and passed away. The treatment they received did not differ significantly from that of most patients with vaccine-associated AIH, but their deaths were attributed to sepsis, which resulted from personal variations. This highlights the importance of careful dosing and medication regimens for patients with vaccine-associated AIH to address any potential treatment-related infections. Therefore, if a bacterial infection is suspected, steroid therapy should be promptly discontinued and antimicrobial therapy initiated.

6. The Potential Mechanism of the Pathogenesis of AIH

While there is currently no concrete evidence of a causal link between the COVID-19 vaccine and AIH, the data we have collected suggest that a possible correlation between vaccination and the occurrence of AIH.

It is plausible that a complex interaction between vaccine components and the vaccinated individual's susceptibility may be responsible for triggering AIH in response to COVID-19 vaccination. One potential mechanism involved in the development of vaccine-related autoimmune disorders is molecular mimicry, which refers to the similarities between peptide sequences in vaccines and those found in the human body's self-peptides [54]. This similarity may be sufficient to lead to immune cross-interactions in which the immune system's response to pathogenic antigens may impair similar human proteins and thus induce autoimmune diseases. The study reported similarities between the small hepatitis B surface antigen (sHBsAg) contained in the vaccine and the MS autoantigens myelin basic protein (MBP) and myelin oligodendrocyte glycoprotein (MOG)—which can be used as targets for immune cross-reaction—by comparing serum samples from 58 adults before and after receiving the HBV vaccine [55,56]. By detecting homology between HPV viral peptides and human proteins, another study indicated a significant overlap between viral and various potential SLE-associated peptides [55,56]. The autoimmune/inflammatory syndrome-induced adjuvant (ASIA) has garnered attention in recent years. Adjuvants are compounds used in the manufacture of vaccines and are designed to enhance the ability of the vaccine to produce an immune response. There are reports suggesting that adjuvants act as ligands for Toll-like receptors (TLRs) through molecular mimicry, triggering the activation of the TLR pathway and the production of type I interferons (IFNs) and proinflammatory cytokines. Moreover, adjuvants activate dendritic cell recruitment through chemotaxis and antigen presentation, resulting in a more robust B cell and T cell response. Ultimately, this leads to an increased adaptive immune response against the antigen [57,58]. To date, the pathogenic mechanism of COVID-19 vaccine-associated AIH is not known. However, recent research indicated that SARS-CoV-2 antibodies produced moderate-to-strong responses with 21 out of 50 tissue antigens [59], suggesting that molecular mimicry likely plays a role. Molecular mimicry results in the production of homologous self-antigens [60], leading to autoimmune diseases [36].

The hypothesized molecular mechanism of autoimmune-mediated liver injury is shown in Figure 4. The presentation of a self-antigenic peptide to the T cell receptor (TCR) of T helper cells (Th0) by antigen-presenting cells (APCs). In healthy conditions, T cells that recognize self-antigens undergo apoptosis by clonal deletion or differentiate into anergic T cells. TGF-β stimulates the differentiation of Th0 cells into regulatory T cells (Tregs), which have immunosuppressive effects [61]. However, in abnormal immune conditions, immune cells against self-antigens remain active and cause autoimmune diseases. The uncommitted Th0 cells differentiate into Th1, Th2, or Th17 cells depending on the cytokine environment [62–64]. Th1 cells secrete interleukin-2 (IL-2) and interferon-γ (IFNγ), stimulating CD8+ cells to recognize the antigen–major histocompatibility complex (MHC) class I complex and activating macrophages to secrete IL-1 and tumor necrosis factor (TNFα) to recognize MCH II, respectively. The Th1 cell proportion and IFN-γ secretion were lower in healthy controls than in patients with AIH [39,63,64]. Th2 cells, on the other hand, secrete cytokines (e.g., IL-4, IL-10, and IL-13) that may stimulate self-antigen reactive B cells that produce autoantibodies [63,64]. Autoantibodies target liver cells and induce damage through natural killer (NK) cells and complement-mediated cytotoxicity. Th17 cells produce proinflammatory cytokines (e.g., IL-17 and IL-22) and TNF-α, leading to the induction of hepatic secretion of IL-6. While the existence of Th17 cells in AIH has been reported, their precise role in disease pathogenesis remains incompletely understood [62,64].

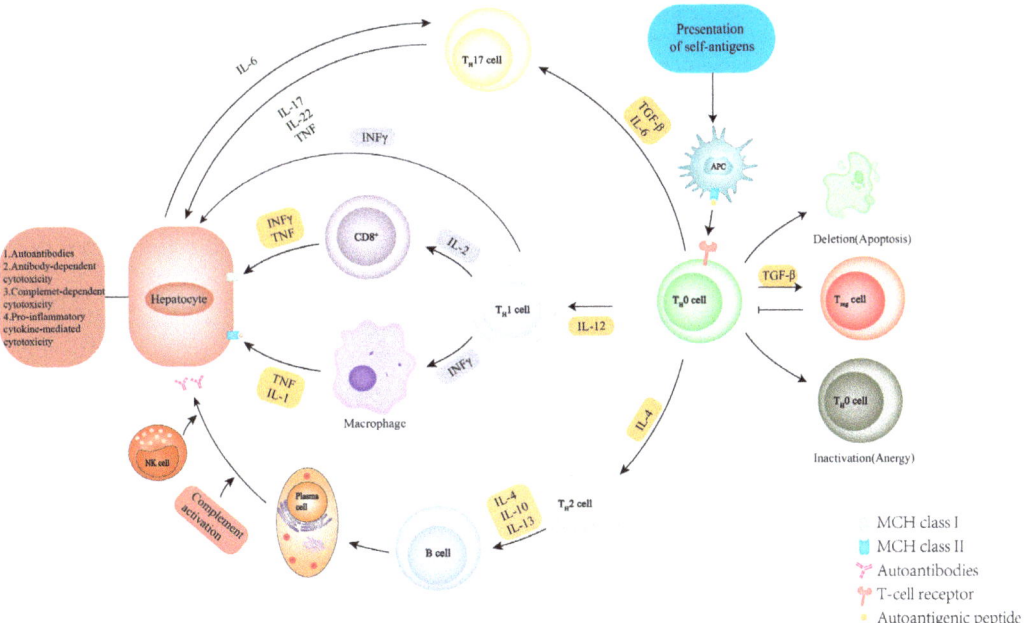

Figure 4. The potential mechanism of the pathogenesis of autoimmune hepatitis. APC, antigen-presenting cell; IFNγ, interferon-γ; MHC, major histocompatibility complex; NK, natural killer; TCR, T cell receptor; TGFβ, transforming growth factor-β; T_H0, naive CD4+ T helper; T_H1, T helper 1; T_H2, T helper 2; T_H17, T helper 17; TNF, tumor necrosis factor; Treg, regulatory T.

7. Limitations

Our study has several limitations that must be acknowledged. First, limited records on the medication and health history of the patients prior to vaccination could have led to oversights of potential risk factors predisposing to AIH. Additionally, incomplete documentation of patient symptoms and laboratory values in the original article resulted in a limited diagnosis of immune-mediated hepatitis following vaccination. Second, due to the possibility of publication bias in case reports and partial asymptomatic patients, it is difficult to accurately determine the incidence of vaccine-related AIH. This could potentially lead to underestimation of the risks involved. Third, as this manuscript lacked data that could be available to examine causal relationships, for example, lack of control data and insufficient number of cases; it is not possible to establish a causal relationship between the vaccine and AIH with the current data.

8. Conclusions

In these 39 cases, the majority of patients were women, over 50 years old, and with potential AIH risk factors, and there are no available data to date to check that AIH occurs after vaccination. Furthermore, vaccine-associated AIH seems to present with consistent clinical features, including clinical symptoms, biochemical features, autoantibodies, and liver biopsy findings, compared to idiopathic AIH. Patients who are asymptomatic after vaccination should be closely monitored, and their liver function should be evaluated. Moreover, while steroid therapy is effective in treating vaccine-associated AIH, it is noteworthy that individual variability may lead to sepsis caused by bacterial infection. Finally, these risk factors should not deter individuals from receiving the COVID-19 vaccine, as a physician has a duty to promote vaccination while being cognizant of potential risks and striving to enhance current medical practice and minimize harm.

Supplementary Materials: The following supporting information can be downloaded at: https://www.mdpi.com/article/10.3390/diseases11020080/s1, Table S1: Clinical information for patients with vaccine-associated AIH.

Author Contributions: Q.Y. devised the conceptual ideas, contributed to the discussion and interpretation of the results, and reviewed the final manuscript. H.Z. drafted the initial manuscript and contributed to manuscript editing. All authors have read and agreed to the published version of the manuscript.

Funding: This study was supported by the Natural Science Foundation of Zhejiang Province (LY22H050001); the National Natural Science Foundation of China (U20A20351); the Key Project of Provincial Ministry Co-Construction, Health Science, and Technology Project Plan of Zhejiang Province (WKJ-ZJ-2128); and Yiluqihang · Shenmingyuanyang's Medical Development and Scientific Research Fund Project on Kidney Diseases (SMYY20220301001).

Institutional Review Board Statement: Not applicable.

Informed Consent Statement: Not applicable.

Data Availability Statement: Not applicable.

Conflicts of Interest: The authors declare that this research was conducted without any commercial or financial relationships that could be construed as a potential conflict of interest.

References

1. Pascarella, G.; Strumia, A.; Piliego, C.; Bruno, F.; Del Buono, R.; Costa, F.; Scarlata, S.; Agrò, F.E. COVID-19 diagnosis and management: A comprehensive review. *J. Intern. Med.* **2020**, *288*, 192–206. [CrossRef] [PubMed]
2. Slaoui, M.; Hepburn, M. Developing Safe and Effective Covid Vaccines-Operation Warp Speed's Strategy and Approach. *N. Engl. J. Med.* **2020**, *383*, 1701–1703. [CrossRef] [PubMed]
3. Ho, R.J.Y. Warp-Speed Covid-19 Vaccine Development: Beneficiaries of Maturation in Biopharmaceutical Technologies and Public-Private Partnerships. *J. Pharm. Sci.* **2021**, *110*, 615–618. [CrossRef] [PubMed]
4. Fiolet, T.; Kherabi, Y.; MacDonald, C.J.; Ghosn; Peiffer-Smadja, N. Comparing COVID-19 vaccines for their characteristics, efficacy and effectiveness against SARS-CoV-2 and variants of concern: A narrative review. *Clin. Microbiol. Infect.* **2022**, *28*, 202–221. [CrossRef] [PubMed]
5. Coronavirus Pandemic (COVID-19). Available online: https://ourworldindata.org/coronavirus#citation (accessed on 16 May 2023).
6. Barda, N.; Dagan, N.; Ben-Shlomo, Y.; Kepten, E.; Waxman, J.; Ohana, R.; Hernán, M.A.; Lipsitch, M.; Kohane, I.; Netzer, D.; et al. Safety of the BNT162b2 mRNA Covid-19 Vaccine in a Nationwide Setting. *N. Engl. J. Med.* **2021**, *385*, 1078–1090. [CrossRef]
7. Baden, L.R.; El Sahly, H.M.; Essink, B.; Kotloff, K.; Frey, S.; Novak, R.; Diemert, D.; Spector, S.A.; Rouphael, N.; Creech, C.B.; et al. Efficacy and Safety of the mRNA-1273 SARS-CoV-2 Vaccine. *N. Engl. J. Med.* **2021**, *384*, 403–416. [CrossRef]
8. Bozkurt, B.; Kamat, I.; Hotez, P.J. Myocarditis With COVID-19 mRNA Vaccines. *Circulation* **2021**, *144*, 471–484. [CrossRef]
9. Long, B.; Bridwell, R.; Gottlieb, M. Thrombosis with thrombocytopenia syndrome associated with COVID-19 vaccines. *Am. J. Emerg. Med.* **2021**, *49*, 58–61. [CrossRef]
10. Garrido, I.; Lopes, S.; Simoes, M.S.; Liberal, R.; Lopes, J.; Carneiro, F.; Macedo, G. Autoimmune hepatitis after COVID-19 vaccine–more than a coincidence. *J. Autoimmun.* **2021**, *125*, 102741. [CrossRef]
11. Avci, E.; Abasiyanik, F. Autoimmune hepatitis after SARS-CoV-2 vaccine: New-onset or flare-up? *J. Autoimmun.* **2021**, *125*, 102745. [CrossRef]
12. Bril, F.; Al Diffalha, S.; Dean, M.; Fettig, D.M. Autoimmune hepatitis developing after coronavirus disease 2019 (COVID-19) vaccine: Causality or casualty? *J. Hepatol.* **2021**, *75*, 222–224. [CrossRef]
13. Ghielmetti, M.; Schaufelberger, H.D.; Mieli-Vergani, G.; Cerny, A.; Dayer, E.; Vergani, D.; Terziroli Beretta-Piccoli, B. Acute autoimmune-like hepatitis with atypical anti-mitochondrial antibody after mRNA COVID-19 vaccination: A novel clinical entity? *J. Autoimmun.* **2021**, *123*, 102706. [CrossRef]
14. Rocco, A.; Sgamato, C.; Compare, D.; Nardone, G. Autoimmune hepatitis following SARS-CoV-2 vaccine: May not be a casuality. *J. Hepatol.* **2021**, *75*, 728–729. [CrossRef]
15. Tan, C.K.; Wong, Y.J.; Wang, L.M.; Ang, T.L.; Kumar, R. Autoimmune hepatitis following COVID-19 vaccination: True causality or mere association? *J. Hepatol.* **2021**, *75*, 1250–1252. [CrossRef]
16. Clayton-Chubb, D.; Schneider, D.; Freeman, E.; Kemp, W.; Roberts, S.K. Autoimmune hepatitis developing after the ChAdOx1 nCoV-19 (Oxford-AstraZeneca) vaccine. *J. Hepatol.* **2021**, *75*, 1249–1250. [CrossRef]
17. Depret, F.; Bouam, S.; Schwarzinger, M.; Mallet, V. Demosthenes research g. Reply to: "Focus on the decisions to forego life-sustaining therapies during ICU stay of patients with cirrhosis and COVID-19: A case control study from the prospective COVID-ICU database". *J. Hepatol.* **2022**, *76*, 744–747. [CrossRef]

18. Lodato, F.; Larocca, A.; D'Errico, A.; Cennamo, V. An unusual case of acute cholestatic hepatitis after m-RNABNT162b2 (Comirnaty) SARS-CoV-2 vaccine: Coincidence, autoimmunity or drug-related liver injury. *J. Hepatol.* **2021**, *75*, 1254–1256. [CrossRef]
19. Ghelfi, J.; Brusset, B.; Thony, F.; Decaens, T. Successful management of refractory ascites in non-TIPSable patients using percutaneous thoracic duct stenting. *J. Hepatol.* **2022**, *76*, 216–218. [CrossRef]
20. Mahalingham, A.; Duckworth, A.; Griffiths, W.J.H. First report of posttransplant autoimmune hepatitis recurrence following SARS-CoV-2 mRNA vaccination. *Transpl. Immunol.* **2022**, *72*, 101600. [CrossRef]
21. Fimiano, F.; D'Amato, D.; Gambella, A.; Marzano, A.; Saracco, G.M.; Morgando, A. Autoimmune hepatitis or drug-induced autoimmune hepatitis following Covid-19 vaccination? *Liver Int.* **2022**, *42*, 1204–1205. [CrossRef]
22. Erard, D.; Villeret, F.; Lavrut, P.M.; Dumortier, J. Autoimmune hepatitis developing after COVID 19 vaccine: Presumed guilty? *Clin. Res. Hepatol. Gastroenterol.* **2022**, *46*, 101841. [CrossRef] [PubMed]
23. Kang, S.H.; Kim, M.Y.; Cho, M.Y.; Baik, S.K. Autoimmune Hepatitis Following Vaccination for SARS-CoV-2 in Korea: Coincidence or Autoimmunity? *J. Korean Med. Sci.* **2022**, *37*, e116. [CrossRef] [PubMed]
24. Shahrani, S.; Sooi, C.Y.; Hilmi, I.N.; Mahadeva, S. Autoimmune hepatitis (AIH) following coronavirus (COVID-19) vaccine-No longer exclusive to mRNA vaccine? *Liver Int.* **2022**, *42*, 2344–2345. [CrossRef] [PubMed]
25. Lasagna, A.; Lenti, M.V.; Cassaniti, I.; Sacchi, P. Development of hepatitis triggered by SARS-CoV-2 vaccination in patient with cancer during immunotherapy: A case report. *Immunotherapy* **2022**, *14*, 915–925. [CrossRef]
26. Goulas, A.; Kafiri, G.; Kranidioti, H.; Manolakopoulos, S. A typical autoimmune hepatitis (AIH) case following COVID-19 mRNA vaccination. More than a coincidence? *Liver Int.* **2022**, *42*, 254–255. [CrossRef]
27. Pinazo-Bandera, J.M.; Hernandez-Albujar, A.; Garcia-Salguero, A.I.; Arranz-Salas, I.; Andrade, R.J.; Robles-Diaz, M. Acute hepatitis with autoimmune features after COVID-19 vaccine: Coincidence or vaccine-induced phenomenon? *Gastroenterol. Rep.* **2022**, *10*, goac014. [CrossRef]
28. Bjornsson, H.K.; Bjornsson, E.S. Reply to: "Can azathioprine prevent infliximab-induced liver injury?". *J. Hepatol.* **2022**, *77*, 555–556. [CrossRef]
29. Londono, M.C.; Gratacos-Gines, J.; Saez-Penataro, J. Another case of autoimmune hepatitis after SARS-CoV-2 vaccination–Still casualty? *J. Hepatol.* **2021**, *75*, 1248–1249. [CrossRef]
30. McShane, C.; Kiat, C.; Rigby, J.; Crosbie, O. The mRNA COVID-19 vaccine—A rare trigger of autoimmune hepatitis? *J. Hepatol.* **2021**, *75*, 1252–1254. [CrossRef]
31. Rela, M.; Jothimani, D.; Vij, M.; Rajakumar, A.; Rammohan, A. Autoimmune hepatitis following COVID vaccination. *J. Autoimmun.* **2021**, *123*, 102688. [CrossRef]
32. Palla, P.; Vergadis, C.; Sakellariou, S.; Androutsakos, T. Letter to the editor: Autoimmune hepatitis after COVID-19 vaccination: A rare adverse effect? *Hepatology* **2022**, *75*, 489–490. [CrossRef]
33. Shroff, H.; Satapathy, S.K.; Crawford, J.M.; Todd, N.J.; VanWagner, L.B. Liver injury following SARS-CoV-2 vaccination: A multicenter case series. *J. Hepatol.* **2022**, *76*, 211–214. [CrossRef]
34. Vuille-Lessard, E.; Montani, M.; Bosch, J.; Semmo, N. Autoimmune hepatitis triggered by SARS-CoV-2 vaccination. *J. Autoimmun.* **2021**, *123*, 102710. [CrossRef]
35. Waldenstrom, J. Liver, blood proteins and food proteins. *Dtsch. Z Verdau Stoffwechselkr.* **1952**, *12*, 113–121.
36. Mieli-Vergani, G.; Vergani, D.; Czaja, A.J.; Manns, M.P.; Krawitt, E.L.; Vierling, J.M.; Lohse, A.W.; Montano-Loza, A.J. Autoimmune hepatitis. *Nat. Rev. Dis. Prim.* **2018**, *4*, 18017. [CrossRef]
37. Manns, M.P.; Lohse, A.W.; Vergani, D. Autoimmune hepatitis—Update 2015. *J. Hepatol.* **2015**, *62*, S100–S111. [CrossRef]
38. Czaja, A.J. Global Disparities and Their Implications in the Occurrence and Outcome of Autoimmune Hepatitis. *Dig. Dis. Sci.* **2017**, *62*, 2277–2292. [CrossRef]
39. Manns, M.P.; Czaja, A.J.; Gorham, J.D.; Krawitt, E.L.; Mieli-Vergani, G.; Vergani, D.; Vierling, J.M. Diagnosis and management of autoimmune hepatitis. *Hepatology* **2010**, *51*, 2193–2213. [CrossRef]
40. European Association for the study of the Liver. EASL Clinical Practice Guidelines: Autoimmune hepatitis. *J. Hepatol.* **2015**, *63*, 971–1004. [CrossRef]
41. van Gerven, N.M.; Verwer, B.J.; Witte, B.I.; van Erpecum, K.J.; van Buuren, H.R.; Maijers, I.; Visscher, A.P.; Verschuren, E.C.; van Hoek, B.; Coenraad, M.J.; et al. Epidemiology and clinical characteristics of autoimmune hepatitis in the Netherlands. *Scand. J. Gastroenterol.* **2014**, *49*, 1245–1254. [CrossRef]
42. Takahashi, H.; Zeniya, M. Acute presentation of autoimmune hepatitis: Does it exist? A published work review. *Hepatol. Res.* **2011**, *41*, 498–504. [CrossRef] [PubMed]
43. Mack, C.L.; Adams, D.; Assis, D.N.; Kerkar, N.; Manns, M.P.; Mayo, M.J.; Vierling, J.M.; Alsawas, M.; Murad, M.H.; Czaja, A.J. Diagnosis and Management of Autoimmune Hepatitis in Adults and Children: 2019 Practice Guidance and Guidelines from the American Association for the Study of Liver Diseases. *Hepatology* **2020**, *72*, 671–722. [CrossRef] [PubMed]
44. Czaja, A.J.; Carpenter, H.A. Optimizing diagnosis from the medical liver biopsy. *Clin. Gastroenterol. Hepatol.* **2007**, *5*, 898–907. [CrossRef] [PubMed]
45. Dienes, H.P.; Erberich, H.; Dries, V.; Schirmacher, P.; Lohse, A. Autoimmune hepatitis and overlap syndromes. *Clin. Liver Dis.* **2002**, *6*, 349–362. [CrossRef] [PubMed]

46. Hennes, E.M.; Zeniya, M.; Czaja, A.J.; Parés, A.; Dalekos, G.N.; Krawitt, E.L.; Bittencourt, P.L.; Porta, G.; Boberg, K.M.; Hofer, H.; et al. Simplified criteria for the diagnosis of autoimmune hepatitis. *Hepatology* **2008**, *48*, 169–176. [CrossRef]
47. Alvarez, F.; Berg, P.A.; Bianchi, F.B.; Bianchi, L.; Burroughs, A.K.; Cancado, E.L.; Chapman, R.W.; Cooksley, W.G.; Czaja, A.J.; Desmet, V.J.; et al. International Autoimmune Hepatitis Group Report: Review of criteria for diagnosis of autoimmune hepatitis. *J. Hepatol.* **1999**, *31*, 929–938. [CrossRef]
48. Komori, A. Recent updates on the management of autoimmune hepatitis. *Clin. Mol. Hepatol.* **2021**, *27*, 58–69. [CrossRef]
49. Harrington, C.; Krishnan, S.; Mack, C.L.; Cravedi, P.; Assis, D.N.; Levitsky, J. Noninvasive biomarkers for the diagnosis and management of autoimmune hepatitis. *Hepatology* **2022**, *76*, 1862–1879. [CrossRef]
50. Beretta-Piccoli, T.; Mieli-Vergani, B.G.; Vergani, D. Autoimmune hepatitis: Standard treatment and systematic review of alternative treatments. *World J. Gastroenterol.* **2017**, *23*, 6030–6048. [CrossRef]
51. Feld, J.J.; Dinh, H.; Arenovich, T.; Marcus, V.A.; Wanless, I.R.; Heathcote, E.J. Autoimmune hepatitis: Effect of symptoms and cirrhosis on natural history and outcome. *Hepatology* **2005**, *42*, 53–62. [CrossRef]
52. Dufour, J.F.; Zimmermann, M.; Reichen, J. Severe autoimmune hepatitis in patients with previous spontaneous recovery of a flare. *J. Hepatol.* **2002**, *37*, 748–752. [CrossRef]
53. Kogan, J.; Safadi, R.; Ashur, Y.; Shouval, D.; Ilan, Y. Prognosis of symptomatic versus asymptomatic autoimmune hepatitis: A study of 68 patients. *J. Clin. Gastroenterol.* **2002**, *35*, 75–81. [CrossRef]
54. Segal Y, Shoenfeld Y: Vaccine-induced autoimmunity: The role of molecular mimicry and immune crossreaction. *Cell. Mol. Immunol.* **2018**, *15*, 586–594. [CrossRef]
55. Segal, Y.; Dahan, S.; Calabrò, M.; Kanduc, D.; Shoenfeld, Y. HPV and systemic lupus erythematosus: A mosaic of potential crossreactions. *Immunol. Res.* **2017**, *65*, 564–571. [CrossRef]
56. Segal, Y.; Calabrò, M.; Kanduc, D.; Shoenfeld, Y. Human papilloma virus and lupus: The virus, the vaccine and the disease. *Curr. Opin. Rheumatol.* **2017**, *29*, 331–342. [CrossRef]
57. Cohen Tervaert, J.W.; Martinez-Lavin, M.; Jara, L.J.; Halpert, G.; Watad, A.; Amital, H.; Shoenfeld, Y. Autoimmune/inflammatory syndrome induced by adjuvants (ASIA) in 2023. *Autoimmun. Rev.* **2023**, *22*, 103287. [CrossRef]
58. Seida, I.; Seida, R.; Elsalti, A.; Mahroum, N. Vaccines and Autoimmunity-From Side Effects to ASIA Syndrome. *Medicina* **2023**, *59*, 364. [CrossRef]
59. Vojdani, A.; Kharrazian, D. Potential antigenic cross-reactivity between SARS-CoV-2 and human tissue with a possible link to an increase in autoimmune diseases. *Clin. Immunol.* **2020**, *217*, 108480. [CrossRef]
60. Hintermann, E.; Holdener, M.; Bayer, M.; Loges, S.; Pfeilschifter, J.M.; Granier, C.; Manns, M.P.; Christen, U. Epitope spreading of the anti-CYP2D6 antibody response in patients with autoimmune hepatitis and in the CYP2D6 mouse model. *J. Autoimmun.* **2011**, *37*, 242–253. [CrossRef]
61. Milojevic, D.; Nguyen, K.D.; Wara, D.; Mellins, E.D. Regulatory T cells and their role in rheumatic diseases: A potential target for novel therapeutic development. *Pediatr. Rheumatol. Online J.* **2008**, *6*, 20. [CrossRef]
62. Muratori, L.; Muratori, P.; Lanzoni, G.; Ferri, S.; Lenzi, M. Application of the 2010 American Association for the study of liver diseases criteria of remission to a cohort of Italian patients with autoimmune hepatitis. *Hepatology* **2010**, *52*, 1857. [CrossRef] [PubMed]
63. Tanaka, A.; Ma, X.; Yokosuka, O.; Weltman, M.; You, H.; Amarapurkar, D.N.; Kim, Y.J.; Abbas, Z.; Payawal, D.A.; Chang, M.L.; et al. Autoimmune liver diseases in the Asia-Pacific region: Proceedings of APASL symposium on AIH and PBC 2016. *Hepatol. Int.* **2016**, *10*, 909–915. [CrossRef] [PubMed]
64. Kim, B.H.; Kim, Y.J.; Jeong, S.H.; Tak, W.Y.; Ahn, S.H.; Lee, Y.J.; Jung, E.U.; Lee, J.I.; Yeon, J.E.; Hwang, J.S.; et al. Clinical features of autoimmune hepatitis and comparison of two diagnostic criteria in Korea: A nationwide, multicenter study. *J. Gastroenterol. Hepatol.* **2013**, *28*, 128–134. [CrossRef] [PubMed]

Disclaimer/Publisher's Note: The statements, opinions and data contained in all publications are solely those of the individual author(s) and contributor(s) and not of MDPI and/or the editor(s). MDPI and/or the editor(s) disclaim responsibility for any injury to people or property resulting from any ideas, methods, instructions or products referred to in the content.

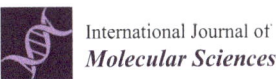

Article

Bioinformatics Analysis of Gene Expression Profiles for Diagnosing Sepsis and Risk Prediction in Patients with Sepsis

Hayoung Choi [1,†], Jin Young Lee [2,†], Hongseok Yoo [2] and Kyeongman Jeon [2,3,*]

1. Division of Pulmonary, Allergy, and Critical Care Medicine, Department of Internal Medicine, Hallym University Kangnam Sacred Heart Hospital, Hallym University College of Medicine, Seoul 07441, Republic of Korea; hychoimd@gmail.com
2. Division of Pulmonary and Critical Care Medicine, Department of Medicine, Samsung Medical Center, Sungkyunkwan University School of Medicine, Seoul 06351, Republic of Korea; yenayein@gmail.com (J.Y.L.); hongseok.yoo@samsung.com (H.Y.)
3. Department of Health Sciences and Technology, SAIHST, Sungkyunkawan University, Seoul 06351, Republic of Korea
* Correspondence: kjeon@skku.edu; Tel.: +82-2-3410-3429; Fax: +82-2-3410-6956
† These authors contributed equally to this work.

Abstract: Although early recognition of sepsis is essential for timely treatment and can improve sepsis outcomes, no marker has demonstrated sufficient discriminatory power to diagnose sepsis. This study aimed to compare gene expression profiles between patients with sepsis and healthy volunteers to determine the accuracy of these profiles in diagnosing sepsis and to predict sepsis outcomes by combining bioinformatics data with molecular experiments and clinical information. We identified 422 differentially expressed genes (DEGs) between the sepsis and control groups, of which 93 immune-related DEGs were considered for further studies due to immune-related pathways being the most highly enriched. Key genes upregulated during sepsis, including S100A8, S100A9, and CR1, are responsible for cell cycle regulation and immune responses. Key downregulated genes, including CD79A, HLA-DQB2, PLD4, and CCR7, are responsible for immune responses. Furthermore, the key upregulated genes showed excellent to fair accuracy in diagnosing sepsis (area under the curve 0.747–0.931) and predicting in-hospital mortality (0.863–0.966) of patients with sepsis. In contrast, the key downregulated genes showed excellent accuracy in predicting mortality of patients with sepsis (0.918–0.961) but failed to effectively diagnosis sepsis. In conclusion, bioinformatics analysis identified key genes that may serve as biomarkers for diagnosing sepsis and predicting outcomes among patients with sepsis.

Keywords: sepsis; biomarkers; diagnosis; genes; bioinformatics

1. Introduction

Sepsis is a life-threatening organ dysfunction caused by a dysregulated host response [1]. Sepsis and septic shock are major healthcare problems that affect millions of patients worldwide each year and kill approximately 17–33% of those affected [2,3]. Unfortunately, the reported incidence of sepsis and its associated healthcare burden are both currently on the rise due to the global trend of population aging and patients having a greater number of comorbidities [4,5]. Biomarker development could serve as a cornerstone of sepsis management and may ameliorate the healthcare burden of sepsis because early recognition is essential for timely treatment and the improvement of sepsis outcomes [6].

Numerous biomarkers for sepsis, including C-reactive protein and procalcitonin, have been investigated previously [7,8]. However, to date no marker has demonstrated sufficient discriminatory power [9,10]. Bioinformatics approaches integrate computational and life sciences to screen molecular and clinical data via data mining, pathway analysis, statistical analysis, and visual processing. These methods can investigate disease on

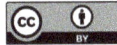

Citation: Choi, H.; Lee, J.Y.; Yoo, H.; Jeon, K. Bioinformatics Analysis of Gene Expression Profiles for Diagnosing Sepsis and Risk Prediction in Patients with Sepsis. *Int. J. Mol. Sci.* **2023**, *24*, 9362. https://doi.org/10.3390/ijms24119362

Academic Editors: Vasso Apostolopoulos, Jack Feehan and Vivek P. Chavda

Received: 10 March 2023
Revised: 19 May 2023
Accepted: 23 May 2023
Published: 27 May 2023

Copyright: © 2023 by the authors. Licensee MDPI, Basel, Switzerland. This article is an open access article distributed under the terms and conditions of the Creative Commons Attribution (CC BY) license (https://creativecommons.org/licenses/by/4.0/).

the molecular level and have been widely used to identify significant biomarkers for sepsis [11–15]. In addition to the previous studies using datasets downloaded from public repositories, some prospective cohort studies also performed bioinformatics analysis to explore potential biomarkers for sepsis diagnosis [16,17]. Although previous studies have provided important insight into biomarkers and the pathophysiology of sepsis, more bioinformatics studies are warranted to validate the study results in association with real-world clinical outcomes.

Thus, the present study aimed to (1) use bioinformatics analyses to explore key differentially expressed genes (DEGs) between patients with sepsis from a prospective cohort and healthy volunteers and (2) validate the accuracy of bioinformatics analyses for diagnosing sepsis and predicting sepsis outcomes by integrating molecular experiments with clinical information.

2. Results

2.1. Clinical Characteristics of Patients with Sepsis

During the study period, we enrolled 133 critically ill patients with sepsis after excluding 63 who were not diagnosed with sepsis and two who withdrew their consent. Of the 133 patients, 90 (67.7%) were male, and the median age of patients was 66 years (interquartile range (IQR), 58–73 years). When patients were admitted to intensive care units, 60 (45.1%) and 69 (51.9%) received mechanical ventilation therapy and vasopressors, respectively. With respect to the severity of illness, the median SAPS 3 score was 55 (IQR, 47–63), the APACHE II score was 24 (IQR, 20–30), and the initial Sequential Organ Failure Assessment score was 9 (IQR, 7–11). The rates of 28-day mortality and in-hospital mortality were 16.5% and 24.8%, respectively (Table 1).

Table 1. Characteristics of patients with sepsis.

Variable	Value (n = 133)
Age (years)	66 (58–73)
Male	90 (67.7)
Comorbidities	
All malignancies	51 (38.3)
Solid organ malignancies	35 (26.3)
Hematologic malignancies	16 (12.0)
Diabetes mellitus	41 (30.8)
Chronic obstructive pulmonary disease	16 (12.0)
Chronic kidney disease	10 (7.5)
Myocardial infarction	8 (6.0)
Congestive heart failure	7 (5.3)
Cerebrovascular disease	8 (6.0)
Chronic liver disease	11 (8.3)
Charlson Comorbidity Index	2 (1–3)
Clinical status on ICU admission	
Mechanical ventilation	60 (45.1)
Vasopressor support	69 (51.9)
Laboratory findings	
WBC (/µL)	13,640 (5060–20,340)
Hemoglobin (g/dL)	10.1 (8.9–11.7)
Platelet (/µL)	136,000 (59,000–214,000)
Albumin (g/dL)	2.9 (2.6–3.2)
CRP (mg/dL)	12.5 (5.8–24.5)
Lactate (mg/dL)	3.0 (2.0–4.4)
PaO_2/FiO_2 ratio	216 (135–323)
Severity of illness	
SAPS 3 score	55 (47–63)
APACHE II score	24 (20–30)
SOFA score, initial	9 (7–11)
Outcome	
28-day mortality	22 (16.5)
In-hospital mortality	33 (24.8)

Data are presented as count (percentage) or median (interquartile range). Abbreviations: APACHE II, Acute Physiology and Chronic Health Evaluation II; COPD, chronic obstructive pulmonary disease; CRP, C-reactive protein; ICU, intensive care unit; PaO_2/FiO_2 ratio, ratio of arterial oxygen pressure to fractional inspired oxygen; SAPS 3, Simplified Acute Physiology Score 3; SOFA, Sequential Organ Failure Assessment.

2.2. Identification of Candidate mRNAs: Bioinformatics Analyses

This study initially identified 422 DEGs between 133 patients with sepsis and 12 healthy volunteers. A principal component analysis (PCA) of global gene expression profiles revealed that sepsis patients were clearly separate from healthy volunteers (Figure 1A). In addition, distinct patterns of gene expression existed in sepsis patients when transcriptomic profiles of sepsis patients were compared to those of healthy volunteers (Figure 1B). Further bioinformatics analyses were conducted to identify key genes related to sepsis. First, enriched gene ontology (GO) functional analysis revealed that the identified DEGs were mainly involved in the immune response (Figure 1C,D).

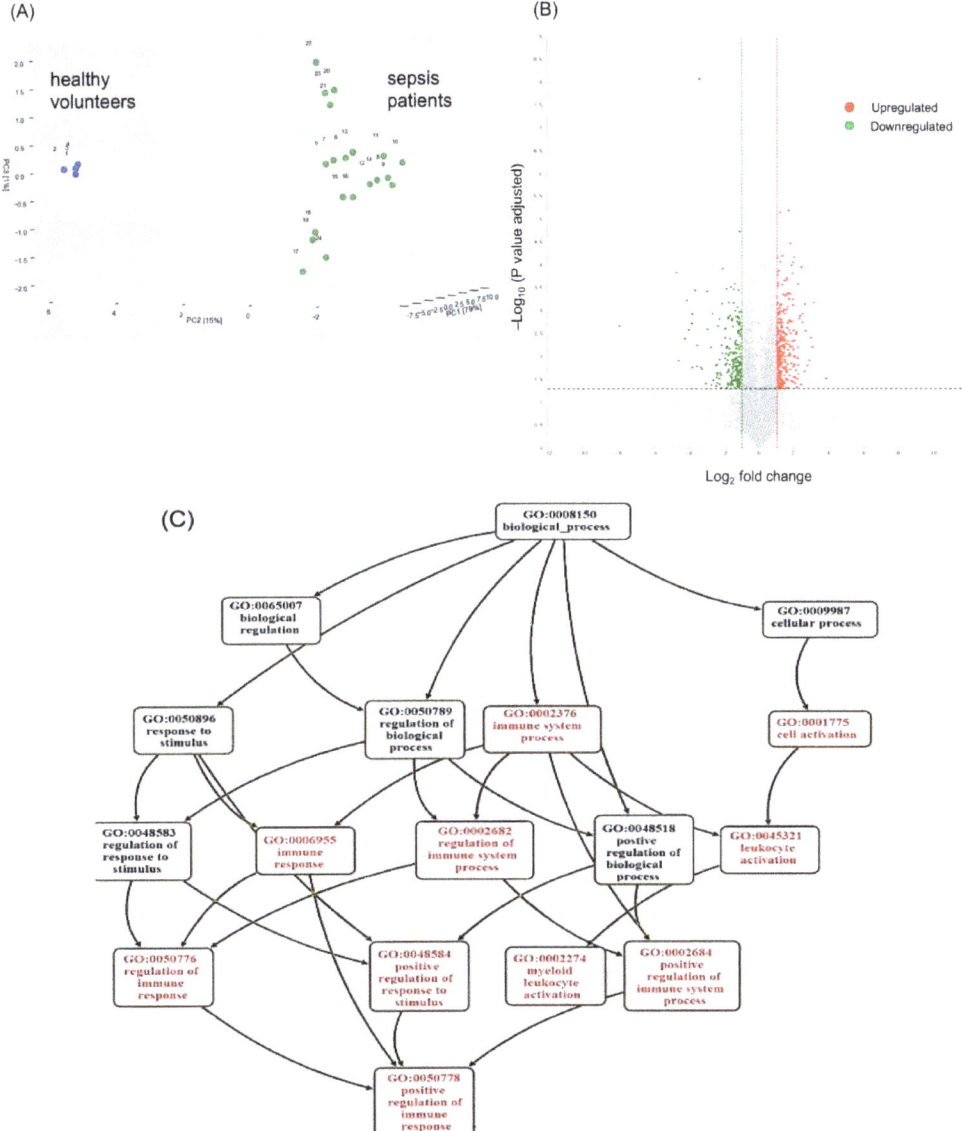

Figure 1. *Cont.*

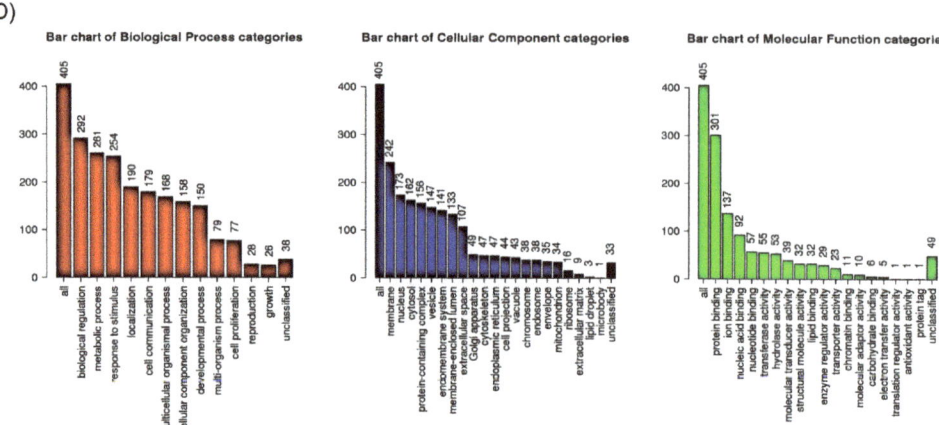

Figure 1. Gene ontology (GO) enrichment analysis of 422 differentially expressed genes (DEGs) between patients with sepsis and healthy volunteers. (**A**) Principal component analysis of the RNA transcriptome from sepsis patients (green) and that from healthy volunteers (blue). (**B**) Volcano plot of DEGs showing upregulated genes in red and downregulated genes in green. (**C**) GO enrichment analysis visualizing main DEGs that are mainly involved in the response to sepsis. (**D**) Number of identified DEGs according to their biological process (red), cellular component (blue), or molecular function (green) categorization.

Second, a protein–protein interaction (PPI) network analysis of the 422 DEGs also showed that the most extensive module was composed of 78 seeds, 1381 nodes, and 1823 edges. Moreover, it appeared to be most strongly enriched in immune-related pathways (Figure 2).

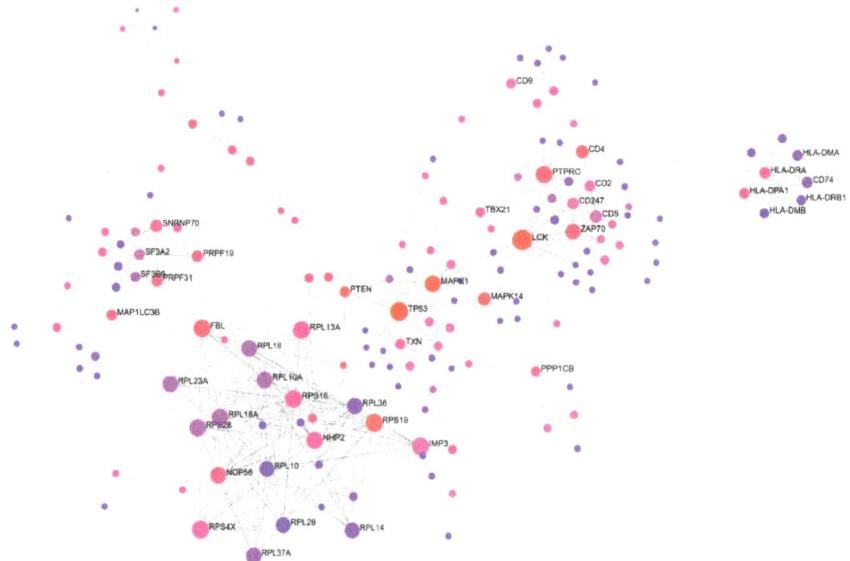

Figure 2. Protein–protein interaction network analysis of all 422 differentially expressed genes between patients with sepsis and healthy volunteers. Immune-related pathways, presented as the largest module (78 seeds, 1381 nodes, and 1823 edges), show the greatest enrichment.

A following PPI network analysis of 93 immune-related DEGs revealed that these enriched immune-related pathways included adaptive immune response, positive regulation of immune response, positive regulation of leukocyte cell–cell adhesion, cell activation, and positive regulation of cytokine production (Figure 3).

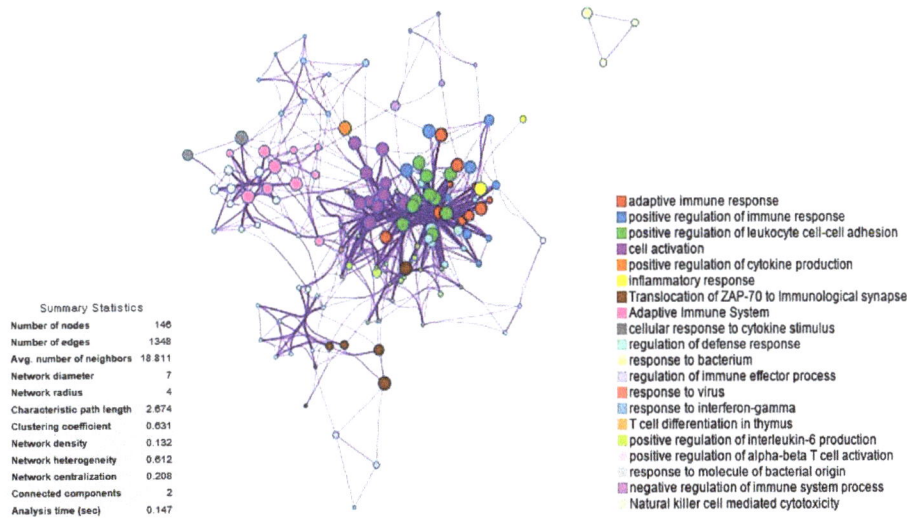

Figure 3. Protein–protein interaction network analysis of 93 immune-related differentially expressed genes between patients with sepsis and healthy volunteers. Enriched pathways are also shown.

Results of a molecular complex detection (MCODE) analysis performed to screen the significant modules of the PPI network are shown in Figure 4.

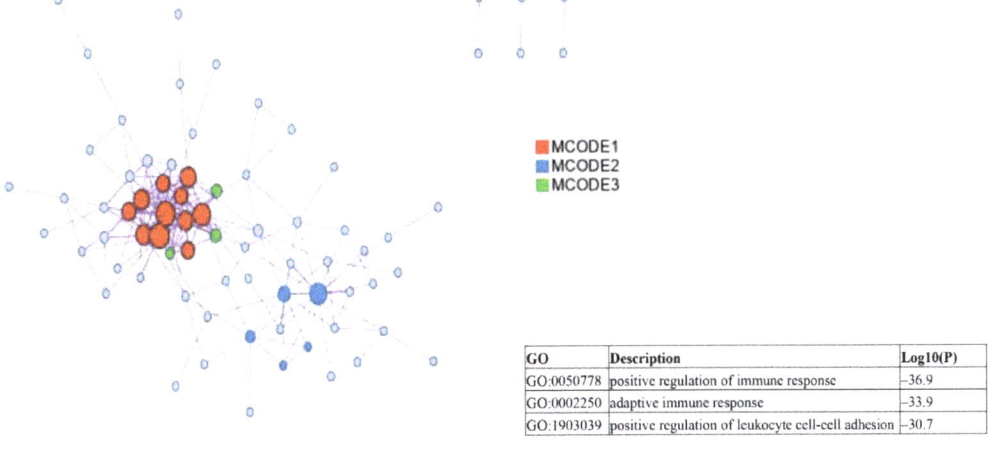

Figure 4. Cont.

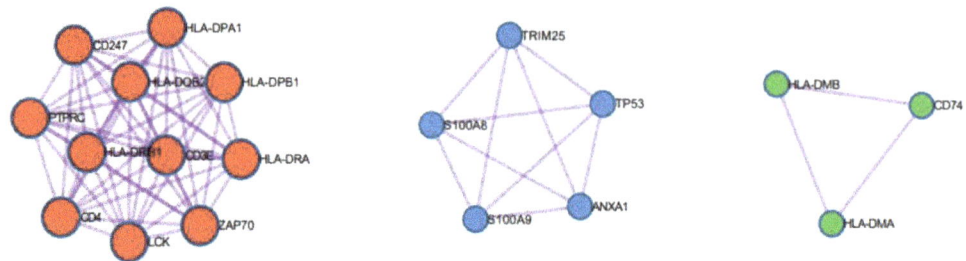

Color	MCODE	GO	Description	Log10(P)
	MCODE_1	R-HSA-202430	Translocation of ZAP-70 to Immunological synapse	−32.2
	MCODE_1	R-HSA-202427	Phosphorylation of CD3 and TCR zeta chains	−31.4
	MCODE_1	R-HSA-202433	Generation of second messenger molecules	−29.1
	MCODE_2	GO:0051238	sequestering of metal ion	−8.5
	MCODE_2	GO:0042063	gliogenesis	−7.7
	MCODE_2	GO:2001244	positive regulation of intrinsic apoptotic signaling pathway	−7.1
	MCODE_3	GO:0019886	antigen processing and presentation of exogenous peptide antigen via MHC class II	−9.1
	MCODE_3	GO:0002495	antigen processing and presentation of peptide antigen via MHC class II	−9
	MCODE_3	GO:0002504	antigen processing and presentation of peptide or polysaccharide antigen via MHC class II	−8

Figure 4. Molecular complex detection analysis results used to screen the significant modules identified in the protein–protein interaction network.

The 93 immune-related DEGs identified here included 51 upregulated and 42 downregulated genes in patients with sepsis compared to healthy volunteers. Table 2 summarizes the top 10 upregulated and downregulated genes in patients with sepsis. Significantly upregulated genes included S100A8, VNN1, HMGB2, and S100A9, whereas significantly downregulated genes included CD79A, HLA-DQB2, PLD4, and CCR7.

Table 2. Top 10 upregulated and downregulated immune-related genes in patients with sepsis relative to healthy volunteers.

Top 10 Upregulated Genes			Top 10 Downregulated Genes		
Entrez ID	Gene Symbol	Fold Change	Entrez ID	Gene Symbol	Fold Change
6279	S100A8	16.17	973	CD79A	0.12
8876	VNN1	7.83	3120	HLA-DQB2	0.13
3148	HMGB2	7.23	122618	PLD4	0.14
6280	S100A9	5.43	1236	CCR7	0.15
301	ANXA1	5.42	259197	NCR3	0.17
665	BNIP3L	4.67	29802	VPREB3	0.18
200315	APOBEC3A	4.61	6932	TCF7	0.199
353514	LILRA5	4.49	933	CD22	0.201
1378	CR1	4.46	10578	GNLY	0.206
1604	CD55	4.29	974	CD79B	0.213

Abbreviations: S100A8, S100 calcium-binding protein A8; VNN1, vanin 1; HMGB2, high-mobility group box 2; S100A9, S100 calcium-binding protein A9; ANXA1, annexin A1; BNIP3L, BCL2 interacting protein 3-like; APOBEC3A, apolipoprotein B mRNA editing enzyme catalytic subunit 3A; LILRA5, leukocyte immunoglobulin-like receptor A5; CR1, complement C3b/C4b receptor 1; CD55, CD55 molecule; CD79A, CD79a molecule; HLA-DQB2, major histocompatibility complex, class II, DQ beta 2; PLD4, phospholipase D family member 4; CCR7, C-C motif chemokine receptor 7; NCR3, natural cytotoxicity triggering receptor 3; VPREB3, V-set pre-B cell surrogate chain 3; TCF7, transcription factor 7; CD22, CD22 molecule; GNLY, granulysin; CD79B, CD79b molecule.

2.3. Experimental and Clinical Validation of Potential Biomarkers from the mRNA Profile

Next, we used quantitative real-time PCR (qPCR) to measure the expression levels of identified DEGs and thereby validate our bioinformatics analyses using molecular data in 133 patients with sepsis and 12 healthy volunteers. Among the 10 upregulated and 10 downregulated genes, 3 upregulated and 4 downregulated genes showed consistent results with bioinformatics analysis. The three upregulated genes, S100A8, S100A9, and CR1, showed significantly higher expression levels in patients with sepsis than in healthy volunteers ($p < 0.001$ for S100A8 and S100A9, and $p = 0.005$ for CR1), whereas the four downregulated genes, CD79A, HLA-DQB2, PLD4, and CCR7, showed significantly lower expression levels in patients with sepsis than in healthy volunteers ($p < 0.001$ for all four genes) (Table 3).

Table 3. Comparisons of the expression levels of differentially expressed genes between patients with sepsis and healthy volunteers, and between patients who died and survived.

		Patients with Sepsis vs. Healthy Volunteers *		
		Patients with Sepsis	Healthy Volunteers	p-Value
Upregulated genes	S100A8	19.8 (11.6–24.2)	7.6 (7.1–8.2)	<0.001
	S100A9	7.6 (3.8–10.3)	3.8 (2.6–4.2)	<0.001
	CR1	5.5 (2.5–8.8)	2.7 (2.3–2.8)	0.005
Downregulated genes	CD79A	0.3 (0.2–0.4)	0.5 (0.5–0.6)	<0.001
	HLA-DQB2	0.2 (0.2–0.2)	0.3 (0.3–0.4)	<0.001
	PLD4	0.5 (0.2–0.7)	0.9 (0.9–1.0)	<0.001
	CCR7	0.3 (0.1–0.4)	0.5 (0.5–0.6)	<0.001
		The Dead vs. Surviving among Patients with Sepsis *		
		Patients (Dead)	Patients (Surviving)	p-Value
Upregulated genes	S100A8	25.9 (24.1–27.8)	17.1 (11.4–21.2)	<0.001
	S100A9	10.7 (9.7–11.8)	6.3 (3.2–8.5)	<0.001
	CR1	10.3 (9.3–11.9)	4.0 (2.0–6.6)	<0.001
Downregulated genes	CD79A	0.5 (0.4–0.6)	0.2 (0.1–0.3)	<0.001
	HLA-DQB2	0.3 (0.2–0.3)	0.2 (0.1–0.2)	<0.001
	PLD4	0.7 (0.6–0.8)	0.4 (0.2–0.6)	<0.001
	CCR7	0.4 (0.4–0.5)	0.2 (0.1–0.3)	<0.001

Data are presented as median (interquartile range). * Values denote fold changes of genes.

A receiver operating characteristic (ROC) curve analysis was then conducted to determine the accuracy of these seven genes in diagnosing sepsis: S100A8 showed very high accuracy (i.e., area under the curve (AUC): 0.931, 95% confidence interval (CI): 0.880–0.982), while both S100A9 (AUC: 0.791, 95% CI: 0.711–0.871) and CR1 (AUC: 0.747, 95% CI: 0.647–0.820) showed fair accuracy. In contrast to the three upregulated genes, all four downregulated genes failed to effectively discriminate between patients with sepsis and healthy volunteers (Table 4).

Further analyses were then performed to compare gene expression in patients with sepsis who died and survived among the 133 with sepsis. All three upregulated genes (S100A8, S100A9, and CR1) and all four downregulated genes (CD79A, HLA-DQB2, PLD4, and CCR7) showed significantly higher expression levels in the dead than in the survivors among patients with sepsis ($p < 0.001$ for all) (Table 3). The ROC curve analysis was then used to assess the accuracy of the seven genes in predicting in-hospital mortality among patients with sepsis. All upregulated and downregulated genes demonstrated excellent accuracy, with CR1 showing the highest accuracy (AUC: 0.966, 95% CI: 0.939–0.993), followed by CD79A (AUC: 0.961, 95% CI: 0.930–0.992) and HLA-DQB2 (AUC: 0.936, 95% CI: 0.895–0.978) (Table 4).

Table 4. Receiver operating characteristic curve analysis and suggested optimal cut-off values of seven mRNAs in diagnosing sepsis and predicting in-hospital mortality among patients with sepsis.

mRNAs	Sepsis Diagnosis					
	AUC	SE	95% CI	Optimal Cut-Off	Sensitivity	Specificity
S100A8	0.931	0.026	0.880–0.982	≥9.0	94.0%	83.3%
S100A9	0.791	0.041	0.711–0.871	≥5.0	69.2%	100%
CR1	0.747	0.037	0.674–0.820	≥3.0	72.9%	100%
CD79A	0.113	0.028	0.059–0.168	NA	NA	NA
HLA-DQB2	0.003	0.003	0–0.009	NA	NA	NA
PLD4	0.013	0.013	0–0.038	NA	NA	NA
CCR7	0.016	0.010	0–0.036	NA	NA	NA
	Mortality Prediction in Sepsis					
	AUC	SE	95% CI	Optimal Cut-Off	Sensitivity	Specificity
S100A8	0.919	0.026	0.868–0.970	≥23.6	84.9%	88.0%
S100A9	0.863	0.033	0.797–0.928	≥9.6	78.8%	85.0%
CR1	0.966	0.014	0.939–0.993	≥9.0	84.9%	95.0%
CD79A	0.961	0.016	0.930–0.992	≥0.42	93.9%	92.0%
HLA-DQB2	0.936	0.021	0.895–0.978	≥0.23	84.9%	88.0%
PLD4	0.918	0.026	0.866–0.969	≥0.64	84.9%	88.0%
CCR7	0.918	0.026	0.866–0.969	≥0.39	78.8%	90.0%

Abbreviations: AUC, area under curve; SE, standard error; CI, confidence interval; NA, not applicable.

3. Discussion

In the present study, bioinformatics analysis revealed that immune-related pathways were strongly enriched in patients with sepsis relative to healthy volunteers. In addition, we identified three key genes that were upregulated in patients with sepsis (S100A8, S100A9, and CR1) as well as four key genes that were downregulated (CD79A, HLA-DQB2, PLD4, and CCR7). Furthermore, validation of these findings by molecular experiments and clinical outcomes determined that the key upregulated genes showed excellent to fair accuracy for both diagnosing sepsis and predicting in-hospital mortality of patients with sepsis. In contrast, the key downregulated genes showed excellent accuracy in predicting in-hospital mortality of patients with sepsis but failed to effectively diagnose sepsis.

Immune-related pathways were the most highly enriched biological pathways in patients with sepsis relative to healthy volunteers; this finding is consistent with previous bioinformatics studies, which also revealed DEGs were significantly enriched in pathways related to neutrophil activation, the TNF signaling pathway, and cytokine secretion [11,13–16,18]. These results suggest that the pathophysiology of sepsis is driven by "an aberrant or dysregulated host response to infection", which is also reflected in the current definition of sepsis [1]. Furthermore, a recent RNA sequencing study provided more insights into the pathophysiology of sepsis. The study compared RNA sequencing results between 18 immunocompromised patients with sepsis and 18 Sequential Organ Failure Assessment score-matched immunocompetent controls, and it demonstrated that patients with sepsis were more likely to show compromised T cell function, decreased T cell diversity, and altered metabolic signaling than controls [19]. In this way, bioinformatics studies will increasingly contribute to unveiling the pathophysiology of sepsis.

Notably, the key genes upregulated during sepsis are responsible for regulating cell cycle progression and differentiation (i.e., S100A8 and S100A9) and immune responses (i.e., ANXA1, APOBEC3A, LILRA5, CR1, and CD55) [20]. In agreement with our findings, one Chinese prospective cohort study also performed a comprehensive transcriptome profile analysis and qPCR validation, and suggested S100A8, S100A9, and ANXA3 as key genes differentially expressed between sepsis patients and healthy controls [16]. Potential underlying mechanisms of upregulated S100A8 and S100A9 may also include altering MyD88-dependent gene programs, which consequently prevent hyperinflammatory responses without impairing pathogen defense [21], and mediating endotoxin-induced cardiomyocyte dysfunction [16,22]. Our qPCR results and ROC curve analyses confirmed the accuracy of S100A8, S100A9, and CR1 in diagnosing sepsis as well as in predicting in-hospital mortality among patients with sepsis. Thus, our results suggest that the expression levels of the key upregulated genes identified here may serve as potential biomarkers of sepsis.

In this study, the key genes downregulated during sepsis also encoded proteins responsible for the immune response, including the expression of antigen-presenting cells, the regulation of cytokine production, and the activation of B and T lymphocytes (i.e., CD79A, HLA-DQB2, PLD4, and CCR7) [20]. This is in line with prior studies showing that genes involving Jak-STAT signaling, T cell receptor signaling, and natural killer cell-mediated pathways were downregulated [23–25]. The results showed that genes participating in the immune response have mixed differential expression patterns of both up- and downregulation. Considering sepsis has been found to manifest a balance between competing pro- and anti-inflammatory pathways [26], the downregulation of immune response genes in patients with sepsis implies the homeostatic regulation of immunity during sepsis. Thus, the failed homeostatic regulation of immunity may have consequently resulted in the development and progression of sepsis. Interestingly, the key downregulated genes revealed an excellent accuracy in predicting in-hospital mortality of patients with sepsis but failed to diagnose sepsis in the ROC curve analyses. Taken together, key downregulated genes helped us understand more about sepsis pathophysiology; however, they may not be useful as sepsis biomarkers compared with key upregulated genes.

This study's most important strength is the validation of key DEGs between patients with sepsis and healthy volunteers via molecular experiments and clinical information from a prospective cohort. These validation methods can elucidate which genes may act as biomarkers of the diagnosis and mortality prediction of sepsis. Nonetheless, two limitations to this study should also be acknowledged. First, the study population was relatively small; thus, future bioinformatics studies, including a larger sample size, are necessary to confirm our findings. Second, this study was conducted in Korea, which might limit the generalizability of our results to other countries or ethnic groups.

4. Materials and Methods

4.1. Study Population

This study included patients with sepsis from the Samsung Medical Center Registry of Critical Illness (SMC-RoCI), a prospective observational study conducted at the Samsung Medical Center (i.e., a 1989-bed, university-affiliated, tertiary referral hospital in Seoul, Republic of Korea) between October 2015 and January 2020 as previously described [27]. Sepsis was defined according to the third edition of the International Consensus Definitions for Sepsis and Septic Shock (Sepsis-3) [1]. Consequently, patients enrolled before the release of this new definition were reclassified according to the Sepsis-3 scheme.

In addition to patients with sepsis, we used a control consisting of 12 healthy volunteers ($\geq$19 years of age) who donated blood specimens for research purposes. Written informed consent was obtained from all participants or their legally authorized representatives before enrollment. This study was conducted according to the Declaration of Helsinki, and all experimental procedures were approved by the institutional review board of the Samsung Medical Center (Application No. 2013-12-033).

4.2. Sample Collection

Blood samples consisted of 19 mL of whole blood collected into ethylenediaminetetraacetic acid tubes within 48 h of enrollment in the SMC-ROCI. Samples were centrifuged at $480\times g$ (Eppendorf Centrifuge 5810 No. 0012529-rotor A-4-81) for 10 min at 4 °C within 4 h of collection. Several plasma aliquots from each study participant were then isolated and stored at -80 °C for further analysis.

4.3. Total RNA Isolation and Quality Analysis

For RNA isolation, whole blood (2 mL) was also collected in PAXgene tubes, using BD PAXgene blood RNA tubes (BD, cat. no. 762165). Total RNA was isolated from whole blood using the TRIzol reagent (Invitrogen, Carlsbad, CA, USA) following the manufacturer's protocol [28]. RNA quantity and purity were measured using a NanoDrop 2000 (Thermo Fisher Scientific, Wilmington, DE, USA). RNA quality, yield, and distribution were determined using an Agilent 2100 Bioanalyzer (Agilent Technologies, Santa Clara, CA, USA) [29]. Blood samples (5 mL) were also collected from healthy volunteers; these samples were also prepared using the method described above.

4.4. Library Preparation and Sequencing

Libraries were prepared from total RNA using a NEBNext Ultra II Directional RNA-Seq Kit (New England BioLabs, UK). Messenger RNA (mRNA) was isolated using a Poly(A) RNA Selection Kit (Lexogen, Inc., Vienna, Austria). Isolated mRNA was then used for cDNA synthesis and shearing by following the manufacturer's instructions. Indexing was performed using Illumina indices 1–12. Enrichment was performed by polymerase chain reaction (PCR). Subsequently, libraries were checked using an Agilent 2100 Bioanalyzer (DNA High Sensitivity Kit) to evaluate the mean fragment size. Quantification was performed using a library quantification kit on a StepOne Real-Time PCR System (Applied Biosystems Life Technologies, Carlsbad, CA, USA). High-throughput sequencing was performed as paired-end 100 bp sequencing on a NovaSeq 6000 sequencing platform (Illumina, Inc., San Diego, CA, USA) [29,30].

4.5. Data Analysis

Quality control of the raw sequencing data was performed using FastQC [31]. Adapter sequences and low-quality reads (<Q20) were removed using the fastx_clipper function implemented in the FASTX_Toolkit and by BBMap [32]. Trimmed reads were then mapped to the reference genome using TopHat [33]. Gene expression levels were estimated as fragments per kilobase of transcript per million (FPKM) mapped reads values as determined by Cufflinks [34]. All FPKM values were normalized based on the quantile normalization method implemented by the EdgeR package for R [35].

4.6. Identification of DEGs

GEO2R was used to screen for DEGs between the sepsis and control groups. GEO2R is an R-based interactive web tool that helps to identify and visualize differential gene expression [36]. PCA of the different groups' samples was performed on the gene expression matrix. We set the threshold of differential expression to the default standard (i.e., |log2 (fold change [FC])| > 1 and adjusted $p < 0.05$) to identify significant DEGs between the two groups. Thus, significantly upregulated DEGs showed log2 FC > 1, and significantly downregulated DEGs showed log2 FC < 1 [37]. Significance was defined as an adjusted p value < 0.05 to control for type I errors in multiple tests.

4.7. Functional and Pathway Enrichment Analyses

To further recognize the underlying biological functions of the DEGs identified in the previous step, we performed GO functional analysis to annotate all DEGs according to the three main GO categories: molecular function, cellular component, and biological process [38]. Furthermore, to further elucidate the DEG pathways, we performed a Kyoto Encyclopedia of Genes and Genomes (KEGG) pathway enrichment analysis [39]. For GO functional annotation and KEGG pathway enrichment analyses, we used the WEB-based Gene SeT AnaLysis Toolkit (WebGestalt), the web-based Database for Annotation, Visualization, and Integrated Discovery (DAVID) tool version 6.8 [37,40], and Metascape [41].

4.8. Protein–Protein Interaction Network Analysis

Because proteins function in a coordinated manner within a complicated and dynamic network, we constructed a PPI network of the target genes using the Search Tool for the Retrieval of Interacting Genes (STRING) database, version 11.0 [42]. In addition, the Cytoscape plug-in Network Analyzer was also used for further analyses. Furthermore, the topological properties of the PPI network, including node degree, were calculated by searching for hub genes using the PPI network [43]. MCODE analysis implemented in Cytoscape was then performed to screen for significant modules of the PPI network using the following cut-off parameters: node score cut-off = 0.2, K-core = 2, and degree cut-off = 2.

4.9. Quantitative Real-Time PCR

To evaluate the expression levels of key genes, we performed qPCR analyses in duplicate. The reaction conditions were as follows: an initial step of 50 °C for 2 min, denaturing at 95 °C for 5 min, followed by 40 cycles of 95 °C for 30 s and 58.5 °C for 1 min. qPCR was performed on an ABI ViiA 7 Real-Time PCR System (Applied Biosystems) and was followed by a melting curve analysis. Glyceraldehyde-3-phosphate dehydrogenase was selected as an internal control. The $2^{-\Delta\Delta CT}$ algorithm (ΔCT = Ct. target − Ct. reference) was employed for downstream data analysis [44].

4.10. Statistical Analysis

Categorical variables were compared using the chi-square or Fisher's exact tests. Continuous variables were compared using Mann–Whitney U tests. For clinical validation of bioinformatics analysis results, an ROC curve was used to analyze the diagnostic accuracy of mRNA expression for (1) discriminating between patients with sepsis and healthy volunteers and (2) predicting in-hospital mortality among patients with sepsis. The sensitivity and specificity were also calculated to suggest the optimal cut-off value of each gene. All tests were two-tailed, and $p < 0.05$ was used as the threshold of statistical significance. Data were analyzed using STATA version 16 (Stata Corp., College Station, TX, USA).

5. Conclusions

Bioinformatics analysis revealed that immune-related pathways were the most enriched in patients with sepsis relative to healthy volunteers. In addition, we identified key genes that were upregulated in sepsis, namely, S100A8, S100A9, and CR1, as well as those that were downregulated, namely, CD79A, HLA-DQB2, PLD4, and CCR7. The key upregulated genes showed excellent to fair accuracy in diagnosing sepsis and predicting in-hospital sepsis mortality; however, the key downregulated genes showed excellent accuracy in predicting in-hospital sepsis mortality but failed to effectively diagnose sepsis.

Author Contributions: Conceptualization, K.J.; methodology, H.C., J.Y.L., H.Y. and K.J.; software, J.Y.L.; validation, H.C. and H.Y.; formal analysis, H.C., J.Y.L. and K.J.; investigation, H.C. and J.Y.L.; resources, J.Y.L. and K.J.; data curation, H.C., J.Y.L., H.Y. and K.J.; writing—original draft preparation, H.C., J.Y.L. and K.J.; writing—review and editing, H.C., J.Y.L., H.Y. and K.J.; visualization, H.C. and J.Y.L.; supervision, K.J.; project administration, K.J.; funding acquisition, K.J. All authors have read and agreed to the published version of the manuscript.

Funding: This work was supported by the Future Medicine 20*30 Project of the Samsung Medical Center (SMX1230441), a National Research Foundation of Korea grant funded by the Korean Government (MSIT) (NRF-2022R1F1A1074855), and a grant from the Korean Academy of Tuberculosis and Respiratory Disease (2022).

Institutional Review Board Statement: The study was conducted according to the guidelines of the Declaration of Helsinki and was approved by the Institutional Review Board of the Samsung Medical Center (IRB no. 2013-12-033).

Informed Consent Statement: Written informed consent was obtained from all patients or their legally authorized representatives prior to enrollment.

Data Availability Statement: The data discussed in this publication have been deposited in NCBI's Gene Expression Omnibus and are accessible through GEO Series accession number GSE232753 (https://www.ncbi.nlm.nih.gov/geo/query/acc.cgi?acc=GSE232753).

Conflicts of Interest: The authors declare no conflict of interest.

References

1. Singer, M.; Deutschman, C.S.; Seymour, C.W.; Shankar-Hari, M.; Annane, D.; Bauer, M.; Bellomo, R.; Bernard, G.R.; Chiche, J.D.; Coopersmith, C.M.; et al. The Third International Consensus Definitions for Sepsis and Septic Shock (Sepsis-3). *JAMA* **2016**, *315*, 801–810. [CrossRef]
2. Fleischmann, C.; Scherag, A.; Adhikari, N.K.; Hartog, C.S.; Tsaganos, T.; Schlattmann, P.; Angus, D.C.; Reinhart, K.; International Forum of Acute Care Trialists. Assessment of Global Incidence and Mortality of Hospital-treated Sepsis. Current Estimates and Limitations. *Am. J. Respir. Crit. Care Med.* **2016**, *193*, 259–272. [CrossRef] [PubMed]
3. Fleischmann-Struzek, C.; Mellhammar, L.; Rose, N.; Cassini, A.; Rudd, K.E.; Schlattmann, P.; Allegranzi, B.; Reinhart, K. Incidence and mortality of hospital- and ICU-treated sepsis: Results from an updated and expanded systematic review and meta-analysis. *Intensive Care Med.* **2020**, *46*, 1552–1562. [CrossRef] [PubMed]
4. Gaieski, D.F.; Edwards, J.M.; Kallan, M.J.; Carr, B.G. Benchmarking the incidence and mortality of severe sepsis in the United States. *Crit. Care Med.* **2013**, *41*, 1167–1174. [CrossRef]
5. Iwashyna, T.J.; Cooke, C.R.; Wunsch, H.; Kahn, J.M. Population burden of long-term survivorship after severe sepsis in older Americans. *J. Am. Geriatr. Soc.* **2012**, *60*, 1070–1077. [CrossRef] [PubMed]
6. Seymour, C.W.; Gesten, F.; Prescott, H.C.; Friedrich, M.E.; Iwashyna, T.J.; Phillips, G.S.; Lemeshow, S.; Osborn, T.; Terry, K.M.; Levy, M.M. Time to Treatment and Mortality during Mandated Emergency Care for Sepsis. *N. Engl. J. Med.* **2017**, *376*, 2235–2244. [CrossRef]
7. Simon, L.; Saint-Louis, P.; Amre, D.K.; Lacroix, J.; Gauvin, F. Procalcitonin and C-reactive protein as markers of bacterial infection in critically ill children at onset of systemic inflammatory response syndrome. *Pediatr. Crit. Care Med.* **2008**, *9*, 407–413. [CrossRef]
8. Yang, Y.; Xie, J.; Guo, F.; Longhini, F.; Gao, Z.; Huang, Y.; Qiu, H. Combination of C-reactive protein, procalcitonin and sepsis-related organ failure score for the diagnosis of sepsis in critical patients. *Ann. Intensive Care* **2016**, *6*, 51. [CrossRef]
9. Pierrakos, C.; Vincent, J.L. Sepsis biomarkers: A review. *Crit. Care* **2010**, *14*, R15. [CrossRef]
10. Yoo, H.; Lee, J.Y.; Park, J.; Yang, J.H.; Suh, G.Y.; Jeon, K. Association of Plasma Level of TNF-Related Apoptosis-Inducing Ligand with Severity and Outcome of Sepsis. *J. Clin. Med.* **2020**, *9*, 1661. [CrossRef]
11. Hu, Y.; Cheng, L.; Zhong, W.; Chen, M.; Zhang, Q. Bioinformatics Analysis of Gene Expression Profiles for Risk Prediction in Patients with Septic Shock. *Med. Sci. Monit.* **2019**, *25*, 9563–9571. [CrossRef] [PubMed]
12. Li, Z.; Huang, B.; Yi, W.; Wang, F.; Wei, S.; Yan, H.; Qin, P.; Zou, D.; Wei, R.; Chen, N. Identification of Potential Early Diagnostic Biomarkers of Sepsis. *J. Inflamm. Res.* **2021**, *14*, 621–631. [CrossRef]
13. Niu, J.; Qin, B.; Wang, C.; Chen, C.; Yang, J.; Shao, H. Identification of Key Immune-Related Genes in the Progression of Septic Shock. *Front. Genet.* **2021**, *12*, 668527. [CrossRef] [PubMed]
14. She, H.; Tan, L.; Zhou, Y.; Zhu, Y.; Ma, C.; Wu, Y.; Du, Y.; Liu, L.; Hu, Y.; Mao, Q.; et al. The Landscape of Featured Metabolism-Related Genes and Imbalanced Immune Cell Subsets in Sepsis. *Front. Genet.* **2022**, *13*, 821275. [CrossRef] [PubMed]
15. Zeng, X.; Feng, J.; Yang, Y.; Zhao, R.; Yu, Q.; Qin, H.; Wei, L.; Ji, P.; Li, H.; Wu, Z.; et al. Screening of Key Genes of Sepsis and Septic Shock Using Bioinformatics Analysis. *J. Inflamm. Res.* **2021**, *14*, 829–841. [CrossRef]
16. Wu, T.; Liang, X.; Jiang, Y.; Chen, Q.; Zhang, H.; Zhang, S.; Zhang, C.; Lv, Y.; Xin, J.; Jiang, J.; et al. Comprehensive Transcriptome Profiling of Peripheral Blood Mononuclear Cells from Patients with Sepsis. *Int. J. Med. Sci.* **2020**, *17*, 2077–2086. [CrossRef] [PubMed]
17. Herwanto, V.; Tang, B.; Wang, Y.; Shojaei, M.; Nalos, M.; Shetty, A.; Lai, K.; McLean, A.S.; Schughart, K. Blood transcriptome analysis of patients with uncomplicated bacterial infection and sepsis. *BMC Res. Notes* **2021**, *14*, 76. [CrossRef] [PubMed]
18. Zhai, J.; Qi, A.; Zhang, Y.; Jiao, L.; Liu, Y.; Shou, S. Bioinformatics Analysis for Multiple Gene Expression Profiles in Sepsis. *Med. Sci. Monit.* **2020**, *26*, e920818. [CrossRef] [PubMed]
19. Cheng, P.L.; Chen, H.H.; Jiang, Y.H.; Hsiao, T.H.; Wang, C.Y.; Wu, C.L.; Ko, T.M.; Chao, W.C. Using RNA-Seq to Investigate Immune-Metabolism Features in Immunocompromised Patients With Sepsis. *Front. Med.* **2021**, *8*, 747263. [CrossRef]
20. National Library of Medicine (US), N.C.f.B.I. Gene. Available online: https://www.ncbi.nlm.nih.gov/gene/ (accessed on 31 January 2023).
21. Ulas, T.; Pirr, S.; Fehlhaber, B.; Bickes, M.S.; Loof, T.G.; Vogl, T.; Mellinger, L.; Heinemann, A.S.; Burgmann, J.; Schöning, J.; et al. S100-alarmin-induced innate immune programming protects newborn infants from sepsis. *Nat. Immunol.* **2017**, *18*, 622–632. [CrossRef]
22. Boyd, J.H.; Kan, B.; Roberts, H.; Wang, Y.; Walley, K.R. S100A8 and S100A9 mediate endotoxin-induced cardiomyocyte dysfunction via the receptor for advanced glycation end products. *Circ. Res.* **2008**, *102*, 1239–1246. [CrossRef] [PubMed]
23. Forel, J.M.; Chiche, L.; Thomas, G.; Mancini, J.; Farnarier, C.; Cognet, C.; Guervilly, C.; Daumas, A.; Vély, F.; Xéridat, F.; et al. Phenotype and functions of natural killer cells in critically-ill septic patients. *PLoS ONE* **2012**, *7*, e50446. [CrossRef]

24. Lv, X.; Zhang, Y.; Cui, Y.; Ren, Y.; Li, R.; Rong, Q. Inhibition of microRNA-155 relieves sepsis-induced liver injury through inactivating the JAK/STAT pathway. *Mol. Med. Rep.* **2015**, *12*, 6013–6018. [CrossRef]
25. Winkler, M.S.; Rissiek, A.; Priefler, M.; Schwedhelm, E.; Robbe, L.; Bauer, A.; Zahrte, C.; Zoellner, C.; Kluge, S.; Nierhaus, A. Human leucocyte antigen (HLA-DR) gene expression is reduced in sepsis and correlates with impaired TNFα response: A diagnostic tool for immunosuppression? *PLoS ONE* **2017**, *12*, e0182427. [CrossRef]
26. Nedeva, C.; Menassa, J.; Puthalakath, H. Sepsis: Inflammation Is a Necessary Evil. *Front. Cell Dev. Biol.* **2019**, *7*, 108. [CrossRef] [PubMed]
27. Choi, H.; Yoo, H.; Lee, J.Y.; Park, J.; Jeon, K. Plasma Mitochondrial DNA and Necroptosis as Prognostic Indicators in Critically Ill Patients with Sepsis. *Biomedicines* **2022**, *10*, 2386. [CrossRef]
28. Li, D.; Ren, W.; Wang, X.; Wang, F.; Gao, Y.; Ning, Q.; Han, Y.; Song, T.; Lu, S. A modified method using TRIzol reagent and liquid nitrogen produces high-quality RNA from rat pancreas. *Appl. Biochem. Biotechnol.* **2009**, *158*, 253–261. [CrossRef]
29. Sp, N.; Kang, D.Y.; Jo, E.S.; Rugamba, A.; Kim, W.S.; Park, Y.M.; Hwang, D.Y.; Yoo, J.S.; Liu, Q.; Jang, K.J.; et al. Tannic Acid Promotes TRAIL-Induced Extrinsic Apoptosis by Regulating Mitochondrial ROS in Human Embryonic Carcinoma Cells. *Cells* **2020**, *9*, 282. [CrossRef] [PubMed]
30. Kukurba, K.R.; Montgomery, S.B. RNA Sequencing and Analysis. *Cold Spring Harb. Protoc* **2015**, *2015*, pdb-top084970. [CrossRef] [PubMed]
31. Wingett, S.W.; Andrews, S. FastQ Screen: A tool for multi-genome mapping and quality control. *F1000Research* **2018**, *7*, 1338. [CrossRef] [PubMed]
32. Bushnell, B.; Rood, J.; Singer, E. BBMerge–Accurate paired shotgun read merging via overlap. *PLoS ONE* **2017**, *12*, e0185056. [CrossRef]
33. Trapnell, C.; Pachter, L.; Salzberg, S.L. TopHat: Discovering splice junctions with RNA-Seq. *Bioinformatics* **2009**, *25*, 1105–1111. [CrossRef] [PubMed]
34. Roberts, A.; Trapnell, C.; Donaghey, J.; Rinn, J.L.; Pachter, L. Improving RNA-Seq expression estimates by correcting for fragment bias. *Genome Biol.* **2011**, *12*, R22. [CrossRef] [PubMed]
35. R Core Team. *R: A Language and Environment for Statistical Computing*; R Foundation for Statistical Computing: Vienna, Austria, 2013. Available online: http://www.R-project.org (accessed on 5 January 2023).
36. Barrett, T.; Wilhite, S.E.; Ledoux, P.; Evangelista, C.; Kim, I.F.; Tomashevsky, M.; Marshall, K.A.; Phillippy, K.H.; Sherman, P.M.; Holko, M. NCBI GEO: Archive for functional genomics data sets—Update. *Nucleic Acids Res.* **2012**, *41*, D991–D995. [CrossRef]
37. Udhaya Kumar, S.; Thirumal Kumar, D.; Bithia, R.; Sankar, S.; Magesh, R.; Sidenna, M.; George Priya Doss, C.; Zayed, H. Analysis of Differentially Expressed Genes and Molecular Pathways in Familial Hypercholesterolemia Involved in Atherosclerosis: A Systematic and Bioinformatics Approach. *Front. Genet.* **2020**, *11*, 734. [CrossRef] [PubMed]
38. Harris, M.; Clark, J.; Ireland, A.; Lomax, J.; Ashburner, M.; Foulger, R.; Eilbeck, K.; Lewis, S.; Marshall, B.; Mungall, C. The Gene Ontology (GO) database and informatics resource. *Nucleic Acids Res.* **2004**, *32*, D258–D261.
39. Huang, D.W.; Sherman, B.T.; Lempicki, R.A. Bioinformatics enrichment tools: Paths toward the comprehensive functional analysis of large gene lists. *Nucleic Acids Res.* **2009**, *37*, 1–13. [CrossRef]
40. Liao, Y.; Wang, J.; Jaehnig, E.J.; Shi, Z.; Zhang, B. WebGestalt 2019: Gene set analysis toolkit with revamped UIs and APIs. *Nucleic Acids Res.* **2019**, *47*, W199–W205. [CrossRef]
41. Zhou, Y.; Zhou, B.; Pache, L.; Chang, M.; Khodabakhshi, A.H.; Tanaseichuk, O.; Benner, C.; Chanda, S.K. Metascape provides a biologist-oriented resource for the analysis of systems-level datasets. *Nat. Commun.* **2019**, *10*, 1523. [CrossRef]
42. Szklarczyk, D.; Gable, A.L.; Lyon, D.; Junge, A.; Wyder, S.; Huerta-Cepas, J.; Simonovic, M.; Doncheva, N.T.; Morris, J.H.; Bork, P.; et al. STRING v11: Protein-protein association networks with increased coverage, supporting functional discovery in genome-wide experimental datasets. *Nucleic Acids Res.* **2019**, *47*, D607–D613. [CrossRef]
43. Wang, J.; Zhong, J.; Chen, G.; Li, M.; Wu, F.X.; Pan, Y. ClusterViz: A Cytoscape APP for Cluster Analysis of Biological Network. *IEEE/ACM Trans. Comput. Biol. Bioinform.* **2015**, *12*, 815–822. [CrossRef] [PubMed]
44. Maru, D.M.; Singh, R.R.; Hannah, C.; Albarracin, C.T.; Li, Y.X.; Abraham, R.; Romans, A.M.; Yao, H.; Luthra, M.G.; Anandasabapathy, S.; et al. MicroRNA-196a is a potential marker of progression during Barrett's metaplasia-dysplasia-invasive adenocarcinoma sequence in esophagus. *Am. J. Pathol.* **2009**, *174*, 1940–1948. [CrossRef] [PubMed]

Disclaimer/Publisher's Note: The statements, opinions and data contained in all publications are solely those of the individual author(s) and contributor(s) and not of MDPI and/or the editor(s). MDPI and/or the editor(s) disclaim responsibility for any injury to people or property resulting from any ideas, methods, instructions or products referred to in the content.

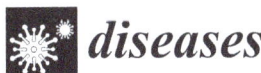 diseases

Review

Scurvy: Rediscovering a Forgotten Disease

Mustafa Gandhi [1], Omar Elfeky [2], Hamza Ertugrul [3], Harleen Kaur Chela [3] and Ebubekir Daglilar [3,*]

1. Department of Internal Medicine, University of Missouri, Columbia, MO 65211, USA
2. Department of Medicine, University of Florida, Leesburg, FL 32611, USA
3. Division of Gastroenterology and Hepatology, Charleston Area Medical Center, West Virginia University, Charleston, WV 25304, USA; he19md@gmail.com (H.E.)
* Correspondence: ebubekir.daglilar@hsc.wvu.edu

Abstract: Scurvy is a nutritional deficiency caused by low vitamin C levels that has been described since ancient times. It leads to a varied presentation, affecting multiple organ systems due to its role in the biochemical reactions of connective tissue synthesis. Common manifestations include gingival bleeding, arthralgias, skin discoloration, impaired wound healing, perifollicular hemorrhage, and ecchymoses. Although there has been a dramatic reduction in the prevalence of scurvy in modern times owing to vitamin C supplementation and intake, sporadic cases still occur. In developed countries, it is mainly diagnosed in the elderly and malnourished individuals and is associated with alcoholism, low socio-economic status, and poor dietary habits. Scurvy has been an unusual cause of gastrointestinal (GI) bleeding among other GI manifestations. It can be adequately treated and prevented via vitamin C supplementation.

Keywords: scurvy; vitamin C deficiency; gastrointestinal bleeding; mucosal ooze; vitamin C supplementation

1. Introduction

First described in 1550 BC in Eber's papyrus, an Egyptian medical scroll, after being reported amongst soldiers and sailors who had minimal access to fruits and vegetables, vitamin C deficiency, also known as scurvy, is an old but not forgotten disease [1]. Scurvy has a deep historical significance and has plagued human populations for centuries. Ancient Egyptian, Greek, and Roman literature all provided detailed descriptions of the clinical signs and symptoms of scurvy. Scurvy decimated the European and British explorers of the Renaissance. During the Great Potato Famine, the American Civil War, the expedition of the North Pole, and the California Gold Rush, scurvy was a significant source of sickness and mortality throughout most of Europe. One of the first to show that sailors who spent months at sea might prevent scurvy by eating a diet high in vegetables was Captain James Cook. In a book titled *Treatise of the Scurvy*, James Lind, a Scottish naval surgeon, detailed his observations and research on scurvy aboard ships and described the effective treatment of scurvy with citrus fruits. As awareness of the importance of fresh fruits and vegetables in the diet increased, there was a decline in the prevalence of scurvy in the 18th century, especially after the establishment of the link between scurvy and vitamin C. Between 1928 and 1931, Szent-Gyorgyi extracted hexuronic acid from various sources such as cabbage, oranges, paprika, and adrenal glands. This substance was later identified as vitamin C and was discovered to have preventive properties against scurvy [2].

Vitamin C, also known as L-ascorbic acid, is a water-soluble nutrient and an essential dietary component that is vulnerable to heat, ultraviolet radiation, and oxygen. Ascorbic acid is involved in various body functions such as the absorption of iron, wound healing, and the formation of collagen. Although there are variations in the prevalence estimates, in some studies, it has been estimated that $7 \pm 0.9\%$ of the population of the United States suffers from scurvy [3]. Some of the risk factors that predispose these patients to the

Citation: Gandhi, M.; Elfeky, O.; Ertugrul, H.; Chela, H.K.; Daglilar, E. Scurvy: Rediscovering a Forgotten Disease. *Diseases* **2023**, *11*, 78. https://doi.org/10.3390/diseases11020078

Academic Editors: Vasso Apostolopoulos, Jack Feehan and Vivek P. Chavda

Received: 14 April 2023
Revised: 19 May 2023
Accepted: 24 May 2023
Published: 26 May 2023

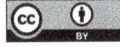

Copyright: © 2023 by the authors. Licensee MDPI, Basel, Switzerland. This article is an open access article distributed under the terms and conditions of the Creative Commons Attribution (CC BY) license (https://creativecommons.org/licenses/by/4.0/).

disease are chronic alcohol use, dietary insufficiency, and obesity [4,5]. Vitamin C is the cofactor for prolyl hydroxylase, which functions to stabilize the collagen molecule, and lysyl hydroxylase, which provides structural strength by cross-linking to the molecule [6]. As there is no long-term vitamin storage mechanism in our bodies, a lack of vitamin C can lead to vitamin C deficiency in as little as 1 to 3 months [7].

Scurvy has a variable clinical presentation due to its role in various bodily functions. Early symptoms can include fatigue, aching pain, irritability, and a loss of appetite. As the deficiency progresses, classic signs may appear, such as swelling of the gums, petechiae, bruising, and abnormal hair growth. Vitamin C deficiency weakens collagen triple-helix structures and fragile capillaries, which can lead to complications such as diffuse mucosal gastrointestinal bleeding [8]. Although coagulation parameters are usually normal, undiagnosed scurvy can result in significant bleeding and hospital burden, especially in post-operative cases [9]. This review article provides an overview of the history, epidemiology, pathophysiology, clinical manifestations, diagnosis, and treatment of scurvy, as well as recent advances in our understanding of this fascinating and important disease while also focusing on the gastrointestinal manifestations of this disease.

2. Biochemistry and Metabolism

Ascorbic acid is the enolic form of alpha-keto lactone, which shares a similar structure to glucose. Vitamin C refers to a group of compounds that have similar biochemical activities to ascorbic acid. Most mammals can synthesize vitamin C using glucose except for primates, fruit bats, and guinea pigs, as they lack the crucial enzyme, L-gluconolactone oxidase, that is necessary for this process.

The body contains a total pool of 1500–2500 mg of vitamin C, and the daily turnover rate is around 45–60 mg, which accounts for approximately 3% of the total amount. The half-life of vitamin C is 10–20 days. The absorption of vitamin C takes place in the ileum via an active transport mechanism The absorption of ascorbic acid occurs in the distal small intestine and relies on an energy-dependent active transport mechanism that can become saturated when the oral intake exceeds 180 mg/day; however, when consumed in typical dietary amounts of up to 100 mg/day, almost all the ascorbic acid is absorbed [10]. However, as dietary intake increases, the absorption rate decreases, and high pharmacologic doses of over 1000 mg/day may result in an absorption rate of less than 50%.

Dehydroascorbic acid is the oxidized form of ascorbic acid metabolism and can passively penetrate cellular membranes [11]. This form of vitamin C is preferred by erythrocytes and leukocytes as it is more readily absorbed by these cells. The ability of dehydroascorbic acid to penetrate cellular membranes plays a crucial role in vitamin C transport and metabolism in the body.

3. Pathophysiology

Ascorbic acid is an essential dietary vitamin for primates. Important dietary sources for humans include fresh fruits and vegetables such as citrus fruits, tomatoes, broccoli, strawberries, cabbage, potatoes, bell peppers, cauliflower, and spinach. Breast milk is an adequate source of vitamin C for infants [12]. Ascorbic acid is a reversible reducing agent that acts as an essential electron donor in several biochemical reactions and enzyme activities. Some of the biological processes that it is involved in are as follows:

- Collagen synthesis: Proline and lysine residues in the collagen structure must be enzymatically hydroxylated to produce the collagen found in the skin, blood vessels, and soft tissues. Prolyl hydroxylase and lysyl hydroxylase are enzymes that catalyze reactions, generating hydroxyproline and hydroxylysine, respectively. This reaction uses ascorbic acid as an electron donor. The inability to finish this step of collagen synthesis has adverse effects on bone and fibroblast functions, tooth development, and wound healing [13]. Furthermore, a deficiency in ascorbic acid causes epigenetic DNA hypermethylation and prevents the transcription of certain collagen types.

- Neurotransmitter synthesis: Ascorbic acid is a necessary cofactor for the enzyme dopamine-beta-monooxygenase, which hydroxylates dopamine to produce norepinephrine [14].
- Nitric oxide synthesis: The production of nitric oxide, a powerful vasodilator, is stimulated by ascorbic acid.
- Fatty acid transport: Ascorbic acid is necessary as an electron donor for the synthesis of carnitine. Long-chain fatty acid transportation across the mitochondrial membrane is a carnitine-dependent process [15].

Considering the widespread involvement of ascorbic acid in the formation and maintenance of soft tissues, scurvy results in numerous manifestations involving the skin and its appendages, impaired wound healing, dental and gingival disease, brittle bones, and hemorrhage relating to the loss of blood vessel integrity.

4. Epidemiology

Scurvy was traditionally described in sailors in older times, but there have been sporadic cases reported in recent times from underdeveloped regions without adequate nutritional support in at-risk populations. Although there is a variation in its global prevalence, the estimated overall prevalence of vitamin C deficiency in the US is about 5.9%, according to the 2017–2018 National Health and Nutrition Examination Survey (NHANES), whose aim was to assess the mean vitamin C serum levels and the prevalence of vitamin C deficiency (defined as a mean serum level of less than 11.4 µmol/L) [16]. The survey study sample consisted of 6740 civilians aged six years and older who were not living in institutions. These individuals were selected from the National Health and Nutrition Examination Survey (NHANES) conducted in 2017–2018 and were representative of 274,157,096 people in the United States. The researchers used multivariable linear and logistic regression analyses to investigate the predictive effects of various factors. They also compared the serum levels of Vitamin C and the prevalence of vitamin C deficiency in this sample with data from NHANES 2005–2006 using Student's t-tests.

They discovered that women had a higher mean vitamin C serum concentration, while current smokers and obese individuals had a lower level. There was a decline in mean serum vitamin C levels without any significant change in the prevalence of vitamin C deficiency since the previous NHANES 2005–2006. The global incidence of scurvy can vary based on the socio-economic status of a region, with underdeveloped areas such as north India having an incidence as high as 73.9% [17].

5. Risk Factors

Given that vitamin C is an essential dietary nutrient for humans, manifestations of its deficiency are mainly related to the inadequate consumption or improper absorption of this nutrient in the small gut. Since 90% of ascorbic acid in the diet is from fruits and vegetables, a lack of these foods commonly leads to a deficiency. Since vitamin C is heat-sensitive, the manner of cooking also plays a role in the bioavailability of this nutrient in food [17]. Based on this, the risk factors or high-risk groups for vitamin C deficiency include the following [6]:

- Individuals with poor dietary habits who consume food of poor nutritional value;
- Limited access to or the inability to afford fresh fruits and vegetables;
- Alcoholism;
- Infants exclusively fed cow's milk;
- Individuals with gastrointestinal disorders such as inflammatory bowel disease;
- Smoking was demonstrated as a significant risk factor in the NHANES [16];
- Low socio-economic status;
- Elderly individuals on a "tea-and-toast" diet;
- Eating disorders and psychiatric illness;
- Long-term use of certain medications such as corticosteroids or proton pump inhibitors, which can alter the absorption and bioavailability of vitamin C in the diet;

- Abdominal surgeries, such as small bowel resection or bariatric surgery, which affect gut absorption;
- Obesity;
- Dialysis [18].

A poor intake of vitamin-C-rich foods is a more obvious cause of deficiency when compared to obesity and abdominal surgeries. When talking about obesity as a cause of vitamin deficiencies, a change in the diet in the past few decades has led to the increased consumption of junk foods and fast foods such as pizzas, burgers, fried foods, and carbonated beverages, with a reduced intake of fresh fruits and vegetables; this has resulted in vitamin deficiencies resurfacing [19].

This change in dietary habits could be attributable to hectic work schedules, convenience, the cost of food, a sedentary lifestyle, and a lack of social support [20]. Bariatric surgeries such as sleeve-gastrectomy or gastric bypass can lead to an alteration in the acidic environment of the gut, causing impaired absorption [21]. The underlying causes of vitamin C deficiency and scurvy in children include psychiatric eating disorders such as avoidant/restrictive food intake disorder and anorexia nervosa, food insecurity, and neglect [22]. Another risk group in which scurvy has been reported is children with autism spectrum disorder who have a diet lacking fruits and vegetables [23]. Scurvy can occur in patients with excess iron secondary to hematological conditions such as thalassemia or sickle cell disease or a prior bone marrow transplantation [24]. Ferric deposition can accelerate the breakdown of ascorbic acid in the body; thus, iron overload can precipitate the manifestation of scurvy [25].

Role of Vitamin C in the Immune System

Vitamin C plays an essential role in the regulation and function of the immune system. It affects the innate and adaptive immune system in a variety of ways.

- Barrier integrity: As previously discussed, vitamin C plays a major role in the synthesis of collagen, which is a component of soft tissue, including the epidermis and dermis. These skin layers actively accumulate ascorbic acid, suggesting that it plays a crucial role in maintaining the integrity of the skin and mucosal barriers to pathogens [26].
- Leukocyte Function: Studies have shown that neutrophils and lymphocytes accumulate ascorbic acid at concentrations 50 to 100 times higher than the plasma concentrations through active transport. The antioxidant properties of ascorbate within the cell are believed to protect the cells from free radicals from the oxidative burst. Additionally, vitamin C is also postulated to play a role in chemotaxis and neutrophil apoptosis [27].

6. Clinical Manifestations

The typical manifestations of scurvy begin to appear after 4 to 12 weeks of inadequate dietary ascorbic acid intake [14]. Non-specific symptoms such as fatigue, anorexia, and irritability may be seen when serum ascorbic acid concentrations dip below 20 µmol/L, but levels below 11.4 µmol/L indicate a substantial deficiency with which the more specific manifestations are observed [3].

Dermatological findings are generally specific for ascorbic acid deficiency and include follicular hyperkeratosis and perifollicular hemorrhage with petechiae and coiled hairs [28]. Ecchymoses, petechiae, and xerosis are other common skin findings. Initially, flat hemorrhagic skin lesions appear which may later coalesce and become palpable, especially on the lower extremities. These findings can be attributed to the reduced integrity of the dermal soft tissues due to impaired collagen synthesis, for which vitamin C is an essential component. Perifollicular hemorrhages usually occur in the lower extremities due to the capillaries' vulnerability to hydrostatic pressure caused by gravity, which leads to "woody edema" [17]. The downregulation of tyrosinase enzyme activity from an ascorbic acid deficiency leads to an inhibition of melanin synthesis and skin discoloration in some patients [29]. Nail findings include koilonychia and splinter hemorrhages.

The musculoskeletal manifestations include arthralgias (typically of the knees, ankles, and wrists), muscle aches, hemarthrosis, and muscular hematomas [28,30]. By virtue of its role in biochemical reactions, vitamin C deficiency leads to alterations in structural collagen, deficient osteoid matrix formation, and increased bone resorption [30]. The musculoskeletal pain can be due to bleeding into the periosteum or muscles. Scurvy also causes the classic oral manifestations of gingivitis with bleeding and receding gums, as well as dental caries.

Fatigue, muscle weakness, malaise, arthralgias, loss of appetite, mood changes, peripheral neuropathy, and vasomotor instability are examples of generalized systemic symptoms that are commonly experienced with vitamin C deficiency. Dyspnea, hypotension, and sudden death have all been described as cardiorespiratory symptoms of scurvy, and it is hypothesized that these symptoms are brought on by a defective vasomotor response (especially given the role of ascorbic acid in nitric oxide synthesis) [30].

In the pediatric population, an acute limp can be the presenting musculoskeletal manifestation of scurvy owing to severe malnutrition [31]. A systematic review conducted by Trapani et al. on scurvy in the pediatric population revealed that 90% of children suffered from musculoskeletal complaints such as arthritis and lower limb pain, while about 33% had a limp and/or refused to walk [31,32]. Magnetic resonance imaging in children with scurvy can demonstrate certain characteristic features, such as a periosteal inflammatory reaction and local soft tissue swelling, in addition to sclerotic and lucent metaphyseal bands [24].

Vitamin C and Lung Function

Ascorbic acid plays an important role in regulating the functioning of the pulmonary system. As an antioxidant, ascorbic acid plays an important role in the protection of lung tissue from reactive oxygen species. Akin to other leukocytes elsewhere in the body, the alveolar macrophages and alveolar type 2 cells concentrate vitamin C and scavenge reactive oxygen species to ameliorate oxidative damage [33].

Studies have shown promising data on the effect of high-dose intravenous ascorbic acid (HDIAA) in improving pulmonary function in those with severe COVID-19 pneumonia. The SARS-CoV infection is associated with a severe inflammatory response and a cytokine storm. Ascorbic acid helps maintain the integrity of the epithelial barrier and mitigates oxidative stress through its antioxidant properties [34].

7. Gastrointestinal Manifestations

The gastrointestinal (GI) tract is supplied by three major unpaired vessels that branch from the abdominal aorta, the celiac trunk, the superior mesenteric artery, and the inferior mesenteric artery. Branches from these major vessels then form anastomotic systems which, in turn, supply the gastrointestinal system and adjoining organs. Due to its high vascularity and large surface area, the GI tract is commonly investigated for bleeding in patients with anemia.

Recent studies have linked vitamin C to vascular function. In a study using cultured epithelial cells, d'Uscio et. al demonstrated the beneficial effect of vitamin C on vascular endothelial function [35]. This effect was mediated in part by the protection of tetrahydrobiopterin and the restoration of endothelial nitric oxide synthase enzymatic activity. There are a few hypothesized mechanisms through which vitamin C modulates vasorelaxation and increases nitric oxide synthesis or bioavailability. Firstly, vitamin C appears to recycle tetrahydrobiopterin, which is a co-factor for endothelial nitric oxide synthase. Endothelial nitric oxide synthase generates nitric oxide, which diffuses into the smooth muscle layer of the vascular wall and interacts with guanylyl cyclase and mediates vasodilation [36]. Secondly, vitamin C appears to regulate the activity of nicotinamide adenine dinucleotide phosphate (NADPH) oxidases and modulates the inflammatory response [37].

There have been infrequent cases reporting scurvy presenting as an overt gastrointestinal bleed. The literature on the gastrointestinal manifestations of scurvy is limited. (Table 1). Ohta et al. described a middle-aged man who had two years of anorexia and a diet deficient in fruits and vegetables when he developed hematochezia [37]. Erythema and intramucosal hemorrhage were discovered in the antrum and duodenum during an upper endoscopic evaluation. Similar observations of several intramucosal hemorrhages and redness in the rectum were found during a colonoscopy; these were biopsied for additional analysis. The rectal erythema was histologically examined, and the results showed inflammatory cell infiltration and fibrin exudation. Scurvy was determined to be the cause after additional testing of vitamin C levels, and hemorrhage was controlled after administration of a high dose of vitamin C. Callus et al. described a case of a 61-year-old man with a history of heavy alcohol use and limited food intake resulting in malnutrition [38]. He presented with upper gastrointestinal bleeding and had multiple bruises, poor dentition with bleeding gums, and telangiectasia upon examination. Blood tests showed low levels of vitamin C (0.21 mg/dL). Another case reported by Antunes et al. described a 40-year-old with a history of alcoholism and an unbalanced diet who presented with symptoms of polyarthralgia, bleeding gums, and episodes of hematochezia [39]. A physical examination revealed severe periodontitis with gingival hypertrophy and purplish areas consistent with necrosis. Blood tests revealed anemia and a vitamin C level of 0.14 mg/dL. A colonoscopy showed multiple intramucosal hemorrhages in the cecum and ascending colon. The patient was diagnosed with scurvy and treated with oral vitamin supplementation and adequate nutrition, resulting in complete clinical recovery within two months. Ertugrul et al. reported a case of refractory upper gastrointestinal bleeding in a morbidly obese patient mimicking portal gastropathy bleeding [40].

Table 1. Summary of cases of gastrointestinal manifestations in scurvy.

	Study	Age (In Years)	Gender	Manifestations
1.	Ohta A. et al. [37]	40	Male	Hematochezia. Antral, duodenal, and rectal erythema and mucosal hemorrhage.
2.	Callus CA et al. [38]	61	Male	Upper gastrointestinal bleeding. Gingivitis and bruising.
3.	Antunes et al. [39]	40	Male	Bleeding gums and episodic hematochezia. Cecal and ascending colon intramucosal hemorrhages.
4.	Ertugrul et al. [40]	56	Female	Refractory upper gastrointestinal bleeding, post-surgical state, mimicking portal gastropathy.

8. Diagnosis

The diagnosis of scurvy can be challenging as its symptoms may mimic those of other conditions. Additionally, individuals with scurvy may not present with all the classic symptoms. A combination of physical examination, medical history, dietary history, and laboratory tests is typically used to diagnose scurvy. During a physical examination, careful attention must be paid to signs of scurvy, such as swollen or bleeding gums, skin discoloration or bruising, and delayed wound healing. A medical history may be taken to determine risk factors for scurvy, such as dietary habits, chronic illness, and lifestyle factors. Laboratory tests can help confirm a diagnosis of scurvy. A blood test can measure vitamin C levels, which are typically low in individuals with scurvy. Symptoms of scurvy occur after the plasma concentration of ascorbic acid falls below 0.2 mg/dL; this value is usually calculated from plasma and leucocyte vitamin C levels [39]. Determining functional vitamin C status is challenging because there are no dependable indicators. Nevertheless, plasma and leukocyte vitamin C levels are commonly used to evaluate the status and are moderately associated with vitamin C consumption. Patients with a vitamin C deficiency commonly exhibit anemia, which may present as either iron-deficiency anemia (microcytic hypochromic) or a normochromic normocytic pattern [28]. In many cases, anemia in vitamin-C-deficient patients can be attributed to acute blood loss caused by defects in collagen synthesis. Such blood loss may occur in various soft tissue sites, including the gastrointestinal tract, joints, and muscles. Additionally, intravascular hemolysis has been observed in some cases, likely due to a decreased lifespan of red blood cells [28]. Overall, anemia is a frequent laboratory finding in patients with vitamin C deficiency and can have various underlying causes. Vitamin C plays a vital role in the absorption and metabolism of several nutrients that impact the production of red blood cells. One of the critical functions of vitamin C is aiding in the conversion of iron from the ferric form to the ferrous form, which is essential for the absorption of iron from the gastrointestinal tract. Moreover, scurvy may be associated with folate deficiency, and vitamin C helps to enhance the effect of folate in the production of red blood cells. Foods that are rich in vitamin C also tend to be high in folic acid, highlighting the importance of a balanced diet in preventing deficiencies in these essential nutrients [41].

Vitamin C deficiency is not commonly encountered in modern medicine. Therefore, a diagnosis of nutritional insufficiency accounting for a severe gastrointestinal bleed can only be considered with high clinical suspicion. Upper gastrointestinal bleeding has a wide range of differential diagnoses that may present similarly to vitamin C deficiency; therefore, it can be easily overlooked. These diagnoses include ulcerative gingivitis, blood dyscrasias, vasculitis and portal hypertensive gastropathy. Therefore, it is crucial to be aware of how uncommon causes of gastrointestinal bleeding, such as scurvy, manifest. The symptomatology can range from minor, non-specific signs to overt bleeding, including ecchymosis, bleeding gums, and a more serious hemorrhage.

In a study by Blee et al., it was found that patients in the hospital or undergoing surgery may have borderline levels of vitamin C which can further decrease due to a lack of oral intake post-surgery or other critical illnesses such as pancreatitis, sepsis, or multiple organ failure [10]. The study was conducted over a 12-month period in a surgical unit to identify patients with bleeding disorders. Out of the 12 patients who experienced widespread bleeding, none had a surgical cause; however, all had normal coagulation parameters but were found to have vitamin C levels below 0.6 mg/dL (the normal range is 0.6–2.0 mg/dL). Most of these patients had undergone abdominal surgeries, but significant bleeding was also observed in the cardiovascular and neurosurgical patients. The patients required a range of 2–13 units of blood transfusions, with 4.8 units being the average. It was also noted that 7 out of 12 of the patients who experienced widespread bleeding had poor oral nutrition prior to surgery.

9. Treatment

The treatment for scurvy is vitamin C supplementation and the reversal of the conditions that led to the deficiency. A wide range of replacement doses have been used successfully. For children, recommended doses are 100 mg of ascorbic acid given three times daily (orally, intramuscularly, or intravenously) for one week, then once daily for several weeks until the patient is fully recovered. Adults are usually treated with 300 to 1000 mg/day for one month [42].

The difficulty in treating hemorrhage caused by scurvy is not in treating the bleeding itself but rather in accurately diagnosing the condition. If scurvy is suspected, it can be effectively treated with high doses of Vitamin C. It has been reported that after just one replacement dose, gastrointestinal bleeding related to vitamin C deficiency will stop, and capillary stability will be established within 24 h. However, it can take up to 2–3 weeks for other symptoms of scurvy, such as skin lesions, to heal. The treatment of scurvy begins with high doses of Vitamin C: replacement is needed to replace the deficit in body stores. A recommended treatment course is an initial dosing of 1000 mg of intravenous ascorbic acid daily for 3 days, followed by further supplementation as needed with a dose of 250 to 500 mg twice daily for 1 month after discharge or longer if vitamin C cannot be to obtained via diet [40].

10. Prevention

Water-soluble vitamins such as vitamin C are stored in the body in very limited amounts and must be replenished through dietary intake. Ascorbic acid is most highly concentrated in certain body parts, including the pituitary gland, adrenal gland, brain, leukocytes, and the eyes. Unlike fat-soluble vitamins, which can be stored for long periods of time, water-soluble vitamins are quickly excreted from the body through urine. Therefore, it is important to ensure that an adequate amount of these nutrients is consumed on a regular basis to maintain healthy levels within the body. The United States RDA recommends the following daily intake amount of vitamin C [12]:

- Up to 6 months: 40 mg, as normally supplied through breastfeeding;
- From 7 to 12 months: 50 mg;
- From 1 to 3 years: 15 mg;
- From 4 to 8 years: 25 mg;
- From 9 to 13 years: 45 mg;
- From 14 to 18 years: 75 mg for males; 65 mg for females;
- From 19 years and older: 90 mg for males; 75 mg for females.

During pregnancy, it is recommended to consume 85 mg of vitamin C per day, increasing the amount to 120 mg during breastfeeding. Smokers require an additional 35 mg of vitamin C daily compared to non-smokers [12,43].

11. Toxicity

The over-supplementation or overconsumption of vitamin C has also been observed in some cases. The literature reports several side effects of ascorbic acid. Ingesting large doses of vitamin C (in gram quantities) can cause false-negative results in stool guaiac tests [44], as well as diarrhea and abdominal bloating. Studies have also found a correlation between vitamin C intake (from diet and supplements) and oxalate kidney stones in males, particularly at high doses [45]. Therefore, routine supplementation with vitamin C is not recommended for males, especially those who are predisposed to form oxalate stones. Such individuals should limit their intake of vitamin C to the recommended dietary allowance (RDA) in the United States.

There have been rare reports of fatal cardiac arrhythmias in patients with iron overload who ingested large amounts of ascorbic acid. This is thought to be due to oxidative injury [46]. Therefore, it may be advisable for patients to avoid taking pharmacologic doses of ascorbic acid supplements. However, there is no reason to discourage the consumption of fresh fruits or vegetables that contain vitamin C.

The LOVIT (Lessening organ dysfunction with Vitamin C) trial concluded that septic ICU patients who received a 4-day course of intravenous vitamin C had a higher risk of death or persistent organ dysfunction compared to those who received a placebo [47]. An interesting paper analyzed the data from the LOVIT trial to attempt to determine the cause of the higher deaths and organ dysfunction in the vitamin C group. They concluded that the increased mortality may be due to the abrupt termination of the ascorbic acid supplementation rather than the administration itself [48]. It is important for clinicians to thus be cognizant that the sudden halt of ascorbic acid supplementation can mimic a severe deficiency and lead to worse outcomes.

12. Limitations

Although this article has attempted to provide a comprehensive and concise review of vitamin C and its deficiency, especially in relation to the gastrointestinal system, we acknowledged certain limitations of this review. The review does not delve into many details about the basic science and biochemistry of vitamin C since we preferred to focus on the clinical implications of the deficiency. Scurvy is primarily still a historical disease, with most of the literature pertaining to it being older, with limited newer literature. Hence, our article contains information from relatively older studies and a limited proportion of recent case reports on scurvy. The demographic data is most relevant to the United States and does not cover the nutritional status of vitamin C in developing countries in Asia and Africa where scurvy would be expected to be most prevalent.

13. Conclusions

In summary, it is crucial for healthcare professionals to recognize and understand the significance of scurvy as a nutritional deficiency that has been prevalent for centuries but is increasingly being diagnosed in modern times. This increase in incidence is mainly due to several factors such as poor dietary habits, alcoholism, low socio-economic status, obesity, and abdominal surgeries. Scurvy can affect various organ systems due to its involvement in several biochemical reactions that affect tissue structure. Therefore, it is important to be aware of its potential gastrointestinal manifestations, particularly gastrointestinal bleeding. In cases in which the cause of gastrointestinal bleeding is an uncontrolled mucosal ooze, a high index of suspicion is necessary. Empirical treatment with vitamin C is a viable option due to its low cost and safety profile, particularly in patients with a high suspicion of scurvy.

In conclusion, scurvy is a preventable disease that can have severe consequences if left untreated. As such, it is crucial to maintain a balanced and healthy diet that includes sufficient amounts of vitamin C. Health professionals should be vigilant about the signs and symptoms of scurvy, especially in at-risk patients, and should consider vitamin C supplementation in suspected cases to prevent further complications.

Author Contributions: Conceptualization, O.E. and E.D.; methodology, M.G.; resources, H.K.C.; data curation, E.D.; writing—original draft preparation, O.E., M.G., H.E. and E.D.; writing—review and editing, H.K.C. and E.D.; visualization, O.E.; supervision, E.D. All authors have read and agreed to the published version of the manuscript.

Funding: This research received no external funding.

Institutional Review Board Statement: Not applicable.

Informed Consent Statement: Not applicable.

Conflicts of Interest: The authors declare no conflict of interest.

References

1. Pimentel, L. Scurvy: Historical Review and Current Diagnostic Approach. *Am. J. Emerg. Med.* **2003**, *21*, 328–332. [CrossRef] [PubMed]
2. Svirbely, J.L.; Szent-Györgyi, A. The chemical nature of vitamin C. *Biochem. J.* **1933**, *27*, 279–285. [CrossRef] [PubMed]
3. Schleicher, R.L.; Carroll, M.D.; Ford, E.S.; Lacher, D.A. Serum vitamin C and the prevalence of vitamin C deficiency in the United States: 2003–2004 National Health and Nutrition Examination Survey (NHANES). *Am. J. Clin. Nutr.* **2009**, *90*, 1252–1263. [CrossRef] [PubMed]
4. Velandia, B.; Centor, R.M.; McConnell, V.; Shah, M. Scurvy is still present in developed countries. *J. Gen. Intern. Med.* **2008**, *23*, 1281–1284. [CrossRef] [PubMed]
5. Hampl, J.S.; Taylor, C.A.; Johnston, C.S. Vitamin C deficiency and depletion in the United States: The Third National Health and Nutrition Examination Survey, 1988 to 1994. *Am. J. Public Health* **2004**, *94*, 870–875. [CrossRef] [PubMed]
6. Doseděl, M.; Jirkovský, E.; Macáková, K.; Krčmová, L.K.; Javorská, L.; Pourová, J.; Mercolini, L.; Remião, F.; Nováková, L.; Mladěnka, P.; et al. Vitamin C-Sources, Physiological Role, Kinetics, Deficiency, Use, Toxicity, and Determination. *Nutrients* **2021**, *13*, 615. [CrossRef]
7. Levine, M.; Rumsey, S.C.; Daruwala, R.; Park, J.B.; Wang, Y. Criteria and recommendations for vitamin C intake. *JAMA* **1999**, *281*, 1415–1423. [CrossRef]
8. Hodges, R.E.; Hood, J.; Canham, J.E.; Sauberlich, H.E.; Baker, E.M. Clinical manifestations of ascorbic acid deficiency in man. *Am. J. Clin. Nutr.* **1971**, *24*, 432–443. [CrossRef]
9. Blee, T.H.; Cogbill, T.H.; Lambert, P.J. Hemorrhage Associated with Vitamin C Deficiency in Surgical Patients. *Surgery* **2002**, *131*, 408–412. [CrossRef]
10. Kallner, A.; Hornig, D.; Pellikka, R. Formation of carbon dioxide from ascorbate in man. *Am. J. Clin. Nutr.* **1985**, *41*, 609–613. [CrossRef]
11. Bigley, R.H.; Stankova, L. Uptake and reduction of oxidized and reduced ascorbate by human leukocytes. *J. Exp. Med.* **1974**, *139*, 1084–1092. [CrossRef]

12. Institute of Medicine. *Dietary Reference Intakes for Vitamin C, Vitamin E, Selenium, and Carotenoids*; The National Academies Press: Washington, DC, USA, 2000. [CrossRef]
13. Ronchetti, I.P.; Quaglino, D., Jr.; Bergamini, G. Ascorbic acid and connective tissue. *Subcell Biochem.* **1996**, *25*, 249–264. [CrossRef] [PubMed]
14. Katsuki, H.; Vitamin, C.; Nervous, T. In Vivo and in Vitro Aspects. In *Subcellular Biochemistry*; Harris, J.R., Ed.; Springer: Boston, MA, USA, 1996; Volume 25. [CrossRef]
15. Rebouche, C.J. Renal handling of carnitine in experimental vitamin C deficiency. *Metabolism* **1995**, *44*, 1639–1643. [CrossRef] [PubMed]
16. Narayanan, S.; Kumar, S.S.; Manguvo, A.; Friedman, E. Current Estimates of Serum Vitamin C and Vitamin C Deficiency in the United States. *Curr. Dev. Nutr.* **2021**, *5* (Suppl. 2), 1067. [CrossRef]
17. Maxfield, L.; Crane, J.S. Vitamin C Deficiency. In *StatPearls*; StatPearls Publishing: Treasure Island, FL, USA, 2022.
18. Panchal, S.; Schneider, C.; Malhotra, K. Scurvy in a hemodialysis patient. Rare or ignored? *Hemodial Int.* **2018**, *22*, S83–S87. [CrossRef]
19. Paeratakul, S.; Ferdinand, D.P.; Champagne, C.M.; Ryan, D.H.; Bray, G.A. Fast-food consumption among US adults and children: Dietary and nutrient intake profile. *J. Am. Diet Assoc.* **2003**, *103*, 1332–1338. [CrossRef]
20. Amisha, F.; Ghanta, S.N.; Kumar, A.; Fugere, T.; Malik, P.; Kakadia, S. Scurvy in the Modern World: Extinct or Not? *Cureus* **2022**, *14*, e22622. [CrossRef]
21. Gasmi, A.; Bjørklund, G.; Mujawdiya, P.K.; Semenova, Y.; Peana, M.; Dosa, A. Micronutrients deficiencies in patients after bariatric surgery. *Eur. J. Nutr.* **2022**, *61*, 55–67. [CrossRef] [PubMed]
22. Pan, T.; Hennrikus, E.F.; Hennrikus, W.L. Modern Day Scurvy in Pediatric Orthopaedics: A Forgotten Illness. *J. Pediatr. Orthop.* **2021**, *41*, e279–e284. [CrossRef]
23. Ma, N.S.; Thompson, C.; Weston, S. Brief Report: Scurvy as a Manifestation of Food Selectivity in Children with Autism. *J. Autism. Dev. Disord.* **2016**, *46*, 1464–1470. [CrossRef]
24. Golriz, F.; Donnelly, L.F.; Devaraj, S.; Krishnamurthy, R. Modern American scurvy-experience with vitamin C deficiency at a large children's hospital. *Pediatr. Radiol.* **2017**, *47*, 214–220. [CrossRef]
25. Wapnick, A.A.; Lynch, S.R.; Krawitz, P.; Seftel, H.C.; Charlton, R.W.; Bothwell, T.H. Effects of iron overload on ascorbic acid metabolism. *Br. Med. J.* **1968**, *3*, 704–707. [CrossRef]
26. Pullar, J.M.; Carr, A.C.; Vissers, M.C.M. The Roles of Vitamin C in Skin Health. *Nutrients* **2017**, *9*, 866. [CrossRef]
27. Carr, A.C.; Maggini, S. Vitamin C and Immune Function. *Nutrients* **2017**, *9*, 1211. [CrossRef] [PubMed]
28. Fain, O. Musculoskeletal manifestations of scurvy. *Jt. Bone Spine* **2005**, *72*, 124–128. [CrossRef]
29. Sanadi, R.M.; Deshmukh, R.S. The effect of Vitamin C on melanin pigmentation—A systematic review. *J. Oral Maxillofac. Pathol.* **2020**, *24*, 374–382. [CrossRef]
30. Hirschmann, J.V.; Raugi, G.J. Adult scurvy. *J. Am. Acad. Dermatol.* **1999**, *41*, 895–910. [CrossRef] [PubMed]
31. Thiemann, S.; Cimorelli, V.; Bajwa, N.M. Case Report: Uncommon cause of limp in the 21st century. *Front. Endocrinol.* **2022**, *13*, 968015. [CrossRef] [PubMed]
32. Trapani, S.; Rubino, C.; Indolfi, G.; Lionetti, P. A Narrative Review on Pediatric Scurvy: The Last Twenty Years. *Nutrients* **2022**, *14*, 684. [CrossRef] [PubMed]
33. Wang, D.; Wang, M.; Zhang, H.; Zhu, H.; Zhang, N.; Liu, J. Effect of Intravenous Injection of Vitamin C on Postoperative Pulmonary Complications in Patients Undergoing Cardiac Surgery: A Double-Blind, Randomized Trial. *Drug Des. Devel. Ther.* **2020**, *14*, 3263–3270. [CrossRef]
34. Sokary, S.; Ouagueni, A.; Ganji, V. Intravenous Ascorbic Acid and Lung Function in Severely Ill COVID-19 Patients. *Metabolites* **2022**, *12*, 865. [CrossRef] [PubMed]
35. d'Uscio, L.V.; Milstien, S.; Richardson, D.; Smith, L.; Katusic, Z.S. Long-term vitamin C treatment increases vascular tetrahydrobiopterin levels and nitric oxide synthase activity. *Circ. Res.* **2003**, *92*, 88–95. [CrossRef] [PubMed]
36. May, J.M.; Harrison, F.E. Role of vitamin C in the function of the vascular endothelium. *Antioxid. Redox Signal.* **2013**, *19*, 2068–2083. [CrossRef] [PubMed]
37. Ohta, A.; Yoshida, S.; Imaeda, H.; Ohgo, H.; Sujino, T.; Yamaoka, M.; Kanno, R.; Kobayashi, T.; Kinoshita, S.; Iida, S.; et al. Scurvy with Gastrointestinal Bleeding. *Endoscopy* **2013**, *45* (Suppl. 2), E147–E148. [CrossRef]
38. Callus, C.A.; Vella, S.; Ferry, P. Scurvy is Back. *Nutr. Metab. Insights* **2018**, *11*, 1178638818809097. [CrossRef]
39. Gião Antunes, A.S.; Peixe, B.; Guerreiro, H. Gastrointestinal Bleeding Secondary to Scurvy in an Alcoholic Malnourished Cirrhotic Patient. *ACG Case Rep. J.* **2017**, *4*, e29. [CrossRef]
40. Ertugrul, H.; Chela, H.K.; Kahveci, A.; Tahan, V.; Daglilar, E. Don't Get Fooled: Scurvy Can Mimic Portal Hypertensive Gastropathy Bleeding. *Am. J. Gastroenterol.* **2022**, *117*, e1696–e1697. [CrossRef]
41. Popovich, D.; McAlhany, A.; Adewumi, A.O.; Barnes, M.M. Scurvy: Forgotten but definitely not gone. *J. Pediatr. Health Care* **2009**, *23*, 405–415. [CrossRef]
42. Weinstein, M.; Babyn, P.; Zlotkin, S. An orange a day keeps the doctor away: Scurvy in the year 2000. *Pediatrics* **2001**, *108*, E55. [CrossRef]
43. Francescone, M.A.; Levitt, J. Scurvy masquerading as leukocytoclastic vasculitis: A case report and review of the literature. *Cutis* **2005**, *76*, 261–266.

44. Jaffe, R.M.; Kasten, B.; Young, D.S.; MacLowry, J.D. False-negative stool occult blood tests caused by ingestion of ascorbic acid (vitamin C). *Ann. Intern. Med.* **1975**, *83*, 824–826. [CrossRef]
45. Ferraro, P.M.; Curhan, G.C.; Gambaro, G.; Taylor, E.N. Total, Dietary, and Supplemental Vitamin C Intake and Risk of Incident Kidney Stones. *Am. J. Kidney Dis.* **2016**, *67*, 400–407. [CrossRef] [PubMed]
46. McLaran, C.J.; Bett, J.H.; Nye, J.A.; Halliday, J.W. Congestive cardiomyopathy and haemochromatosis—Rapid progression possibly accelerated by excessive ingestion of ascorbic acid. *Aust. N. Z. J. Med.* **1982**, *12*, 187–188. [CrossRef] [PubMed]
47. Adhikari, N.K.; Pinto, R.; Day, A.G.; Masse, M.H.; Ménard, J.; Sprague, S. Lessening Organ Dysfunction With Vitamin C (LOVIT) Trial: Statistical Analysis Plan. *JMIR Res. Protoc.* **2022**, *11*, e36261. [CrossRef] [PubMed]
48. Hemilä, H.; Chalker, E. Abrupt termination of vitamin C from ICU patients may increase mortality: Secondary analysis of the LOVIT trial. *Eur. J. Clin. Nutr.* **2023**, *77*, 490–494. [CrossRef] [PubMed]

Disclaimer/Publisher's Note: The statements, opinions and data contained in all publications are solely those of the individual author(s) and contributor(s) and not of MDPI and/or the editor(s). MDPI and/or the editor(s) disclaim responsibility for any injury to people or property resulting from any ideas, methods, instructions or products referred to in the content.

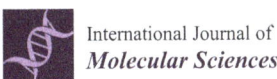

International Journal of
Molecular Sciences

Article

A Protocol for Simultaneous In Vivo Imaging of Cardiac and Neuroinflammation in Dystrophin-Deficient MDX Mice Using [^{18}F]FEPPA PET

Joanne M. Tang [1,2], Andrew McClennan [1,2], Linshan Liu [2], Jennifer Hadway [2], John A. Ronald [1,3], Justin W. Hicks [1,2], Lisa Hoffman [1,2,4,†] and Udunna C. Anazodo [1,2,5,*,†]

1. Department of Medical Biophysics, Western University, London, ON N6A 3K7, Canada
2. Lawson Health Research Institute, London, ON N6A 4V2, Canada
3. Robarts Research Institute, Western University, London, ON N6A 3K7, Canada
4. Department of Anatomy and Cell Biology, Western University, London, ON N6A 3K7, Canada
5. Department of Neurology and Neurosurgery, Montreal Neurological Institute, McGill University, Montreal, QC H3A 0G4, Canada
* Correspondence: udunna.anazodo@mcgill.ca
† These authors contributed equally to this work.

Abstract: Duchenne muscular dystrophy (DMD) is a neuromuscular disorder caused by dystrophin loss—notably within muscles and the central neurons system. DMD presents as cognitive weakness, progressive skeletal and cardiac muscle degeneration until pre-mature death from cardiac or respiratory failure. Innovative therapies have improved life expectancy; however, this is accompanied by increased late-onset heart failure and emergent cognitive degeneration. Thus, better assessment of dystrophic heart and brain pathophysiology is needed. Chronic inflammation is strongly associated with skeletal and cardiac muscle degeneration; however, neuroinflammation's role is largely unknown in DMD despite being prevalent in other neurodegenerative diseases. Here, we present an inflammatory marker translocator protein (TSPO) positron emission tomography (PET) protocol for in vivo concomitant assessment of immune cell response in hearts and brains of a dystrophin-deficient mouse model [*mdx:utrn*(+/−)]. Preliminary analysis of whole-body PET imaging using the TSPO radiotracer, [^{18}F]FEPPA in four *mdx:utrn*(+/−) and six wildtype mice are presented with ex vivo TSPO-immunofluorescence tissue staining. The *mdx:utrn*(+/−) mice showed significant elevations in heart and brain [^{18}F]FEPPA activity, which correlated with increased ex vivo fluorescence intensity, highlighting the potential of TSPO-PET to simultaneously assess presence of cardiac and neuroinflammation in dystrophic heart and brain, as well as in several organs within a DMD model.

Keywords: Duchenne muscular dystrophy; [^{18}F]FEPPA; positron emission tomography (PET); cardiac inflammation; neuroinflammation; *mdx:utrn*(+/−) mice

1. Introduction

Duchenne muscular dystrophy (DMD) is a progressive neuromuscular degenerative disease, affecting approximately 1 in 3600 live male births worldwide [1]. Individuals with DMD are unable to produce functional Dystrophin protein which is found systemically across various tissues, notably in skeletal and cardiac muscle, and neurons in the central nervous system (CNS). As a result, DMD is clinically characterized by progressive skeletal and cardiac muscle degeneration along with cognitive impairment [2–4]. These multi-organ degenerations are exacerbated by fibrosis, ischemia, and chronic inflammation until an early death from cardiac or respiratory complications [5–7]. Although there is still no cure for DMD, recent advancements in experimental therapies have prolonged both ambulation and life expectancy to 30–40 years [8,9].

With increased longevity in DMD patients, the clinical relevance of heart disease and cognitive impairment is becoming more apparent. More than 90% of DMD patients over

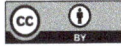

the age of 18 show signs of cardiac involvement, with nearly 60% of DMD patients dying from cardiac complications by age 19 [9,10]. Currently, it is known that the dystrophin loss in cardiac muscles leads to membrane integrity destabilization of striated cardiac muscle fibers, which in turn contributes to increased intracellular calcium levels and subsequent muscle fiber deterioration [11,12]. As with skeletal muscle, it is suspected that this initiates the pathological cycle of chronic inflammation, fibrosis, and necrosis, leading to damage in regions of high contractility and movement (e.g., left ventricle). The loss of viable myocardium leads to further fibrosis, and the clinical emergence of cardiomyopathy and eventually heart failure [6,7,13–15].

In the brain, dystrophin plays a role in brain development and aging. The lack of intrinsic dystrophin gene products within CNS—namely Dp427, Dp140, and Dp71—are thought to contribute to cognitive weakness by causing functional and morphological abnormalities to occur [3,4,16]. However, the underlying mechanisms are not well-understood. Cognitive and behavioural symptoms usually manifest in the form of lowered intelligence quotient (IQ) scores, learning difficulties, memory deficits, and higher incidences of neuropsychiatric disorders [16]. Recent investigations also report the delayed emergence of cerebral infarcts and progressive cognitive decline within older DMD subjects, leading to the possible paradigm of neurodegeneration in the later stages of disease progression [13,17,18].

There is growing evidence that inflammation may be an inciting factor in skeletal and cardiac muscle degeneration in DMD. Inflammation is thought to exacerbate symptoms and promote muscular degeneration [5,7,14] and we have demonstrated that the degree of inflammatory cell infiltration is associated with disease progression within dystrophin-deficient murine models [19]. Despite neuroinflammation being a prime component of several pediatric and adult neurodegenerative disorders [20], the role of inflammation within the dystrophic brain is relatively unexplored. To the best of our knowledge, immune cell infiltration in the brain has yet to be demonstrated within DMD patients or dystrophin-deficient animals. However, in brain tissue from *mdx* mice, heightened levels of pro-inflammatory interleukin (IL)-1β and tumor necrosis factor (TNF)-α associated with several neurological diseases [21] have been found and several cognitive deficits have also been observed [22]. Considering the well-known consequences of unchecked inflammation potentially leading to cardiac and neurodegeneration, there is an unmet need to better understand the role of inflammation in multi-organ degeneration, as it may lead to the development of effective therapeutic strategies that targets multiple tissues systems especially brain and heart resilience in DMD patients.

Recent advancements in non-invasive molecular imaging techniques for assessing inflammatory load have inspired interest in understanding the role of inflammation in multi-organ degeneration in several disease systems. In particular, Thackeray et al. [23] demonstrated evidence of concomitant inflammation in both the hearts and brains of ischemic heart disease mice and patients using positron emission tomography (PET) imaging targeting mitochondrial translocator protein (TSPO). TSPOs are highly expressed on activated microglia and macrophages [24], making it a promising tool for in vivo multi-organ imaging when combined with positron emission tomography (PET). Thus, this exploratory study sought to probe the capacity of TSPO-PET imaging in assessing in vivo inflammatory involvement in the dystrophic heart and brain, and across several organs. Specifically, we used [^{18}F]-N-(2-(2-fluoroethoxy)benzyl)-N-(4-phenoxypyridin-3-yl)acetamide ([^{18}F]FEPPA), a second-generation TSPO tracer, to simultaneously assess cardiac and neural inflammation in a dystrophin-deficient *mdx:utrn*(+/−) mouse model with one functional utrophin protein (Figure 1), known to exhibit moderate to severe disease phenotypes that better mimic human cardiomyopathy symptoms [24]. Our primary aim was to design an experimental protocol to test the hypothesis that *mdx:utrn*(+/−) mice will have increased inflammation levels in dystrophic cardiac and neural tissues, which will be exhibited as heightened TSPO-PET signal and correlative histological TSPO expression.

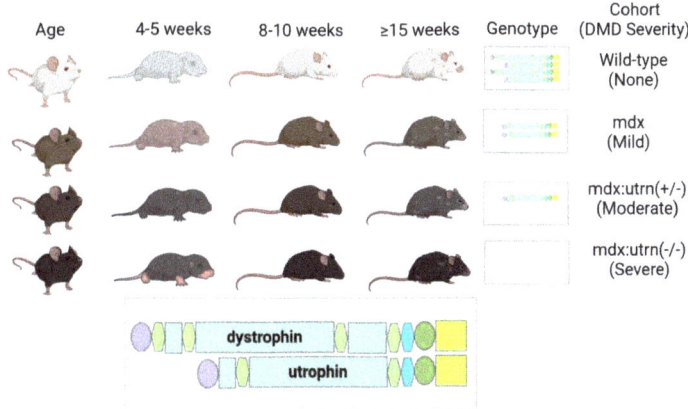

Figure 1. Murine models of DMD including the dystrophin-deficient mdx:utrn(+/−) mouse model used in this pilot study and the feasibility of modeling DMD symptom severity longitudinally with consideration for age-related effects.

2. Results

We explored our experimental design and imaging approach (Figure 2) in a pilot study of four *mdx:utrn*(+/−) (MDX) (two females, two males) and six wild-type (WT) (two females, four males) mice aged 8–10 weeks old to estimate the sample size to adequately test the hypothesis. All mice were both able to take up [^{18}F]FEPPA throughout the entire body—notably binding to our tissues of interest, the heart and brain (Figure 3). Although there were not sufficient tissue samples to measure differences in [^{18}F]FEPPA binding using autoradiography and biodistribution, the preliminary results demonstrate [^{18}F]FEPPA activity occurring body-wide within the heart and brain as well as in several other tissues, such as skeletal muscles, aorta, diaphragm, etc., as shown in Appendix A Figures A1–A3.

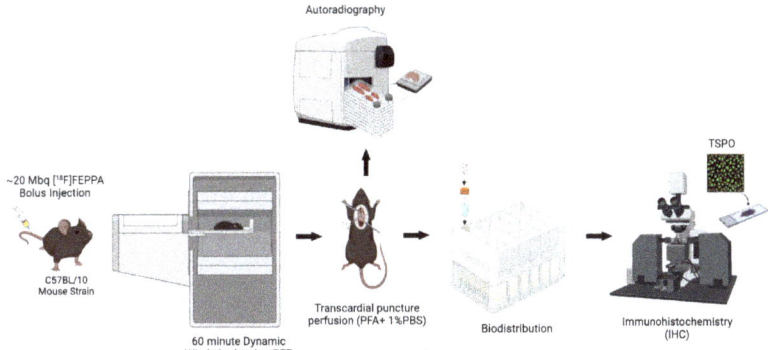

Figure 2. Experimental protocol for simultaneous in vivo [^{18}F]FEPPA PET imaging and ex vivo histopathology confirmation for assessing multi-organ inflammatory involvement in DMD mice models. PFA = paraformaldehyde; PBS = phosphate-buffered saline; TSPO = (18 kDa) translocator protein.

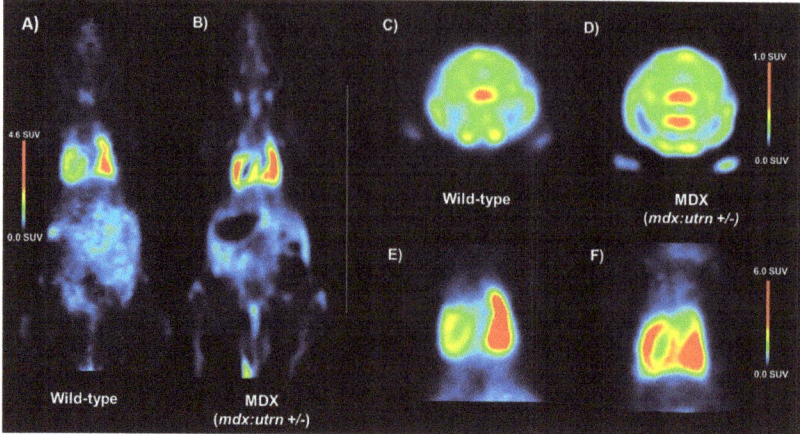

Figure 3. [^{18}F]FEPPA SUV images of representative 8–10 week wild-type (**A,C,E**) and age-matched MDX dystrophy (**B,D,F**) mice. Coronal whole-body (**A,B**), axial whole brain slices (**C,D**), and heart images (**E,F**) were generated from PET time-activity curves at 30–60 min (n = 4–6 mice/genotype). MDX = dystrophin-deficient *mdx:utrn*(+/−) mouse model, SUV = standardized uptake values.

2.1. Elevation of In Vivo Inflammation-Targeted Radiotracer Binding in DMD Models

To assess the influence of inflammation on dystrophic cardiac and neural tissue, inflammation was quantified from the [^{18}F]FEPPA PET images as mean standard uptake values (SUV). In the thoracic region, left-ventricle-to-lung mean SUV ratios indicated that MDX mice had significantly higher [^{18}F]FEPPA uptake (Figure 4; t = 2.58, p = 0.0338), as these left-ventricle-to-lung ratios increased from 0.63 ± 0.10 in WT mice to 0.99 ± 0.06 in the MDX cohort. In neural tissue, similar accumulations of inflammatory tracer were also observed in MDX mice. The WT brains demonstrated [^{18}F]FEPPA uptake of 0.34 ± 0.08 SUV, while MDX brains experienced 82.4% more uptake at 0.62 ± 0.08 SUV.

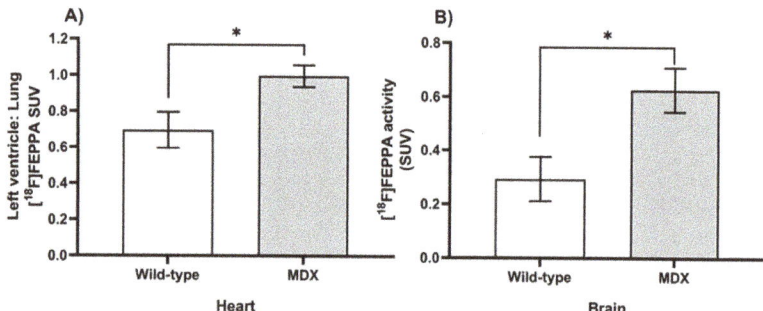

Figure 4. Quantified [^{18}F]FEPPA activity in hearts (**A**) and brains (**B**) of age-matched MDX and wild-type mice. Standardized uptake values were generated from PET time-activity curves at 30–60 min using manually drawn regions of interest (ROIs) segmented for the left ventricle, lung, and whole brain (n = 3–4 slices/mouse/genotype). Significant differences (p < 0.05; indicated by *) were observed between wild-type (white bars) and *mdx:utrn*(+/−) mice (gray bars) for both left ventricle-to-lung ratio (**A**) and whole brain (**B**) SUVs using Welch's two-way *t*-test. Data are depicted as mean ± standard error. TSPO = (18 kDa) Translocator protein, MDX = dystrophin-deficient *mdx:utrn*(+/−) mouse model, SUV = standardized uptake values.

2.2. Ex Vivo TSPO Signal Indicates Heightened Cardiac and Neuroinflammation in DMD

Fluorescence immunostaining of heart and brain slices demonstrated the presence of TSPO in age-matched MDX mice. Although both groups expressed a modest baseline level of TSPO (Figure 5), MDX mice consistently expressed significantly higher TSPO fluorescence intensity in both cardiac (Figure 6; t = 2.35, p = 0.025) and neural tissue (Figure 6; t = 5.15, p < 0.001). Within cardiac tissue, MDX mice experienced a 63.9% increase in fluorescence intensity when compared to age-matched wild-type mice; as dystrophic hearts demonstrated TSPO fluorescence intensities of 1261.57 ± 307.76 arbitrary unit (AU) compared to those of wild-type mice at 454.59 ± 63.93 AU. Similarly, in neural tissue, TSPO fluorescence intensity was remarkably 68.3% lower in WT compared to MDX mice. Dystrophic brain tissues displayed fluorescence intensities of 1149.74 ± 148.35 AU, which is lower than the 364.84 ± 73.71 AU observed in WT brains. Histological myocardium TSPO signal significantly correlated with [^{18}F]FEPPA uptake in the left ventricle (Figure 7; r = 0.75, p = 0.01). This was also observed between neural tissue TSPO fluorescence intensity in histology and in vivo whole brain TSPO-PET tracer SUV values (Figure 7; r = 0.57, p = 0.042). Analysis of the H&E staining (Appendix A, Figure A4) showed infiltration within heart tissue and higher nuclei counts in the MDX brain compared to age-matched WT mice (t = 3.17, p = 0.01).

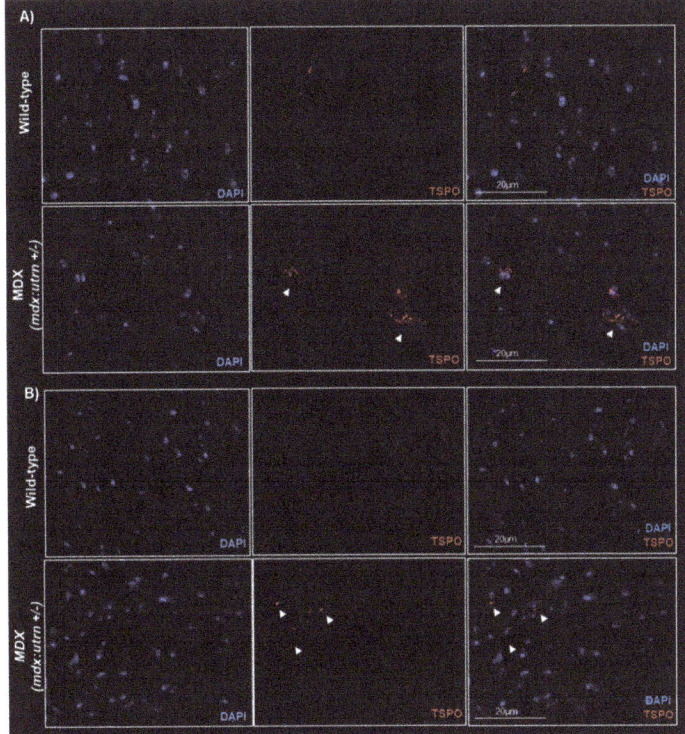

Figure 5. Ex vivo histology of TSPO-bound microglial and macrophages in an MDX and wild-type mice cardiac (**A**) and neural tissues (**B**). Representative fluorescence immunostained images of microglial and macrophages with TSPO (red) and DAPI (blue) in 8–10 weeks old *mdx:utrn*(+/−) mice depict qualitatively more prevalent TSPO expression in the dystrophin-deficient mice. White arrow heads indicate regions of TSPO signal. Scale bar overlaid on merged (DAPI and TSPO) images = 20 μm in length. Translocator protein, MDX = dystrophin-deficient *mdx:utrn*(+/−) mouse model.

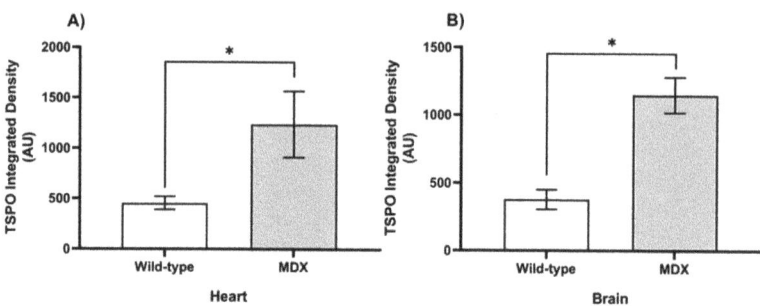

Figure 6. Quantified fluorescence immunohistochemical images of microglial and macrophages with TSPO in 8–10 weeks old MDX and wild-type subjects. Data (mean ± SE) depict higher TSPO in *mdx:utrn*(+/−) mice (gray bars) than wild-type controls (white bars) (*n* = 3 mice/genotype). Significant differences (*p* < 0.05), indicated by *, were observed for slices of cardiac (**A**) and neural (**B**) tissue when compared using Welch's two-way *t*-test (*n* = 5–10 images/mouse/genotype). AU = arbitrary units. Other abbreviations as described in prior figures.

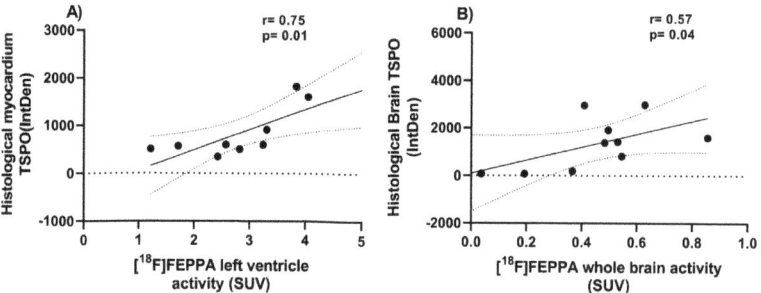

Figure 7. Correlation of [^{18}F]FEPPA activity with histological TSPO fluorescence intensity. Data depict the strong correlation of the left ventricle (**A**) or whole brain (**B**) PET avtivity, with quantified TSPO myocardium or neural tissue fluorescence signal. Pearson product-moment correlation coefficients (r) were calculated on all animals imaged with PET (*n* = 9 for heart association with 1 outlier excluded and *n* = 10 for brain associations, no outlier detected). Significance was considered when *p* < 0.05. IntDen = Integrated Density, the product of the mean fluorescence intensity and area of selected cell.

2.3. Sample Size Estimation

Given that findings from cardiac tissue fluorescence immunostaining showed the least between group differences in TSPO levels across modalities and in comparison, to the brain, and more importantly required ex vivo analysis, its results were used to estimate the number of samples per group required to detect the minimum difference in TSPO signal for a larger scale study. A minimum of seven 8–10 weeks old *mdx:utrn*(+/−) and seven age-matched WT mice are required to detect at least 63% differences in TSPO levels.

3. Discussion

The goal of this exploratory study was to evaluate [^{18}F]FEPPA PET as a tool to assess inflammation in vivo in multiple organs of mice with dystrophic disease. We found 8–10 weeks old dystrophin-deficient mice had elevated [^{18}F]FEPPA uptake in cardiac and neural tissues compared to healthy controls, which mirrored heightened ex vivo TSPO levels in our histological data. These results, while preliminary support our hypothesis that subjects with dystrophic deficiency demonstrate significant inflammation in their heart and brains, which can be confirmed in a larger experimental study using TSPO-PET.

To the best of our knowledge, our study is the first to observe significantly elevated TSPO-PET in the heart and brains of MDX mice. Interestingly, these increases seem to be occurring body-wide within several other tissues, akin to other diseases linked to chronic inflammation (e.g., atherosclerosis, myocardial infarctions, etc.) [25–27]. As such, it is likely that this heightened TSPO activity may be a consequence of activated macrophages and microglia within regions of tissue injury or dysfunction [27]. For example, immunohistostaining of mice one-week post-myocardial infarction indicated colocalization of TSPO to CD68+ microglia and cardiac monocytes within the brain cortex and infarcted myocardium respectively [25]. Interestingly, no colocalization was found between TSPO and GFAP-stained astrocytes at that time point. TSPO-tracers were also found to localize to magnetic resonance imaging (MRI)-identified ischemic lesions within ischemic stroke patients, further demonstrating the tracer's feasibility to map inflammation after tissue damage [28]. Thus, as DMD pathophysiology is known to be associated with contraction-induced damage and severe immune cell infiltration, it is likely that TSPO is upregulated within regions of injury—manifesting as the displayed [^{18}F]FEPPA tracer uptake within the dystrophic heart and brain. Our preliminary biodistribution and autoradiography observations support these claims, as the TSPO-tracer accumulated notably within regions associated with dystrophic symptoms (i.e., heart, brain, skeletal muscles, etc.). Although this exploratory study demonstrated the feasibility of [^{18}F]FEPPA PET to assess in vivo inflammation simultaneously within the heart and the brain, our study cannot provide a definite answer to whether [^{18}F]FEPPA PET can demonstrate inflammatory load within other tissues—despite the promising trends—due to the small sample sizes of our autoradiography and biodistribution data. To answer this question, a study using a larger sample size of seven or more mice per group along with quantification of tracer uptake in the other tissues within the PET data is needed.

In contrast to our results, three previous 2-deoxy-2-[^{18}F]fluoro-D-glucose ([^{18}F]FDG) PET studies reported lower mean cardiac SUV and highlighted select neural regions of hypometabolism in canine models of DMD [29–31]. While [^{18}F]FDG can be used as an analogue of inflammation in several neurological and cardiac diseases, it should be noted that these specific studies were focused on investigating the metabolic functionality of dystrophin-deficient tissue regions rather than its associated peripheral inflammation [32,33]. Because of the heart and the brain's disposition as highly metabolically-active organs, there is naturally a higher accumulation of [^{18}F]FDG tracer within those regions, which makes it difficult to detect inflammatory infiltrates without being potentially obscured by background activity or alterations in myocardial/neuronal function [34,35]. Additionally, a multi-tracer study longitudinally tracking microglial activation and glucose hypometabolism simultaneously in a transgenic mouse model of Alzheimer's disease observed discrepancies between the data trend of the TSPO-tracer [^{18}F]GE-180 and [^{18}F]FDG [36]. The authors observed progressive increases in [^{18}F]GE-180 uptake throughout the entire course of the disease (5–16 months), which differed from the life-course kinetics of [^{18}F]FDG which peaked at ~8 months of age before decreasing for the remaining 8 months, suggesting that the incidences of hypometabolism demonstrated within the dementia animals are occurring much later in life and as disease progressed. Interestingly, this early hypermetabolism may be capturing increased glial activity as it matches the peak of [^{18}F]GE-180 at 8 months—indicating the potential early onset of inflammation prior to rampant hypometabolism (and with it, the neurodegenerative symptoms) [37]. Taken together, although prior [^{18}F]FDG studies in DMD models show known indications of late-life brain and cardiac degeneration/dysfunction, our data highlight the potential role of inflammation in contributing to these metabolic deficiencies within dystrophin-deficient mice. Further longitudinal multi-tracer studies on dystrophic animal models using both [^{18}F]FEPPA and [^{18}F]FDG would greatly improve our understanding of the time course and interaction of inflammation and glucose hypometabolism onset.

The increased in vivo [^{18}F]FEPPA activity within the heart of our 8–10 weeks old MDX mice correlated with increases in ex vivo histology. We suspect that the [^{18}F]FEPPA uptake is localized to the activated macrophages present in the dystrophic myocardium, increasing TSPO expression above baseline. Thus, making [^{18}F]FEPPA a viable candidate for PET imaging of cardiac inflammation. Although we acknowledge that TSPO is constitutively expressed within cardiac tissue, the mRNA profile of TSPO typically remains at a steady moderate state within normal healthy tissue [38,39]. Importantly, TSPO is found to be overexpressed in inflammatory cardiac foci, seemingly being upregulated in activated immune cells [40,41]. TSPO-PET has similarly been used as a marker of cardiac macrophage infiltration in previous studies of myocarditis, and myocardial infarction [25,40]. As such, it is suggested that these heightened [^{18}F]FEPPA activities may indicate activated macrophage presence within the murine dystrophic heart.

Our data, highlighting the presence of TSPO-bound ligands in MDX mice and the histological evidence of M1-like (proinflammatory) and M2-like (reparative) macrophage infiltration into the sites of dystrophin-related injury support this hypothesis [42–45]. Interestingly, these suspected elevations in inflammatory load are observed quite early at 8–10 weeks—when the *mdx:utrn*(+/−) model heart function is relatively stable. This agrees with earlier reports that indicate a certain degree of inflammation, cellular necrosis, and fibrosis within their myocardium at 10 weeks of age [45]. However, it should be noted that one cardiac dystrophin-deficient murine study found a lack of macrophage infiltration into cardiac tissue until 6 months of age—in contrast to our results [46]. This delayed inflammatory onset might be due to the authors' use of a comparatively less severe *mdx* model than ours, as it is known to demonstrate minimal—if any—cardiac dysfunction [47,48]. Within studies pertaining the same murine model—*mdx:utrn*(+/−)—evidence of ventricular dysfunction (i.e. impaired stroke volume, decreased ejection fraction, and elevated heart rate) were observed far later at 10 months, compared to our observed onset of cardiac inflammation at 8–10 weeks [49]. Thus, the present findings may indicate an early inflammatory onset prior to the onset of cardiac symptoms. Considering that *mdx:utrn*(+/−) mice who were started on an anti-inflammatory quercetin-enriched diet at 8 weeks old have comparatively minimal cardiac damage than those without, the early detection and intervention to modulate cardiac inflammation may be vital in possibly attenuating downstream DMD cardiac degenerative symptoms [50]. A more extensive explanation of this mechanism is outside of the scope of this paper. However, a further longitudinal study pairing this [^{18}F]FEPPA PET protocol with an anatomical or morphological modality (such as MRI), may be undertaken to better assess how this early inflammatory response may contribute to dystrophic cardiac tissue pathology.

In vivo [^{18}F]FEPPA SUV has been correlated with post-mortem pro-inflammatory markers histologically in other neuroinflammatory or disease models, validating its use as an analogue of activated microglia cells [51]. In this study, in vivo [^{18}F]FEPPA signal within the whole brain correlated with ex vivo TSPO immunofluorescence intensity, suggesting the possible localization of activated microglia to the dystrophic neural tissue. To the best of our knowledge, there are no other studies demonstrating the presence of immune cell infiltration into the dystrophic brain. However, in support of our observations, heightened levels of IL-1β and TNF-α have been found within *mdx* murine brains, who also displayed cognitive impairment similar to those in DMD patients [22]. Recent literature has also speculated that these specific cytokines may participate in the emergence of DMD cognitive dysfunction symptoms by altering several features in synaptic transmission (see review in Rae and O'Malley [52] and Stephenson et al. [53]. Considering that activated microglia are known to upregulate TSPO expression and release pro-inflammatory cytokines (e.g., IL-1β, IL-6, TNF-α), it is possible that activated microglia may contribute to the dystrophic brain's impairment [25,54,55]. Additionally, the activated microglia may also predict cognitive deterioration [56] as multiple studies regarding neurodegenerative diseases (e.g., Alzheimer's dementia) reported that the degree of neuroinflammation can predict longitudinal cognitive decline [57]. While the underlying mechanism on how activated microglia contributes to downstream neurodegeneration is still under debate, the early observation of neuroinflammation within our study and the knowledge of late-onset cognitive decline within both older DMD patients (occurring at 30 years of age) [58] and aged murine models (occurring at 18 months) [17,22] suggests a possible similar association. As such, a future study using TSPO-PET to longitudinally assess neuroinflammation in these MDX murine models—alongside cognitive testing—is suggested to better delineate the relationship between early neuroinflammation and late-onset cognitive decline.

A possible explanation for this microglia activation within the brain may, in part, be due to pro-inflammatory cytokines—which are abundant in DMD circulation—passing through the "leaky" dystrophin-deficient blood-brain barrier (BBB) [59]. Within the brain, dystrophin—specifically Dp71—is located in the perivascular end-feet of astrocytes, normally participating in the stabilization and regulation of molecules transporting through the BBB [60]. In *mdx* mice, the reduction in Dp71 demonstrates severe alteration of endothelial and glial cells, as well as a reduction in the expression of zonula occludens and Aquaporin-4. As a result, *mdx* mice shows increased vascular permeability and by proxy, increased BBB permeability [60–62]. Increased BBB permeability and IL-6 levels within the brain were shown when systemic inflammation was induced by a peripheral lipopolysaccharide injection to an Alzheimer's APP transgenic mouse, resulting in more severe cognitive symptoms [63]. Thus we speculate that the nature of this neural [^{18}F]FEPPA uptake and subsequent TSPO overexpression may be a result of a similar incidence. However, it should be noted that within a study investigating the permeability of the BBB in *mdx* mice, CD4-, CD8-, CD20- and CD68-positive cells were not histologically observed within the BBB perivascular stroma [64]. These observations, while contrasting, do not conflict with our findings as alternate passages of cytokines through the BBB has already been extensively investigated [65,66]. A possible source of systemic inflammation/pro-inflammatory cytokines within our study include the dystrophin-deficient cardiac and skeletal muscles—which as stated before are known to sustain critical damage upon sarcolemma contraction and release pro-inflammatory cytokines into circulation. The concomitant cardiac and neural TSPO-tracer uptake and our autoradiography and biodistribution results (i.e. trends towards heightened binding across almost all tissue types) speaks to the systemic nature of inflammation within a dystrophin-deficient disorder, while hinting its possible contribution to both downstream cardiac and neurodegeneration damage. It will be interesting to investigate if the neuroinflammation observed in this murine model of DMD is widespread across the whole brain, or specific to certain regions, especially in the hippocampus where atrophy within this region has been linked to progressive cognitive impairment in *mdx* mice [17]. Further PET/MRI studies linking [^{18}F]FEPPA PET to regional MRI volumetry and functional MRI network changes will help shed more light.

The strengths of our proposed protocol include: (1) the utility of non-invasive inflammation imaging using second generation TSPO radioligand [^{18}F]FEPPA, (2) the use of a high-resolution (1.4–1.5 mm) small animal PET scanner capable of multi-organ/whole-body image data acquisition, and (3) the showcase of tissue-specific dosimetry and molecular colocalization capabilities via biodistribution and autoradiography respectively in a murine model of DMD—allowing for the additional in vitro histopathological validation of our in vivo imaging studies. While the pilot study demonstrated that our imaging approach is well-tolerated and may not be burdensome for longitudinal studies across age groups, the pilot study does have several limitations. Firstly, the study sample size (Appendix B) is relatively small and uses a mixed sex murine cohort despite DMD being a X-linked genetic disorder and thus, primarily appearing in only human male patients. While this is a common notion in DMD pre-clinical literature since both sexes can express this phenotype through mutations in their dystrophic and utrophin genes, there have been reports that female patients and rodents express constitutively higher levels of TSPO in both cardiac and neural tissue [48,67–69]. Due to low sample sizes, we could not account for these potential sex differences with this study; however, a fair balance between sexes were used (wild-type: 2 females, 4 males; MDX: 2 females, 2 males). This relatively small cohort could underpower our sample size estimation since analysis of covariates such as sex differences were not included in the sample size analysis. The use of male-only or female-only mice for the larger study could reduce the likelihood of underpowered studies. Consequently, future studies using same-sex subjects are strongly recommended. Secondly, similar to other TSPO-PET literature, [^{18}F]FEPPA is unable to differentiate between macrophage/microglia morphological states (i.e. pro-inflammatory and anti-inflammatory). Further studies including in-depth histopathological analysis using H&E staining and immunohistochemistry of dedicated inflammatory antibodies (CD68 or F4-80) co-localized to TSPO could reveal contributions of pro-inflammatory macrophage and microglia phenotypes, as well as the extent of inflammation in MDX heart and brain tissues. Lastly, while [^{18}F]FEPPA is commonly used to assess activated microglia, it is difficult to discern the true sensitivity of this tracer within DMD as TSPO is also present in astrocytes, pericytes, and endothelial cells, among other structures within the brain at low levels and within injured cardiomyocytes. During DMD, astrocytes may be activated due to a lack of functional dystrophin, as its absence can precipitate a series of complex signaling cascades that leads to glutamate toxicity in the CNS [70]. However, it should be noted that the percentage of cells expressing TSPO are reported to be ~7 times higher for microglia than for astrocytes, as measured by scRNA-seq—suggesting a preference for the TSPO radiotracer to bind to microglia [71]. Thus, it is suggested that further multi-tracer studies using both [^{18}F]FEPPA and specific PET tracers targeting solely activated macrophages or microglia such as triggering receptor expressed on myeloid cells (TREM) can be used to further validate the use of [^{18}F]FEPPA as a multi-organ inflammation assessment tool in DMD [72].

4. Materials and Methods

The pilot study for protocol development of a larger scale study was conducted at Lawson Health Research Institute at St. Joseph's Health Care in London, Ontario, Canada. All animal protocols were approved by the Animal Use Subcommittee at Western University, London, Ontario, Canada and were conducted in accordance with guidelines set by the Canadian Council on Animal Care (CCAC).

4.1. Study Population

Breeding pairs of wild-type and functional dystrophin-deficient mdx:utrn(+/−) (a point mutation in dystrophin gene and a single utrophin allele lost) mice [73] were purchased from Charles River and Jackson Laboratories (Bar Harbor, ME, USA). The C57BL/10 (Jax stock #000665) substrain widely used in immunological research was used as wild-type while the mdx:utrn(+/−) mice were on a C57BL/10ScSnJ genetic background (Jax stock #000476). The C57BL/10ScSnJ substrain are similar to C57BL/10 except for minor known behavioural differences and a propensity for lower brain glutamic acid decarboxylase [74,75]. However, there is no evidence that the C57BL/10ScSnJ strain have altered inflammatory response and unlike the C57BL/c10, both strains are not known to have the spontaneous Toll-like receptor 4 (Tlr4) deletion that could produce hyposensitivity to microglia/macrophage [76]. Colonies were maintained under controlled conditions (19–23 °C, 12-h light/dark cycles), and were allowed water and food ad libitum. Two separate groups of eight- to ten-week-old mice were used in this study where the in vivo imaging ($n = 4$–6 mice/genotype) and ex vivo histology cohorts ($n = 3$ mice/genotype) are the PET and immunohistochemistry (IHC) cohort, respectively.

4.2. PET Imaging Protocol

All PET mice were induced in a chamber with 3% oxygen-balanced isoflurane mixture and then anesthetized with 1.5–2%; both mixtures were delivered at a constant rate of 1 L/min via a nose cone. After induction, these mice were imaged using a micro-PET scanner (eXplore VISTA, GE Healthcare, Chicago, IL, USA; Inveon DPET, Siemens, Munich, Germany). To assess whole-body inflammation accumulation, TSPO-targeted PET images were obtained after [^{18}F]FEPPA tracer injection. 30 s following the start of the scan, a dose of approximately 20 MBq of prepared [^{18}F]FEPPA in saline (approximately 5 µg/kg) was administered via tail vein catheter for dynamic acquisition. Summarily, 60-min whole-body dynamic scans in list-mode were acquired using the Inveon system or the eXplore VISTA scanner. Because of the limited field-of-view of the eXplore VISTA scanner not fully encompassing the whole mice, dynamic imaging was performed from head-to-chest followed by a 30-min full-body static scan. Injected dose did not exceed 0.3 mL to ensure proper animal health conditions.

4.3. PET Image Analysis

For each mouse, the dynamic PET list mode data were reconstructed into the following time frames: 12 × 10 s, 60 × 30 s, 5 × 60 s, 5 × 120 s, 8 × 300 s using ordered subset expectation maximization (OSEM, Shoham, Israel) algorithm with no scatter and attenuation correction. Data were corrected to injected dose and decay corrected to start of PET scan using in-house MATLAB v2019a scripts (Mathworks, Natick, MA, USA). Standardized Uptake Values (SUV) were generated from PET data 30–60 min post-injection in PMOD 3.9 (PMOD Technologies, Zurich, Switzerland). Using manually drawn regions of interest (ROI), mean SUV were calculated for the left ventricle, lung, and whole brain covering 3–4 slices spanning each whole organ. Left ventricle-to-heart ratio—used to offset lung [^{18}F]FEPPA activity and act as a correlative of cardiac events—was calculated from mean SUV within each animal [77].

4.4. Biodistribution and Autoradiography

The mice were sacrificed immediately after imaging through 5% oxygen-balanced isoflurane gas euthanasia followed by cervical dislocation. To preserve tissue anatomy, the mice underwent whole animal perfusion fixation via an intracardiac infusion of 4% paraformaldehyde (Sigma-Aldrich), and then phosphate-buffered saline (PBS) as directed in Gage et al. [78] before the heart and brain were dissected. Each heart was bisected twice—once transversely and once along the septum—and each brain were bisected along the central sulcus to ensure that exactly half of each tissue was fixed in 10% Formalin or frozen in Optimal Cutting Temperature solution (VWR) for biodistribution and autoradiography use respectively. Biodistribution was conducted for the heart, brain, thoracic aorta, diaphragm, gastrocnemius, soleus, tibialis anterior, large/small intestines, tibia/fibula, kidney, liver, and lungs; each organ was weighed for quantitative estimation of gamma counts from the ^{18}F conjugate using the ORETC DSPEC50 Spectrometer. Radioactivity obtained from different organs was calculated as the percentage of the injected dose per gram of the tissue (%ID/g) and decay corrected to time of injection. Radioactivity was standardized to the dose injected into each animal. For autoradiography, frozen tissue samples were cryosectioned into a thickness of 20 μm with a Leica Clinical Cryostat (CM1850, Leica Biosystems, Wetzlar, Germany). Autoradiographic images of the heart, brain, thoracic aorta, diaphragm, gastrocnemius, tibialis anterior, kidney and liver were acquired for 12 h using a digital autoradiography system (BeaQuant AI4R, Nantes, France) fitted with a positron holder.

4.5. Histology Tissue Preparation

To supplement data from acute imaging for immunohistochemistry and histopathological analysis, a cohort of 8–10-week-old mice were sacrificed through cervical dislocation following CO_2 gas euthanasia without PET imaging. The heart and brain were dissected and fixed in 10% formalin for 24–48 h. These tissues were embedded in paraffin for immunohistochemistry and histopathology by the Molecular Pathology facility (Robarts Research Institute, London, ON, Canada) and cut into 10 μm thick sections. Care was taken to ensure that the tissues were embedded in the same orientation within each block.

4.6. Immunohistochemistry Protocol

Following a modified protocol based on Abcam standards, tissue sections were deparaffinized and rehydrated in a series of xylene and ethanol washes prior to heat-mediated antigen retrieval in a citrate buffer for 30 min. Slides were then cooled slowly to room temperature, and Background Sniper (Biocare Medical, Concord, CA, USA) was applied for 8 min to reduce nonspecific background staining. Sections were incubated overnight at 4 °C with either primary anti-PBR (1:200, Abcam), primary anti-α-SMA (1:500, Abcam), or no antibodies—the latter acting as the positive and negative control. All antibodies were diluted in 1% bovine serum albumin (BSA) PBS. Following thorough washing with 1 × PBS, Alexafluor IgG (Life Technologies, 1:500) secondary antibodies were used to visualize the primary antibodies: anti-PBR sections were incubated with 594 Goat anti-rabbit IgG, and anti-α-SMA sections with 488 Goat anti-mouse IgG for 2 h at room temperature. For heart tissue, a solution of $Cu_2SO_4 \bullet 5H_2O$ (10 mM copper sulfate, 50 mM ammonium acetate buffer, pH 5.0) was applied thereafter to prevent red blood cell autofluorescence. Additional 1 × PBS washes and an immersion in 0.1% Sudan Black B was performed to quench autofluorescence in both heart and brain tissue sections. Lastly, ProLong Gold anti-fade with DAPI (Life Technologies) was added to all sections to visualize the nuclei and to mount the coverslips onto glass slides.

4.7. Microscopy and Image Analysis

Fluorescent images were acquired on an epifluorescence microscope (Nikon Eclipse Ts2R) using NIS Elements Microscope Image Software. Non-overlapping fields of view at 60x magnification were taken for each tissue section (n = 5–10 images/slide). Quantitative assessment of TSPO fluorescent signal in both wild-type and *mdx:utrn*(+/−) (henceforth named MDX) mice —while minimizing image exposure and auto-fluorescence (i.e. background signal)—was performed using an in-house semi-automatic grey scale thresholding protocol in ImageJ (LOCI, Madison, WI, USA) with FIJI package v2.0.0 [29].

4.8. Hematoxylin and Eosin (H&E) Staining

Routine H&E staining were applied on deparaffinized heart and brain tissue samples cut to 5 μm slices to show the extent of inflammation and visualize changes in tissue morphology. H&E stained images were captured using a Zeiss Axioskop Fluorescence microscope (Carl Zeiss Jena GmbH, Jena, Germany) and nuclei counts were determined using ImageJ [79].

4.9. Statistical Analysis

Analyses were performed using RStudio v1.0.136 (Boston, MA, USA) or SPSS 26 (IBM, Armonk, NY, USA) software. Data results are expressed as mean ± standard error (SE). Comparisons between groups were performed using Welch's two-tailed t-test. No statistical analyses were conducted on autoradiography and biodistribution data due to low sample sizes. Negative biodistribution values for which measurement errors resulted in negative tissue weights (i.e., stemming from weight of empty tube exceeding the weight of tube and tissue) were removed from the data set. One-tailed Pearson correlation coefficients were calculated between [^{18}F]FEPPA left ventricle/whole brain uptake, and myocardium/neural tissue histological TSPO fluorescence intensity using GraphPad Prism version 9.3.1 for Windows (San Diego, CA, USA). Outliers were identified using the ROUT coefficient Q method implemented in GraphPad Prism and excluded from the correlational analysis. p-values of less than 0.05 were considered significant. Replicate numbers are indicated in the figure legends.

4.10. Sample Size Estimation

The sample size for a larger scale study was estimated using the p-value method [80] for two independent samples, as described in the equation below.

$$N = \left[\left(\frac{Z_\pi \pm Z_{1-\frac{\alpha}{2}}}{Z_{1-\frac{p}{2}}}\right)\right]^2 N_{ref}$$

where Z_π is the z-value from the standard normal distribution for power (π) of 80% = 0.84, and $Z_{1-\alpha/2}$ is the z-value from the standard normal distribution for the two-sided significance level (α) of 0.05 = 1.96, $Z_{1-P/2}$ is the z-value from the standard normal distribution for the *p*-value from the between group comparison performed using the Welsh's two-tailed *t*-test on the pilot study data. The between group comparison of the fluorescence immunostaining of the heart slices was used, since it showed the least effect (minimum detectable difference) compared to PET or autoradiography findings. Based on this, $Z_{1-P/2}$ for the *p*-value of 0.025 = 2.24.

5. Conclusions

In general, this exploratory study suggested that dystrophin-deficient mice were associated with higher inflammatory [^{18}F]FEPPA radiotracer binding, mirroring ex vivo histological TSPO data within both their hearts and their brains, indicating a potential presence of early-onset cardiac- and neuroinflammation. While preliminary, the results highlight the feasibility for TSPO-PET imaging in the in vivo assessment of chronic inflammation in several organs simultaneously, particularly within a dystrophic disease. A larger longitudinal study across age groups (immature, mature, aged) and DMD disease severity (normal, mild, moderate, severe) using our protocol in same-sex subjects will confirm whether TSPO-PET can track multi-organ activated immune cells to better understand their contribution to dysfunctional outcomes.

Author Contributions: Conceptualization, L.H.; methodology, J.M.T., A.M., L.H. and U.C.A.; formal analysis, J.M.T., A.M., L.L. and U.C.A.; investigation, J.M.T., L.H., J.H. and U.C.A.; resources, J.W.H. and J.A.R.; data curation, J.M.T. and A.M.; writing—original draft preparation, J.M.T., L.H. and U.C.A.; writing—review and editing, J.M.T., A.M., L.L., J.A.R., J.W.H., L.H. and U.C.A.; visualization, J.M.T., A.M., L.L. and U.C.A.; supervision, L.H. and U.C.A.; project administration, L.H.; funding acquisition, L.H. and U.C.A. All authors have read and agreed to the published version of the manuscript.

Funding: This research was funded by Canadian Institutes of Health Research (CIHR), grant number PJT-152990 and Heart and Stroke Foundation of Canada (HSFC), grant number G-20-0029408. The APC was funded by Natural Sciences and Engineering Research Council of Canada (NSERC), grant number DGECR-2022-00136.

Institutional Review Board Statement: The animal study protocol was approved by the Animal Use Subcommittee of the University of Western Ontario (protocol code AUP 2018-140 and approved on 1 July 2019.

Informed Consent Statement: Not applicable.

Data Availability Statement: Not applicable.

Acknowledgments: The authors thank Matthew Fox, Haris Smailovic, and Lise Desjardins who assisted in PET/autoradiography operations. The authors acknowledge Vasiliki Economopoulos for valuable insight in neuroimmunology. Figures 1 and 2 were created with BioRender.com.

Conflicts of Interest: The authors declare no conflict of interest.

Appendix A

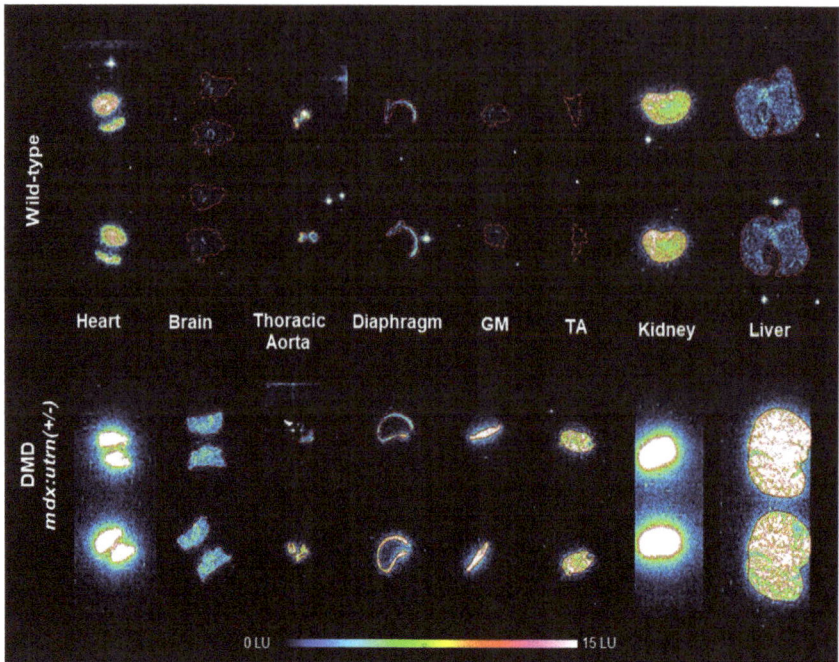

Figure A1. Autoradiography images of the heart, brain, and multiple tissues excised from a representative MDX and wild-type mice injected with [^{18}F]FEPPA. LU = light units. MDX = dystrophin-deficient *mdx:utrn*(+/−) mouse models.

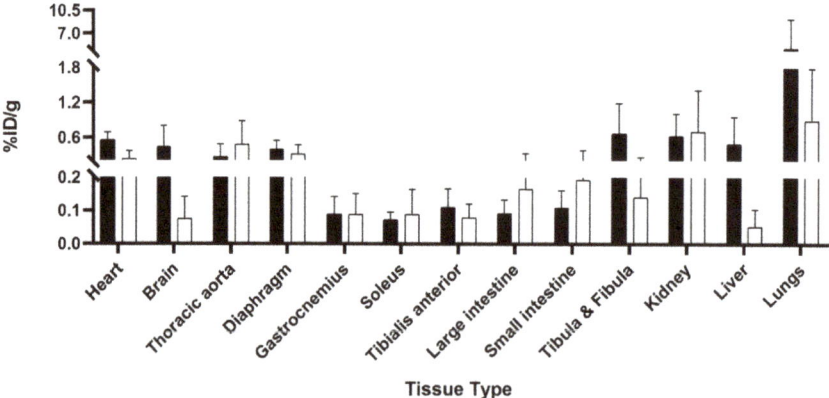

Figure A2. Multi-organ Biodistribution of [^{18}F]FEPPA within murine models. Data (±SE) shows the differences in radiotracer uptake as across multiple tissues as the percentage of the injected dose per gram of the tissue (%ID/g) of MDX (*mdx:utrn*(+/−)) (black bars; n = 4 mice) and age-matched wild-type controls (white bars; n = 2 mice). No statistical analyses were conducted due to low sample sizes.

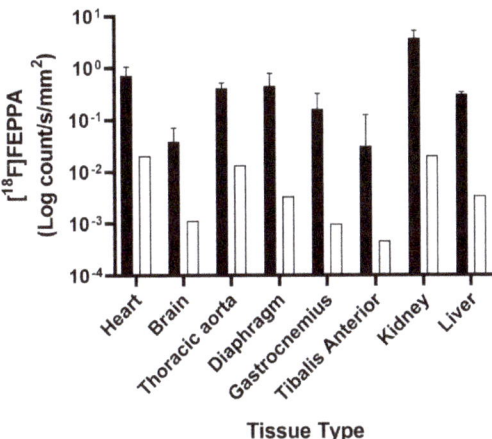

Figure A3. Quantified autoradiography of [^{18}F]FEPPA activity in MDX and wild-type mice. Data (±SE) depicts the log counts per second per millimetre squared area of [^{18}F]FEPPA activity within slices of heart, brain, thoracic aorta, diaphragm, skeletal muscles, kidney and liver for MDX (black bars; n = 3 mice) and an age-matched wild-type control (white bars; n = 1 mouse). No statistical analyses were conducted due to low sample sizes. MDX = dystrophin-deficient $mdx{:}utrn(+/-)$ mouse models.

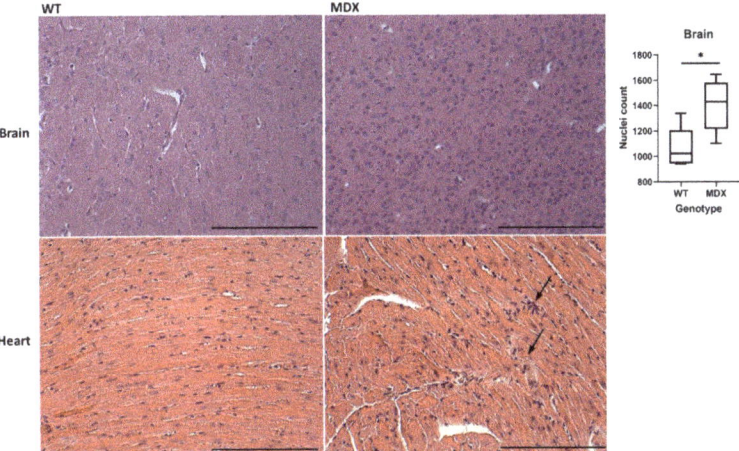

Figure A4. Representative Hematoxylin and Eosin (H&E) stained images from heart and brain tissue sections of an 8–10 week dystrophin-deficient $mdx{:}utrn(+/-)$ mouse (MDX) and age-matched C57bl/10 wild-type (WT) mouse. Heart tissue obtained from MDX mouse show infiltrate (black arrows) within heart tissue and higher nuclei counts (mean (±SE)) in brain tissues. Heart image filter chosen to highlight myocardial fibers. Images scale bar = 100 μm; one biological and 3 technical replicates were used for the heart and one biological, and 6 technical replicates were used for the brain. Significant difference ($p < 0.05$), indicated by *.

Appendix B

Table A1. Sample size for the number of unique wild-type and MDX mice successfully completed for each protocol cohort.

	PET	Biodistribution	Autoradiography	Immunohistochemistry	H&E
Wild-type C57Bl10	6	2	2	3	1
MDX mdx:utrn(+/−)	4	4	1	3	1

References

1. Dooley, J.; Gordon, K.E.; Dodds, L.; Macsween, J. Duchenne muscular dystrophy: A 30-year population-based incidence study. *Clin. Pediatr. (Phila)* **2010**, *49*, 177–179. [CrossRef] [PubMed]
2. Bushby, K.; Finkel, R.; Birnkrant, D.J.; Case, L.E.; Clemens, P.R.; Cripe, L.; Kaul, A.; Kinnett, K.; McDonald, C.; Pandya, S.; et al. Diagnosis and management of Duchenne muscular dystrophy, part 1: Diagnosis, and pharmacological and psychosocial management. *Lancet Neurol.* **2010**, *9*, 77–93. [CrossRef] [PubMed]
3. Ueda, Y. Cognitive Function and Quality of Life of Muscular Dystrophy. In *Muscular Dystrophies*; Sakuma, K., Ed.; IntechOpen: Rijeka, Croatia, 2019; p. 3. [CrossRef]
4. Doorenweerd, N. Combining genetics, neuropsychology and neuroimaging to improve understanding of brain involvement in Duchenne muscular dystrophy—A narrative review. *Neuromuscul. Disord.* **2020**, *30*, 437–442. [CrossRef] [PubMed]
5. Rosenberg, A.S.; Puig, M.; Nagaraju, K.; Hoffman, E.P.; Villalta, S.A.; Rao, V.A.; Wakefield, L.M.; Woodcock, J. Immune-mediated pathology in Duchenne muscular dystrophy. *Sci. Transl. Med.* **2015**, *7*, 299rv4. [CrossRef]
6. D'amario, D.; Amodeo, A.; Adorisio, R.; Tiziano, F.D.; Leone, A.M.; Perri, G.; Bruno, P.; Massetti, M.; Ferlini, A.; Pane, M.; et al. A current approach to heart failure in Duchenne muscular dystrophy. *Heart* **2017**, *103*, 1770–1779. [CrossRef]
7. Shin, J.; Tajrishi, M.M.; Ogura, Y.; Kumar, A. Wasting mechanisms in muscular dystrophy. *Int. J. Biochem. Cell Biol.* **2013**, *45*, 2266–2279. [CrossRef]
8. Eagle, M.; Baudouin, S.V.; Chandler, C.; Giddings, D.R.; Bullock, R.; Bushby, K. Survival in Duchenne muscular dystrophy: Improvements in life expectancy since 1967 and the impact of home nocturnal ventilation. *Neuromuscul. Disord.* **2002**, *12*, 926–929. [CrossRef]
9. Nigro, G.; Comi, L.; Politano, L.; Bain, R. The incidence and evolution of cardiomyopathy in Duchenne muscular dystrophy. *Int. J. Cardiol.* **1990**, *26*, 271–277. [CrossRef]
10. Ballard, E.; Grey, N.; Jungbluth, H.; Wraige, E.; Kapetanakis, S.; Davidson, C.; Hart, N. Observation cohort study of cause of death in patients with Duchenne muscular dystrophy (DMD). *Eur. Respir. J.* **2012**, *40* (Suppl. 56), P1720.
11. Kamdar, F.; Garry, D.J. Dystrophin-Deficient Cardiomyopathy. *J. Am. Coll. Cardiol.* **2016**, *67*, 2533–2546. [CrossRef]
12. Dubinin, M.V.; Belosludtsev, K.N. Ion Channels of the Sarcolemma and Intracellular Organelles in Duchenne Muscular Dystrophy: A Role in the Dysregulation of Ion Homeostasis and a Possible Target for Therapy. *Int. J. Mol. Sci.* **2023**, *24*, 2229. [CrossRef]
13. Johnstone, V.P.A.; Viola, H.M.; Hool, L.C. Dystrophic Cardiomyopathy—Potential Role of Calcium in Pathogenesis, Treatment and Novel Therapies. *Genes* **2017**, *8*, 108. [CrossRef]
14. Nitahara-Kasahara, Y.; Takeda, S.; Okada, T. Inflammatory predisposition predicts disease phenotypes in muscular dystrophy. *Inflamm. Regen.* **2016**, *36*, 14. [CrossRef]
15. Meyers, T.A.; Townsend, D. Cardiac Pathophysiology and the Future of Cardiac Therapies in Duchenne Muscular Dystrophy. *Int. J. Mol. Sci.* **2019**, *20*, 4098. [CrossRef]
16. Snow, W.M.; Anderson, J.E.; Jakobson, L.S. Neuropsychological and neurobehavioral functioning in Duchenne muscular dystrophy: A review. *Neurosci. Biobehav. Rev.* **2013**, *37*, 743–752. [CrossRef]
17. Bagdatlioglu, E.; Porcari, P.; Greally, E.; Blamire, A.M.; Straub, V.W. Cognitive impairment appears progressive in the *mdx* mouse. *Neuromuscul. Disord.* **2020**, *30*, 368–388. [CrossRef]
18. Winterholler, M.; Holländer, C.; Kerling, F.; Weber, I.; Dittrich, S.; Türk, M.; Schröder, R. Stroke in Duchenne Muscular Dystrophy: A Retrospective Longitudinal Study in 54 Patients. *Stroke* **2016**, *47*, 2123–2126. [CrossRef]
19. Mavrogeni, S.; Papavasiliou, A.; Spargias, K.; Constandoulakis, P.; Papadopoulos, G.; Karanasios, E.; Georgakopoulos, D.; Kolovou, G.; Demerouti, E.; Polymeros, S.; et al. Myocardial inflammation in Duchenne Muscular Dystrophy as a precipitating factor for heart failure: A prospective study. *BMC Neurol.* **2010**, *10*, 33. [CrossRef]
20. Chen, W.-W.; Zhang, X.; Huang, W.-J. Role of neuroinflammation in neurodegenerative diseases (Review). *Mol. Med. Rep.* **2016**, *13*, 3391–3396. [CrossRef]
21. Aarli, J.A. Role of cytokines in neurological disorders. *Curr. Med. Chem.* **2003**, *10*, 1931–1937. [CrossRef]
22. Comim, C.M.; Ventura, L.; Freiberger, V.; Dias, P.; Bragagnolo, D.; Dutra, M.L.; Amaral, R.A.; Camargo-Fagundes, A.L.S.; Reis, P.A.; Castro-Faria-Neto, H.C.; et al. Neurocognitive Impairment in *mdx* Mice. *Mol. Neurobiol.* **2019**, *56*, 7608–7616. [CrossRef] [PubMed]

23. Thackeray, J.T.; Hupe, H.C.; Wang, Y.; Bankstahl, J.P.; Berding, G.; Ross, T.L.; Bauersachs, J.; Wollert, K.C.; Bengel, F.M. Myocardial Inflammation Predicts Remodeling and Neuroinflammation After Myocardial Infarction. *J. Am. Coll. Cardiol.* **2018**, *71*, 263–275. [CrossRef] [PubMed]
24. Wilson, A.A.; Garcia, A.; Parkes, J.; McCormick, P.; Stephenson, K.A.; Houle, S.; Vasdev, N. Radiosynthesis and initial evaluation of [^{18}F]-FEPPA for PET imaging of peripheral benzodiazepine receptors. *Nucl. Med. Biol.* **2008**, *35*, 305–314. [CrossRef] [PubMed]
25. Thackeray, J.T.; Bengel, F. Molecular Imaging of Myocardial Inflammation with Positron Emission Tomography Post-Ischemia: A Determinant of Subsequent Remodeling or Recovery. *JACC Cardiovasc. Imaging* **2018**, *11*, 1340–1355. [CrossRef] [PubMed]
26. Cuhlmann, S.; Gsell, W.; Van der Heiden, K.; Habib, J.; Tremoleda, J.L.; Khalil, M.; Turkheimer, F.; Meens, M.J.; Kwak, B.R.; Bird, J.; et al. In vivo mapping of vascular inflammation using the translocator protein tracer ^{18}F-FEDAA1106. *Mol. Imaging* **2014**, *13*, 1–10. [CrossRef]
27. Largeau, B.; Dupont, A.-C.; Guilloteau, D.; Santiago-Ribeiro, M.-J.; Arlicot, N. TSPO PET Imaging: From Microglial Activation to Peripheral Sterile Inflammatory Diseases? *Contrast Media Mol. Imaging* **2017**, *2017*, 6592139. [CrossRef]
28. Gerhard, A.; Neumaier, B.; Elitok, E.; Glatting, G.; Ries, V.; Tomczak, R.; Ludolph, A.C.; Reske, S.N. In vivo imaging of activated microglia using [^{11}C]PK11195 and positron emission tomography in patients after ischemic stroke. *Neuroreport* **2000**, *11*, 2957–2960. [CrossRef]
29. Schneider, S.M.; Sridhar, V.; Bettis, A.K.; Heath-Barnett, H.; Balog-Alvarez, C.J.; Guo, L.-J.; Johnson, R.; Jaques, S.; Vitha, S.; Glowcwski, A.C.; et al. Glucose Metabolism as a Pre-clinical Biomarker for the Golden Retriever Model of Duchenne Muscular Dystrophy. *Mol. Imaging Biol.* **2018**, *20*, 780–788. [CrossRef]
30. Lee, J.S.; Pfund, Z.; Juhász, C.; Behen, M.E.; Muzik, O.; Chugani, D.C.; Nigro, M.A.; Chugani, H.T. Altered regional brain glucose metabolism in Duchenne muscular dystrophy: A pet study. *Muscle Nerve* **2002**, *26*, 506–512. [CrossRef]
31. Bresolin, N.; Castelli, E.; Comi, G.; Felisari, G.; Bardoni, A.; Perani, D.; Grassi, F.; Turconi, A.C.; Mazzucchelli, F.; Gallotti, D.; et al. Cognitive impairment in Duchenne muscular dystrophy. *Neuromuscul. Disord.* **1994**, *4*, 359–369. [CrossRef]
32. Basu, S.; Zhuang, H.; Torigian, D.A.; Rosenbaum, J.; Chen, W.; Alavi, A. Functional imaging of inflammatory diseases using nuclear medicine techniques. *Semin. Nucl. Med.* **2009**, *39*, 124–145. [CrossRef]
33. Jeong, Y.J.; Yoon, H.J.; Kang, D.-Y. Assessment of change in glucose metabolism in white matter of amyloid-positive patients with Alzheimer disease using F-18 FDG PET. *Medicine* **2017**, *96*, e9042. [CrossRef]
34. MacRitchie, N.; Frleta-Gilchrist, M.; Sugiyama, A.; Lawton, T.; McInnes, I.B.; Maffia, P. Molecular imaging of inflammation—Current and emerging technologies for diagnosis and treatment. *Pharmacol. Ther.* **2020**, *211*, 107550. [CrossRef]
35. Lange, P.S.; Avramovic, N.; Frommeyer, G.; Wasmer, K.; Pott, C.; Eckardt, L.; Wenning, C. Routine ^{18}F-FDG PET/CT does not detect inflammation in the left atrium in patients with atrial fibrillation. *Int. J. Cardiovasc. Imaging* **2017**, *33*, 1271–1276. [CrossRef]
36. Brendel, M.; Probst, F.; Jaworska, A.; Overhoff, F.; Korzhova, V.; Albert, N.L.; Beck, R.; Lindner, S.; Gildehaus, F.-J.; Baumann, K.; et al. Glial Activation and Glucose Metabolism in a Transgenic Amyloid Mouse Model: A Triple-Tracer PET Study. *J. Nucl. Med.* **2016**, *57*, 954–960. [CrossRef]
37. Zimmer, E.R.; Parent, M.J.; Souza, D.G.; Leuzy, A.; Lecrux, C.; Kim, H.-I.; Gauthier, S.; Pellerin, L.; Hamel, E.; Rosa-Neto, P. [^{18}F]FDG PET signal is driven by astroglial glutamate transport. *Nat. Neurosci.* **2017**, *20*, 393–395. [CrossRef]
38. Giatzakis, C.; Papadopoulos, V. Differential utilization of the promoter of peripheral-type benzodiazepine receptor by steroidogenic versus nonsteroidogenic cell lines and the role of Sp1 and Sp3 in the regulation of basal activity. *Endocrinology* **2004**, *145*, 1113–1123. [CrossRef]
39. Gavish, M.; Bachman, I.; Shoukrun, R.; Katz, Y.; Veenman, L.; Weisinger, G.; Weizman, A. Enigma of the peripheral benzodiazepine receptor. *Pharmacol. Rev.* **1999**, *51*, 629–650.
40. Kim, G.R.; Paeng, J.C.; Jung, J.H.; Moon, B.S.; Lopalco, A.; Denora, N.; Lee, B.C.; Kim, S.E. Assessment of TSPO in a Rat Experimental Autoimmune Myocarditis Model: A Comparison Study between [^{18}F]Fluoromethyl-PBR28 and [^{18}F]CB251. *Int. J. Mol. Sci.* **2018**, *19*, 276. [CrossRef]
41. Qi, X.; Xu, J.; Wang, F.; Xiao, J. Translocator protein (18 kDa): A promising therapeutic target and diagnostic tool for cardiovascular diseases. *Oxid. Med. Cell. Longev.* **2012**, *2012*, 162934. [CrossRef]
42. Villalta, S.A.; Nguyen, H.X.; Deng, B.; Gotoh, T.; Tidball, J.G. Shifts in macrophage phenotypes and macrophage competition for arginine metabolism affect the severity of muscle pathology in muscular dystrophy. *Hum. Mol. Genet.* **2008**, *18*, 482–496. [CrossRef] [PubMed]
43. Bridges, L. The association of cardiac muscle necrosis and inflammation with the degenerative and persistent myopathy of MDX mice. *J. Neurol. Sci.* **1986**, *72*, 147–157. [CrossRef] [PubMed]
44. Nitahara-Kasahara, Y.; Hayashita-Kinoh, H.; Chiyo, T.; Nishiyama, A.; Okada, H.; Takeda, S.; Okada, T. Dystrophic *mdx* mice develop severe cardiac and respiratory dysfunction following genetic ablation of the anti-inflammatory cytokine IL-10. *Hum. Mol. Genet.* **2013**, *23*, 3990–4000. [CrossRef] [PubMed]
45. Hainsey, T.; Senapati, S.; Kuhn, D.; Rafael, J. Cardiomyopathic features associated with muscular dystrophy are independent of dystrophin absence in cardiovasculature. *Neuromuscul. Disord.* **2003**, *13*, 294–302. [CrossRef] [PubMed]
46. Van Erp, C.; Loch, D.; Laws, N.; Trebbin, A.; Hoey, A.J. Timeline of cardiac dystrophy in 3-18-month-old *MDX* mice. *Muscle Nerve* **2010**, *42*, 504–513. [CrossRef]
47. Yucel, N.; Chang, A.C.; Day, J.W.; Rosenthal, N.; Blau, H.M. Humanizing the mdx mouse model of DMD: The long and the short of it. *NPJ Regen. Med.* **2018**, *3*, 4. [CrossRef]

48. Gutpell, K.M.; Hrinivich, W.T.; Hoffman, L.M. Skeletal muscle fibrosis in the mdx/utrn+/− mouse validates its suitability as a murine model of Duchenne muscular dystrophy. *PLoS ONE* **2015**, *10*, e0117306. [CrossRef]
49. Verhaart, I.E.; van Duijn, R.J.; Adel, B.D.; Roest, A.A.; Verschuuren, J.J.; Aartsma-Rus, A.; van der Weerd, L. Assessment of cardiac function in three mouse dystrophinopathies by magnetic resonance imaging. *Neuromuscul. Disord.* **2012**, *22*, 418–426. [CrossRef]
50. Ballmann, C.; Denney, T.S.; Beyers, R.J.; Quindry, T.; Romero, M.; Amin, R.; Selsby, J.T.; Quindry, J.C. Lifelong quercetin enrichment and cardioprotection in Mdx/Utrn$^{+/-}$ mice. *Am. J. Physiol. Circ. Physiol.* **2017**, *312*, H128–H140. [CrossRef]
51. Zammit, M.; Tao, Y.; Olsen, M.E.; Metzger, J.; Vermilyea, S.C.; Bjornson, K.; Slesarev, M.; Block, W.F.; Fuchs, K.; Phillips, S.; et al. [^{18}F]FEPPA PET imaging for monitoring CD68-positive microglia/macrophage neuroinflammation in nonhuman primates. *EJNMMI Res.* **2020**, *10*, 93. [CrossRef]
52. Rae, M.G.; O'Malley, D. Cognitive dysfunction in Duchenne muscular dystrophy: A possible role for neuromodulatory immune molecules. *J. Neurophysiol.* **2016**, *116*, 1304–1315. [CrossRef]
53. Stephenson, K.A.; Rae, M.G.; O'Malley, D. Interleukin-6: A neuro-active cytokine contributing to cognitive impairment in Duchenne muscular dystrophy? *Cytokine* **2020**, *133*, 155134. [CrossRef]
54. Sawada, M.; Kondo, N.; Suzumura, A.; Marunouchi, T. Production of tumor necrosis factor-alpha by microglia and astrocytes in culture. *Brain Res.* **1989**, *491*, 394–397. [CrossRef]
55. Hanisch, U. Microglia as a source and target of cytokines. *Glia* **2002**, *40*, 140–155. [CrossRef]
56. Ponomarev, E.D.; Shriver, L.P.; Maresz, K.; Dittel, B.N. Microglial cell activation and proliferation precedes the onset of CNS autoimmunity. *J. Neurosci. Res.* **2005**, *81*, 374–389. [CrossRef]
57. Malpetti, M.; Kievit, R.A.; Passamonti, L.; Jones, P.S.; Tsvetanov, K.A.; Rittman, T.; Mak, E.; Nicastro, N.; Bevan-Jones, W.R.; Su, L.; et al. Microglial activation and tau burden predict cognitive decline in Alzheimer's disease. *Brain* **2020**, *143*, 1588–1602. [CrossRef]
58. Cotton, S.; Voudouris, N.J.; Greenwood, K.M. Intelligence and Duchenne muscular dystrophy: Full-scale, verbal, and performance intelligence quotients. *Dev. Med. Child Neurol.* **2001**, *43*, 497–501. [CrossRef]
59. Nico, B.; Frigeri, A.; Nicchia, G.P.; Quondamatteo, F.; Herken, R.; Errede, M.; Ribatti, D.; Svelto, M.; Roncali, L. Role of aquaporin-4 water channel in the development and integrity of the blood-brain barrier. *J. Cell Sci.* **2001**, *114*, 1297–1307. [CrossRef]
60. Naidoo, M.; Anthony, K. Dystrophin Dp71 and the Neuropathophysiology of Duchenne Muscular Dystrophy. *Mol. Neurobiol.* **2019**, *57*, 1748–1767. [CrossRef]
61. Nico, B.; Tamma, R.; Annese, T.; Mangieri, D.; De Luca, A.; Corsi, P.; Benagiano, V.; Longo, V.; Crivellato, E.; Salmaggi, A.; et al. Glial dystrophin-associated proteins, laminin and agrin, are downregulated in the brain of mdx mouse. *Lab. Investig.* **2010**, *90*, 1645–1660. [CrossRef]
62. Nico, B.; Nicchia, G.P.; Frigeri, A.; Corsi, P.; Mangieri, D.; Ribatti, D.; Svelto, M.; Roncali, L. Altered blood–brain barrier development in dystrophic MDX mice. *Neuroscience* **2004**, *125*, 921–935. [CrossRef] [PubMed]
63. Takeda, S.; Sato, N.; Ikimura, K.; Nishino, H.; Rakugi, H.; Morishita, R. Increased blood–brain barrier vulnerability to systemic inflammation in an Alzheimer disease mouse model. *Neurobiol. Aging* **2013**, *34*, 2064–2070. [CrossRef] [PubMed]
64. Nico, B.; Frigeri, A.; Nicchia, G.P.; Corsi, P.; Ribatti, D.; Quondamatteo, F.; Herken, R.; Girolamo, F.; Marzullo, A.; Svelto, M.; et al. Severe alterations of endothelial and glial cells in the blood-brain barrier of dystrophic mdx mice. *Glia* **2003**, *42*, 235–251. [CrossRef] [PubMed]
65. Gutierrez, E.G.; Banks, W.A.; Kastin, A.J. Murine tumor necrosis factor alpha is transported from blood to brain in the mouse. *J. Neuroimmunol.* **1993**, *47*, 169–176. [CrossRef]
66. Banks, W.A.; Kastin, A.J.; Broadwell, R.D. Passage of cytokines across the blood-brain barrier. *Neuroimmunomodulation* **1995**, *2*, 241–248. [CrossRef]
67. Gutpell, K.M.; Tasevski, N.; Wong, B.; Hrinivich, W.T.; Su, F.; Hadway, J.; Desjardins, L.; Lee, T.-Y.; Hoffman, L.M. ANG1 treatment reduces muscle pathology and prevents a decline in perfusion in DMD mice. *PLoS ONE* **2017**, *12*, e0174315. [CrossRef]
68. Fairweather, D.; Coronado, M.J.; Garton, A.E.; Dziedzic, J.L.; Bucek, A.; Cooper, L.; Brandt, J.; Alikhan, F.S.; Wang, H.; Endres, C.J.; et al. Sex differences in translocator protein 18 kDa (TSPO) in the heart: Implications for imaging myocardial inflammation. *J. Cardiovasc. Transl. Res.* **2014**, *7*, 192–202. [CrossRef]
69. Tuisku, J.; Plavén-Sigray, P.; Gaiser, E.C.; Airas, L.; Al-Abdulrasul, H.; Brück, A.; Carson, R.E.; Chen, M.-K.; Cosgrove, K.P.; Ekblad, L.; et al. Effects of age, BMI and sex on the glial cell marker TSPO—A multicentre [^{11}C]PBR28 HRRT PET study. *Eur. J. Nucl. Med.* **2019**, *46*, 2329–2338. [CrossRef]
70. Patel, A.M.; Wierda, K.; Thorrez, L.; van Putten, M.; De Smedt, J.; Ribeiro, L.; Tricot, T.; Gajjar, M.; Duelen, R.; Van Damme, P.; et al. Dystrophin deficiency leads to dysfunctional glutamate clearance in iPSC derived astrocytes. *Transl. Psychiatry* **2019**, *9*, 200. [CrossRef]
71. Notter, T.; Schalbetter, S.M.; Clifton, N.E.; Mattei, D.; Richetto, J.; Thomas, K.; Meyer, U.; Hall, J. Neuronal activity increases translocator protein (TSPO) levels. *Mol. Psychiatry* **2020**, *26*, 2025–2037. [CrossRef]
72. Liu, Q.; Johnson, E.M.; Lam, R.K.; Wang, Q.; Ye, H.B.; Wilson, E.N.; Minhas, P.S.; Liu, L.; Swarovski, M.S.; Tran, S.; et al. Peripheral TREM1 responses to brain and intestinal immunogens amplify stroke severity. *Nat. Immunol.* **2019**, *20*, 1023–1034. [CrossRef]
73. Grady, R.; Teng, H.; Nichol, M.C.; Cunningham, J.C.; Wilkinson, R.S.; Sanes, J.R. Skeletal and cardiac myopathies in mice lacking utrophin and dystrophin: A model for Duchenne muscular dystrophy. *Cell* **1997**, *90*, 729–738. [CrossRef]

74. Fiebich, B.L.; Batista, C.R.A.; Saliba, S.W.; Yousif, N.M.; De Oliveira, A.C.P. Role of Microglia TLRs in Neurodegeneration. *Front. Cell. Neurosci.* **2018**, *12*, 329. [CrossRef]
75. Cui, W.; Sun, C.; Ma, Y.; Wang, S.; Wang, X.; Zhang, Y. Inhibition of TLR4 Induces M2 Microglial Polarization and Provides Neuroprotection via the NLRP3 Inflammasome in Alzheimer's Disease. *Front. Neurosci.* **2020**, *14*, 444. [CrossRef]
76. Wang, Z.; Dong, B.; Feng, Z.; Yu, S.; Bao, Y. A study on immunomodulatory mechanism of Polysaccharopeptide mediated by TLR4 signaling pathway. *BMC Immunol.* **2015**, *16*, 34. [CrossRef]
77. Homma, S.; Kaul, S.; Boucher, C.A. Correlates of lung/heart ratio of thallium-201 in coronary artery disease. *J. Nucl. Med.* **1987**, *28*, 1531–1535.
78. Gage, G.J.; Kipke, D.R.; Shain, W. Whole animal perfusion fixation for rodents. *J. Vis. Exp.* **2012**, *65*, e3564. [CrossRef]
79. Rasband, W.S. *ImageJ*; U.S. National Institutes of Health: Bethesda, MD, USA, 1997. Available online: https://imagej.nih.gov/ij/ (accessed on 25 February 2023).
80. Borm, G.F.; Bloem, B.R.; Munneke, M.; Teerenstra, S. A simple method for calculating power based on a prior trial. *J. Clin. Epidemiol.* **2010**, *63*, 992–997. [CrossRef]

Disclaimer/Publisher's Note: The statements, opinions and data contained in all publications are solely those of the individual author(s) and contributor(s) and not of MDPI and/or the editor(s). MDPI and/or the editor(s) disclaim responsibility for any injury to people or property resulting from any ideas, methods, instructions or products referred to in the content.

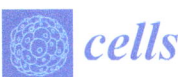

Article

Distinct Responses to IL4 in Macrophages Mediated by JNK

Luís Arpa [1], Carlos Batlle [1], Peijin Jiang [1], Carme Caelles [2,3], Jorge Lloberas [1,*,†] and Antonio Celada [1,*,†]

1. Biology of Macrophages Group, Department of Cellular Biology, Physiology and Immunology, Universitat de Barcelona, 08007 Barcelona, Spain; luisarpa@hotmail.com (L.A.); carlos.batlle3@gmail.com (C.B.); jin.jiang017@gmail.com (P.J.)
2. Institute of Biomedicine, Universitat de Barcelona (IBUB), 08028 Barcelona, Spain; ccaelles@ub.edu
3. Department of Biochemistry and Physiology, School of Pharmacy and Food Sciences, Universitat de Barcelona, 08028 Barcelona, Spain
* Correspondence: jlloberas@ub.edu (J.L.); acelada@ub.edu (A.C.); Tel.: +34-934037165 (A.C.)
† These authors contributed equally to this work.

Abstract: IL(Interleukin)-4 is the main macrophage M2-type activator and induces an anti-inflammatory phenotype called alternative activation. The IL-4 signaling pathway involves the activation of STAT (Signal Transducer and Activator of Transcription)-6 and members of the MAPK (Mitogen-activated protein kinase) family. In primary-bone-marrow-derived macrophages, we observed a strong activation of JNK (Jun N-terminal kinase)-1 at early time points of IL-4 stimulation. Using selective inhibitors and a knockout model, we explored the contribution of JNK-1 activation to macrophages' response to IL-4. Our findings indicate that JNK-1 regulates the IL-4-mediated expression of genes typically involved in alternative activation, such as *Arginase 1* or *Mannose receptor*, but not others, such as *SOCS* (suppressor of cytokine signaling) *1* or $p21^{Waf-1}$ (cyclin dependent kinase inhibitor 1A). Interestingly, we have observed that after macrophages are stimulated with IL-4, JNK-1 has the capacity to phosphorylate STAT-6 on serine but not on tyrosine. Chromatin immunoprecipitation assays revealed that functional JNK-1 is required for the recruitment of co-activators such as CBP (CREB-binding protein)/p300 on the promoter of *Arginase 1* but not on $p21^{Waf-1}$. Taken together, these data demonstrate the critical role of STAT-6 serine phosphorylation by JNK-1 in distinct macrophage responses to IL-4.

Keywords: monocytes/macrophages; chemokines; cytokines; kinases/phosphatases; inflammation

Citation: Arpa, L.; Batlle, C.; Jiang, P.; Caelles, C.; Lloberas, J.; Celada, A. Distinct Responses to IL4 in Macrophages Mediated by JNK. *Cells* **2023**, *12*, 1127. https://doi.org/10.3390/cells12081127

Academic Editors: Vasso Apostolopoulos, Jack Feehan and Vivek P. Chavda

Received: 10 February 2023
Revised: 20 March 2023
Accepted: 6 April 2023
Published: 11 April 2023

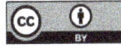

Copyright: © 2023 by the authors. Licensee MDPI, Basel, Switzerland. This article is an open access article distributed under the terms and conditions of the Creative Commons Attribution (CC BY) license (https://creativecommons.org/licenses/by/4.0/).

1. Introduction

Interleukin-4 (IL-4) is a cytokine with functional pleiotropy that plays an important role in host defense in cells involved in innate (macrophages) and acquired immunity (T and B lymphocytes) [1].

Macrophages play a critical role in the resolution of inflammation. During the initial inflammatory reaction, macrophages, under the effects of Th (T helper) 1-type cytokines such as IFN (Interferon)-γ, become pro-inflammatory and secrete a large number of harmful molecules (e.g., NO (Nitric oxide), reactive oxygen species (ROS), enzymes, and immunomodulatory cytokines such as TNF (Tumor necrosis factor)-α). This process has been named classical activation or the acquisition of an M1 phenotype [2]. During the later stages of inflammation, macrophages become anti-inflammatory and constructive [3]. They are activated by Th2-type cytokines, such as IL-4, and through the degradation of arginine they produce proline and polyamines, the latter of which serve to rebuild the extracellular matrix. This process is known as alternative activation or the acquisition of an M2 phenotype [4].

Upon ligand binding, IL-4 signals through a receptor comprising either the IL-4 receptor α (IL-4Rα) and CD132 (γc) chains (type I receptor) or IL-4Rα and IL-13Rα1 chains (type II receptor) [1]. Both types of chains oligomerize and, subsequently, JAK (Janus kinase) -1 and -3 are activated, inducing the phosphorylation of the IL-4 receptor. This process provides a docking site for STAT-6, which induces the phosphorylation of tyrosine 641 (Y641). This leads to its dimerization, translocation to the nucleus, and binding to specific response elements on target genes [1]. In addition, previous data have revealed that multiple serine residues are susceptible to phosphorylation on the STAT-6 transactivation domain (TAD) [5,6].

Several publications have shown that MAPK family members were activated by IL-4. Depending on the cell type, ERK (Extracellular signal-regulated kinase) in T cells [7,8], p38 in B cells [9], and JNK in fibroblasts [10] have been involved in signal transduction to this cytokine.

MAPKs are conserved serine/threonine kinases involved in the transduction of signaling that regulate cell growth, differentiation, and apoptosis [11–13]. These kinases include ERK-1 and -2, JNK-1 and -2, and p38. Through phosphorylation, MAPKs directly regulate downstream targets, including protein kinases, cytoskeleton components, phospholipase A2, and transcription factors or complexes, such as Ets (E-twenty-six)-1, Elk/TCF, and AP-1 (activating protein-1). In turn, these transcription factors promote immediate early gene expression.

In this study, we observed an early and strong activation of JNK-1 during macrophage response to IL-4 as well as the weak and late activation of ERKs and p38. The inhibition of JNK-1 activation resulted in the decreased expression of a number of genes typically induced by IL-4, such as *Arginase 1* or *Mannose receptor*, but not others, such as *SOCS1* or *p21^{Waf-1}*. We have observed that STAT6 was phosphorylated at Y641 and serine. Tyrosine phosphorylation is independent of JNK-1, while serine phosphorylation is dependent on the aforementioned kinase. By using chromatin immunoprecipitation assays, STAT-6 and JNK-1 were detected in some promoters but not in others. This finding demonstrates the critical role of the serine phosphorylation of STAT-6 by JNK-1 in macrophages' response to IL-4.

2. Materials and Methods

2.1. Reagents

Recombinant IL-4 and M-CSF were purchased from R&D Systems. SP600125, PD98059, and SB203580 were obtained from Calbiochem. Actinomycin D (Act D) and 5,6-dichlorobenzimidazole 1-β-D-ribofuranoside (DBR) were obtained from Sigma-Aldrich. The following antibodies used were used: anti-ERK-1/2, anti-phospho-p38 (Thr180/Tyr182), anti-JNK1, anti-STAT-6, phosphorylated anti-STAT-6 (Tyr 641), anti-phosphoserine, anti-CBP/p300, and anti-β-actin (Supplementary Materials Table S1).

2.2. Cell Culture and Animal Models

Bone-marrow-derived macrophages (BMDMs) were obtained from 8-week-old C57BL/6 female mice (Charles River Laboratories, Wilmington, MA, USA), as described previously [14]. Bone marrow cells were extracted from femora, tibia, and humerus. The obtained cells were grown on plastic tissue culture dishes (150 mm) in DMEM (Cultek, Madrid, Spain) containing 20% FCS (GIBCO, Thermo Fisher Scientific, Waltham, MA, USA) and 20 ng/mL of recombinant M-CSF (Thermo Fisher, Loughborough, England) supplemented with 100 U/mL of penicillin and 100 µg/mL of streptomycin. In a humidified atmosphere, cells were incubated at 37 °C with 5% CO_2. After 7 days of culture, a homogeneous population (99.34 ± 0.52% CD11b/CD18 and 98.41 ± 0.93% F4/80) of adherent macrophages was obtained. BMDMs were left for 16 h in medium without M-CSF to allow for synchronization of cell cycles prior to stimulation. Mice deficient in JNK-1 (JNK-1$^{-/-}$) [15] were donated by Dr. R. A. Flavell (Yale University School of Medicine, New Haven, CT, USA). The Animal Research Committee of the University of Barcelona approved use of animals (number 2523).

2.3. RNA Extraction, Reverse Transcription PCR, and qPCR

RNA extraction was achieved using a method previously described by our group [16]. To clone the reporter plasmids and perform PCR, total RNA from cells was purified using the ReliaPrep RNA Miniprep System (Promega, Madison, WI, USA). To remove contaminating DNA, RNA was treated with DNase (Roche, Basel, Switzerland). Using the Moloney murine leukemia virus (MMLV) reverse transcriptase, RNase H Minus (Promega, Madison, WI, USA), RNA was retrotranscribed into cDNA according to the manufacturer's indications. Quantitative PCR (qPCR) was performed using the SYBR Green Master Mix (Applied Biosystems, Waltham, MA, USA). To design the primers, we used Primer3Plus (https://www.bioinformatics.nl/cgi-bin/primer3plus/primer3plus.cgi (accessed on 12 June 2022). For each gene, water was used as negative control. When a signal was detected in these negative controls (at 40 Ct), the primer pairs were replaced with alternative ones. By making a standard curve from serially diluted cDNA samples, we calculated the amplification efficiency for each pair of primers. We only used primer pairs with an amplification efficiency of 100 ± 10%. Supplementary Material Table S2 provides a list of the primers used (Sigma Aldrich, St. Louis, MO, USA). The ΔΔCt method [17] was used to analyze the data. This was performed using the Biogazelle Qbase$^+$ software. Gene expression of the three housekeeping genes, namely, *Hprt1*, *L14*, and *Sdha*, was used to normalize data to address the one-sample problem. The reference genes' stability was determined by establishing that their geNorm M value was inferior by 0.5 [18].

2.4. Protein Extraction and Western Blot Analysis

Protein extraction was accomplished as described in our previous work [19]. In cold PBS, cells were washed twice and lysed on ice using lysis solution (1% Triton X-100, 10% glycerol, 50 mM HEPES at pH 7.5, 250 mM NaCl, 1 µg/mL aprotinin, 1 µg/mL of leupeptin, 1 µg/mL of iodoacetamide, 1 mM PMSF, and 1 mM sodium orthovanadate). Then, through centrifugation at 13,000× g for 8 min at 4 °C, we removed the insoluble material. In Laemli SDS-loading buffer, cell lysates (50–100 µg) were boiled at 95 °C. Subsequently, cell lysates were separated by 10% SDS-PAGE. Then, proteins were transferred electrophoretically to nitrocellulose membranes (Hybond-ECL, Amersham, England). Next, for 1 h at room temperature, membranes were blocked in 5% dry milk in TBS-0.1% Tween 20 (TBS-T). When using the anti-phosphoserine antibody, we did not employ milk as a blocking agent because milk casein is phosphorylated at several serine residues. Instead, we used bovine serum albumin as recommended by the supplier (Abcam, Cambridge, UK). Membranes were incubated with primary antibody overnight at 4 °C (Supplementary Materials Table S1). Subsequently, membranes were washed three times in TBS-T. This was followed by incubation with horseradish-peroxidase (HRP)-conjugated secondary antibody for 1 h at room temperature. After three 5 min washes with TBS-T, chemiluminescence detection was performed (Amersham), and the membranes were exposed to X-ray films (Amersham).

2.5. JNK Activity Assay

JNK activity was measured as previously described [20]. Nuclear extracts were obtained from cells and then immune-precipitated with protein A-sepharose and anti-JNK-1 antibody. After five washes, the reaction was performed with 1 µg of cytosolic glutathione S-transferases (GST)-c-jun (1-169) (MBL) as JNK substrate, 20 µM ATP and 1 µCi µ^{32}P-ATP. In Figure 6, protein A-sepharose and anti-STAT-6 antibodies immune-precipitate total protein extracts (150 µg) from macrophages. Subsequently, immune-precipitates were washed, and used as substrate for JNK-1 instead of GST-c-jun. Then, SDS-PAGE electrophoresis was performed, and the gel was exposed to Agfa X-ray films.

2.6. Chromatin Immunoprecipitation Assay

The ChIP assays were performed as described in our previous work [21,22]. BMDMs were incubated with the recommended stimuli and time. Subsequently, 20 × 10^6 cells were cultured in a 150 mm plate and fixed in paraformaldehyde. After 10 min at room temperature, to stop fixation, glycine (2 M) was added. After 5 min, the plates were washed, and the cells were then scraped and recovered. The precipitate was washed in 1 mL of PBS, Buffer I (10 mM HEPES at pH 6.5, 0.25% Triton X-100, 10 mM EDTA, and 0.5 mM EGTA), and Buffer II (10 mM HEPES at pH 6.5, 20 mM NaCl, 1 mM EDTA, and 0.5 mM EGTA). A protease inhibitor cocktail (1 mM PMSF, 1 mM iodoacetamide, 1 mM sodium orthovanadate, 10 µg/mL of aprotinin, and 1 µg/mL of leupeptin) was added before centrifugation to Buffer I and Buffer II. A total of 300 µL of lysis buffer (1% SDS, 10 mM EDTA, 0.5 mM Tris-HCl at pH 8.1, and the protease inhibitor cocktail) was added to the pellet of cells and incubated at RT. Then, the samples were sonicated for 10 min in high mode (30″ on/30″ off) using Bioruptor Twin (Diagenode; Liege, Belgium). The procedure was repeated 5 times. Subsequently, to confirm a good degree of sonication of the samples (the DNA fragments should have a size of 200 bp to 1200 bp), DNA agarose gel electrophoresis was performed. The soluble chromatin was centrifuged at $16,000\times g$ for 10 min and diluted to a final volume of 1.1 mL in the following buffer (1% Triton X-100, 2 mM EDTA, 150 mM NaCl, and 20 mM Tris-HCl at pH 8.1, and a protease inhibitor cocktail). For control or INPUT, 100 µL was separated and stored at 4 °C. To reduce the number of non-specific bindings, the remaining sample was incubated overnight at 4 °C with 2 µg of sonicated salmon sperm DNA (Amersham), 2.6 µg of non-specific IgGs (Sigma Aldrich, St. Louis, MO, USA), and 20 µg of Magna ChIP protein A magnetic beads (Millipore, Burlington, MA, USA). To remove the beads, the sample was centrifuged at $16,000\times g$ for 10 s. Then, the sample was diluted to a volume of 2 mL (1 mL of the specific precipitate and 1 mL of the control). The two precipitates were incubated for 6 h with the same amount of either antibody (phosphorylated anti-STAT-6 (Tyr 641) or anti-CBP/p300) or a non-specific IgG. Then, the samples were incubated at 4 °C overnight with 20 µL of magnetic beads. The following day, the samples were centrifuged ($16,000\times g$ for 10 s), and the beads were washed and incubated for 10 min in 1 mL of TSE I (150 mM NaCl, 0.1% SDS, 1% Triton X-100, 2 mM EDTA, and 20 mM Tris HCl at pH 8.1); in 1 mL of TSE II (500 mM NaCl, 0.1% SDS, 1% Triton X-100, 2 mM EDTA, and 20 mM Tris HCl at pH 8.1); and finally in 1 mL of Buffer III (0.25 M LiCl, 1% NP-40, 1% w/v deoxycholate, 1 mM EDTA, and 10 mM Tris HCl at pH 8.1). After these washes, the beads were cleaned with 1 mL of PBS (4 °C), and the immune precipitates were eluted with 300 µL of the following solution (0.1 M NaHCO3 and 1% SDS). The elution was performed in three steps. First, the beads were incubated for 20 min in 100 µL of the elution solution. Subsequently, the samples were centrifuged at $16,000\times g$ for 10 s. The resulting supernatant was recovered in a 1.5 mL Eppendorf tube. This procedure was repeated two more times and a final volume of 300 µL was obtained. Before DNA purification, a "reverse crosslinking" step was required, wherein the samples (non-specific and immune precipitates) and INPUTs were incubated overnight at 65 °C. The following day, the QIAquick PCR Purification Kit (Qiagen, Hilden, Germany) was used to purify the DNA of the samples. The final elution volume was 30 µL. These samples were analyzed by qPCR using the primers of the *Arginase 1* promoter: forward, 5′-GCATTGTTCAGACTTCCTTATGCTT-3′; reverse, 5′-TGTTGGCTAATACAGCCTG-TTCAT-3′ [23]. For the control, we used a non-promoter region of an unrelated gene, the *36B4* gene encoding a ribosomal protein. The following primers were used: 5′-AGATGCAGCAGATCCGCAT-3′ and 5′-GTTCTTGCCCATCAGCACC-3′. Primers used for PCR amplification of the $p21^{Waf-1}$ promoter were 5′-TTAACGCGCGCCGGTTCTA-3′ and 5′-AGCGCATTGCTACGGGGAA-3′ [24,25].

To obtain the final results, we performed two normalization steps. The first step involved the specific INPUTs and the second one involved the results obtained from the analysis of the *36B4* gene encoding a ribosomal protein, which was located outside the promoter region of *Arginase 1* or $p21^{Waf-1}$.

2.7. Statistical Analysis

Data were analyzed using the Student's *t*-test. Statistical analysis was performed with the GraphPad Prism 9.1 software.

3. Results

3.1. IL-4 Induces Early and Short Activation of JNK-1 but Not of ERK or p38

A number of publications have shown that depending on the cell type, ERK in T cells [7], p38 in B cells [26], and JNK in fibroblasts [27] are involved in signal transduction to IL-4. Based on these findings, we addressed whether MAPK activation is involved in the IL-4-mediated alternative activation of bone-marrow-derived macrophages. For this purpose, primary macrophages obtained from murine bone marrow were deprived of their specific growth factor (M-CSF) for 18 h to minimize MAPK activity; then, they were stimulated with IL-4 for the indicated periods of time (Figure 1). The activity of JNK-1, reported as glutathione S-transferase (GST)-c-jun, was strongly induced after 5 min of IL-4 treatment and was maintained for only 15 min (Figure 1A), thereby suggesting that JNK-1 participates in the alternative activation of macrophages. The activity of JNK-2 was also measured but was undetectable in in vitro kinase assays (data not shown). In contrast to JNK-1, the Western blot analysis of both phospho-ERK-1/2 and phospho-p38 revealed no activation at early stages but a significant induction of both kinases after 60 min of IL-4 stimulation (Figure 1B,C).

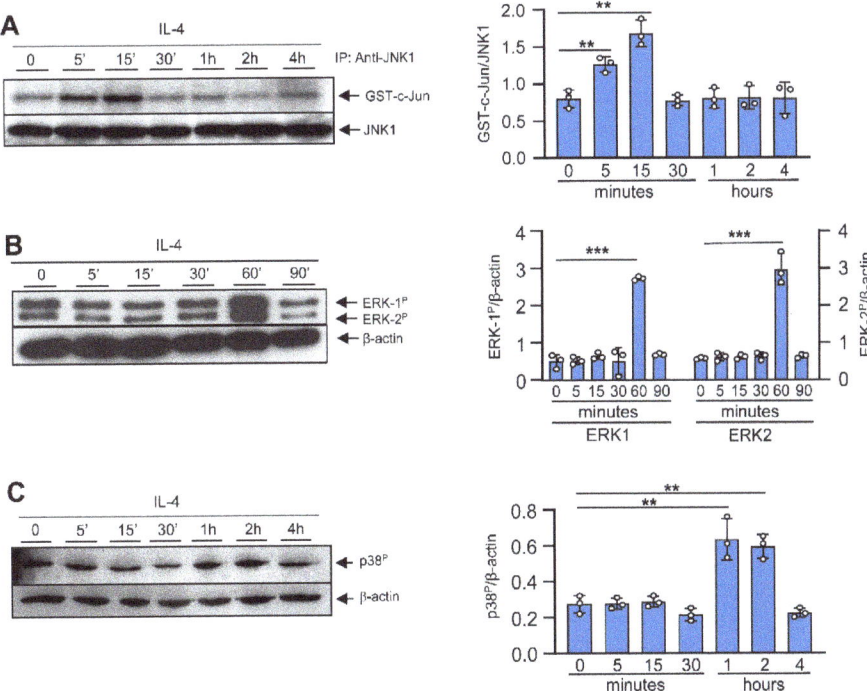

Figure 1. Effects of IL-4 on MAPK activation. Bone-marrow-derived macrophages were cultured for 6 days in the presence of M-CSF. Then, to render the cells quiescent, they were deprived of M-CSF for 18 h. At this point, IL-4 (10 ng/mL) or M-CSF (10 ng/mL) was added for the indicated periods of time. (**A**) JNK-1 activity was studied after immunoprecipitation and then an in vitro kinase assay was performed on recombinant c-Jun. An immunoblot for JNK-1 was performed in parallel as a loading control for the kinase assay. (**B,C**) Activation of MAPK ERK-1/2 and the phosphorylated form of p38 were analyzed via Western blot using the corresponding antibodies. In parallel, as a loading control, an immunoblot for β-actin was performed. Images on the right depict quantification by densitometry of 3 independent experiments. The results are shown as the mean ± SD. ** $p < 0.01$ and *** $p < 0.001$ in relation to the corresponding treatments with IL-4 after all the independent experiments had been compared. Data were analyzed using Student's *t*-test.

To determine whether there is a negative feedback mechanism induced by IL-4 to regulate MAPK activity, we analyzed the expression of MAPK phosphatases (MKP) 1, 2, and 5 as well as PAC1 and CPG 21. In contrast to M-CSF, which activates MAPKs and induces the expression of several members of the MKP family, IL-4 was only able to induce the expression of MKP-2 and, very transiently, MKP-5 (Figure 2). These results show a correlation between the dephosphorylation state of JNK and the induction of some specific MKPs [28,29].

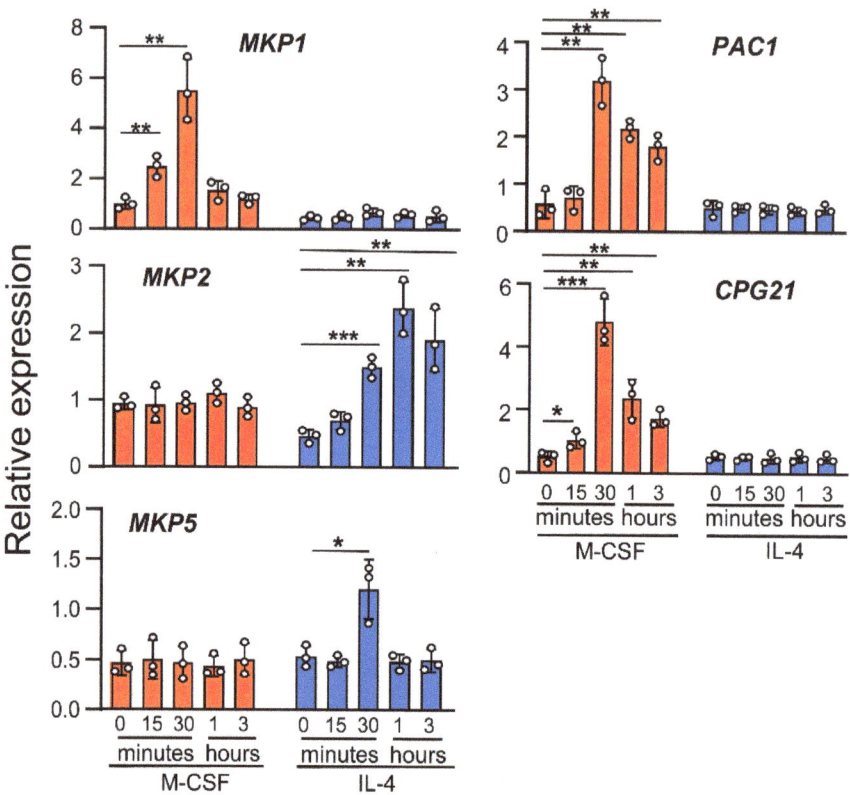

Figure 2. Effects of IL-4 on MKP expression. Macrophages were treated with M-CSF (control) or IL-4 for the indicated periods of time. MKP expression was analyzed by qPCR. The results are shown as the mean ± SD of 3 independent experiments. * $p < 0.05$, ** $p < 0.01$, and *** $p < 0.001$ in relation to the corresponding treatments after all the independent experiments had been compared. Data were analyzed using Student's t-test.

3.2. IL-4-Induced JNK-1 Activation Contributes to the Regulation of Selective Genes

Next, we evaluated the involvement of JNK-1 in the alternative activation of macrophages mediated by IL-4. For this objective, we analyzed the expression levels of several genes, including *Arginase 1*, chemokines such as *CCL22* (a macrophage-derived chemokine) and *CCL24* (eotaxin-2), the cytokine *IL-10*, the *Mannose Receptor*, the *scavenger receptor CD163*, the *suppressor of cytokine signaling (SOCS)-1*, and the regulators of the cell cycle $p21^{Waf-1}$ and *c-myc*. In previous studies [30], we determined the time course of the induction of these genes by IL-4. Most were induced at high levels within 3 h after IL-4 treatment and maximal induction was detected after 6 h. The expression of *c-myc* and *SOCS1*, in contrast to the other genes, was detected early, namely, within the first 1 to 3 h after treatment.

To determine the role of JNK-1 in IL-4-induced gene expression, we used the selective inhibitor SP600125 and the JNK-1 knockout mouse model. Previous studies conducted by our group demonstrated that the dose of SP600125 used in the macrophages in this study blocks JNK activity without inducing cellular toxicity [31]. Surprisingly, the inhibition of JNK with SP600125 resulted in the efficient blockage of the expression of a subset of genes, including *Arginase 1*, *Mannose Receptor*, *CD163*, and *c-myc*; the chemokines *CCL22* and *CCL24*; and the cytokine *IL-10* (Figure 3A), whereas the expression of *SOCS1* or $p21^{Waf-1}$ was not significantly reduced (Figure 3B), thereby suggesting that the link between JNK-1 and IL-4 responses may be promoter-dependent. We also performed similar experiments using SB203580 to inhibit p38 and PD98059 to block MEK and, therefore, ERK-1/2 activity; however, none of these inhibitors significantly reduced the expression of the genes tested (Supplementary Materials Figure S1). To confirm the role of JNK-1, we also used macrophages from JNK1$^{-/-}$ mice. In these cells, the expression of *Arginase 1*, *CCL22*, *CCL24*, and *c-myc* was drastically downregulated (Figure 4A). However, the levels of *SOCS1* or $p21^{Waf-1}$ were not affected (Figure 4B).

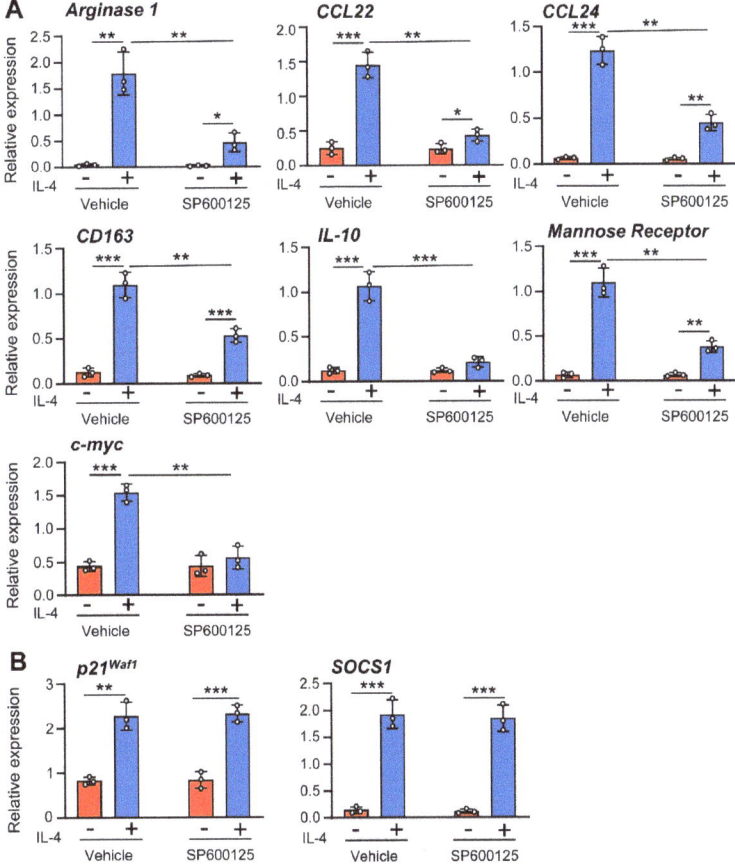

Figure 3. (**A,B**) Different effects of JNK-1 on IL-4-induced gene expression. Macrophages were pre-incubated for 1 h with the JNK inhibitor SP600125 (5 µM) or vehicle (DMSO) as a control. The cells were then stimulated for 6 h with IL-4 except when gene expression of *SOCS1* (3 h) and *c-myc* and $p21^{Waf1}$ (1 h) were analyzed by qPCR. The results are shown as the mean ± SD of 3 independent experiments. * $p < 0.05$, ** $p < 0.01$, and *** $p < 0.001$ in relation to the corresponding treatments after all the independent experiments had been compared. Data were analyzed using Student's *t*-test.

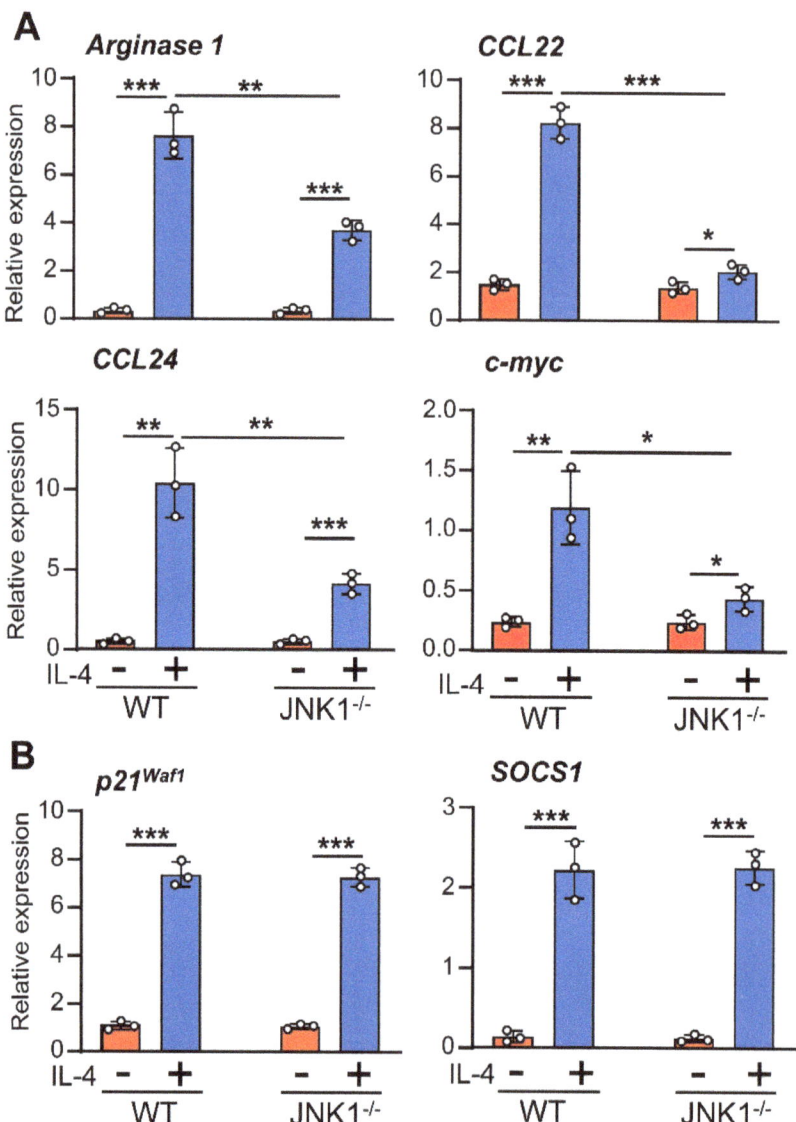

Figure 4. (**A**,**B**) Different effects of JNK-1 on IL-4-induced gene expression. Macrophages derived from WT or *JNK-1*-deficient mice (*JNK-1*$^{-/-}$) were stimulated with IL-4 for 6h except when the gene expression of *SOCS1* (3 h), *p21*$^{Waf-1}$ (1 h), and c-*Myc* (1 h) was analyzed by qPCR. Control cells from each genotype were left untreated. The results are shown as the mean ± SD of 3 independent experiments. * $p < 0.05$, ** $p < 0.01$, and *** $p < 0.001$ in relation to the corresponding treatments after all the independent experiments had been compared. Data were analyzed using Student's *t*-test.

3.3. JNK-1 Does Not Affect mRNA Stability

Previous studies reported that MAPKs perform posttranscriptional regulation by affecting the stability of specific mRNAs [31,32]. Therefore, we tested whether the effects observed on the expression levels of the genes studied herein were due to the JNK-dependent modulation of their mRNA stability. We first induced the expression of IL-4-regulated genes and then blocked further mRNA synthesis by using a cocktail of Actinomycin D and

5,6-dichlorobenzimidazole 1-β-D-ribofuranoside (DBR) [33], at a concentration sufficient to block all further RNA synthesis, as determined by [^{3}H]UTP incorporation [34]. We then measured the remaining mRNA for each gene after different periods of time. To normalize the results of each time point, for each treatment, we set the level of expression at 100% in the absence of an inhibitor. We did not detect any significant variation in the mRNA stability of the genes when the cells were pretreated for 1 h with the JNK inhibitor SP600125 before the addition of IL-4 (Figure 5). This observation suggests that JNK-1 affects the expression of these genes at the transcriptional level rather than their mRNA stability.

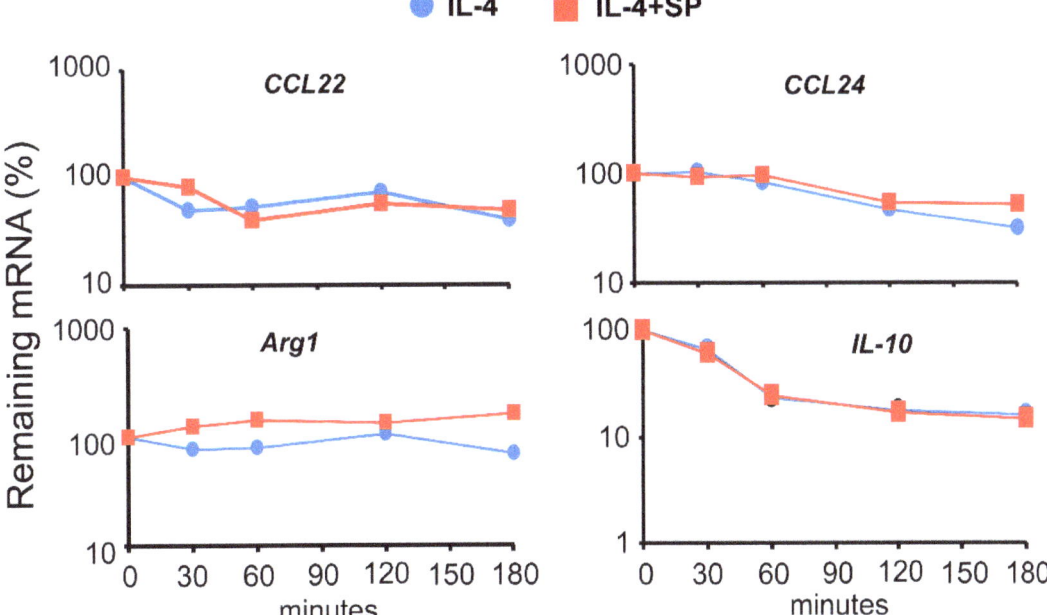

Figure 5. Effects of JNK-1 on the mRNA stability of IL-4-induced genes. Macrophages were pre-incubated with SP600125 for 1 h; then, IL-4 was added, and incubation proceeded for 6 h. At this point, a combination of the RNA synthesis inhibitors 5,6-dichlorobenzimidazole 1-β-D-ribofuranoside (DBR) (20 μg/mL) and actinomycin D (Act D) (5 μg/mL) was added for the indicated periods of time. The levels of gene expression were evaluated using qPCR. To evaluate the rate of mRNA degradation, the mRNA remaining after treatment with inhibitors of RNA synthesis was calculated as a percentage of the expression of the gene in the cells stimulated with IL-4 (+/− SP600125) in the absence of RNA synthesis inhibitors. These experiments were performed three times, and the results from the mean are shown. Data were analyzed using Student's *t*-test, and no significant differences were found.

3.4. JNK-1 Phosphorylates STAT-6 on Serine Residues without Affecting Its Binding to DNA

STAT-6 must be phosphorylated on Y641 to induce its dimerization, translocation to the nucleus, and binding to target genes [1]. To determine the degree of phosphorylation on Y641, we checked whether the activity of JNK-1 toward STAT-6 interfered with the JAK-mediated tyrosine phosphorylation of STAT-6. For this purpose, we stimulated cells with IL-4 for 15 min in the presence or absence of the JNK-1 inhibitor SP600125. Having stimulated the cells, we immunoprecipitated STAT-6 and performed an immune-blotting assay against STAT6 phosphorylated on Y641. No variations were observed in the phosphorylation of STAT-6 on tyrosines (Figure 6A). The DNA-binding capacity of STAT-6 was tested through chromatin immunoprecipitation assays using the promoter of *Arginase 1*. As described previously [35,36], STAT-6 bonded to the *Arginase 1* promoter (Figure 6B). No impaired binding of STAT-6 was observed when JNK-1 was inhibited in the IL-4-stimulated cells (Figure 6B). These data demonstrate that Y641 phosphorylation is not mediated by JNK; therefore, this kinase could be involved in another phosphorylation process.

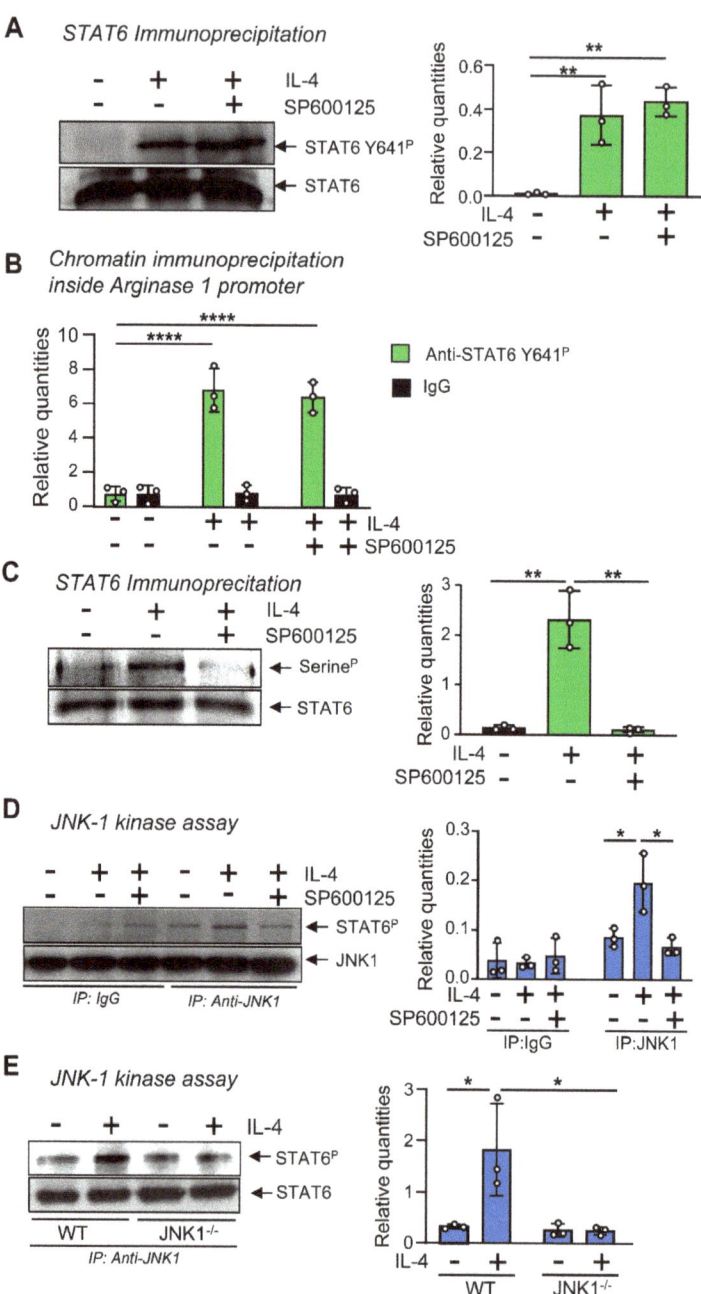

Figure 6. JNK-1 phosphorylates STAT-6 on serine without affecting its capacity to bind DNA. For A to C, macrophages were pretreated with the JNK inhibitor SP600125 (SP) for 1 h and then stimulated with IL-4 for 15 min. (**A**) Phosphorylation of STAT-6 (Y641) was analyzed by immunoprecipitation of STAT-6 and then via immunoblotting with an antibody, namely, either anti-phospho-Stat6 (Y641) or

anti-STAT-6. (**B**) Chromatin immunoprecipitation assay (CHIP) was performed using the antibodies indicated. The presence of STAT6 Y641P in the *Arginase 1* promoter was evaluated using qPCR and normalized with the level of expression of a *36B4* exon and the inputs of each sample as a loading control. (**C**) Phosphorylation of STAT-6 on serine was analyzed by immunoprecipitating STAT-6 and then via immunoblotting with an antibody against phospho-serine or anti-STAT6. (**D**) Quiescent macrophages were stimulated with IL-4 for 15 min to reach maximum JNK-1 activity and then total protein extraction was performed. STAT-6 from quiescent macrophages (to avoid any basal kinase activity on STAT) was immunoprecipitated (150 μg of total protein extracts) and used as substrate in an in vitro kinase assay for JNK-1. As control for immunoprecipitation, IgG was used. An immunoblot for JNK1 was performed in parallel as a load control for the kinase assay. (**E**) An experiment similar to (**D**) but in which macrophages derived from WT or JNK-1 deficient mice (JNK-1$^{-/-}$) were used. As a control for charge, a sample of total protein extracts was used for immunoblotting with an antibody (anti-STAT6). The results are shown as the mean ± SD of 3 independent experiments. * $p < 0.05$, ** $p < 0.01$, and **** $p < 0.0001$ in relation to the corresponding treatments after all the independent experiments had been compared. Data were analyzed using Student's *t*-test.

Regarding STAT6's activation, it has recently been described that in addition to Y641, STAT6 requires the phosphorylation of S407, which is located in the DBD (DNA-binding domain) [37]. Therefore, we examined whether STAT-6 is a substrate for JNK-1. Due to the lack of commercial antibodies that can detect STAT-6 phosphorylated on specific serines, we tested whether JNK-1 could phosphorylate STAT-6 on serine. For this purpose, we immunoprecipitated STAT-6 from IL-4-stimulated cells in the presence or absence of SP600125 and immunoblotted it with an anti-phophoserine antibody. The STAT-6 from cells induced with IL-4 showed strong phosphorylation on serine (Figure 6C). Interestingly, in cells treated with both IL-4 and SP600215, we did not detect any serine phosphorylation on STAT-6. This observation suggests that JNK is responsible for this phosphorylation. Moreover, to confirm these data, we immunoprecipitated STAT-6 from quiescent macrophages and used it as substrate in a JNK-1 kinase assay (Figure 6D). Based on the time course of JNK activation (Figure 1A), JNK-1 was immunoprecipitated from cells stimulated with IL-4 for 15 min. In the cells treated with IL-4, phosphorylated STAT-6 co-immunoprecipitated with JNK. Treatment with SP600125 reduced this effect (Figure 6D), which was more evident when we used the JNK-1$^{-/-}$ cells (Figure 6E). So far, all these data suggest that although JNK-1 mediates the serine phosphorylation of STAT-6, it does not modify the phosphorylation of STAT-6 on tyrosine or its capacity to bind DNA.

3.5. JNK-1 Is Required for Promoting the Recruitment of CBP/p300 to the Arginase 1 Promoter

The phosphorylation of serine 727 of STAT-1 is responsible for the recruitment of cofactors at the promoter level [38]. IL-4 induces the phosphorylation of the IL-4α receptor, which recruits JAK and STAT6 for phosphorylation. Phosphorylated STAT6 triggers the formation of dimers and, subsequently, the translocation of dimerized STAT6 into the nucleus for transcriptional regulation after the recruitment of coactivators to the transcriptosome, such as CBP/p300 or the nuclear receptor coactivator 3 (NCOA3) [39,40]. Since the interaction between JNK-1 and STAT-6 resulted in the serine phosphorylation of STAT-6, we evaluated whether this interaction could also be a mechanism for cofactor recruitment. For this purpose, we performed chromatin immunoprecipitation assays.

First, we tested whether CBP/p300 binds to the *Arginase 1* promoter in our macrophage model, as described before in other types of cells [41,42]. We stimulated quiescent macrophages with IL-4 for 15 min. Using chromatin immunoprecipitation assays, we observed that the treatment with IL-4 induced the binding of CBP/p300 to the *Arginase 1* promoter, which was reversed by SP600125 (Figure 7A). To confirm these results, we used the JNK-1$^{-/-}$ model. We stimulated the cells with IL-4 for 15 min and performed chromatin immunoprecipitation assays. In JNK-1$^{-/-}$ cells, after stimulation with IL-4, no increase in the binding of CBP/p300 to the Arginase 1 promoter was observed (Figure 7B). Moreover, we also examined the recruitment of CBP/p300 in the promoter of $p21^{Waf-1}$, whose expression is not inhibited in the absence of JNK-1 (Figure 3). In this case, we still detected the binding of CBP/p300 in the JNK-$1^{-/-}$ cells treated with IL-4 (Figure 7B). These data suggest that JNK-1 activity is required for the recruitment of cofactors in some IL-4-induced genes.

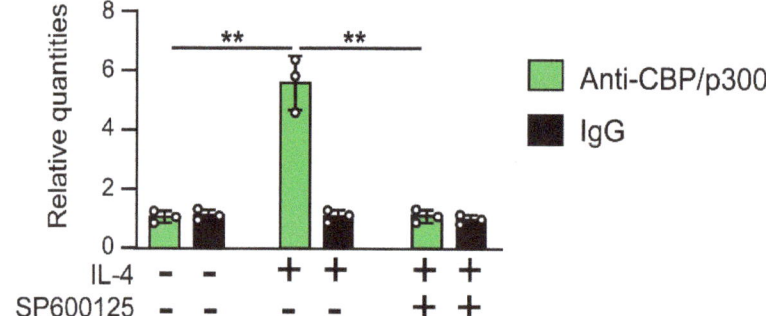

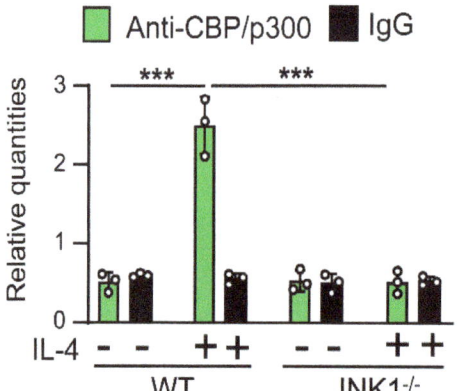 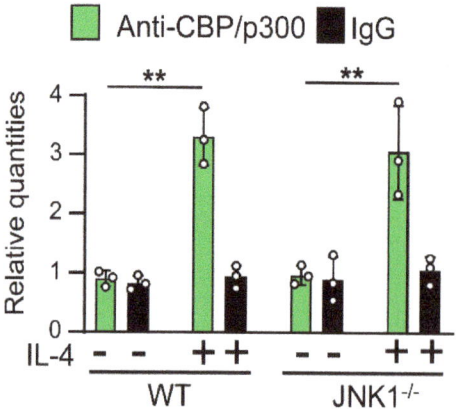

Figure 7. JNK-1 activity is required for the binding of the cofactor CBP/p300 to the *Arginase 1* promoter in response to IL-4 but not to the $p21^{Waf-1}$ promoter. Quiescent macrophages were treated with IL-4 for 15 min. In A, the cells were pretreated for 1 h with the JNK inhibitor SP600125 (SP) or the vehicle (DMSO) before the addition of IL-4. (A,B) Chromatin immunoprecipitation assay was performed with the antibodies indicated. The expression of the promoters was evaluated by quantitative PCR and normalized with the level of expression of a 36B4 exon and the inputs of each sample as a control for loading. The results are shown as the mean ± SD of 3 independent experiments. ** $p < 0.01$, and *** $p < 0.001$ in relation to the corresponding treatments after all the independent experiments had been compared. Data were analyzed using Student's *t*-test.

4. Discussion

The involvement of MAPKs in the cell-type-dependent-signaling of IL-4 by ERK in T cells [7], p38 in B cells [26], and JNK in fibroblasts [27] has been previously documented. In our study, we determined the activation of MAPKs in macrophages activated by IL-4 and how JNK regulates the macrophage response to this cytokine. We did not explore the upstream regulators of JNK-1 in response to IL-4. However, we found that STAT-6, a critical mediator of IL-4 signaling, is phosphorylated at tyrosine 641, which occurs through the action of the kinase JNK-1 in serine. Due to a lack of commercially available reagents, we were unable to determine the exact serine phosphorylation site on STAT-6. However, although the activation of JNK-1 is required for the maximal expression of several genes, it is not necessary for STAT-6 translocation to the nucleus and DNA binding. The cross-talk between STAT-6 and JNK-1 provides a mechanistic link through which cytokine signaling can be modulated.

In our studies, the involvement of JNK-1 appears to play a critical role in the regulation of the expression of several genes induced by IL-4, as demonstrated by the relatively broad effects of the JNK-1 inhibitor SP600125. The effect of some MAPKs, such as p38 in IFN-γ-inducible genes, has been associated with the regulation of mRNA stability [31,43]. Using synthetic blockers of RNA synthesis, we have demonstrated that this is not the case for the effects of JNK-1 on the IL-4-dependent genes studied herein. Therefore, these observations suggest that during the macrophage response to IL-4, JNK-1 serves to modulate transcriptional events and enhance the expression of selective targets. Studies in STAT-6-deficient mice [44,45] showed that STAT-6 is involved in a highly confined manner in the signaling carried out by IL-4, playing a critical role in generating many of the responses induced by IL-4. However, whereas IL-4-induced differentiation appears to be largely dependent on STAT-6, IL-4-induced proliferation and survival have been shown to be at least partially independent of STAT-6 [44,45]. This finding suggests that IL-4 uses additional pathways other than STAT-6 to regulate gene expression. This does not seem to be the case here, as the genes whose regulation is affected by JNK-1 depend only on STAT-6 activation [30].

Our results confirm and extend the previous observations of Haoa et al. [46], showing the involvement of JNK signaling in IL-4. However, these authors used the two cell lines RAW264.7 and THP-1 as a cellular model of macrophages, while we used primary cultures of macrophages. In addition, we showed the critical role of the serine phosphorylation of STAT6 in the transactivation of several genes. Finally, we confirmed our previous observations showing that gene induction by IL-4 does not have a common signaling mechanism. Thus, as we reported previously, the deacetylation of C/EBPβ inhibited the IL-4-induced expression of *Arginase-1*, *Fizz1*, and *Mannose receptor*, while in other genes, such as *Ym1*, *Mgl1*, and *Mgl2*, expression was not affected [47].

One question that remains to be resolved is the location of the phosphorylated serine in STAT-6. In the literature, the IL-4-induced serine phosphorylation of STAT-6 is a highly controversial topic whose conclusions greatly depend on the experimental conditions and, in particular, the cell type used. Using Ramos cells (a B cell originating from Burkitt's lymphoma), Pesu et al. [48] showed that IL-4-induced transcription requires the serine phosphorylation of STAT-6. In HeLa cells (a human cell derived from adenocarcinoma), Shirakawa et al. [49] demonstrated that the cytokine IL-1 mediated by JNK induces STAT-6 phosphorylation at serine 707. This phosphorylation decreases the DNA-binding ability of IL-4-stimulated STAT6, which has been reported to be a mechanism controlling the balance between IL-1 and IL-4 signals.

Recently, using multiple human cell lines of fibroblasts, the activation of STAT6 has been shown to be critical in antiviral innate immunity [37]. In this case, the phosphorylation of serine 407 located in the DNA-binding region plays a determining role. However, studies of the structural basis for DNA recognition by STAT6 show that the residue S407 is not likely to be accessible for phosphorylation by any kinase in the conformations of the protein observed in the crystal structures where STAT-6 is bound to DNA [50]. This controversy intensified when the same authors used luciferase-reporter-based assays to show that the

S407 mutation nullifies the IL-4 response [50]. In fact, a large number of proteins, including CBP/P300, CD28, C/EBPβ, Detergent-sensitive factor, Ets-1, glucocorticoid receptor (GR), IFNαRI, IL-4Rα, IRF4, LITAF, NF-kB, p100, PU.1, SRC-1, and STAT-2, have been reported to interact with STAT-6 [51], and the binding of some of these proteins may undergo conformational changes to STAT-6 that render S407 capable of being phosphorylated.

The mechanism of JNK-1-enhanced gene expression remains elusive. However, we have demonstrated that the binding of CBP/p300 to the *Arginase 1* promoter was increased in the presence of JNK-1. It has been described that CBP/p300 must be serine-phosphorylated to act as a co-activator [52,53], and in some studies, this phosphorylation was carried out by members of the MAPK family [54]. It has been proposed that STAT-6 is acetylated by CBP/p300 [55]. The acetylation of STAT-6 was shown to be required for the STAT-6-mediated activation of expression [55,56].

The binding of STAT-6 to DNA alone is not normally sufficient to stimulate a specific locus. The initiation of transcription requires the interplay of STAT-6 with the basic transcription machinery, which is dependent on different groups of transcriptional co-regulatory proteins. STAT-6 interacts with co-factors through its transactivation domain [57]. Although a direct physical interaction between STAT-6 and CBP/p300 has been demonstrated in some studies, the binding relies on the adaptor protein p100 [58]. p100 is another co-activator protein that recruits histone acetyltransferase activity to STAT6 and enhances STAT-6-mediated transcriptional activation and gene expression [59]. CBP/p300 binds to the p300/CBP co-integrating protein (p/CIP), also known as the nuclear receptor co-activator-3 (NCoA-3), thereby recruiting it into the STAT-6 transcriptional activation complex [40]. p/CIP belongs to the family of p160/SRC co-activator proteins and was found to be a positive regulator of transcriptional activation by STAT-6. A member of the p160/SRC family, SRC-1 (NCoA-1), was found to be crucial for activation by STAT-6. Unlike p/CIP, SRC-1 interacts directly with STAT-6. Finally, a collaborator of STAT-6 (CoaSt6)-associated Poly(ADP-ribose) polymerase activity has been shown to modulate STAT-6-dependent gene transcription [60]. On the basis of our results, we have demonstrated that JNK-1, a signal transduction molecule, is required to initiate the activation of some genes by IL-4.

5. Conclusions

In macrophages, after the interaction of IL-4 with its receptor, the phosphorylation of the STAT-6 molecule is induced in tyrosine 641, leading to its dimerization and translocation to the nucleus. For the induction of certain genes, such as *Arginase 1* or the *Mannose receptor*, the activation of JNK-1 and the phosphorylation of STAT-6 in serines are also required. Similarly, JNK-1 activation is necessary to recruit co-activators such as CREB-binding protein (CBP)/p300 to the promoters of these genes. However, for other genes, such as $p21^{waf1}$ or *SOCS1*, STAT-6 does not require serine phosphorylation nor the recruitment of co-activators. In conclusion, the transcription machinery induced by IL-4 is not the same for all genes.

Supplementary Materials: The following supporting information can be downloaded at: https://www.mdpi.com/article/10.3390/cells12081127/s1, Supplementary Material Figure S1: Effects of MAPK inhibition on IL-4-mediated gene expression. Supplementary Material Table S1: Antibodies—identification, source, application, and dilution used. Table S2: Primer sequences for the various quantitative PCRs performed.

Author Contributions: L.A., C.B. and P.J. performed research and analyzed data; C.C. performed research, analyzed data, and provided critical reagents; J.L. designed research and wrote the paper; and A.C. supervised research and wrote the paper. All authors have read and agreed to the published version of the manuscript.

Funding: This work was supported by the Ministerio de Ciencia e Innovación Grant BFU2017-85353 (J.L. and A.C.) and PID2020-1872 1RB-I00 (J.L.). LA was supported by a predoctoral fellowship ("Formació Personal Investigador, Generalitat de Catalunya").

Institutional Review Board Statement: The animal study protocol was approved by the Animal Research Committee of the University of Barcelona and the Institutional Ethics Committee of Catalonia government (protocol number 2523 and 20 January 2020).

Informed Consent Statement: Not applicable.

Data Availability Statement: MDPI Research Data Policies.

Acknowledgments: We thank R.A. Flavell (Yale University School of Medicine) for the JNK-1 knockout mice.

Conflicts of Interest: The authors declare no conflict of interest.

Abbreviations

Act D: Actinomycin D; DBR, 5,6-dichlorobenzimidazole 1-β-D-ribofuranoside; WT, wildtype.

References

1. Nelms, K.; Keegan, A.D.; Zamorano, J.; Ryan, J.J.; Paul, W.E. The IL-4 receptor: Signaling mechanisms and biologic functions. *Annu. Rev. Immunol.* **1999**, *17*, 701–738. [CrossRef]
2. Murray, P.J. Macrophage Polarization. *Annu. Rev. Physiol.* **2017**, *79*, 541–566. [CrossRef]
3. Wynn, T.A.; Vannella, K.M. Macrophages in Tissue Repair, Regeneration, and Fibrosis. *Immunity* **2016**, *44*, 450–462. [CrossRef]
4. Gordon, S.; Martinez, F.O. Alternative Activation of Macrophages: Mechanism and Functions. *Immunity* **2010**, *32*, 593–604. [CrossRef]
5. Wick, K.R.; Berton, M.T. IL-4 induces serine phosphorylation of the STAT6 transactivation domain in B lymphocytes. *Mol. Immunol.* **2000**, *37*, 641–652. [CrossRef]
6. Wang, Y.; Malabarba, M.G.; Nagy, Z.S.; Kirken, R.A. Interleukin 4 Regulates Phosphorylation of Serine 756 in the Transactivation Domain of Stat6. Roles for Multiple Phosphorylation Sites and Stat6 Function. *J. Biol. Chem.* **2004**, *279*, 25196–25203. [CrossRef]
7. So, E.-Y.; Oh, J.; Jang, J.-Y.; Kim, J.-H.; Lee, C.-E. Ras/Erk pathway positively regulates Jak1/STAT6 activity and IL-4 gene expression in Jurkat T cells. *Mol. Immunol.* **2007**, *44*, 3416–3426. [CrossRef] [PubMed]
8. Tripathi, P.; Sahoo, N.; Ullah, U.; Kallionpää, H.; Suneja, A.; Lahesmaa, R.; Rao, K.V.S. A novel mechanism for ERK-dependent regulation of *IL4* transcription during human Th2-cell differentiation. *Immunol. Cell Biol.* **2012**, *90*, 676–687. [CrossRef]
9. Kawano, A.; Ariyoshi, W.; Yoshioka, Y.; Hikiji, H.; Nishihara, T.; Okinaga, T. Docosahexaenoic acid enhances M2 macrophage polarization via the p38 signaling pathway and autophagy. *J. Cell. Biochem.* **2019**, *120*, 12604–12617. [CrossRef] [PubMed]
10. Levings, M.K.; Bessette, D.C.; Schrader, J.W. Interleukin-4 synergizes with Raf-1 to promote long-term proliferation and activation of c-jun N-terminal kinase. *Blood* **1999**, *93*, 3694–3702. [CrossRef] [PubMed]
11. Seger, R.; Krebs, E.G. The MAPK signaling cascade. *FASEB J.* **1995**, *9*, 726–735. [CrossRef] [PubMed]
12. Comalada, M.; Lloberas, J.; Celada, A. MKP-1: A critical phosphatase in the biology of macrophages controlling the switch between proliferation and activation. *Eur. J. Immunol.* **2012**, *42*, 1938–1948. [CrossRef]
13. Sun, Y.; Liu, W.-Z.; Liu, T.; Feng, X.; Yang, N.; Zhou, H.-F. Signaling pathway of MAPK/ERK in cell proliferation, differentiation, migration, senescence and apoptosis. *J. Recept. Signal Transduct. Res.* **2015**, *35*, 600–604. [CrossRef] [PubMed]
14. Celada, A.; Gray, P.W.; Rinderknecht, E.; Schreiber, R.D. Evidence for a gamma-interferon receptor that regulates macrophage tumoricidal activity. *J. Exp. Med.* **1984**, *160*, 55–74. [CrossRef] [PubMed]
15. Kim, C.; Sano, Y.; Todorova, K.; Carlson, B.A.; Arpa, L.; Celada, A.; Lawrence, T.; Otsu, K.; Brissette, J.L.; Arthur, J.S.C.; et al. The kinase p38α serves cell type–specific inflammatory functions in skin injury and coordinates pro- and anti-inflammatory gene expression. *Nat. Immunol.* **2008**, *9*, 1019–1027. [CrossRef] [PubMed]
16. Tur, J.; Pereira-Lopes, S.; Vico, T.; Marín, E.A.; Muñoz, J.P.; Hernández-Alvarez, M.; Cardona, P.-J.; Zorzano, A.; Lloberas, J.; Celada, A. Mitofusin 2 in Macrophages Links Mitochondrial ROS Production, Cytokine Release, Phagocytosis, Autophagy, and Bactericidal Activity. *Cell Rep.* **2020**, *32*, 108079. [CrossRef]
17. Bustin, S.A.; Benes, V.; Garson, J.A.; Hellemans, J.; Huggett, J.; Kubista, M.; Mueller, R.; Nolan, T.; Pfaffl, M.W.; Shipley, G.L.; et al. The MIQE Guidelines: Minimum Information for Publication of Quantitative Real-Time PCR Experiments. *Clin. Chem.* **2009**, *55*, 611–622. [CrossRef]
18. Hellemans, J.; Mortier, G.; De Paepe, A.; Speleman, F.; Vandesompele, J. qBase relative quantification framework and software for management and automated analysis of real-time quantitative PCR data. *Genome Biol.* **2007**, *8*, R19. [CrossRef]
19. Valledor, A.F.; Comalada, M.; Xaus, J.; Celada, A. The Differential Time-course of Extracellular-regulated Kinase Activity Correlates with the Macrophage Response toward Proliferation or Activation. *J. Biol. Chem.* **2000**, *275*, 7403–7409. [CrossRef]
20. Caelles, C.; González-Sancho, J.M.; Muñoz, A. Nuclear hormone receptor antagonism with AP-1 by inhibition of the JNK pathway. *Genes Dev.* **1997**, *11*, 3351–3364. [CrossRef]
21. Sebastián, C.; Herrero, C.; Serra, M.; Lloberas, J.; Blasco, M.A.; Celada, A. Telomere Shortening and Oxidative Stress in Aged Macrophages Results in Impaired STAT5a Phosphorylation. *J. Immunol.* **2009**, *183*, 2356–2364. [CrossRef] [PubMed]

22. Vico, T.; Youssif, C.; Zare, F.; Comalada, M.; Sebastian, C.; Lloberas, J.; Celada, A. GM-CSF Protects Macrophages from DNA Damage by Inducing Differentiation. *Cells* **2022**, *11*, 935. [CrossRef] [PubMed]
23. Sharda, D.R.; Yu, S.; Ray, M.; Squadrito, M.L.; De Palma, M.; Wynn, T.A.; Morris, S.M., Jr.; Hankey, P.A. Regulation of Macrophage Arginase Expression and Tumor Growth by the Ron Receptor Tyrosine Kinase. *J. Immunol.* **2011**, *187*, 2181–2192. [CrossRef] [PubMed]
24. Prince, S.; Carreira, S.; Vance, K.W.; Abrahams, A.; Goding, C.R. Tbx2 Directly Represses the Expression of the p21WAF1 Cyclin-Dependent Kinase Inhibitor. *Cancer Res.* **2004**, *64*, 1669–1674. [CrossRef] [PubMed]
25. Al Bitar, S.; Gali-Muhtasib, H. The Role of the Cyclin Dependent Kinase Inhibitor p21cip1/waf1 in Targeting Cancer: Molecular Mechanisms and Novel Therapeutics. *Cancers* **2019**, *11*, 1475. [CrossRef]
26. Canfield, S.; Lee, Y.; Schröder, A.; Rothman, P. Cutting Edge: IL-4 Induces Suppressor of Cytokine Signaling-3 Expression in B Cells by a Mechanism Dependent on Activation of p38 MAPK. *J. Immunol.* **2005**, *174*, 2494–2498. [CrossRef]
27. Hashimoto, S.; Gon, Y.; Takeshita, I.; Maruoka, S.; Horie, T. IL-4 and IL-13 induce myofibroblastic phenotype of human lung fibroblasts through c-Jun NH2-terminal kinase–dependent pathway. *J. Allergy Clin. Immunol.* **2001**, *107*, 1001–1008. [CrossRef]
28. Robinson, C.J.; Sloss, C.M.; Plevin, R. Inactivation of JNK activity by mitogen-activated protein kinase phosphatase-2 in EAhy926 endothelial cells is dependent upon agonist-specific JNK translocation to the nucleus. *Cell Signal.* **2001**, *13*, 29–41. [CrossRef]
29. Jiao, H.; Tang, P.; Zhang, Y. MAP Kinase Phosphatase 2 Regulates Macrophage-Adipocyte Interaction. *PLoS ONE* **2015**, *10*, e0120755. [CrossRef]
30. Arpa, L.; Valledor, A.F.; Lloberas, J.; Celada, A. IL-4 blocks M-CSF-dependent macrophage proliferation by inducing p21Waf1 in a STAT6-dependent way. *Eur. J. Immunol.* **2009**, *39*, 514–526. [CrossRef]
31. Valledor, A.F.; Sánchez-Tilló, E.; Arpa, L.; Park, J.M.; Caelles, C.; Lloberas, J.; Celada, A. Selective Roles of MAPKs during the Macrophage Response to IFN-γ. *J. Immunol.* **2008**, *180*, 4523–4529. [CrossRef] [PubMed]
32. Sze, K.-L.; Lui, W.-Y.; Lee, W.M. Post-transcriptional regulation of *CLMP* mRNA is controlled by tristetraprolin in response to TNFα via c-Jun N-terminal kinase signalling. *Biochem. J.* **2008**, *410*, 575–583. [CrossRef] [PubMed]
33. Poele, R.H.T.; Okorokov, A.L.; Joel, S.P. RNA synthesis block by 5,6-dichloro-1-β-D-ribofuranosylbenzimidazole (DRB) triggers p53-dependent apoptosis in human colon carcinoma cells. *Oncogene* **1999**, *18*, 5765–5772. [CrossRef] [PubMed]
34. Celada, A.; Klemsz, M.J.; Maki, R.A. Interferon-γ activates multiple pathways to regulate the expression of the genes for major histocompatibility class II I-Aβ, tumor necrosis factor and complement component C3 in mouse macrophages. *Eur. J. Immunol.* **1989**, *19*, 1103–1109. [CrossRef] [PubMed]
35. Wei, L.H.; Jacobs, A.T., Jr.; Morris, S.M., Jr.; Ignarro, L.J. IL-4 and IL-13 upregulate arginase I expression by cAMP and JAK/STAT6 pathways in vascular smooth muscle cells. *Am. J. Physiol. Physiol.* **2000**, *279*, C248–C256. [CrossRef]
36. Gray, M.J.; Poljakovic, M.; Kepka-Lenhart, D.; Morris, S.M., Jr. Induction of arginase I transcription by IL-4 requires a composite DNA response element for STAT6 and C/EBPβ. *Gene* **2005**, *353*, 98–106. [CrossRef]
37. Chen, H.; Sun, H.; You, F.; Sun, W.; Zhou, X.; Chen, L.; Yang, J.; Wang, Y.; Tang, H.; Guan, Y.; et al. Activation of STAT6 by STING Is Critical for Antiviral Innate Immunity. *Cell* **2011**, *147*, 436–446. [CrossRef]
38. Varinou, L.; Ramsauer, K.; Karaghiosoff, M.; Kolbe, T.; Pfeffer, K.; Müller, M.; Decker, T. Phosphorylation of the Stat1 Transactivation Domain Is Required for Full-Fledged IFN-γ-Dependent Innate Immunity. *Immunity* **2003**, *19*, 793–802. [CrossRef]
39. Mikita, T.; Daniel, C.; Wu, P.; Schindler, U. Mutational Analysis of the STAT6 SH2 Domain. *J. Biol. Chem.* **1998**, *273*, 17634–17642. [CrossRef]
40. Arimura, A.; van Peer, M.; Schröder, A.J.; Rothman, P.B. The Transcriptional Co-activator p/CIP (NCoA-3) Is Up-regulated by STAT6 and Serves as a Positive Regulator of Transcriptional Activation by STAT6. *J. Biol. Chem.* **2004**, *279*, 31105–31112. [CrossRef]
41. Gingras, S.; Simard, J.; Groner, B.; Pfitzner, E. p300/CBP is required for transcriptional induction by interleukin-4 and interacts with Stat6. *Nucleic Acids Res.* **1999**, *27*, 2722–2729. [CrossRef]
42. Bao, L.; Alexander, J.B.; Zhang, H.; Shen, K.; Chan, L.S. Interleukin-4 Downregulation of Involucrin Expression in Human Epidermal Keratinocytes Involves Stat6 Sequestration of the Coactivator CREB-Binding Protein. *J. Interf. Cytokine Res.* **2016**, *36*, 374–381. [CrossRef] [PubMed]
43. Sun, D.; Ding, A. MyD88-mediated stabilization of interferon-γ-induced cytokine and chemokine mRNA. *Nat. Immunol.* **2006**, *7*, 375–381. [CrossRef] [PubMed]
44. Shimoda, K.; van Deursent, J.; Sangster, M.Y.; Sarawar, S.R.; Carson, R.T.; Tripp, R.A.; Chu, C.; Quelle, F.W.; Nosaka, T.; Vignali, D.A.A.; et al. Lack of IL-4-induced Th2 response and IgE class switching in mice with disrupted Stat6 gene. *Nature* **1996**, *380*, 630–633. [CrossRef] [PubMed]
45. Takeda, K.; Tanaka, T.; Shi, W.; Matsumoto, M.; Minami, M.; Kashiwamura, S.-I.; Nakanishi, K.; Yoshida, N.; Kishimoto, T.; Akira, S. Essential role of Stat6 in IL-4 signalling. *Nature* **1996**, *380*, 627–630. [CrossRef]
46. Hao, J.; Hu, Y.; Li, Y.; Zhou, Q.; Lv, X. Involvement of JNK signaling in IL4-induced M2 macrophage polarization. *Exp. Cell Res.* **2017**, *357*, 155–162. [CrossRef]
47. Serrat, N.; Pereira-Lopes, S.; Comalada, M.; Lloberas, J.; Celada, A. Deacetylation of C/EBPβ is required for IL-4-induced *arginase-1* expression in murine macrophages. *Eur. J. Immunol.* **2012**, *42*, 3028–3037. [CrossRef]
48. Pesu, M.; Takaluoma, K.; Aittomäki, S.; Lagerstedt, A.; Saksela, K.; Kovanen, P.E.; Silvennoinen, O. Interleukin-4-induced transcriptional activation by Stat6 involves multiple serine/threonine kinase pathways and serine phosphorylation of Stat6. *Blood* **2000**, *95*, 494–502. [CrossRef]

49. Shirakawa, T.; Kawazoe, Y.; Tsujikawa, T.; Jung, D.; Sato, S.-I.; Uesugi, M. Deactivation of STAT6 through Serine 707 Phosphorylation by JNK. *J. Biol. Chem.* **2011**, *286*, 4003–4010. [CrossRef]
50. Li, J.; Rodriguez, J.P.; Niu, F.; Pu, M.; Wang, J.; Hung, L.-W.; Shao, Q.; Zhu, Y.; Ding, W.; Liu, Y.; et al. Structural basis for DNA recognition by STAT6. *Proc. Natl. Acad. Sci. USA* **2016**, *113*, 13015–13020. [CrossRef]
51. Hebenstreit, D.; Wirnsberger, G.; Horejs-Hoeck, J.; Duschl, A. Signaling mechanisms, interaction partners, and target genes of STAT6. *Cytokine Growth Factor Rev.* **2006**, *17*, 173–188. [CrossRef] [PubMed]
52. Huang, W.-C.; Chen, C.-C. Akt Phosphorylation of p300 at Ser-1834 Is Essential for Its Histone Acetyltransferase and Transcriptional Activity. *Mol. Cell. Biol.* **2005**, *25*, 6592–6602. [CrossRef] [PubMed]
53. Liu, Y.; Denlinger, C.E.; Rundall, B.K.; Smith, P.W.; Jones, D.R. Suberoylanilide Hydroxamic Acid Induces Akt-mediated Phosphorylation of p300, Which Promotes Acetylation and Transcriptional Activation of RelA/p65. *J. Biol. Chem.* **2006**, *281*, 31359–31368. [CrossRef] [PubMed]
54. Chen, Y.-J.; Wang, Y.-N.; Chang, W.-C. ERK2-mediated C-terminal Serine Phosphorylation of p300 Is Vital to the Regulation of Epidermal Growth Factor-induced Keratin 16 Gene Expression. *J. Biol. Chem.* **2007**, *282*, 27215–27228. [CrossRef]
55. Shankaranarayanan, P.; Chaitidis, P.; Kühn, H.; Nigam, S. Acetylation by Histone Acetyltransferase CREB-binding Protein/p300 of STAT6 Is Required for Transcriptional Activation of the 15-Lipoxygenase-1 Gene. *J. Biol. Chem.* **2001**, *276*, 42753–42760. [CrossRef]
56. Razeto, A.; Ramakrishnan, V.; Litterst, C.M.; Giller, K.; Griesinger, C.; Carlomagno, T.; Lakomek, N.; Heimburg, T.; Lodrini, M.; Pfitzner, E.; et al. Structure of the NCoA-1/SRC-1 PAS-B Domain Bound to the LXXLL Motif of the STAT6 Transactivation Domain. *J. Mol. Biol.* **2004**, *336*, 319–329. [CrossRef]
57. Goenka, S.; Marlar, C.; Schindler, U.; Boothby, M. Differential Roles of C-terminal Activation Motifs in the Establishment of Stat6 Transcriptional Specificity. *J. Biol. Chem.* **2003**, *278*, 50362–50370. [CrossRef]
58. Välineva, T.; Yang, J.; Palovuori, R.; Silvennoinen, O. The Transcriptional Co-activator Protein p100 Recruits Histone Acetyltransferase Activity to STAT6 and Mediates Interaction between the CREB-binding Protein and STAT6. *J. Biol. Chem.* **2005**, *280*, 14989–14996. [CrossRef]
59. Yang, J.; Aittomäki, S.; Pesu, M.; Carter, K.; Saarinen, J.; Kalkkinen, N.; Kieff, E.; Silvennoinen, O. Identification of p100 as a coactivator for STAT6 that bridges STAT6 with RNA polymerase II. *EMBO J.* **2002**, *21*, 4950–4958. [CrossRef]
60. Goenka, S.; Cho, S.H.; Boothby, M. Collaborator of Stat6 (CoaSt6)-associated Poly(ADP-ribose) Polymerase Activity Modulates Stat6-dependent Gene Transcription. *J. Biol. Chem.* **2007**, *282*, 18732–18739. [CrossRef]

Disclaimer/Publisher's Note: The statements, opinions and data contained in all publications are solely those of the individual author(s) and contributor(s) and not of MDPI and/or the editor(s). MDPI and/or the editor(s) disclaim responsibility for any injury to people or property resulting from any ideas, methods, instructions or products referred to in the content.

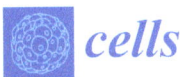

Article

Lung Inflammation Induced by Inactivated SARS-CoV-2 in C57BL/6 Female Mice Is Controlled by Intranasal Instillation of Vitamin D

William Danilo Fernandes de Souza [1,*], Sofia Fernanda Gonçalves Zorzella-Pezavento [1], Marina Caçador Ayupe [2], Caio Loureiro Salgado [2], Bernardo de Castro Oliveira [2], Francielly Moreira [2], Guilherme William da Silva [2], Stefanie Primon Muraro [3], Gabriela Fabiano de Souza [3], José Luiz Proença-Módena [3], Joao Pessoa Araujo Junior [1], Denise Morais da Fonseca [2,*,†] and Alexandrina Sartori [1,†]

[1] Department of Chemical and Biological Sciences, Institute of Biosciences, São Paulo State University (UNESP), Botucatu 18618-689, SP, Brazil
[2] Laboratory of Mucosal Immunology, Department of Immunology, Institute of Biomedical Sciences, University of São Paulo (USP), São Paulo 05508-000, SP, Brazil
[3] Laboratory of Emerging Viruses, Department of Genetics, Evolution, Microbiology and Immunology, Institute of Biology, University of Campinas (UNICAMP), Campinas 13083-862, SP, Brazil
* Correspondence: wdansouza@hotmail.com (W.D.F.d.S.); denisefonseca@usp.br (D.M.d.F.)
† These authors contributed equally to this work.

Abstract: The COVID-19 pandemic was triggered by the coronavirus SARS-CoV-2, whose peak occurred in the years 2020 and 2021. The main target of this virus is the lung, and the infection is associated with an accentuated inflammatory process involving mainly the innate arm of the immune system. Here, we described the induction of a pulmonary inflammatory process triggered by the intranasal (IN) instillation of UV-inactivated SARS-CoV-2 in C57BL/6 female mice, and then the evaluation of the ability of vitamin D (VitD) to control this process. The assays used to estimate the severity of lung involvement included the total and differential number of cells in the bronchoalveolar lavage fluid (BALF), histopathological analysis, quantification of T cell subsets, and inflammatory mediators by RT-PCR, cytokine quantification in lung homogenates, and flow cytometric analysis of cells recovered from lung parenchyma. The IN instillation of inactivated SARS-CoV-2 triggered a pulmonary inflammatory process, consisting of various cell types and mediators, resembling the typical inflammation found in transgenic mice infected with SARS-CoV-2. This inflammatory process was significantly decreased by the IN delivery of VitD, but not by its IP administration, suggesting that this hormone could have a therapeutic potential in COVID-19 if locally applied. To our knowledge, the local delivery of VitD to downmodulate lung inflammation in COVID-19 is an original proposition.

Keywords: SARS-CoV-2; COVID-19; lung; inflammation; mice; vitamin D

1. Introduction

SARS-CoV-2, a newly identified β-coronavirus, is the causative agent of the pandemic respiratory pathology known as COVID-19, whose peak occurred in 2020 and 2021. Even though most affected individuals are asymptomatic or develop mild symptoms, a minor proportion evolves towards a severe pathology. A plethora of factors related to the host, the environment, and the virus itself can affect the disease outcome [1]. Although the lung is considered the primary target of SARS-CoV-2, the virus can spread to many other organs such as the kidneys, intestine, liver, pancreas, spleen, muscles, and the nervous system [2,3]. Pulmonary manifestations vary from asymptomatic or mild pneumonia to a severe disease accompanied by hypoxia, shock, respiratory failure, and multiorgan deterioration or death [4]. The complexity of SARS-CoV-2 infection includes its aggravation by other comorbidities as hypertension, diabetes, and cardiovascular diseases [5] and

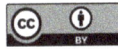

by the adverse outcomes that may manifest after an acute illness and that are known as long COVID. In addition, there are emerging data on an extensive spectrum of sequelae associated with long COVID, mainly characterized by cardiovascular, pulmonary, and neuropsychiatric manifestations [6].

It is well established that the innate immune system works as the first line of response against pathogens, including SARS-CoV-2. This initial response is intended to limit viral infection and to promote the development of adaptive immunity. Pathogens, danger and damage-derived signals are detected by pattern-recognition receptors (PRRs) present in the surface, cytosol, or nucleus of epithelial cells, macrophages, monocytes, dendritic cells (DCs), neutrophils, and innate lymphoid cells (ILCs), which recognize PAMPs (pathogen-associated molecular patterns) and DAMPs (danger-associated molecular patterns). Several PRRs are able to mediate signaling pathways in response to an interaction with SARS-CoV-2 or to the products resulting from the viral infection, including Toll-like receptors (TLRs), retinoic acid-inducible gene-I-like receptors (RLRs), and nucleotide-binding oligomerization domain (NOD)-like receptors (NLRs). A detailed description of this interaction was recently published [7]. A growing body of clinical data have suggested that COVID-19 severity is mostly determined by inflammation and the associated cytokine storm [8,9]. The use of appropriate animal models allows a better understanding of infection and pathogenesis triggered by SARS-CoV-2. Most of the experimental in vivo studies have been conducted using macaques, cats, ferrets, hamsters, and mice, with hamsters and genetically modified mice being widely employed. Recently, it has been demonstrated that hamsters inoculated with SARS-CoV-2 by the intranasal (IN) route developed a viral pneumonia and systemic illness, showing histological evidence of lung injury, increased pulmonary permeability, acute inflammation, and hypoxemia [10].

Many of the findings described in mice are consistent with severe COVID-19 in patients. For example, the IN inoculation of SARS-CoV-2 in transgenic mice expressing the ACE2 receptor driven by cytokeratin-18 resulted in high virus levels in the lungs. An accentuated deterioration in the pulmonary function, which coincided with a local infiltration of monocytes, neutrophils, and activated T cells, was identified a few days later. Such inflammatory infiltrate displayed an impressive up-regulation of innate immunity markers, characterized by signatures of type I and II IFN and leukocyte activation pathways [11]. Standard laboratory mice strains and non-infectious virus components have also been used to establish models of lung inflammation. For instance, the intratracheal inoculation of SARS-CoV-2 N protein in C57BL/6, C3H/HeJ, and C3H/HeN mice induces an acute lung injury associated with inflammation through NF-kB activation [12]. Recently, a model of pulmonary inflammation induced by the lung coadministration of aerosolized SARS-CoV-2 spike (S) protein together with bacterial lipopolysaccharide (LPS) in C57BL/6 mice has also been described [13]. In particular, this procedure significantly increased the NF-kB activation, the number of inflammatory macrophages and polymorphonuclear cells (PMNs) in the BALF, and also triggered pathognomonic changes in the lungs. BALF analysis revealed an increased level of inflammatory cytokines and chemokines resembling a cytokine storm. In this context, the first objective of our investigation was to characterize the inflammatory lung process induced by the IN instillation of UV-inactivated SARS-CoV-2.

Most therapeutic strategies in clinical trials against COVID-19 consist of repurposing existing drugs already used for other infectious or inflammatory pathologies. Anti-viral drugs, monoclonal antibodies, high-titer convalescent plasma, and immunomodulators are frequently investigated [14–16]. Observational studies have shown that serum vitamin D (VitD) levels were inversely correlated with COVID-19 incidence and severity, suggesting that supplementation with this hormone could be explored to prevent or treat COVID-19 patients [17]. Since then, VitD has been tested, alone or associated with other pharmaceuticals, as a potential prophylactic, immunoregulatory, and even neuroprotective measure for this infection [18,19]. According to ClinicalTrials.gov, there are 31 completed studies involving tests with VitD in COVID-19 patients. Some of these trials aimed to assess the effects of VitD on the lungs indicated that one single dose did not prevent the respiratory worsening of hospitalized patients [20], nor did it reduce hospital length in moderate to severe COVID-19 [21]. On the other hand, other reports have been more promising, mainly by using multiple doses of this vitamin. For instance, multiple doses of VitD treatment have resulted in shorter lengths of stay, lower oxygen requirements, and a reduction in inflammatory markers status in COVID-19 patients [22]. Additionally, a 5000 IU daily supplementation for 15 days in VitD-deficient patients reduced the time to recovery for cough and gustatory sensory loss [23].

To the best of our knowledge, most of these trials were conducted by administering VitD orally, which is, considering some limitations, a route that allows a systemic drug distribution [24]. In this context, our second objective was to investigate if the lung inflammatory process induced by inactivated SARS-CoV-2 could be downmodulated by VitD administered by both intraperitoneal (IP) and IN routes. The choice of the IP route was based on our previous experience, showing that vitD was able to control the central nervous system (CNS) inflammation in an experimental murine model of multiple sclerosis [25]. The decision to test VitD administered via the IN route was adopted considering different reasons. Initially, we thought about practical issues as, for example, non-invasiveness, where there may be a possible immediate effect considering that VitD would be applied directly at the inflammatory site, and even the possibility of self-administration. We also considered the fact that previous reports indicate that VitD has a remarkable anti-inflammatory effect when locally applied to the respiratory system. This has already been demonstrated in some lung experimental conditions such as rhinitis [26] and asthma [27]. In addition, the in situ application of VitD has also been effective in other localized pro-inflammatory diseases, for example, vitiligo [28] and psoriasis [29]. The fact that IN VitD could theoretically control, at least partially, some of the immediate or late neurological alterations caused by the dissemination of SARS-CoV-2 to the nervous system was also pondered. This possibility was based on reports showing that VitD attenuates blood–brain barrier disruption [30], therefore decreasing the entry of inflammatory cells into the central nervous system. In addition, the nose-to-brain route has been proposed as a promising strategy for drug delivery to the brain [31].

2. Materials and Methods

2.1. General Experimental Design

In this investigation, we initially characterized a model of pulmonary inflammation induced by the intranasal (IN) administration of 3 doses of inactivated SARS-CoV-2 in C57BL/6 mice. Then, we evaluated the ability of VitD, administered by intraperitoneal (IP) (4 doses) or IN (3 doses) routes, to control or modify this process. The following methodologies were used: the total and differential count of cells in the broncho-alveolar lavage fluid (BALF), histopathological analysis of the target tissue, determination of lymphocyte subpopulations and inflammatory mediators by RT-PCR, flow cytometric analysis of cells recovered from the lung, and cytokine quantification in pulmonary homogenates. These analyses were performed on the seventh day after the administration of the first virus dose. The induction of lung inflammation and the evaluation of VitDs therapeutic potential are outlined in Supplementary Figure S1—General experimental design, A and B, respectively, provided in the supplementary data section (Supplementary Figure S1). Body weight loss and serum calcium levels were also determined to assess the possible side effects of VitD.

2.2. Animals

Female C57BL/6 mice were acquired from the Animal Facility of the Animal Research and Production Center (ARPC/IBTECH), UNESP, Botucatu, or from the Animal Facility of the University of Sao Paulo. The animals were housed in polypropylene cages with a maximum capacity for 4–5 animals on a rack with individual ventilation (Alesco). The temperature was controlled by air conditioning and was maintained at about 22 °C. The animals received water and commercial feed ad libitum and were handled according to the standards of the ethics committee in animal experimentation of IB, UNESP, Botucatu (CEUA

Protocol No. 1959140820, ID: 000129) and the ethics committee in animal experimentation of the ICB, USP (CEUA Protocol 3147240820).

2.3. SARS-CoV-2 Propagation and Inactivation

This study used a B lineage isolate of SARS-CoV-2 (SARS-CoV-2/SP02.2020, GenBank accession number MT126808) kindly provided by Edison Luiz Durigon (PhD, Institute of Biomedical Sciences–University of São Paulo–São Paulo-Brazil), recovered from a sample collected on 28 February 2020 in Brazil. The virus was propagated in Vero cells (CCL-81; ATCC, Manassas, VA, USA) according to the previously described protocol [32] in a biosafety level 3 laboratory (BSL-3) located in the University of Campinas. All the viral stocks used in the study were titrated using a plaque-forming assay according to previously published studies [33]. Briefly, decimal serially diluted samples were incubated with Vero cells into 24-well plates for 1 h at 37 °C and 5% CO_2. After adsorption, the cells were overlaid and maintained with a semi-solid medium (1% w/v carboxymethylcellulose) in DMEM supplemented with 5% fetal bovine serum (FBS) for 4 days. After fixation with 8% formaldehyde solution and staining with 1% methylene blue (Sigma-Aldrich, St. Louis, MO, USA), the viral titer was determined by dividing the average number of plates by the value obtained from the multiplication between the dilution factor and the volume of the viral suspension added to the plate. The results were expressed as the viral plaque-forming units (PFU)/mL of the sample. The virus used in this study, with a titer of 8×10^6 PFU/mL, was inactivated by exposure to 7560 mJ/cm^2 of UVC (30 min) according to what has been described previously [34]. The supernatant of non-infected Vero cells, inactivated by UVC, was used as a negative control. The inactivation efficacy was determined by inoculating the UVC-inactivated product into Vero cells. The Vero cells infected with UVC-inactivated SARS-CoV-2 showed no cytopathic effect. In addition, no virus was detected in the supernatant of these cells by a plaque-forming assay or quantitative RT-PCR.

2.4. Induction and Characterization of Pulmonary Inflammation by SARS-CoV-2

We adopted a protocol which has been previously described [35]. Briefly, the animals received 3 doses of 4×10^5 PFU/50 μL, administered on days 1, 3, and 5 and dispensed with a tip connected to a pipette. The pulmonary inflammatory response was analyzed on the 7th day by using 5 methodologies: total and differential cell counts performed in the BALF, RT-PCR for the quantification of the transcription factors, cytokines and inflammasome genes, flow cytometry for the identification of cells present in the parenchyma, histopathological analysis, and cytokine quantification in lung homogenates.

2.5. Bronchoalveolar Lavage Procedure

The bronchoalveolar washes were obtained from mice previously euthanized with ketamine and xylazine. The animal's trachea was exposed with the help of scissors and tweezers, and a catheter was introduced through which 1 mL of sterile PBS was injected and then aspirated. This PBS injection/aspiration process was repeated 3 consecutive times and the samples were centrifuged at 4 °C for 10 min, 1500 rpm. The pellets were pooled and resuspended in 300 μL, and the total cell concentration was determined using a Neubauer chamber. Smears for differential cell counts were prepared by cytocentrifugation at 600 rpm for 5 min and then stained with the Rapid Pannotic Kit (Laborclin, Paraná, Brazil).

2.6. Quantitative Real-Time PCR (RT-qPCR) Analysis

The total RNA from the lung samples was extracted with the reagent TRIZOL (Invitrogen, Carlsbad, CA, USA) and the synthesis of cDNA (High-Capacity RNA-to-cDNA Converter Kit Applied Biosystems, Foster City, CA, USA), according to the manufacturer's recommendations. The quantitative expression of mRNA for the transcription factors *Tbx21* (Mm00450960_m1), *GATA3* (Mm00484683_m1), *RORc* (Mm01261022_m1) and *Foxp3* (Mm00475162_m1), cytokines *IL-6* (Mm00446190_m1), *TNF-α* (Mm0043258_m1), *IFN-γ* (Mm01168134_m1), *IL-12* (Mm00434169_m1), *IL-17* (Mm00439618_m1), inflammasome components as *NLRP3* (Mm09840904_m1), *IL-1β* (Mm00434228_m1), and *Caspase-1* (Mm00438023_m1), and other inflammatory markers *iNOS* (Mm00440502_m1), *CPA3* (Mm00483940_m1), and *Arginase* (Mm00475988_m1) were analyzed by real-time PCR, using the TaqMan system with primers and probes sold by Life Technologies (Applied Biosystems) according to the manufacturer's recommendations. The gene expression was based on GAPDH (Mm99999915_g1), a reference gene, and presented as a relative change in the fold ($2^{-\Delta\Delta ct}$), using the control group as a calibrator.

2.7. Lung Histopathological Analysis

Left lung samples were collected on the seventh day after the beginning of IN instillations and then they were washed with PBS, fixed in 10% buffered formalin for 24 h, and washed and stored in 70% ethanol until inclusion. Then, 5 μm thick sections from the control (saline), culture medium, and SARS-CoV-2 groups were obtained using a Leica RM2245 microtome and they were stained with H&E. Histopathological alterations were evaluated in a Carl Zeiss microscope GmbH, Oberkochen, Germany, attached to a digital camera (AxioCamHRc, Carl Zeiss, Oberkochen, Germany).

2.8. Isolation of Lung Cells and Flow Cytometry Analysis

In order to differentiate the parenchyma-infiltrating leukocytes from the vascular-associated fraction, the mice were intravenously injected with 3 μg of FITC-labeled anti-CD45 antibody (Biolegend, San Diego, CA, USA) in 200 μL of sterile saline solution. After 3 min, the mice were euthanized, and the lungs were perfused and collected for tissue processing. The vascular fraction of leukocytes was identified based on the anti-CD45 FITC staining and they were excluded from the analysis.

The right lungs, which were removed soon after euthanasia, were shredded, processed in digestion buffer (incomplete RPMI medium (Sigma, St. Louis, MO, USA)) containing 0.5 mg/mL of DNAse I (Sigma-Aldrich, USA) and 1 mg/mL of collagenase IV (Sigma Aldrich, USA) and incubated at 37 °C for 30 min at 180 rpm. Once homogenized, the digested samples were passed through 70 μm cell strainers, transferred to conical centrifuge tubes containing 8 mL of complete RPMI (3% FBS (Sigma-Aldrich, St. Louis, MO, USA)), 10 mg/mL of penicillin + 10,000 units/mL streptomycin (Hyclone, Logan, UT, USA), 0.3 g/mL of L-glutamine (Sigma-Aldrich, USA), 0.0040 g/mL of beta-mercaptoethanol (Sigma-Aldrich, USA), 0.0089 g/mL of non-essential amino acids (Sigma-Aldrich, USA), 0.0089 g/mL of sodium pyruvate (Sigma-Aldrich, USA), and then centrifuged at 4 °C for 8 min at 1600 rpm. The supernatants were discarded, and the cells were resuspended in 500 μL of ACK erythrocyte lysis buffer and incubated on ice. After 2 min, 10 mL of complete RPMI were added and the samples were centrifuged again at 4 °C for 8 min at 1600 rpm. Then the supernatant was discarded, and the cells were resuspended in 1 mL of complete RPMI, counted, and prepared for cytometry analysis. Two million lung cells were stained for surface markers or for transcription factors, according to Table S1 (available in the supplementary data section). All the antibodies and intranuclear staining were conducted according to the manufacturer's instructions using an eBioscience Transcription Factor Buffer set.

Alternatively, 2 million cells were used for the intracellular cytokine detection. For the labeling of cytokine-producing cells, the cells were incubated for 4 h with 100 μL of complete RPMI containing 50 ng/mL of phorbol myristate acetate (PMA) (Sigma Aldrich, USA), 500 ng/mL of ionomycin (Sigma-Aldrich, USA), and 1 μL/mL of GolgiPlug (BD Biosciences, San Jose, CA, USA). The cytokines, transcription factors, and cells from innate and specific immunity were then labeled with fluorochrome-conjugated antibodies. Prior to the addition of the antibody mix, as specified in Table S1, all samples from all panels were incubated for 20 min at 4 °C with 30 μL of live dead, 1:1000 (LD, Thermo Fisher Scientific, USA), followed by surface staining and intracellular staining (BD-Citofix-Citoperm kit, USA). The data were acquired in the BD LSRFortessa X-20 flow cytometer (BD Biosciences, USA) and the compensation and data analyses were performed using the FlowJo software. The gate strategies are described in Supplementary Figures S2–S4.

2.9. VitD Administration by IP and IN Routes

1α,25-dihydroxyvitamin D3 (1,25-VitD3, Sigma-Aldrich, USA) was administered by IP or IN routes. The 2 therapeutic protocols with 1α,25-dihydroxyvitamin D3 (VitD) were carried out using different strategies. In the IN protocol, each animal was treated with 3 doses of VitD (0.1 µg/dose), which were administered simultaneously with the SARS-CoV-2 inoculum (4×10^5 PFU/each inoculum) in a final volume of 57 µL. This volume was divided between the 2 nostrils on days 1, 3, and 5. In the IP protocol, each animal was treated with 4 doses of VitD (0.1 µg/100 µL/dose) that were delivered on days 0, 2, 4, and 6 to mice that were instilled with 50 µL of SARS-CoV-2 on days 1, 3, and 5. In both cases, euthanasia was performed at the seventh day after the beginning of the protocol.

2.10. Measurement of Serum Calcium Levels

The blood samples collected after anesthesia were centrifuged, and the sera were stored at $-20\ °C$ until further analyses. The serum levels of calcium were measured according to the instructions of the manufacturer (Cálcio Arsenazo III, Bioclin-Quibasa Química Básica Ltda, Belo Horizonte, MG, Brazil). In this technique, calcium quantification was based on a colorimetric reaction in which calcium reacts with arsenazo III, in an acidic medium, generating a blue complex whose intensity is proportional to the calcium concentration in the sample.

2.11. Statistical Analysis

In the case of parametric variables, the values were presented as the mean and standard error of the mean (SEM), and the comparison between the two groups was performed using an unpaired *t*-test and, among three or more groups, an ANOVA was performed followed by Tukey's test. When the variables were non-parametric, the results were presented in median and interquartile intervals and the comparison between the groups was performed using Kruskal–Wallis' test followed by Dunn's test. The level of significance adopted was 5%. The data were analyzed using the SigmaPlot for Windows version 2.0 statistical package (1995, Jandel, Corporation, CA, USA). For t-distributed stochastic neighbor embedding (t-SNE) algorithm analysis, 100,000 or 50,000 events per sample, were downsampled from the live parenchymal leukocytes gate (Supplementary Figure S2) and concatenated. The t-SNE algorithm was applied in the concatenated samples using 2000 interactions and perplexity 80. After that, the cell clusters were identified based on the main cell subsets gated according to Supplementary Figure S2, and the percentage of each cell subset was calculated after segregating the groups based on the sample IDs.

3. Results

3.1. Cell Infiltration in the BALF Suggests Pulmonary Inflammation in Mice Intranasally Instilled with Inactivated SARS-CoV-2

The ability of inactivated SARS-CoV-2 to trigger a lung inflammatory process was initially investigated by analyzing the amount and identity of white blood cells (WBCs) obtained from the broncho-alveolar lavage fluid (BALF). Two control groups were included in all the initial experimental procedures and were identified as the control and culture medium, which corresponded to animals that were anesthetized and instilled with 0.9% saline or with the culture medium used for virus propagation in VERO cells, respectively. The total number of WBCs and specific cell populations were identified in cytospin smears, are shown in Figure 1A, and they indicate a significant increase in the total cell number, as well as in lymphocytes and neutrophils in animals that received SARS-CoV-2 in comparison to the control groups. The percentage alterations observed in the SARS-CoV-2 group included a significant decrease in macrophages and a significant increase in neutrophils, as illustrated in Figure 1B. This lower percentage of macrophages in the SARS-CoV-2 group, in comparison to the control groups, indicates an increment of other cell types as lymphocytes (discreet) and PMNs (significant) associated with the cellular influx to the lungs triggered by the virus. Even though the proportion of macrophages was smaller, the total number of this cell type was almost double in the SARS-CoV-2 group, in comparison to the control groups (Figure 1A). Animals injected with saline or culture medium displayed a similar profile, characterized by a smaller number of all cell types, indicating that the culture medium present in SARS-CoV-2 preparation was not triggering a significant pulmonary airway inflammation.

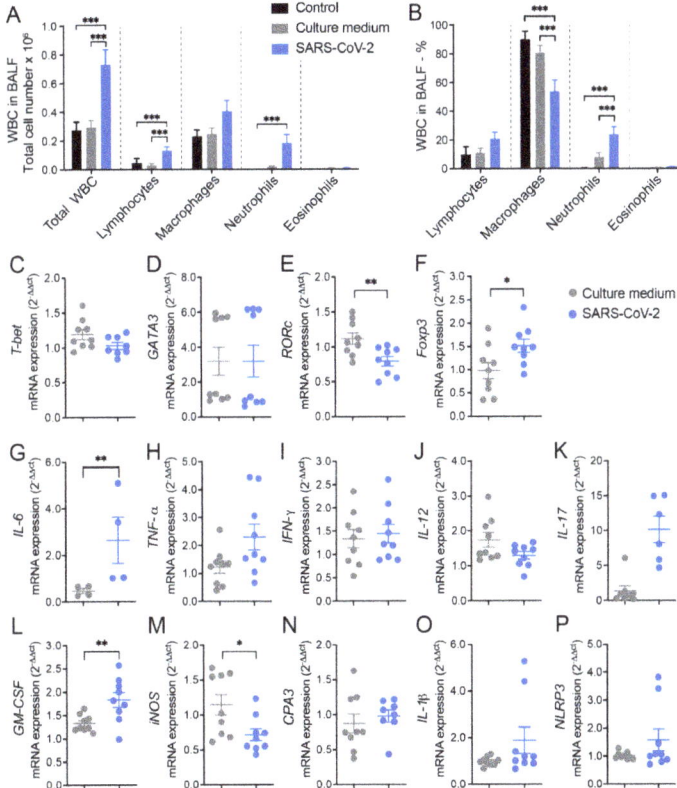

Figure 1. Cell counts in the BALF and lung mRNA transcripts for T cell subsets, cytokines, and other indicators of inflammation in mice intranasally instilled with UV-inactivated SARS-CoV-2. C57BL/6 mice were instilled with the virus (3 doses of 4×10^5 PFU/each) on days 1, 3, and 5. On the 7th day, the BALF and the left lower lobe were collected for WBCs differential count and mRNA transcript determinations, respectively. Total number (**A**) and percentage (**B**) of WBCs: *T-bet* (**C**), *GATA3* (**D**), *RORc* (**E**), *Foxp3* (**F**), *IL-6* (**G**), *TNF-α* (**H**), *IFN-γ* (**I**), *IL-12* (**J**), *IL-17* (**K**), *GM-CSF* (**L**), *iNOS* (**M**), *CPA3* (**N**), *IL-1β* (**O**), *NLRP3* (**P**). In figure (**A**,**B**), the results are expressed as mean ± SEM and the statistical significance of the differences was analyzed using ANOVA followed by Tukey's test. In figures (**C**–**P**), the results were expressed in median and interquartile intervals and the comparison between the groups was performed using the *t*-test. Data shown in (**A**,**B**) and (**C**–**P**) are derived from two experiments with similar results which were combined (n = 9), except *Tbet* (n = 8), *IL-17* (n = 6), and *IL-6* (n = 4). * $p < 0.05$; ** $p < 0.01$; *** $p < 0.001$.

3.2. RT-qPCR from Lung Homogenates Shows Alterations in T Cell Subsets, Cytokines, and Other Inflammatory Mediators

Next, we measured the relative expression of several genes by RT-q PCR which revealed differences between culture medium and SARS-CoV-2 groups. In the SARS-CoV-2 group, there was a significantly higher expression of *Foxp3* (Figure 1F), *IL-6* (Figure 1G), and *GM-CSF* (Figure 1L) transcripts and a higher, even though not statistically significant, expression of *TNF-α* (Figure 1H), *IL-17* (Figure 1K), *IL-1β* (Figure 1O), and *NLRP3* (Figure 1P) transcripts. On the other hand, we found a significant decrease in the expression of *RORc* (Figure 1E) and *iNOS* (Figure 1M) in the lungs of the SARS-CoV-2 group compared to the culture medium control. Other genes, such as *T-bet*, *GATA-3*, *IFN-γ*, *IL-12*, and *CPA3* (Figure 1C,D,I,J,N, respectively), were similarly expressed in the culture medium and SARS-CoV-2 groups.

3.3. Histopathology and Cytometric Analysis Reveal an Impressive Infiltration of Inflammatory Cells into the Pulmonary Parenchyma

According to the histopathological evaluation illustrated in Figure 2A, the lung architecture was preserved in the animals from the control group, allowing the visualization of alveoli and longitudinally and transversally sectioned blood vessels and bronchi. The culture medium and SARS-CoV-2 groups displayed inflammatory foci; however, the ones found in the virus-instilled animals were clearly more numerous and intense. These inflammatory foci were, in both cases, located around the vessels and bronchi, as indicated by black and green arrows, respectively. The presence of neutrophilic infiltrates (green arrowhead), macrophage infiltrates (blue arrowhead), and lymphocytic infiltrates (yellow arrowhead) are indicated in the microphotographs. Numerous consolidation areas were present in the lungs of SARS-CoV-2-instilled animals, but they were rare and absent in the culture medium and saline control groups, respectively. To confirm these findings, we evaluated the leukocytes infiltrating the lung parenchyma by using cells isolated from mice previously injected with FITC-labeled anti-CD45 antibodies to distinguish circulating cells from the tissue infiltrate. Indeed, confirming the histopathological findings, the quantification of total and parenchymal infiltrating CD45$^+$ leukocytes revealed a significant increase in the cell number in the group of mice that received UV-inactivated SARS-CoV-2 compared to both control groups (Figure 2B).

Next, we characterized the tissue-infiltrating leukocytes based on the surface molecules expression using flow cytometry, and the t-SNE algorithm was used for dimension reduction (Figure 2C and Supplementary Figure S2). In the lungs of mice exposed to the inactivated virus, we found an enrichment in the clusters of cells that indicate the presence of neutrophils, eosinophils, macrophages (tissue-resident), and monocytes in the CD103$^-$CD11b$^+$ DC subset (Figure 2C). On the other hand, the frequency of other cell subsets, such as CD103$^+$CD11b$^-$ DCs, alveolar macrophages, and B cells, were reduced (Figure 2C). Furthermore, the frequency of proinflammatory cytokine-producing cells was also increased in the SARS-CoV-2 group, in particular, the frequency of IFN-γ- and TNF-α-producing TCRβ$^+$ T cells and IL-6- and TNF-α-producing CD11b$^+$ myeloid cells (Figure 2D). The quantification of each cell subset number is shown in Figure 2F–Q. The predominant profile of all the tested cells was characterized by a significantly higher number of cells enriched in the t-SNE analysis in the SARS-CoV-2 group in comparison to the control group. This was the case for the total number of neutrophils (Figure 2F), eosinophils (Figure 2G), inflammatory monocytes (Figure 2I), resident macrophages (Figure 2K), dendritic cells (DCs) (Figure 2L), CD11b$^+$CD103$^-$ DCs (Figure 2M), IFN-γ$^+$- and TNF-α$^+$-producing T cells (Figure 2N–O and Supplementary Figure S3), and TNF-α$^+$- and IL-6-producing myeloid cells (Figure 2P–Q and Supplementary Figure S3). Contrastingly, the total number of each cell population in the culture medium-instilled animals was intermediate between the control and SARS-CoV-2 groups (data not shown). Therefore, these data show that the IN instillation of the inactivated virus is sufficient to promote a proinflammatory lung milieu that resembles most of the markers of the infection with SARS-CoV-2.

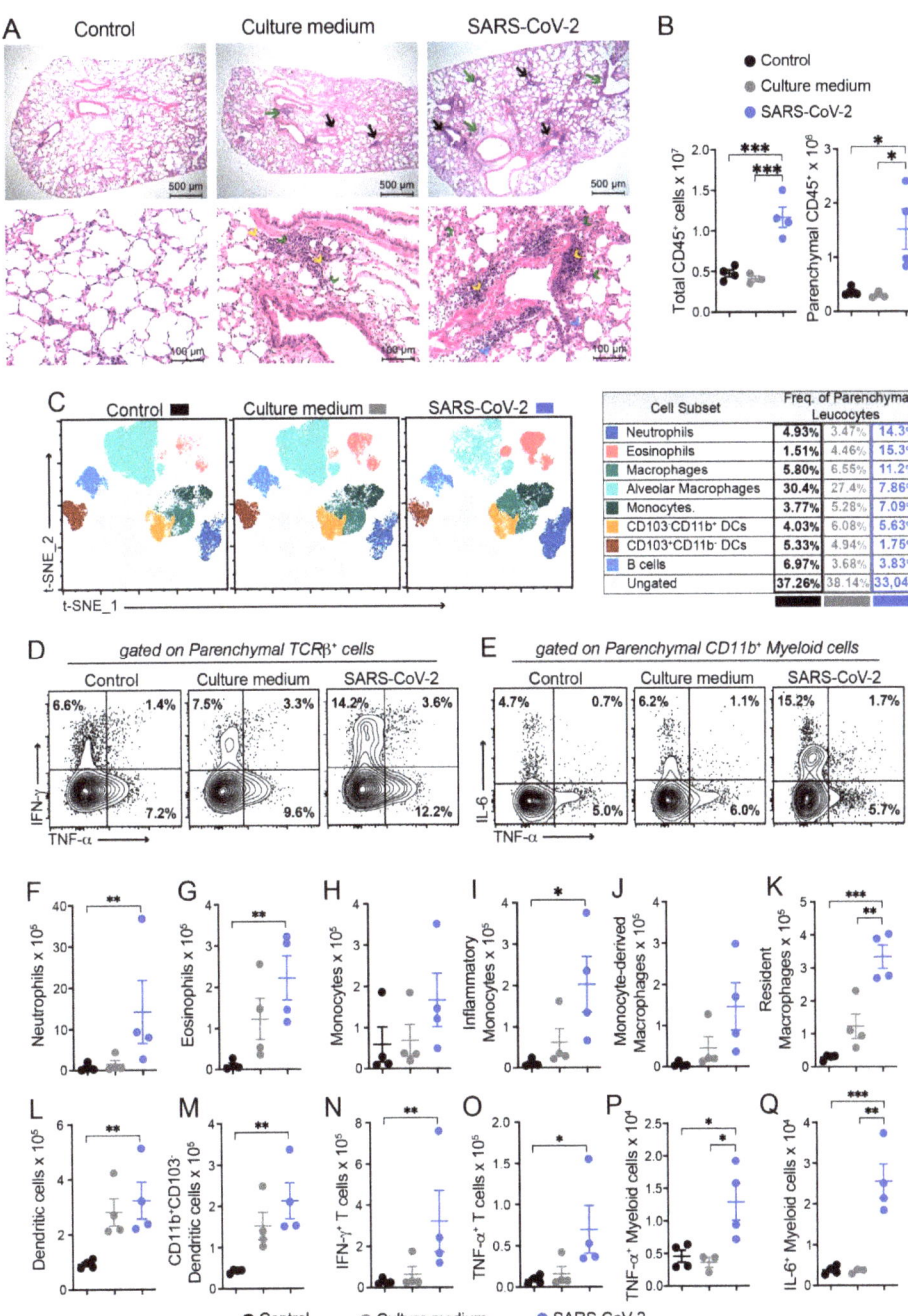

Figure 2. Characterization of the inflammatory process induced by IN instillation of inactivated SARS-CoV-2 by histopathological and cytometry analyses. C57BL/6 mice were instilled with the virus (3 doses of 4×10^5 PFU/each) on days 1, 3, and 5. On the 7th day, the upper left lobe and whole right lung were collected for histopathological and cytometric analyses, respectively. For histopathological evaluation, the samples were washed, fixed, stained with H&E, and then evaluated

concerning the presence of inflammatory foci. Then, 5 um thick sections from the control (saline), culture medium, and SARS-CoV-2 groups were analyzed, and the representative images are shown in (**A**). Inflammatory foci around the vessels (black arrows) and around the bronchi (green arrows), neutrophilic infiltrates (green arrow head), macrophage infiltrates (blue arrow head), and lymphocystic infiltrates (yellow arrow head). The cells were isolated from the lung tissue and total $CD45^+$ leukocytes or the parenchymal infiltrating leukocyte fraction (identified based on anti-CD45 intravenous injection) were quantified by flow cytometry (**B**) and specific cells subsets were evaluated according to the gating strategy described in Supplementary Figure S2. t-distributed stochastic neighbor embedding (t-SNE) analysis illustrating the distribution of cell clusters in each experimental group (**C**) according to the gate strategy described in Supplementary Figure S2. The table on the right side indicates the frequency of each cell cluster relative to the $CD45^+$ parenchyma-infiltrating leukocyte in the control (black), culture medium (grey), and SARS-CoV-2 (blue) groups. The representative contour plots of IL-6, TNF-α, or IFN-γ staining in parenchymal TCRβ^+ T cells (**D**) or $CD11b^+$ myeloid cells (**E**), according to gate strategy described in Supplementary Figure S3. The total cell numbers of each parenchymal-infiltrating cell subsets are expressed in mean $\pm$ SEM, including neutrophils (**F**), eosinophils (**G**), monocytes (**H**), inflammatory monocytes (**I**), monocyte-derived macrophages (**J**), resident macrophages (**K**), dendritic cells (**L**), $CD11b^+CD103^-$ dendritic cells (**M**), IFN-γ^+ TCRβ^+ cells (**N**), TNF-α^+ TCRβ^+ cells (**O**), TNF-α^+ CD11b+ myeloid cells (**P**), and IL-6$^+$CD11b$^+$ myeloid cells (**Q**). Data are derived from one experiment between two showing similar findings (n = 4). The results are presented in median and interquartile intervals and the comparison between the groups was performed using the Kruskal–Wallis test, followed by Dunn's test. * $p < 0.05$; ** $p < 0.01$; *** $p < 0.001$.

3.4. BALF and Cytokine Levels in Lung Homogenates Suggest That in VitD Modulates Pulmonary Inflammation Induced by SARS-CoV-2

Considering that VitD has a strong effect on the immune system and that it is considered for prophylactic or therapeutic application in COVID-19 patients [18,19], we tested its IP and IN effectiveness to control experimental lung inflammation induced by inactivated SARS-CoV-2. As already observed in previous studies, IP VitD administration triggered a significant loss of body weight (Figure 3A) and also significant hypercalcemia (Figure 3B) in comparison to all the other experimental groups. Even though VitD also significantly increased serum calcium levels, it only slightly increased body weight loss, as illustrated in Figure 3A,B, respectively. Concerning the BALF, the comparison among SARS-CoV-2, SARS-CoV-2/VitD (IP), and SARS-CoV-2/VitD (IN) showed no differences in the total number of WBCs, macrophages, and lymphocytes. However, a significant decrease in PMNs was detected in the SARS-CoV-2/VitD (IN)-treated group in comparison to the non-treated groups. Additionally, the number of eosinophils in the SARS-CoV-2/VitD (IP) group was significantly higher than in the IN-treated one. Concerning the percentage of these cells, a higher percent of macrophages was found in the IN-treated group in comparison with the two other groups, and a decreased percentage of PMNs and eosinophils was observed in the IN-treated group in relation to the non-treated one. The percent of eosinophils in the IN-treated mice was also significantly reduced in comparison to the IP-treated ones. To analyze if the SARS-CoV-2-induced lung inflammation model was also mimicking the cytokine storm-like phenomenon and to reinforce the presumed down-modulatory effect of VitD, we tested the presence of pro-inflammatory and regulatory cytokines in lung homogenates. As can be observed in Figure 3E, IN VitD decreased TNF-α and IL-6 and IP VitD decreased IL-6 levels; however, these alterations were not significant. No changes were detected in IL-17A and IFN-γ (Figure 3E) or in the other tested cytokines as IL-2, IL-4, and IL-10 (data not shown).

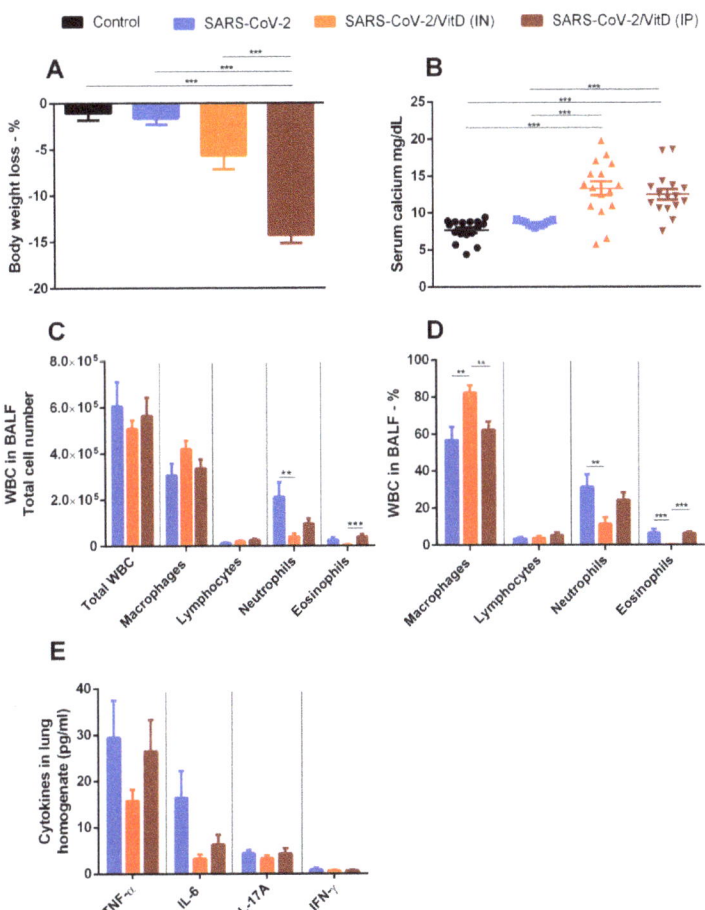

Figure 3. VitD effects on body weight, serum calcium levels, BALF cell counts, and cytokine levels in lung homogenates form mice of mice instilled with inactivated SARS-CoV-2. C57BL/6 mice were instilled with the virus (3 doses of 4×10^5 PFU/each) on days 1, 3, and 5. Body weight was checked daily and, at the 7th day, we collected blood samples for calcium measurement, BALF for WBCs analysis, and lower left lobe for cytokine quantification. Body weight loss (**A**), serum calcium levels (**B**), total WBCs, and WBCs subsets in BALF (**C**), percentage of WBCs in BALF (**D**), and cytokines in lung homogenates (**E**). Data shown in (**A,B,D**) derive from 3 experiments which were combined (n = 5 mice/experimental group). Data shown in (**A,C–E**) derive from 2 experiments with similar results which were combined (n = 16 mice/experimental group). The results are expressed as mean ± SEM and the comparison between the groups was performed using an ANOVA followed by Tukey's test. The results shown in (**B**) are expressed as median and interquartile intervals and the comparison between the groups was performed by the Kruskal–Wallis test followed by Dunn's test. ** $p < 0.01$; *** $p < 0.001$.

3.5. Differential Effects of VitD Delivered by IN and IP Routes on RORc and Inflammasome Genes Expression

The expression of various genes in the lungs of mice IN challenged with UV-inactivated SARS-CoV-2 was similar in the three compared groups, as was the case of *T-bet*, *GATA3*, *Foxp3*, *TNF-α*, *IFN-γ*, *IL-12*, *GM-CSF*, and *INOs* (Figure 4A,B,D–J, respectively). In contrast, the expression of *RORC* (Figure 4C) was significantly higher in the IP VitD-treated mice compared to the SARS-CoV-2 group, and the expression of *IL-1β*, and *NLRP3* was significantly higher in the IP VitD-treated group in comparison to the IN VitD-treated one (Figure 4C,K,L), respectively. A significantly reduction in the *ARG* expression was observed in the SARS-CoV-2/VitD (IN) group in comparison to the SARS-CoV-2 group (Figure 4J). In order to clarify whether these slight changes in gene expression would be reflected in the inflammatory infiltrate, we next performed flow cytometry of tissue infiltrating cells to better define the immunological changes associated with VitD treatment.

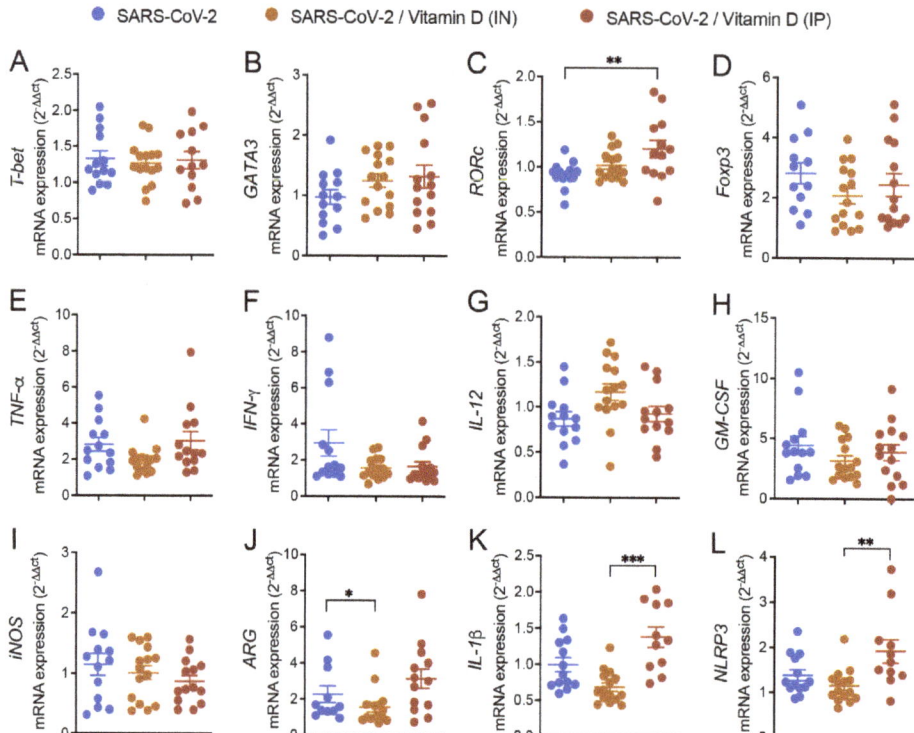

Figure 4. Effect of IN and IP VitD delivery on T cell transcription factors, cytokines, and inflammasome gene transcripts in lungs of mice IN challenged with UV-inactivated SARS-CoV-2. C57BL/6 mice were instilled with the virus (3 doses of 4×10^5 PFU/each) on days 1, 3, and 5. In the IN protocol, mice were treated with 3 VitD doses (0.1 µg/dose) simultaneously with the SARS-CoV-2 inoculum. In the IP protocol, each animal was treated with 4 VitD doses delivered on days 0, 2, 4, and 6. On the 7th day, the lower left lobe was removed, and the RNA extracted and submitted to RT-PCR. Tested genes included *T-bet* (**A**), *GATA3* (**B**), *RORc* (**C**), *Foxp3* (**D**), *TNF-α* (**E**), *IFN-γ* (**F**), *IL-12* (**G**), *GM-CSF* (**H**), *iNOS* (**I**), *ARG* (**J**), *IL-1β* (**K**), *NLRP3* (**L**). Data derive from three experiments with similar results which were combined (n = 11–15 mice/experimental group). The results are presented in median and interquartile intervals and the comparison between the groups was performed by the Kruskal–Wallis test followed by Dunn's test. * $p < 0.05$; ** $p < 0.01$; *** $p < 0.001$.

3.6. IN VitD Treatment Efficiently Controls Pulmonary Inflammation

The analysis of the histological sections clearly indicates the strong ability of IN VitD, in contrast to IP VitD, to control lung inflammation. In this case, there was a convincing interruption of the accumulation of inflammatory cells in the lung parenchyma of IN VitD-treated mice that were exposed to the inactivated virus. These findings can be clearly observed in Figure 5A. Inflammatory foci are easily observed around the vessels (black arrows) and bronchi (green arrows) in SARS-CoV-2 and SARS-CoV-2/VitD IP groups. The presence of neutrophilic (green arrowhead), macrophage (blue arrowhead), and lymphocytic infiltrates (yellow arrowhead) are also numerous in these two experimental groups, but rare in animals treated with VitD through the IN route.

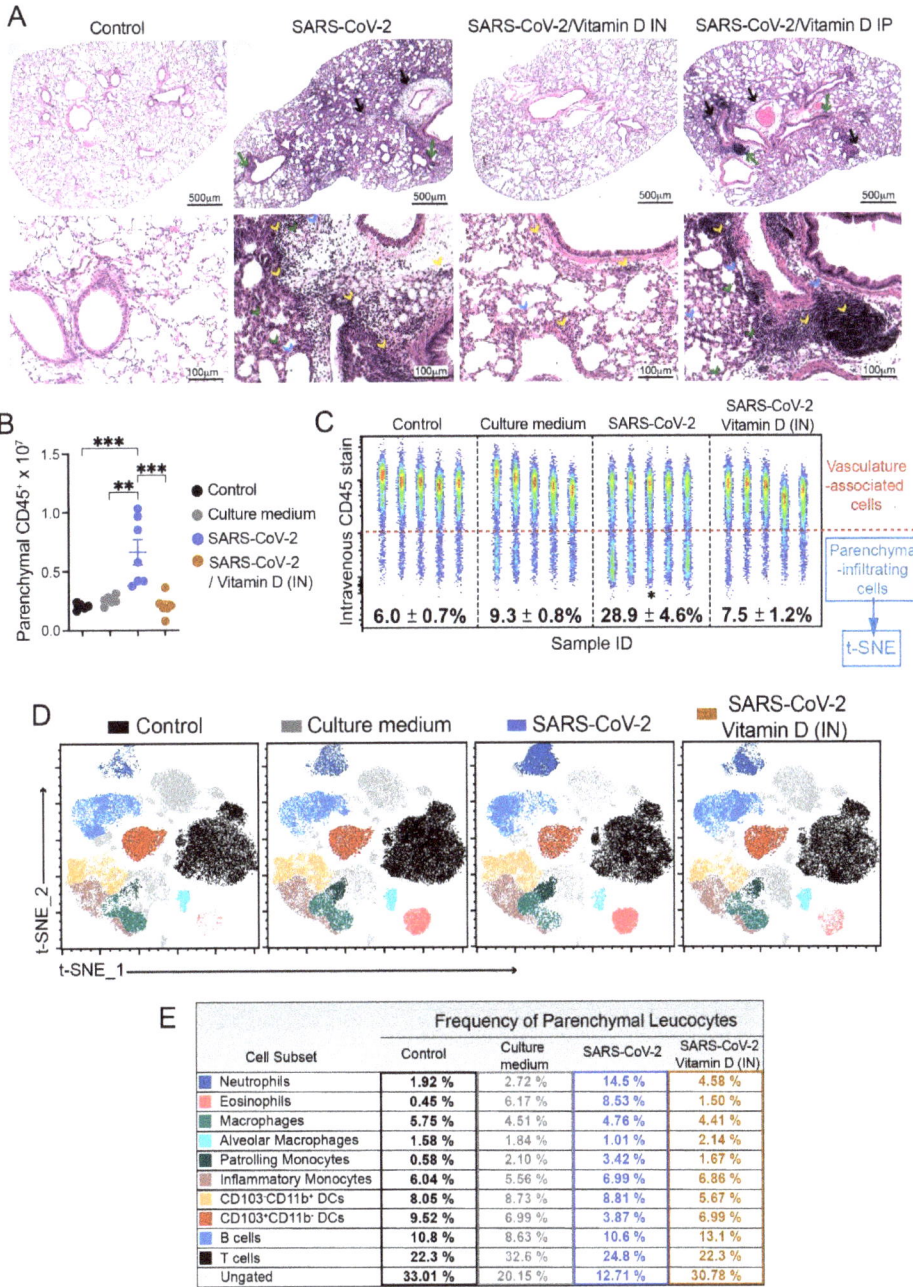

Figure 5. Effect of IN and IP VitD on lung histopathology (**A**) and effect of IN VitD on lung infiltration of pro-inflammatory cells (**B**–**E**) triggered by IN instillation of UV-inactivated SARS-CoV-2. C57BL/6 mice were instilled with the virus (3 doses of 4×10^5 PFU/each) on days 1, 3, and 5. In the IN protocol,

mice were treated with 3 VitD doses (0.1 µg/dose) simultaneously with the SARS-CoV-2 inoculum. In the IP protocol, each animal was treated with 4 VitD doses delivered on days 0, 2, 4, and 6. On the 7th day, the upper left lobe and the right lung were collected for histopathological and flow cytometry analyses, respectively. The upper left lobe was washed, fixed, and stained with H&E, and then evaluated concerning the presence of inflammatory foci (**A**) around the vessels (black arrows) and around the bronchi (green arrows), neutrophilic infiltrates (green arrow head), macrophage infiltrates (blue arrow head), and lympho-cystic infiltrates (yellow arrow head). Cells from lung parenchyma were eluted and analyzed after labeling with an array of specific antibodies (**B–E**). (**B**) Total numbers of CD45$^+$ parenchymal infiltrating leukocyte fraction (identified based on anti-CD45 intravenous injection). (**C**) Representative dot plot of 5 concatenated samples from all groups illustrating the average and SEM of % CD45-negative cells (parenchymal fraction) in lungs from all experimental groups. The specific cell subsets quantified by flow cytometry were evaluated according to the gating strategy described in Supplementary Figure S2. (**D**) t-distributed stochastic neighbor embedding (t-SNE) analysis illustrating the distribution of cell clusters in each experimental group according to gate strategy described in the Supplementary Figure S2. (**E**) Table indicating the frequency of each cell cluster relative to the CD45$^+$ parenchyma-infiltrating leukocytes in the control (black), culture medium (grey), SARS-CoV-2 (blue) groups and SARS-CoV-2 IN VitD-treated group (orange). Data shown in A are derived from one experiment (n = 5 animals/experimental group) and data shown in (**B–E**) are derived from one experiment (n = 7–8 animals/group). Results are presented in median and interquartile intervals and the comparison between the groups was performed using the Kruskal–Wallis test followed by the Dunn's test. ** $p < 0.01$; *** $p < 0.001$.

To clarify whether this anti-inflammatory effect of IN VitD was involved in the modulation of specific cell types, including myeloid, DCs, ILCs, and lymphocytes, we used flow cytometry to identify the cells infiltrating in the lung parenchyma, as described above. The total number and the frequency of CD45$^+$ cells infiltrating the lung parenchyma of mice instilled with inactivated SARS-CoV-2 was significantly increased compared to both control groups (control and culture medium) (Figure 5B,C). Notably, the IN VitD treatment significantly reduced the number and frequency of leukocytes infiltrating the lung parenchyma of mice receiving the inactivated virus (Figure 5B,C).

Next, to better understand the modulatory effects of VitD in the virus-induced parenchymal lung inflammation, we analyzed the frequency of distinct cell subsets by t-SNE and found that the VitD treatment reverted the recruitment of neutrophils, eosinophils, patrolling monocytes, and CD103$^-$CD11b$^+$ DCs induced by the inoculation of inactivated SARS-CoV-2 (Figures 5D,E and 6C). Notably, the VitD treatment increased the percentage of B cells and CD103$^+$CD11b$^-$ DCs in the lung parenchyma in comparison to the SARS-CoV-2 group (Figures 5E and 6C), suggesting that the treatment might be selectively controlling the inflammatory immune tone in the lung.

In addition, the functional impact of an IN VitD treatment on inflammatory cytokine production was analyzed using flow cytometry in myeloid, B, Tγδ, ILCs, and TCD4$^+$ cells (Figure 6). Concerning cytokine production by myeloid cells, while the inactivated virus promoted the production of TNF-α and IL-6 by myeloid lung cells, the IN VitD treatment controlled the frequency of cytokine-producing cells (Figure 6A). When we quantified the number of cytokine-producing myeloid cells, the only population displaying a significant difference was the one producing both cytokines. Even though the percentage of TNF-α$^+$IL-6$^+$CD11b$^+$ cells was similar in SARS-CoV-2 and SARS-CoV-2/VitD groups (Figure 6E), the total number of these cells was significantly lower in the VitD-treated animals, as shown in Figure 6D. These data could be explained by the consistent reduction in total cell recruitment to the lung parenchyma in the VitD-treated mice.

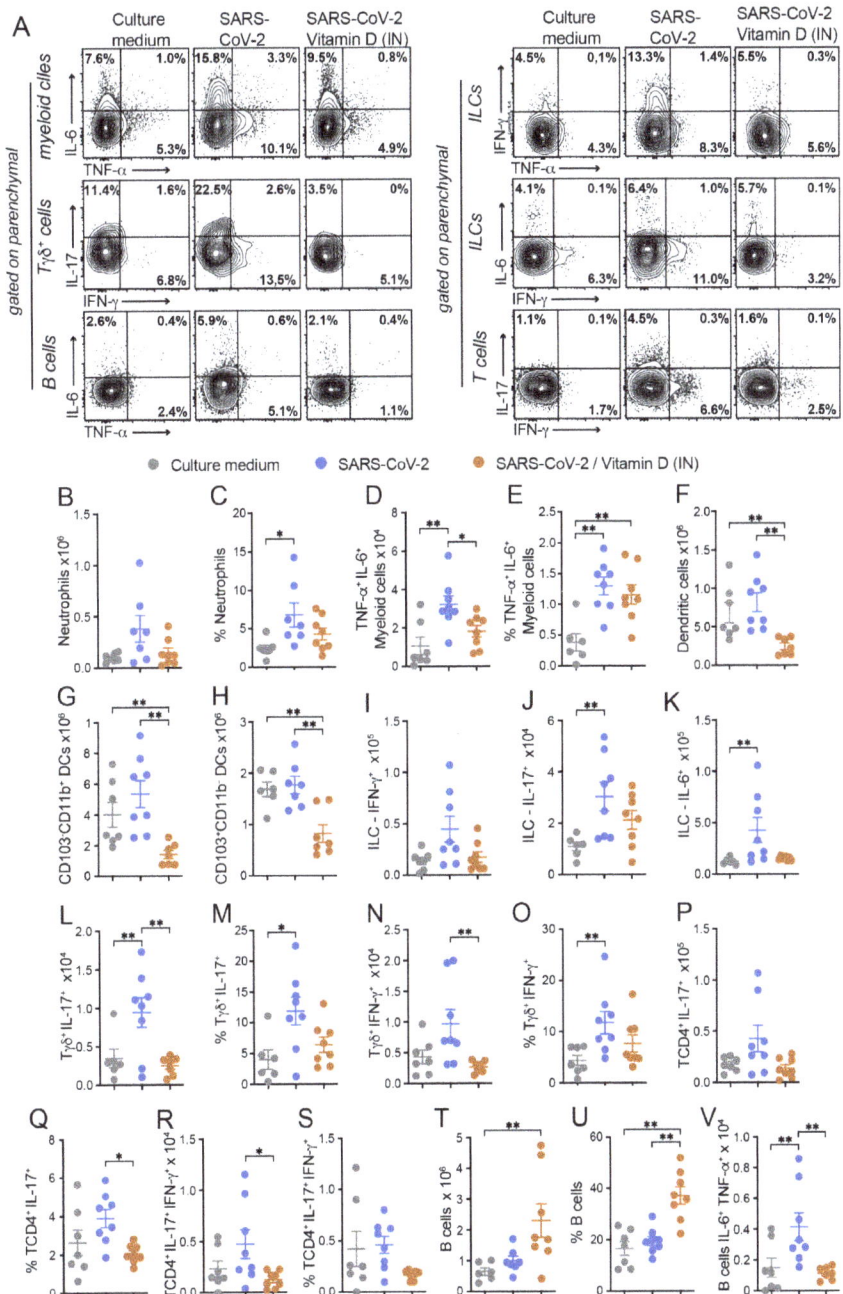

Figure 6. Effect of IN VitD on cell infiltration triggered by IN instillation of UV-inactivated SARS-CoV-2. C57BL/6 mice were instilled with the virus (3 doses of 4×10^5 PFU/each) on days 1, 3, and 5. Mice were treated with 3 VitD doses (0.1 µg/dose) simultaneously with the SARS-CoV-2 inoculum. On the 7th day, the upper left lobe and the right lung were collected for flow cytometry analyses. In order to differentiate the parenchyma-infiltrating leukocytes from the vasculature-associated fraction, mice were intravenously injected with FITC-labeled anti-CD45 antibody 3 min before euthanasia.

Specific cell subsets infiltrating the lungs of mice were analyzed according to the gate strategy described in Supplementary Figures S2–S4. Intracellular cytokine production was detected by flow cytometry in PMA/Ionomycin/brefeldin in vitro stimulated cells. (**A**) Representative contour plots of each experimental group indicating the frequency of cytokine production by each parenchymal cell subset, as indicated in the *y* axis of the figure. (**B–V**) Absolute numbers and/or percentage of each cell subset or cytokine-producing cell as indicated in each graph *y* axis. Data derive from one experiment (n = 7–8 animals/group), results are presented in median and interquartile intervals, and the comparison between the groups was performed using the Kruskal–Wallis test followed by Dunn's test. * $p < 0.05$ ** $p < 0.01$.

The frequency of DCs was only slightly reduced by VitD (data not shown). As already observed during the characterization phase of the lung inflammatory process, the amount of DCs was very similar in SARS-CoV-2 and its respective control group (culture medium). In spite of this, VitD therapy was able to significantly reduce the total number of DCs (Figure 6F) and also of the two evaluated subsets, $CD103^-CD11b^+$ (Figure 6G) and $CD103^+CD11b^-$ (Figure 6H), but not the frequency of $CD103^+CD11b^-$ (Figure 5B,D). Once again, this inconsistency in the modulation of the cell number but not in its frequency could be attributed to the considerable reduction in leukocyte recruitment to the lung parenchyma of VitD-treated animals (Figure 5B).

The total numbers of IL-17- and IL-6-producing ILCs were usually increased in the SARS-CoV-2 group in comparison to the control that received the culture medium, and VitD therapy triggered a clear tendency to decrease the total number of theses cytokine-producing cells, as shown in Figure 6A,J,K. Concerning the Tγδ lymphocytes, the most relevant alterations were detected in the cells that were producing IL-17 or IFN-γ. As shown in Figure 6A,L,N, VitD significantly downregulated the total cell number of IL-17- and IFN-γ-producing cells. VitD also downmodulated, although not significantly, their percentages, as illustrated in Figure 6M,O, for IL-17 and IFN-γ, respectively. In regard to $TCD4^+$ lymphocytes, the most pronounced differences were also observed in IL-17- and IL-17/IFN-γ-producing cells. The % of these cells was reduced by treatment with VitD, making this reduction statistically significant in the case of $TCD4^+IL17^+$ (Figure 6A,Q). The total amount of these two cell subsets was also decreased by VitD therapy, making this reduction statistically significant regarding $TCD4^+IL-17^+IFN-\gamma^+$ (Figure 6R). The % and the total number of B cells were similar in the culture medium and SARS-CoV-2 groups (Figure 6T,U). However, a significant increase in these two parameters was triggered by a local IN VitD administration, as shown in figures T and U. Interestingly, the number of $IL-6^+TNF-\alpha^+$ B cells, which was increased in the SARS-CoV-2 group, was significantly downregulated by IN VitD (Figure 6V).

Taken together, our data suggest that the local administration of VitD was sufficient to suppress the recruitment of inflammatory cells to the lung parenchyma induced by the exposure to inactivated SARS-CoV-2.

4. Discussion

This investigation was conducted considering that COVID-19 can be a lethal disease and which the treatment for is not well established. Initially, we used female C57BL/6 mice, instilled with UV-inactivated SARS-CoV-2, to establish a working model of inflammation in the lung, the initial and main target of COVID-19 [36]. We then employed this model to investigate the potential of VitD to control local inflammation. The choice of the C57BL/6 mice strain and inactivated virus would, in our view, make the model more accessible to a greater number of researchers and laboratory facilities and allow for a further use of transgenic mice to answer specific questions about the inflammatory response during SARS-CoV-2 infection.

The initial results obtained by analyzing the cell influx to the BALF revealed the ability of inactivated SARS-CoV-2 to trigger a local inflammatory process characterized by an increase in WBCs, including in lymphocytes and neutrophils. As the BALF obtained from the culture medium group presented a profile very similar to the other control group (saline), most of the inflammatory process can be attributed to the virus and not to the content of the medium used to grow the virus. Altogether, the total number of WBCs along with their different cell types presented a clear and more direct idea of the inflammatory extension. On the other hand, the calculation of the percentage of each cell type presented an idea of the pattern of the immune response recruited to this compartment. In our experimental model, the immune tone of the airways was shifted towards a neutrophilic inflammatory profile in the detriment of a mononuclear or eosinophilic infiltrate. Therefore, we found an increase in both the percentage and total counts of neutrophils, but not in the other cell subsets.

Even though the subsequent analyses provided much more enlightening information about this model, these preliminary data were considered relevant because BALF procedures have been largely employed as a tool to study a plethora of experimental and human lung diseases [37,38]. In addition, this technique has been explored in experimental and clinical investigations involving the SARS-CoV-2 virus itself [39].

The analysis of the lung RNA expression reinforced the initial findings, showing an increased expression of *GM-CSF* and *Foxp3* and a tendency towards increased values for *IL-17*, *IL-1β*, and *NLRP3* mRNA expression. The possible contribution of the inflammasome activation to COVID-19 immunopathogenesis is highly supported by the literature. It has been reported that inflammasome activation is triggered by SARS-CoV-2 components [40,41], that its higher activation is possibly involved in COVID-19 severity [42], and that the specific inhibition of the NLRP3 inflammasome was able to decrease the intensity of a COVID-19-like pathology in mice [43]. In addition, NLRP3 inflammasome activation during COVID-19 can also be induced by DAMPs released as a result of the initial innate inflammatory process that follows the exposure to SARS-CoV-2 components [44]. For instance, the inflammatory process that drives cell damage and extracellular ATP release can activate the purinergic P2X7 receptor, resulting in K+ efflux and, consequently, NLRP3 inflammation [44,45]. Notably, the inflammasome activation throughout this process does not require the active infection of the virus, but this could be induced by the inflammation resulting from viral components exposure. Considering this scenario, it seems plausible to hypothesize that this could be one of the pathways for NLRP3 activation in our inflammation experimental model triggered by inactivated SARS-CoV-2 instillation. Another possibility for NLRP3 activation by viral components could be the accumulation of angiotensin II in the cell which results from the interaction of SARS-CoV-2 protein with ACE2 in the cell surface. This process reduces angiotensin II degradation and its subsequent accumulation in the cell [44].

Histopathological analysis, together with the flow cytometry analysis of the cells obtained from the lung parenchyma, allowed a better evaluation of the intensity and quality of the inflammatory process triggered by the exposition to the virus. H&E-stained sections clearly showed that the IN instillation of inactivated SARS-CoV-2 induced a multifocal and interstitial pneumonia characterized by perivascular and perialveolar inflammation. Flow cytometric evaluation performed with the cells isolated from the lung parenchyma allowed a more precise identification of the cells involved in local inflammation. A plethora of cell types, such as PMNs, eosinophils, lymphocytes, and macrophages, including monocyte-derived macrophages and parenchyma-resident macrophages, were identified using this methodology [46]. All these cellular types have been associated with COVID-19, and their contribution to disease immunopathogenesis has been apprised in pre-clinical and clinical studies [39–41]. An increased amount of PMNs is described in the bloodstream and the lungs of COVID-19 patients, and strong evidence indicates that they play a paramount role in disease pathophysiology [47]. A neutrophilic mucositis involving the entire lower respiratory tract has been described in lung autopsies from COVID-19 deceased patients [48]. Moreover, a neutrophil activation signature predicted critical illness and mortality in COVID-19 [49]. Most of the damage triggered by PMNs has been attributed to their extensive and prolonged activation, which leads to an excessive ROS release composed of superoxide radicals and H_2O_2 [50]. In addition, according to [51], PMNs have been seen as drivers of hyperinflammation by enhanced degranulation and pro-inflammatory cytokine production. The release of neutrophil extracellular traps (NETs) by PMNs is also pointed as a major promotor of damage in COVID-19 by causing endothelial injury and necroinflammation via complement activation, and by promoting the formation of venous thrombi [52]. This activation of PMNs could be directly determined by the virus. It was recently described [53] that single-strand RNAs from the SARS-CoV-2 genome are able to activate human neutrophils via TLR8, triggering a remarkable production of TNF-α, IL-1ra, and CXCL8, apoptosis delay, the modulation of CD11b and CD62L expression, and the release of NETs. Additionally, the tissue damage induced by the neutrophilic infiltration can activate the inflammasome, as described above, resulting in more inflammation and neutrophil recruitment, perpetuating, therefore, the inflammatory process. This exuberant contribution of PMNs to the interstitial pneumonia that occurs in COVID-19 was, in many aspects, reproduced in an h-ACE2 mouse model infected with SARS-CoV-2 [54].

The presence of dendritic cells (DCs) in the pulmonary parenchyma also deserves attention considering that they are fundamental for both an innate and specific anti-viral immune response, but they can also contribute to viral dissemination and immunopathogenesis during COVID-19 [55]. In this regard, by analyzing circulating DCs and monocyte subsets from hospitalized COVID-19 patients, [56] described their impaired function and delayed regeneration. Flow cytometry also allowed the identification of lymphoid and myeloid cells producing cytokines such as TNF-α, IFN-γ, and IL-17, which are among the most important mediators of COVID-19 immunopathogenesis [57].

The validation of our model as an adequate tool to investigate other procedures to control lung inflammation is supported by another investigation ongoing in our research group. The histological changes that we found after the instillation of the UV-inactivated SARS-CoV-2 are comparable to the lung inflammation that h-ACE2 mice develop after the active infection. The profile of inflammatory cells eluted from the lung parenchyma is also very similar to the one described in our investigation (Aype et al., unpublished data).

This validation is also reinforced by the data described by [58]. These authors developed a model of SARS-CoV-2-induced acute respiratory distress syndrome by the intratracheal instillation of formaldehyde-inactivated SARS-CoV-2. Their described histopathological alterations and profile of cells infiltrated in the lungs are also similar to our findings.

Having confirmed that SARS-CoV-2 IN instillation triggered a pulmonary inflammation similar to that developed by the instillation of active or inactivated SARS-CoV-2 in h-ACE2 transgenic mice, our model employing UV-inactivated SARS-CoV-2 was used to test the ability of VitD to modulate the lung inflammatory process. The option for VitD was based on the extensive literature, attesting the powerful immunomodulatory property of this hormone [59], the robust evidences linking its low levels with poor COVID-19 outcomes [60], and our own previous experience, indicating its ability to counteract the inflammatory process that damages the central nervous system (CNS) in a multiple sclerosis (MS) murine model [25,61]. As indicated by the results, only IN VitD was capable of controlling pulmonary inflammation by downmodulating the presence of proinflammatory cytokine-producing cells. The effectiveness of IN VitD was confirmed by histopathological and flow cytometry analyses. The H&E sections from these animals revealed well-preserved lung structures, similar to those observed in the animals from the control group which were instilled with saline. The flow cytometry analysis indicated that, in this case, VitD was able to impair the recruitment of several cell types, as neutrophils, DCs, and lymphocytes, such as TCD4$^+$ and T$\gamma\delta$, in the lungs of mice challenged with SARS-CoV-2. This approach also allowed the identification of various cell subsets whose cytokine production was decreased by VitD, including myeloid (CD11b+), ILCs, T$\gamma\delta$, TCD4$^+$, and B cells. These findings were considered especially relevant because the main detected cytokines, TNF-α, IL-6, IL-17, and IFN-γ, have been identified as some of the major villains of the cytokine storm associated with COVID-19 severity and were significantly downmodulated by VitD.

The possible association between COVID-19 and VitD levels has been investigated from different perspectives, including the possible role of its deficiency and worst disease outcomes [62] and its prophylactic, immune regulatory, and protective role in COVID-19 [19]. Its therapeutic benefit is also being widely pursued, but a final conclusion is not possible yet due to the discordant results reported so far [63,64]. As far as we know, there are no publications concerning the administration of IN VitD to control lung inflammation triggered by SARS-CoV-2 in animal models or patients up to now. In this context, and considering the efficacy of its IN instillation demonstrated here, we believe that once this effect had also been proven in SARS-CoV-2-infected animals, it would be worth going to clinical trials.

Our initial hypothesis predicting a superior efficacy of IN VitD was based, among other information, on the fact that other lung inflammatory pathologies, such as experimental asthma and rhinitis, were efficiently controlled by local (IN) vitD delivery [26,27]. We also considered the fact that it is increasingly recognized that local synthesis of active VitD is more relevant for many of its immune effects on respiratory diseases than its systemic production [65]. We did not investigate in detail the mechanism by which the IN route, in contrast to the IP one, effectively controlled lung inflammation. We could speculate that the IN protocol, which theoretically allows the local availability of VitD during the initial interaction of the virus with pulmonary immune cells, could decrease the intensity of this interaction by, for example, locally decreasing the TLR expression. This effect, which has already been demonstrated after the exposition of peripheral blood mononuclear cells to VitD, decreased the production of pro-inflammatory cytokines [66]. We could also theorize that local VitD instillation is in the lung-draining lymph nodes and in the lungs themselves considering that this is one of the goals of local drug delivery [67]. However, future studies are necessary to measure the local vitD bioavailability and the optimal dose–response kinetics following its IN administration.

Based on the literature, we expected results supporting the more classical mechanisms attributed to immunomodulation by VitD as an induction of tolerogenic DCs [65], the expansion of Tregs (Ma et al., 2021), and reduced Th1/Th17 polarization [68]. Even though these canonical mechanisms were not observed, the cytometry results clearly showed the reduced production of pro-inflammatory cytokines by different cell types, which has been considered a relevant mechanism by which VitD could control elicitation and resolution phases of acute inflammation [19]. A possible reduction in the TLR expression, as proposed above, could additionally decrease the initial tissue damage by the early blocking of the release of chemokines, and therefore control the subsequent movement of leukocytes towards the lung. In line with this hypothesis, VitD is also capable of inhibiting NLRP3 inflammasome [69]. As discussed before, NLRP3 activation could be one of the main drivers for the innate inflammation after the virus exposure. Indeed, we found a reduction, even though not statistically significant, in the IL-1β expression in the lungs of IN VitD-treated animals. In addition, this treatment reduced the production of the inflammatory cytokines that we have evaluated using flow cytometry and could initiate the leukocyte influx to the lung tissue. In this context, we cannot exclude a direct impact of VitD in the lung epithelial mucosa [70]. Possibly, by interfering in the initial response of the epithelial cells to the interaction with the virus, IN VitD could control the initial release of chemokines and cytokines that will initiate the inflammatory loop driven by the virus. Therefore, we strongly believe that VitD is blocking the initial innate signals that drive the influx of inflammatory cells to the lung parenchyma instead of reversing or suppressing an already established inflammation. Notably, as stated before and supporting this hypothesis, we found no increase in Tregs or IL-10 production in the lungs of IN VitD-treated mice. In addition to the blockage of inflammasome activation, classical immunomodulatory mechanisms involving the innate immunity as the inhibition of DC maturation and blockage of antigen presentation to T helper cells could also occur. In addition, VitD suppresses the release of a plethora of pro-inflammatory cytokines [19], which seem, considering our results, to play a major role in its therapeutic effect when delivered intranasally. The model of inflammation limited to the lung, used in this work, does not allow us to predict whether IN VitD would control extrapulmonary inflammatory processes triggered by SARS-CoV-2 infection. As IN VitD was able to attenuate LPS-induced acute lung inflammation [71], it is expected that its application by this route would also be effective to control the pulmonary inflammatory processes triggered by other infectious agents or substances.

Even though the IP administration of VitD triggered a few downmodulatory effects, this procedure was not able to control lung inflammation. Conversely, this protocol increased the IL-1β, NLRP3, and RORc expression, suggesting a possible toxic proinflammatory activity associated with an excess of VitD. Actually, some authors have raised the possibility that VitD excess could trigger inflammation through T-cell stimulation via hypercalcemia. In this sense, serum calcium levels and body weight loss have been frequently employed to indicate VitD toxicity [72,73]. In healthy individuals, exogenous VitD toxicity is generally associated with the continuous use of high VitD doses [74]. Even though only a few VitD doses were employed in our protocols, calcium levels were similarly altered in IP- and IN-treated mice, possibly excluding the extracellular hypercalcemia in IP VitD-treated mice as the cause of inflammasome activation [75]. Of note, the IP VitD-treated animals also lost significantly more weight than the ones treated by IN VitD. If this accentuated body weight loss, which is also indicative of VitD toxicity, is somehow related to IP VitD ineffectiveness in controlling lung inflammation, it is not known yet. As body weight loss during VitD treatment has been attributed to its effect in the brain [63], a simple explanation for the finding that VitD IP causes much more weight loss than IN VitD is that IP VitD determines a higher concentration of this vitamin in the brain. A pharmacodynamic study of the tissue distribution of VitD administered by these two routes, especially in the CNS and in the lungs, will be necessary to understand this differential effect.

We believe that the most relevant contribution of this investigation is the proof of concept that IN VitD can significantly control the lung inflammatory process triggered by the local presence of the virus. Our study seems to be the first report suggesting that IN VitD administration has the potential to control inflammation induced by viral components. Future studies are indeed required to compare the efficacy in relation to the oral route, to define a better dose–response, and also to understand the pharmacokinetics and possible reduction in systemic side effects associated with both delivery routes. In addition, we have already observed that inflammation triggered by viable SARS-CoV-2 closely resembles the one induced by the inactivated virus (manuscript in preparation). The efficacy of VitD to control inflammation during an active SARS-CoV-2 infection requires a future and careful investigation and will possibly demand the association to virucidal drugs.

Even though the focus of our work has been the control of lung inflammation, we conceive that the possible adoption of IN VitD could bring additional advantages to COVID-19 patients. In this sense, we highlight the stabilizing activity towards the blood–brain barrier (BBB) disruption and the anti-fibrotic property of VitD considering that an increased BBB [76] and lung fibrosis had been associated with more severe COVID-19 cases.

Our study is mainly limited by the fact that we did not show that this anti-inflammatory effect of VitD also occurs during experimental SARS-CoV-2 infection. However, considering its adjunct therapeutic potential for COVID-19, we understand that this anti-inflammatory activity determined by IN VitD deserves to be further and fully investigated in preclinical and clinical assays.

5. Conclusions

The results provided by our investigation suggest a promising potential of VitD delivery by the IN route to control the pulmonary inflammation associated with the presence of SARS-CoV-2 antigens/components in the lungs. Further preclinical and clinical investigations will be essential to determine if these experimental findings can be translated to SARS-CoV-2 infection in humans.

Supplementary Materials: The following supporting information can be downloaded at: https://www.mdpi.com/article/10.3390/cells12071092/s1.

Author Contributions: Conceptualization, W.D.F.d.S., J.L.P.-M., J.P.A.J., D.M.d.F. and A.S.; methodology, S.P.M., G.F.d.S. and J.L.P.-M.; formal analysis, W.D.F.d.S., B.d.C.O. and D.M.d.F.; investigation, W.D.F.d.S., S.F.G.Z.-P., M.C.A., C.L.S., B.d.C.O., F.M., G.W.d.S., D.M.d.F. and A.S.; resources, S.P.M., G.F.d.S., J.L.P.-M. and D.M.d.F.; writing—original draft, W.D.F.d.S. and A.S.; writing—review and editing, J.L.P.-M. and J.P.A.J.; supervision, D.M.d.F. and A.S.; project administration, A.S.; funding acquisition, D.M.d.F. and A.S. All authors have read and agreed to the published version of the manuscript.

Funding: This study was supported by JBS S.A. and the scholarships of the Coordination for the Improvement of Higher Education Personnel (CAPES), WDFS master's scholarship 88882.495054/2020-01; São Paulo Research Support Foundation (FAPESP, scholarship 2020/04558-0); DMF is supported by CNPq scholarship 313429/2020-0 and FAPESP 2021/06881-5 grant; J.L.P.-M. is supported by CNPq scholarship 305628/2020-8; A.S. is supported by the CNPq 307269/2017-5 grant; MCA, CSL, BCO, GWS were supported by FAPESP scholarships 2019/12691-4, 2019/13916-0, 2019/07771-9 and 2021/12768-7, respectively.

Institutional Review Board Statement: The animal study protocol was approved by the ethics committee in the animal experimentation of IB, UNESP, Botucatu (CEUA Protocol No. 1959140820, ID: 000129) and the ethics committee in animal experimentation of the ICB, USP (CEUA Protocol 3147240820).

Informed Consent Statement: Not applicable.

Data Availability Statement: Not applicable.

Acknowledgments: Edison Luiz Durigon (IBS-USP) for the donation of SARS-CoV-2, Maria Luisa Cotrim Sartor de Oliveira (Pathology laboratory UNESP/SP) for the use of the equipment, and Flow Cytometry and Imaging Research FLUIR-CEFAP/USP core facility for the support on the flow cytometry experiments.

Conflicts of Interest: The authors declare that the research was conducted in the absence of any commercial or financial relationships that could be construed as a potential conflict of interest.

References

1. Samadizadeh, S.; Masoudi, M.; Rastegar, M.; Salimi, V.; Shahbaz, M.B.; Tahamtan, A. COVID-19: Why Does Disease Severity Vary among Individuals? *Respir. Med.* **2021**, *180*, 106356. [CrossRef]
2. Machhi, J.; Herskovitz, J.; Senan, A.M.; Dutta, D.; Nath, B.; Oleynikov, M.D.; Blomberg, W.R.; Meigs, D.D.; Hasan, M.; Patel, M.; et al. The Natural History, Pathobiology, and Clinical Manifestations of SARS-CoV-2 Infections. *J. Neuroimmune Pharmacol.* **2020**, *15*, 359–386. [CrossRef]
3. Khreefa, Z.; Barbier, M.T.; Koksal, A.R.; Love, G.; Del Valle, L. Pathogenesis and Mechanisms of SARS-CoV-2 Infection in the Intestine, Liver, and Pancreas. *Cells* **2023**, *12*, 262. [CrossRef]
4. Gavriatopoulou, M.; Korompoki, E.; Fotiou, D.; Ntanasis-Stathopoulos, I.; Psaltopoulou, T.; Kastritis, E.; Terpos, E.; Dimopoulos, M.A. Organ-Specific Manifestations of COVID-19 Infection. *Clin. Exp. Med.* **2020**, *20*, 493–506. [CrossRef]
5. Zhou, Y.; Yang, Q.; Chi, J.; Dong, B.; Lv, W.; Shen, L.; Wang, Y. Comorbidities and the Risk of Severe or Fatal Outcomes Associated with Coronavirus Disease 2019: A Systematic Review and Meta-Analysis. *Int. J. Infect. Dis.* **2020**, *99*, 47–56. [CrossRef]
6. Kobusiak-Prokopowicz, M.; Fułek, K.; Fułek, M.; Kaaz, K.; Mysiak, A.; Kurpas, D.; Beszłej, J.A.; Brzecka, A.; Leszek, J. Cardiovascular, Pulmonary, and Neuropsychiatric Short- and Long-Term Complications of COVID-19. *Cells* **2022**, *11*, 3882. [CrossRef]
7. Diamond, M.S.; Kanneganti, T.-D. Innate Immunity: The First Line of Defense against SARS-CoV-2. *Nat. Immunol.* **2022**, *23*, 165–176. [CrossRef]
8. Hu, B.; Huang, S.; Yin, L. The Cytokine Storm and COVID-19. *J. Med. Virol.* **2021**, *93*, 250–256. [CrossRef]
9. Karki, R.; Sharma, B.R.; Tuladhar, S.; Williams, E.P.; Zalduondo, L.; Samir, P.; Zheng, M.; Sundaram, B.; Banoth, B.; Malireddi, R.K.S.; et al. Synergism of TNF-α and IFN-γ Triggers Inflammatory Cell Death, Tissue Damage, and Mortality in SARS-CoV-2 Infection and Cytokine Shock Syndromes. *Cell* **2021**, *184*, 149–168.e17. [CrossRef]
10. Bednash, J.S.; Kagan, V.E.; Englert, J.A.; Farkas, D.; Tyurina, Y.Y.; Tyurin, V.A.; Samovich, S.N.; Farkas, L.; Elhance, A.; Johns, F.; et al. Syrian Hamsters as a Model of Lung Injury with SARS-CoV-2 Infection: Pathologic, Physiologic, and Detailed Molecular Profiling. *Transl. Res.* **2022**, *240*, 1–16. [CrossRef]
11. Winkler, E.S.; Bailey, A.L.; Kafai, N.M.; Nair, S.; McCune, B.T.; Yu, J.; Fox, J.M.; Chen, R.E.; Earnest, J.T.; Keeler, S.P.; et al. SARS-CoV-2 Infection of Human ACE2-Transgenic Mice Causes Severe Lung Inflammation and Impaired Function. *Nat. Immunol.* **2020**, *21*, 1327–1335. [CrossRef]

12. Xia, J.; Tang, W.; Wang, J.; Lai, D.; Xu, Q.; Huang, R.; Hu, Y.; Gong, X.; Fan, J.; Shu, Q.; et al. SARS-CoV-2 N Protein Induces Acute Lung Injury in Mice via NF-κB Activation. *Front. Immunol.* **2021**, *12*, 791753. [CrossRef]
13. Puthia, M.; Tanner, L.; Petruk, G.; Schmidtchen, A. Experimental Model of Pulmonary Inflammation Induced by SARS-CoV-2 Spike Protein and Endotoxin. *ACS Pharmacol. Transl. Sci.* **2022**, *5*, 141–148. [CrossRef]
14. Alunno, A.; Najm, A.; Mariette, X.; De Marco, G.; Emmel, J.; Mason, L.; McGonagle, D.G.; Machado, P.M. Immunomodulatory Therapies for the Treatment of SARS-CoV-2 Infection: An Update of the Systematic Literature Review to Inform EULAR Points to Consider. *RMD Open* **2021**, *7*, e001899. [CrossRef]
15. Majumder, J.; Minko, T. Recent Developments on Therapeutic and Diagnostic Approaches for COVID-19. *AAPS J.* **2021**, *23*, 14. [CrossRef]
16. ŞiMşek Yavuz, S.; Komşuoğlu ÇeliKyurt, İ. An Update of Anti-Viral Treatment of COVID-19. *Turk. J. Med. Sci.* **2021**, *51*, 3372–3390. [CrossRef]
17. Mercola, J.; Grant, W.B.; Wagner, C.L. Evidence Regarding Vitamin D and Risk of COVID-19 and Its Severity. *Nutrients* **2020**, *12*, 3361. [CrossRef]
18. Alexander, J.; Tinkov, A.; Strand, T.A.; Alehagen, U.; Skalny, A.; Aaseth, J. Early Nutritional Interventions with Zinc, Selenium and Vitamin D for Raising Anti-Viral Resistance against Progressive COVID-19. *Nutrients* **2020**, *12*, 2358. [CrossRef]
19. Xu, Y.; Baylink, D.J.; Chen, C.-S.; Reeves, M.E.; Xiao, J.; Lacy, C.; Lau, E.; Cao, H. The Importance of Vitamin d Metabolism as a Potential Prophylactic, Immunoregulatory and Neuroprotective Treatment for COVID-19. *J. Transl. Med.* **2020**, *18*, 322. [CrossRef]
20. Mariani, J.; Antonietti, L.; Tajer, C.; Ferder, L.; Inserra, F.; Sanchez Cunto, M.; Brosio, D.; Ross, F.; Zylberman, M.; López, D.E.; et al. High-Dose Vitamin D versus Placebo to Prevent Complications in COVID-19 Patients: Multicentre Randomized Controlled Clinical Trial. *PLoS ONE* **2022**, *17*, e0267918. [CrossRef]
21. Murai, I.H.; Fernandes, A.L.; Antonangelo, L.; Gualano, B.; Pereira, R.M.R. Effect of a Single High-Dose Vitamin D3 on the Length of Hospital Stay of Severely 25-Hydroxyvitamin D-Deficient Patients with COVID-19. *Clinics* **2021**, *76*, e3549. [CrossRef] [PubMed]
22. Ohaegbulam, K.C.; Swalih, M.; Patel, P.; Smith, M.A.; Perrin, R. Vitamin D Supplementation in COVID-19 Patients: A Clinical Case Series. *Am. J. Ther.* **2020**, *27*, e485–e490. [CrossRef]
23. Sabico, S.; Enani, M.A.; Sheshah, E.; Aljohani, N.J.; Aldisi, D.A.; Alotaibi, N.H.; Alshingetti, N.; Alomar, S.Y.; Alnaami, A.M.; Amer, O.E.; et al. Effects of a 2-Week 5000 IU versus 1000 IU Vitamin D3 Supplementation on Recovery of Symptoms in Patients with Mild to Moderate COVID-19: A Randomized Clinical Trial. *Nutrients* **2021**, *13*, 2170. [CrossRef]
24. Lou, J.; Duan, H.; Qin, Q.; Teng, Z.; Gan, F.; Zhou, X.; Zhou, X. Advances in Oral Drug Delivery Systems: Challenges and Opportunities. *Pharmaceutics* **2023**, *15*, 484. [CrossRef] [PubMed]
25. de Oliveira, L.R.C.; Mimura, L.A.N.; de Campos Fraga-Silva, T.F.; Ishikawa, L.L.W.; Fernandes, A.A.H.; Zorzella-Pezavento, S.F.G.; Sartori, A. Calcitriol Prevents Neuroinflammation and Reduces Blood-Brain Barrier Disruption and Local Macrophage/Microglia Activation. *Front. Pharmacol.* **2020**, *11*, 161. [CrossRef] [PubMed]
26. Cho, S.-W.; Zhang, Y.-L.; Ko, Y.K.; Shin, J.M.; Lee, J.H.; Rhee, C.-S.; Kim, D.-Y. Intranasal Treatment with 1, 25-Dihydroxyvitamin D3 Alleviates Allergic Rhinitis Symptoms in a Mouse Model. *Allergy Asthma Immunol. Res.* **2019**, *11*, 267. [CrossRef]
27. Feng, J.; Meng, T.; Qi, Y.; Athari, S.S.; Chen, X. Study Effect of Vitamin D on the Immunopathology Responses of the Bronchi in Murine Model of Asthma. *Iran. J. Allergy Asthma Immunol.* **2021**, *20*(5), 509. [CrossRef]
28. Forschner, T.; Buchholtz, S.; Stockfleth, E. Current State of Vitiligo Therapy? Evidence-Based Analysis of the Literature. *JDDG J. Dtsch. Dermatol. Ges.* **2007**, *5*, 467–475. [CrossRef]
29. Kieffer, M.A. Topical Vitamin D Analogs. *Dermatol. Nurs.* **2004**, *16*, 89–90, 93, 100.
30. Enkhjargal, B.; McBride, D.W.; Manaenko, A.; Reis, C.; Sakai, Y.; Tang, J.; Zhang, J.H. Intranasal Administration of Vitamin D Attenuates Blood–Brain Barrier Disruption through Endogenous Upregulation of Osteopontin and Activation of CD44/P-Gp Glycosylation Signaling after Subarachnoid Hemorrhage in Rats. *J. Cereb. Blood Flow Metab.* **2017**, *37*, 2555–2566. [CrossRef] [PubMed]
31. Wang, Z.; Xiong, G.; Tsang, W.C.; Schätzlein, A.G.; Uchegbu, I.F. Nose-to-Brain Delivery. *J. Pharmacol. Exp.* **2019**, *370*, 593–601. [CrossRef] [PubMed]
32. Wölfel, R.; Corman, V.M.; Guggemos, W.; Seilmaier, M.; Zange, S.; Müller, M.A.; Niemeyer, D.; Jones, T.C.; Vollmar, P.; Rothe, C.; et al. Virological Assessment of Hospitalized Patients with COVID-2019. *Nature* **2020**, *581*, 465–469. [CrossRef] [PubMed]
33. Coimbra, L.D.; Borin, A.; Fontoura, M.; Gravina, H.D.; Nagai, A.; Shimizu, J.F.; Bispo-dos-Santos, K.; Granja, F.; Oliveira, P.S.L.; Franchini, K.G.; et al. Identification of Compounds with Antiviral Activity Against SARS-CoV-2 in the MMV Pathogen Box Using a Phenotypic High-Throughput Screening Assay. *Front.Virol.* **2022**, *2*, 854363. [CrossRef]
34. Bispo-dos-Santos, K.; Barbosa, P.P.; Granja, F.; Martini, M.C.; Oliveira, C.F.S.; Schuck, D.C.; Brohem, C.A.; Arns, C.W.; Hares Junior, S.J.; Sabino, C.P.; et al. Ultraviolet Germicidal Irradiation Is Effective against SARS-CoV-2 in Contaminated Makeup Powder and Lipstick. *J. Photochem. Photobiol.* **2021**, *8*, 100072. [CrossRef]
35. Roberts, A.; Deming, D.; Paddock, C.D.; Cheng, A.; Yount, B.; Vogel, L.; Herman, B.D.; Sheahan, T.; Heise, M.; Genrich, G.L.; et al. A Mouse-Adapted SARS-Coronavirus Causes Disease and Mortality in BALB/c Mice. *PLoS Pathog.* **2007**, *3*, e5. [CrossRef]
36. Bösmüller, H.; Matter, M.; Fend, F.; Tzankov, A. The Pulmonary Pathology of COVID-19. *Virchows Arch.* **2021**, *478*, 137–150. [CrossRef] [PubMed]

37. Meyer, K.C.; Raghu, G. Bronchoalveolar Lavage for the Evaluation of Interstitial Lung Disease: Is It Clinically Useful? *Eur. Respir. J.* **2011**, *38*, 761–769. [CrossRef]
38. Van Hoecke, L.; Job, E.R.; Saelens, X.; Roose, K. Bronchoalveolar Lavage of Murine Lungs to Analyze Inflammatory Cell Infiltration. *J. Vis. Exp.* **2017**, *123*, 55398. [CrossRef]
39. Liao, M.; Liu, Y.; Yuan, J.; Wen, Y.; Xu, G.; Zhao, J.; Cheng, L.; Li, J.; Wang, X.; Wang, F.; et al. Single-Cell Landscape of Bronchoalveolar Immune Cells in Patients with COVID-19. *Nat. Med.* **2020**, *26*, 842–844. [CrossRef]
40. Pan, P.; Shen, M.; Yu, Z.; Ge, W.; Chen, K.; Tian, M.; Xiao, F.; Wang, Z.; Wang, J.; Jia, Y.; et al. SARS-CoV-2 N Protein Promotes NLRP3 Inflammasome Activation to Induce Hyperinflammation. *Nat. Commun.* **2021**, *12*, 4664. [CrossRef]
41. Albornoz, E.A.; Amarilla, A.A.; Modhiran, N.; Parker, S.; Li, X.X.; Wijesundara, D.K.; Aguado, J.; Zamora, A.P.; McMillan, C.L.D.; Liang, B.; et al. SARS-CoV-2 Drives NLRP3 Inflammasome Activation in Human Microglia through Spike Protein. *Mol. Psychiatry* **2022**, 1–16. [CrossRef]
42. Rodrigues, T.S.; de Sá, K.S.G.; Ishimoto, A.Y.; Becerra, A.; Oliveira, S.; Almeida, L.; Gonçalves, A.V.; Perucello, D.B.; Andrade, W.A.; Castro, R.; et al. Inflammasomes Are Activated in Response to SARS-CoV-2 Infection and Are Associated with COVID-19 Severity in Patients. *J. Exp. Med.* **2021**, *218*, e20201707. [CrossRef] [PubMed]
43. Zeng, J.; Xie, X.; Feng, X.-L.; Xu, L.; Han, J.-B.; Yu, D.; Zou, Q.-C.; Liu, Q.; Li, X.; Ma, G.; et al. Specific Inhibition of the NLRP3 Inflammasome Suppresses Immune Overactivation and Alleviates COVID-19 like Pathology in Mice. *eBioMedicine* **2022**, *75*, 103803. [CrossRef]
44. Zhao, N.; Di, B.; Xu, L. The NLRP3 Inflammasome and COVID-19: Activation, Pathogenesis and Therapeutic Strategies. *Cytokine Growth Factor Rev.* **2021**, *61*, 2–15. [CrossRef] [PubMed]
45. Carta, S.; Penco, F.; Lavieri, R.; Martini, A.; Dinarello, C.A.; Gattorno, M.; Rubartelli, A. Cell Stress Increases ATP Release in NLRP3 Inflammasome-Mediated Autoinflammatory Diseases, Resulting in Cytokine Imbalance. *Proc. Natl. Acad. Sci. USA* **2015**, *112*, 2835–2840. [CrossRef] [PubMed]
46. Hou, F.; Xiao, K.; Tang, L.; Xie, L. Diversity of Macrophages in Lung Homeostasis and Diseases. *Front. Immunol.* **2021**, *12*, 753940. [CrossRef]
47. Reusch, N.; De Domenico, E.; Bonaguro, L.; Schulte-Schrepping, J.; Baßler, K.; Schultze, J.L.; Aschenbrenner, A.C. Neutrophils in COVID-19. *Front. Immunol.* **2021**, *12*, 652470. [CrossRef] [PubMed]
48. Barnes, B.J.; Adrover, J.M.; Baxter-Stoltzfus, A.; Borczuk, A.; Cools-Lartigue, J.; Crawford, J.M.; Daßler-Plenker, J.; Guerci, P.; Huynh, C.; Knight, J.S.; et al. Targeting Potential Drivers of COVID-19: Neutrophil Extracellular Traps. *J. Exp. Med.* **2020**, *217*, e20200652. [CrossRef] [PubMed]
49. Meizlish, M.L.; Pine, A.B.; Bishai, J.D.; Goshua, G.; Nadelmann, E.R.; Simonov, M.; Chang, C.-H.; Zhang, H.; Shallow, M.; Bahel, P.; et al. A Neutrophil Activation Signature Predicts Critical Illness and Mortality in COVID-19. *Blood Adv.* **2021**, *5*, 1164–1177. [CrossRef]
50. Cavalcante-Silva, L.H.A.; Carvalho, D.C.M.; de Almeida Lima, É.; Galvão, J.G.F.M.; da Silva, J.S.D.F.; de Sales-Neto, J.M.; Rodrigues-Mascarenhas, S. Neutrophils and COVID-19: The Road so Far. *Int. Immunopharmacol.* **2021**, *90*, 107233. [CrossRef]
51. Parackova, Z.; Zentsova, I.; Bloomfield, M.; Vrabcova, P.; Smetanova, J.; Klocperk, A.; Mesežnikov, G.; Casas Mendez, L.F.; Vymazal, T.; Sediva, A. Disharmonic Inflammatory Signatures in COVID-19: Augmented Neutrophils' but Impaired Monocytes' and Dendritic Cells' Responsiveness. *Cells* **2020**, *9*, 2206. [CrossRef] [PubMed]
52. Tomar, B.; Anders, H.-J.; Desai, J.; Mulay, S.R. Neutrophils and Neutrophil Extracellular Traps Drive Necroinflammation in COVID-19. *Cells* **2020**, *9*, 1383. [CrossRef] [PubMed]
53. Gardiman, E.; Bianchetto-Aguilera, F.; Gasperini, S.; Tiberio, L.; Scandola, M.; Lotti, V.; Gibellini, D.; Salvi, V.; Bosisio, D.; Cassatella, M.A.; et al. SARS-CoV-2-Associated SsRNAs Activate Human Neutrophils in a TLR8-Dependent Fashion. *Cells* **2022**, *11*, 3785. [CrossRef]
54. Liang, Y.; Li, H.; Li, J.; Yang, Z.-N.; Li, J.-L.; Zheng, H.-W.; Chen, Y.-L.; Shi, H.-J.; Guo, L.; Liu, L.-D.; et al. Role of Neutrophil Chemoattractant CXCL5 in SARS-CoV-2 Infection-Induced Lung Inflammatory Innate Immune Response in an in vivo HACE2 Transfection Mouse Model. *Zool. Res.* **2020**, *41*, 621–631. [CrossRef] [PubMed]
55. Marongiu, L.; Valache, M.; Facchini, F.A.; Granucci, F. How Dendritic Cells Sense and Respond to Viral Infections. *Clin. Sci.* **2021**, *135*, 2217–2242. [CrossRef] [PubMed]
56. Winheim, E.; Rinke, L.; Lutz, K.; Reischer, A.; Leutbecher, A.; Wolfram, L.; Rausch, L.; Kranich, J.; Wratil, P.R.; Huber, J.E.; et al. Impaired Function and Delayed Regeneration of Dendritic Cells in COVID-19. *PLoS Pathog.* **2021**, *17*, e1009742. [CrossRef]
57. Darif, D.; Hammi, I.; Kihel, A.; El Idrissi Saik, I.; Guessous, F.; Akarid, K. The Pro-Inflammatory Cytokines in COVID-19 Pathogenesis: What Goes Wrong? *Microb. Pathog.* **2021**, *153*, 104799. [CrossRef]
58. Bi, Z.; Hong, W.; Que, H.; He, C.; Ren, W.; Yang, J.; Lu, T.; Chen, L.; Lu, S.; Peng, X.; et al. Inactivated SARS-CoV-2 Induces Acute Respiratory Distress Syndrome in Human ACE2-Transgenic Mice. *Signal Transduct. Target.* **2021**, *6*, 439. [CrossRef]
59. Sassi, F.; Tamone, C.; D'Amelio, P. Vitamin D: Nutrient, Hormone, and Immunomodulator. *Nutrients* **2018**, *10*, 1656. [CrossRef]
60. Karonova, T.L.; Andreeva, A.T.; Golovatuk, K.A.; Bykova, E.S.; Simanenkova, A.V.; Vashukova, M.A.; Grant, W.B.; Shlyakhto, E.V. Low 25(OH)D Level Is Associated with Severe Course and Poor Prognosis in COVID-19. *Nutrients* **2021**, *13*, 3021. [CrossRef]
61. Mimura, L.A.N.; de Campos Fraga-Silva, T.F.; de Oliveira, L.R.C.; Ishikawa, L.L.W.; Borim, P.A.; de Moraes Machado, C.; Júnior, J.D.A.D.C.E.H.; da Fonseca, D.M.; Sartori, A. Preclinical Therapy with Vitamin D3 in Experimental Encephalomyelitis: Efficacy and Comparison with Paricalcitol. *Int. J. Mol. Sci.* **2021**, *22*, 1914. [CrossRef] [PubMed]

62. Radujkovic, A.; Hippchen, T.; Tiwari-Heckler, S.; Dreher, S.; Boxberger, M.; Merle, U. Vitamin D Deficiency and Outcome of COVID-19 Patients. *Nutrients* **2020**, *12*, 2757. [CrossRef] [PubMed]
63. Entrenas Castillo, M.; Entrenas Costa, L.M.; Vaquero Barrios, J.M.; Alcalá Díaz, J.F.; López Miranda, J.; Bouillon, R.; Quesada Gomez, J.M. "Effect of Calcifediol Treatment and Best Available Therapy versus Best Available Therapy on Intensive Care Unit Admission and Mortality among Patients Hospitalized for COVID-19: A Pilot Randomized Clinical Study". *J. Steroid Biochem. Mol. Biol.* **2020**, *203*, 105751. [CrossRef] [PubMed]
64. Marcinkowska, E.; Brown, G. Editorial: Vitamin D and COVID-19: New Mechanistic and Therapeutic Insights. *Front. Pharmacol.* **2022**, *13*, 882046. [CrossRef]
65. Hansdottir, S.; Monick, M.M. Vitamin D Effects on Lung Immunity and Respiratory Diseases. In *Vitamins & Hormones*; Elsevier: Amsterdam, The Netherlands, 2011; Volume 86, pp. 217–237. ISBN 978-0-12-386960-9.
66. Adamczak, D. The Role of Toll-Like Receptors and Vitamin D in Cardiovascular Diseases—A Review. *Int. J. Mol. Sci.* **2017**, *18*, 2252. [CrossRef]
67. Labiris, N.R.; Dolovich, M.B. Pulmonary Drug Delivery. Part I: Physiological Factors Affecting Therapeutic Effectiveness of Aerosolized Medications: Physiological Factors Affecting the Effectiveness of Inhaled Drugs. *Br. J. Clin. Pharmacol.* **2003**, *56*, 588–599. [CrossRef]
68. Zeitelhofer, M.; Adzemovic, M.Z.; Gomez-Cabrero, D.; Bergman, P.; Hochmeister, S.; N'diaye, M.; Paulson, A.; Ruhrmann, S.; Almgren, M.; Tegnér, J.N.; et al. Functional Genomics Analysis of Vitamin D Effects on CD4$^+$ T Cells in Vivo in Experimental Autoimmune Encephalomyelitis. *Proc. Natl. Acad. Sci. USA* **2017**, *114*, E1678–E1687. [CrossRef]
69. Rao, Z.; Chen, X.; Wu, J.; Xiao, M.; Zhang, J.; Wang, B.; Fang, L.; Zhang, H.; Wang, X.; Yang, S.; et al. Vitamin D Receptor Inhibits NLRP3 Activation by Impeding Its BRCC3-Mediated Deubiquitination. *Front. Immunol.* **2019**, *10*, 2783. [CrossRef]
70. Schrumpf, J.A.; van der Does, A.M.; Hiemstra, P.S. Impact of the Local Inflammatory Environment on Mucosal Vitamin D Metabolism and Signaling in Chronic Inflammatory Lung Diseases. *Front. Immunol.* **2020**, *11*, 1433. [CrossRef]
71. Serré, J.; Mathyssen, C.; Ajime, T.T.; Heigl, T.; Verlinden, L.; Maes, K.; Verstuyf, A.; Cataldo, D.; Vanoirbeek, J.; Vanaudenaerde, B.; et al. Local Nebulization of 1α,25(OH)2D3 Attenuates LPS-Induced Acute Lung Inflammation. *Respir. Res.* **2022**, *23*, 76. [CrossRef]
72. DeLuca, H.F.; Prahl, J.M.; Plum, L.A. 1,25-Dihydroxyvitamin D Is Not Responsible for Toxicity Caused by Vitamin D or 25-Hydroxyvitamin D. *Arch. Biochem. Biophys.* **2011**, *505*, 226–230. [CrossRef]
73. Häusler, D.; Torke, S.; Weber, M.S. High-Dose Vitamin D-Mediated Hypercalcemia as a Potential Risk Factor in Central Nervous System Demyelinating Disease. *Front. Immunol.* **2020**, *11*, 301. [CrossRef] [PubMed]
74. Marcinowska-Suchowierska, E.; Kupisz-Urbańska, M.; Łukaszkiewicz, J.; Płudowski, P.; Jones, G. Vitamin D Toxicity–A Clinical Perspective. *Front. Endocrinol.* **2018**, *9*, 550. [CrossRef]
75. Rossol, M.; Pierer, M.; Raulien, N.; Quandt, D.; Meusch, U.; Rothe, K.; Schubert, K.; Schöneberg, T.; Schaefer, M.; Krügel, U.; et al. Extracellular Ca^{2+} Is a Danger Signal Activating the NLRP3 Inflammasome through G Protein-Coupled Calcium Sensing Receptors. *Nat. Commun.* **2012**, *3*, 1329. [CrossRef] [PubMed]
76. Krasemann, S.; Haferkamp, U.; Pfefferle, S.; Woo, M.S.; Heinrich, F.; Schweizer, M.; Appelt-Menzel, A.; Cubukova, A.; Barenberg, J.; Leu, J.; et al. The Blood-Brain Barrier Is Dysregulated in COVID-19 and Serves as a CNS Entry Route for SARS-CoV-2. *Stem Cell Rep.* **2022**, *17*, 307–320. [CrossRef] [PubMed]

Disclaimer/Publisher's Note: The statements, opinions and data contained in all publications are solely those of the individual author(s) and contributor(s) and not of MDPI and/or the editor(s). MDPI and/or the editor(s) disclaim responsibility for any injury to people or property resulting from any ideas, methods, instructions or products referred to in the content.

Review

Influence of Immune System Abnormalities Caused by Maternal Immune Activation in the Postnatal Period

Yo Shimizu [1,2], Hiromi Sakata-Haga [2], Yutaka Saikawa [3] and Toshihisa Hatta [2,*]

1. Department of Pediatrics, Daido Hospital, Nagoya 457-8511, Japan
2. Department of Anatomy, Kanazawa Medical University, Kahoku 920-0265, Japan
3. Department of Pediatrics, Kanazawa Medical University, Kahoku 920-0265, Japan
* Correspondence: thatta@kanazawa-med.ac.jp

Abstract: The developmental origins of health and disease (DOHaD) indicate that fetal tissues and organs in critical and sensitive periods of development are susceptible to structural and functional changes due to the adverse environment in utero. Maternal immune activation (MIA) is one of the phenomena in DOHaD. Exposure to maternal immune activation is a risk factor for neurodevelopmental disorders, psychosis, cardiovascular diseases, metabolic diseases, and human immune disorders. It has been associated with increased levels of proinflammatory cytokines transferred from mother to fetus in the prenatal period. Abnormal immunity induced by MIA includes immune overreaction or immune response failure in offspring. Immune overreaction is a hypersensitivity response of the immune system to pathogens or allergic factor. Immune response failure could not properly fight off various pathogens. The clinical features in offspring depend on the gestation period, inflammatory magnitude, inflammatory type of MIA in the prenatal period, and exposure to prenatal inflammatory stimulation, which might induce epigenetic modifications in the immune system. An analysis of epigenetic modifications caused by adverse intrauterine environments might allow clinicians to predict the onset of diseases and disorders before or after birth.

Keywords: maternal infection; maternal immune activation; immune disorders; immune overreaction; immune response failure; epigenetic modification

1. Introduction

Postnatal disorders are significantly influenced by the prenatal environment [1]. During World War II, Barker et al. were the first to report that maternal malnutrition was associated with adverse effects on adult health and resulted in an increased risk of cardiovascular diseases in adulthood [2]. A positive correlation between low birth weight and mortality rate from ischemic heart disease was observed. Based on several investigations, they proposed a hypothesis of the developmental origins of health and disease (DOHaD) [3]. This hypothesis indicates that the fetal tissues and organs experience structural and functional changes during critical and sensitive developmental periods due to adverse environments in utero. The association between the risk factors of the maternal environment, such as exposure to adverse intrauterine factors including infection, allergens, oxidative stress, and medicine and disease development, such as ischemic heart disease, has also been reported [4–9]. The postnatal disability caused by adverse environments in the fetuses may result in neonatal or infant death or impact on their health as adults [1,2]. These damages affect not only the individual but multiple organs of the whole body and are inherited by the next generation. Maternal immune activation (MIA) is a DOHaD mechanism. It is a phenomenon in which maternal infections, autoimmune diseases, allergies, asthma, atherosclerosis, malignancy, hyperhomocysteinemia, and alcohol consumption activate maternal immune response [10–13]. An inflammatory response due to cytokine production during gestation is common in these diseases. According to epidemiologic studies on humans, maternal infection during pregnancy causes various disorders associated with abnormal immunity in the offspring, including type 1 diabetes, allergy diseases, psychosis, and neurodevelopmental abnormalities [7,14,15]. Increased plasma levels of cytokines such as interleukin (IL)-1, IL-6, IL-8, IL-12p40, IL-13, and tumor necrosis factor (TNF)-α, as well as the immune system's activation in response to inflammatory stimuli in monocyte cell culture, have been linked to abnormal immunity in patients with autism-like disorders [10,16,17]. Thus, MIA induces abnormal immunity in offspring. Previous studies have reported that MIA causes alterations in epigenetics, neurotrophin expression, brain structure and function, gut microbiota, oxidative stress response, and mitochondrial dysfunction in the fetus as well as neurodevelopmental disorders, psychosis, cardiovascular diseases, metabolic diseases, and immune disorders in the offspring (Figure 1) [18,19]. Therefore, MIA is a very critical factor associated with the onset of various diseases in offspring.

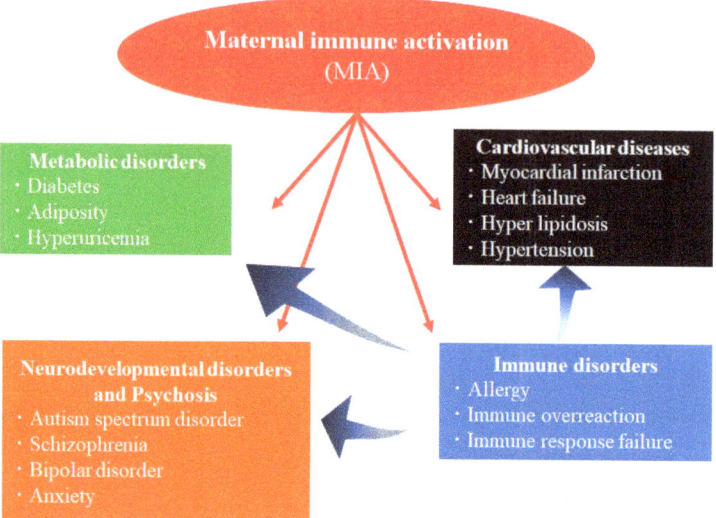

Figure 1. Effects of exposure to MIA in offspring. Exposure to MIA in the prenatal period induces various diseases, such as metabolic, neurodevelopmental, immune system disorders, and cardiovascular diseases. MIA is one of the risk factors for developing these diseases and disorders in the postnatal period. Immune system disorders might cause these diseases due to MIA exposure in the prenatal period.

This review aims to clarify the relationship between the gestational period of exposure to maternal inflammation induced by MIA, the severity of maternal inflammation, the type of cytokine or signaling pathway stimulation, and postnatal immune dysregulation reactions based on the current literature. A new form of severe acute respiratory syndrome coronavirus 2 (SARS-CoV-2) has been spreading worldwide, and maternal infection's postnatal effects in gestation are of great concern. Although limited, the current reported maternal coronavirus disease 2019 (COVID-19) infection and its postnatal effects are described. Some mechanisms of diseases and disorders associated with MIA have already been reported. Epigenetic alterations caused by MIA directly affect the immune system and might prospect to applicate the treatment and diagnosis using epigenetic technology. The potential application of epigenetic technology in the future is explained. We also reviewed how genes, prenatal environment, and postnatal environment influence the development of postnatal immune disorders, and the positioning of MIA among them is summarized.

2. Immunological Disorders Caused by MIA in Humans

2.1. Diseases Associated with an Abnormal Immunity Induced by Maternal Infection in Humans

Genetic factors play a critical role in inducing diseases and disorders, with the prenatal environment being a key factor. In epidemiological studies of humans, maternal infection during pregnancy evoked several diseases associated with abnormal immunity, including type 1 diabetes mellitus, allergic diseases, and neurodevelopmental disorders in offspring. The mechanisms include the autoimmune response in type 1 diabetes mellitus, immune hypersensitivity in allergic diseases, and immune overreaction in neurodevelopmental disorders [7,14,15] (Figure 2). Abnormal immunity originating in the prenatal period continues to influence the tissues and organs after birth. It ultimately results in several diseases, such as allergic diseases caused by exposure to postnatal risk factors in offspring. It is necessary to clarify the mechanism of abnormal immunity induced by MIA in offspring.

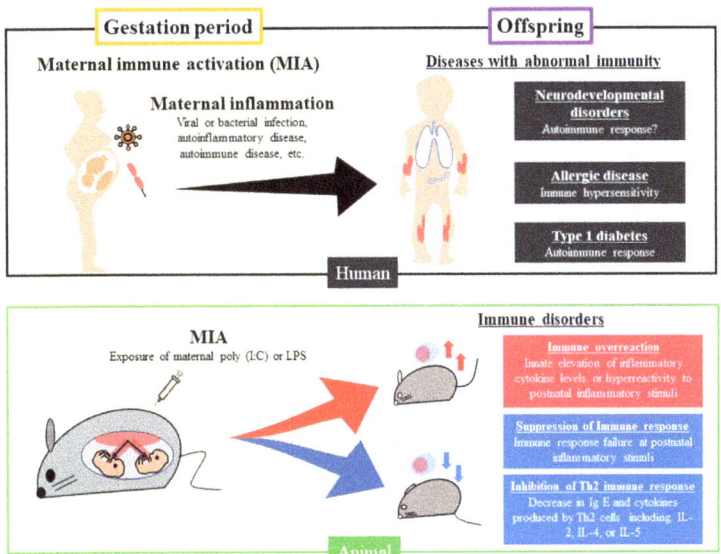

Figure 2. Epidemiologic and experimental data associated with MIA and immune disorders in human and animal models.

2.2. Mechanism of Diseases and Disorders with Abnormal Immunity Caused by Maternal Infection

2.2.1. Diabetes Mellitus

In a previous meta-analysis, maternal infection was significantly associated with type 1 diabetes mellitus [15]. Maternal infection is driven by T cell response in the fetus and leads to the development of pathogen-specific T cells implicated in autoimmune response. Moreover, maternal infection leads to the production of antibodies and transmission to the fetus through the placenta [20,21]. These immune system alterations in the prenatal period could produce proinflammatory cytokines after birth, resulting in β-cell dysfunction in offspring.

2.2.2. Allergic Diseases

Exposure to maternal infection in utero may cause allergic diseases, including asthma, eczema, and hay fever, to develop. Previous research has shown that the complex process underlying asthma, an allergic disease, involves prenatal and postnatal risk factors, including genetic variables and prenatal and postnatal environments, including human rhinoviruses and respiratory syncytial virus infections [7]. The prenatal environments, such as maternal viral or bacterial infections, allergen, tobacco smoke, and air pollution, induce epigenetic alterations associated with airway function, mucosal immune response, systemic immune response, and atopic sensitization in offspring [7]. As a result, immunological hypersensitivity and the development of allergy diseases such as asthma, eczema, and hay fever are caused by genetic factors and prenatal exposure to MIA. Farm exposure during gestation may protect infants against allergic diseases, including asthma, hay fever, and eczema [22]. The frequency of contact with farm environments by the mother during gestation correlates inversely with the incidence of allergic diseases in offspring. Contact with live stocks or drinking fresh milk can lead to exposure to multiple bacteria, endotoxin, and fungi. When compared to neonates who had no maternal farm contact, those with a history of maternal farm contact had weaker immune responses. The interferon (IFN)-γ/IL-13 ratio increased after lipopolysaccharide (LPS) stimulation in the farming mother group, and the immune response tended to be Th1 dominant. Moreover, the number of Th9 cells increased in patients with allergies. IL-9 production decreased after LPS stimulation in cord blood mononuclear cells from neonates exposed to maternal farm contact and may be implicated in the suppression of Th9 function. Alterations in the quality and function of neonatal Tregs induced an imbalance in the immune response, causing a Th1-dominant state and suppressing Th9 cell function and IL-9 production [23].

2.2.3. Neurodevelopmental Disorders and Psychosis

Previous reports have suggested that maternal inflammation may play a role in neurodevelopmental disorders in children, such as autism spectrum disorder, attention deficit hyperactivity disorder, specific learning disorders, communication disorders, intellectual disability, and psychosis such as schizophrenia or anxiety in offspring [18,19,24–28]. The risk of neurodevelopmental diseases may depend on infectious agents, gestation period, and infection site [29]. Numerous investigations on inflammatory disorders in children with autism have revealed that several proinflammatory cytokines were elevated in plasma and whole blood cell mRNA, whereas anti-inflammatory cytokines, including IL-4 or IL-10, were unchanged compared with the control group [16,17,30–37]. Thus, anti-inflammatory cytokines are weakly associated with patients with autism. TNF-α levels correlated positively with autism severity, and decreased expression of immunoregulatory genes is related to TNF-α [34]. Although the mechanism underlying abnormal immunity in neurodevelopmental disorders is still poorly understood, dysregulated peripheral blood cell toll-like receptor response to inflammatory stimulation during the postnatal period has been observed in these patients [38]. After birth, maternal inflammation causes abnormal immunity, such as immune overreaction or autoimmunity. This results in damage to the fetal brain caused by neuron impairment because of the continuous production of proinflammatory cytokines. An increased copy number of long interspersed nuclear element-1 (L1) has been identified in induced pluripotent stem cells derived from neurons in the brains of patients with schizophrenia with a 22q11 deletion. An increased L1 copy number was also found in the offspring of mice exposed to polyriboinosinic-polyribocytidylic acid [poly(I:C)]-induced MIA, which exhibit schizophrenia-like behavior [39]. This suggests that the increase in L1 copy number in neurons induced by environmental factors is involved in schizophrenia susceptibility and pathogenesis [39].

Exposure to maternal inflammation from a viral or bacterial infection and autoinflammatory, autoimmune, and allergic diseases cause neurodevelopmental disorders, allergic diseases, and type 1 diabetes with immunological abnormality in humans. A rodent MIA model using poly(I:C) or LPS during the gestation period affected the immune system, resulting in immune overreaction, suppression of immune response, or inhibition of Th2 immune response, in offspring.

3. The Impact of Exposure to SARS-CoV-2 Infections in the Prenatal and Postnatal Period

3.1. Possible Relationship between Prenatal Environment and COVID-19 Infection in the Postnatal Period

A new form of SARS-CoV-2 has been spreading worldwide, which has caused many deaths. This disease was named COVID-19 [40] and has a wide range of symptoms, including cold symptoms for mild cases and multiple organ failure for severe cases [41,42]. There are many reports about the risk factors of severe COVID-19. First, postnatal risk factors include aging and comorbidities, including diabetes mellitus, hypertension, obesity, asthma, chronic obstructive pulmonary disease, and chronic kidney disease [43–46]. Second, there are genetic variants of SARS-CoV-2 entry cytoplasm-related mechanisms and abnormal immunity [47]. Third, epigenetic modifications with clinical severity of COVID-19 are related to virus entry and innate immune systems, such as IFN signaling, angiotensin-converting enzyme-2, inflammasome component absent in melanoma 2, and major histocompatibility complex class IC candidates [47,48]. These epigenetic alterations might be related to prenatal stimulation in the fetus or changes caused by COVID-19 in the postnatal period. The association between epigenetic modifications and the prenatal environments in patients with severe COVID-19 needs to be clarified. Thus, an analysis of the association between epigenome changes and the prenatal environment in various diseases, such as COVID-19, is expected to benefit future clinical practice.

3.2. Adverse Effects in Infants Exposed to COVID-19 Infection in the Prenatal Period

3.2.1. Neurodevelopmental Disorders

The mechanism of neurodevelopmental disorders, including autism, schizophrenia, learning disability, and ADHD, remains unclear. However, the relationship between maternal viral and bacterial infections in pregnancy and neurodevelopmental disorders in the postnatal period is well known in epidemiologic studies [18,19]. Recently, fetal developmental disorders due to maternal SARS-CoV-2 infection in pregnancy were a primary concern because the inflammatory cytokines implicated in maternal and placental inflammation damage the fetal brain in the prenatal period. As expected, recent studies have suggested that infants of mothers with SARS-CoV-2 infection during pregnancy develop neurodevelopmental disorders at one year of age [49]. Neurodevelopmental disorders, such as autism, schizophrenia, learning disabilities, and ADHD, are often diagnosed after one year and require long-term follow-up beyond the neonatal period.

Additionally, the dysfunction of organs and tissues other than the brain needs to be examined. There are concerns about the direct effects of COVID-19, such as pneumonia or organ failure, and the impact on future generations. Further epidemiological investigations and mechanistic studies are warranted.

3.2.2. Immune Dysfunction

Recent studies reported immune abnormalities caused by SARS-CoV-2 infection in the prenatal period. The immune abnormalities in newborn babies from maternal SARS-CoV-2 infection are affected by maternal infection status. The babies born from mothers with recent or ongoing infection have high cytokine levels in the serum and increase the percentage of natural killer (NK) and regulatory T cells compared with those born from mothers with recovered or uninfected. However, B cells, $CD4^+$ T cells, and $CD8^+$ T cells had similar percentages in both groups. The serology test of babies does not show a vertical infection from the mother [50,51]. Therefore, immune abnormalities might be associated not with direct fetal infection but with the immune response of maternal SARS-CoV-2 infection. This study evaluates the immune system at birth and has limited results because no other study performed this examination. Furthermore, there are no reports of long-term alteration in the immune system, such as during infancy, childhood, or adolescence. However, long-term changes in the immune system due to maternal infection are expected along with other infections, and further investigation is crucial.

3.2.3. Endothelial Cell Dysfunction

SARS-CoV-2 infection induces endothelial cell dysfunction because of endothelium-related deleterious molecules, including alterations of oxidative stress, inflammation, glycocalyx damage, thrombosis, and vascular tone. The endothelial cells maintain function involved in circulating blood and various tissues or organs homeostasis. Therefore, maternal SARS-CoV-2 infection in the gestation period leads to adverse effects associated with endothelial cell dysfunction. First, severe cases of maternal SARS-CoV-2 infection progress multiple organ failure due to hypercytokinemia and lead to blood flow disturbance from mother to fetus through the placenta because of circulatory failure by the septic shock of SARS-CoV-2 infection [52,53]. Second, previous studies reported that the histopathology findings of maternal SARS-CoV-2 infection in the third trimester detected both fetal vascular and maternal malperfusion. These findings included inflammation in the placenta without SARS-CoV-2 vertical infection via the placenta [54]. Epidemiological studies indicate that maternal SARS-CoV-2 infection causes preterm birth, low birth weight, and stillbirth [55–57]. These adverse influences might be associated with blood flow disturbance caused by endothelial cell dysfunction; however, its status is implicated with complicated factors, such as the direct effects of infection or indirect effects of a respiratory disorder, liver injury, kidney injury, and myocardial injury [53].

4. Immune Dysfunction Caused by MIA in Animal Models

4.1. Immune Dysfunction Caused by Prenatal Exposure to Poly (I:C)

Numerous studies have revealed that immunological disorders are associated with MIA. According to a previous meta-analysis of the association between MIA and immunological dysfunction, midgestational maternal exposure to poly (I:C) caused immune overreaction from the perinatal period through preweaning without inducing inflammatory stimulation after birth (Figure 2) [58–61]. IL-1β and TNF-α levels in offspring are slightly elevated in the absence of inflammatory stimuli. Although cytokines such as IL-1 or TNF-α are a more immediate inflammatory response to poly (I:C) than to IL-6, the IL-6 level increased significantly [61]. These results showed that immune hypersensitivity acquired during the prenatal period caused the continuous production of inflammatory cytokines after birth without any postnatal inflammatory stimulation. Anti-inflammatory cytokines, including IL-4 and IL-10, were unchanged, and poly (I:C)-induced MIA might not affect anti-inflammatory cytokine levels in offspring [62]. The mechanisms of immune dysfunction caused by maternal infection are associated with altered cellular stress response, gut microbiota, neurotrophin expression, brain structure and function, and neuroimmune regulation [14,15,63]. MIA induced changes in species and distribution in gut microbiota, inflammatory cytokines, such as TNF-α, and the cerebellum associated with gut microbiota; it also plays a critical role in regulating neuroinflammatory response [62]. Furthermore, mouse or human commensal bacteria, which induce Th17 cell response, cause neurodevelopmental disorders in mice [63]. Therefore, the condition or modification of gut microbiota caused by MIA is associated with immune dysfunction implicated in the Th17 immune response or regulation of the neuroinflammatory response.

Few reports using animal models have examined how offspring exposed to maternal inflammatory stimuli in utero respond when exposed to a second inflammatory stimulus after birth. In a case exposed to poly (I:C) prenatally, the serum IL-6, IL-17, and TNF-α levels increased much higher than those in offspring not exposed to poly (I:C) in vivo during the postnatal period; liver necrosis as an organ injury was also detected in this case [58]. The mRNA expression of the binding immunoglobulin protein and activating transcription factor 4, a major regulator and key transcription factor of the unfolded stress response (UPR), was low compared with controls, suggesting that the UPR defect is induced by prenatal MIA exposure. UPR defects cause an inability for tissue and organ homeostasis maintenance due to excess unfolding proteins, leading to excessive activation of the immune response to inflammatory stimuli [58]. The mechanisms of immune overreaction also include an increase in macrophage 1 polarization, activation of innate immunity, and deficit in T regulatory cells [59,60,64]. Cells derived from offspring exposed to poly (I:C) prenatally exhibited increases in IL-1 and IL-12 levels following LPS stimulation in vitro [59,60] (Table 1). These results suggest that prenatal exposure to inflammation due to MIA is an important event associated with postnatal immune dysfunction. The second attack of inflammatory stimulation after birth enhances the MIA-induced immune overreaction in offspring. Moreover, these second-hit models may be involved in various diseases, such as severe infections or autoinflammatory diseases with an immune hypersensitivity to inflammatory stimuli [65,66]. The most common diseases in children are caused by viral infections, which sometimes progress to severe conditions with multiple organ failure (encephalopathy, cardiomyopathy, liver failure, kidney failure, or respiratory failure) because of cytokine storm. The brain has not detected the influenza virus in encephalopathy caused by an influenza virus, a representative disease of organ failure induced by a viral infection. Immune overreaction against a viral infection induces apoptosis due to cytokine storm. The pathology of aggravating viral infection is the immune overreaction to inflammation rather than direct damage of the virus [65,67–69]. Inflammatory stimulations can easily aggravate patients with autoinflammatory diseases because of the constitution of immune hypersensitivity [66]. A child's immune system is the most sensitive, indicating that immune overreaction in children may be the most adverse effect of MIA.

Table 1. Association between MIA caused by poly (I:C) and immune disorders caused by postnatal inflammatory stimuli.

Literature Authors (Year) (Ref#)	Species	Treatment of Pregnant Dam		Postnatal Treatment of Offspring				
		First Stimulation (mg/kg BW)	Period (Gestational Day, GD)	Second Stimulation	Period (Postnatal Day, PD)	Findings	Histopathology	Assumed Pathogenesis
Charity et al. (2014) [68]	Mouse	Poly (I:C) (20)	Third trimester (GD12.5)	LPS and IFN-γ	PD 21	Increase in IL-1, and IL12 in vitro	NE	Macrophage 1 polarization
Destanie et al. (2017) [67]	Monkey	Poly (I:C) (2500)	First and second trimester (GD 43,44, 46, 100,101, and 103)	LPS or Poly (I:C)	1 year	Increase in IL-1, IL-2, IL4, IL6, IL12, and TNF-α in vitro	NE	Activation of innate and Th2 immune response
Shimizu et al. (2021) [66]	Mouse	Poly (I:C) (20)	Third trimester (GD 12.5, 14.5, and 16.5)	Poly (I:C)	PD 21-28	Increase in IL-6, IL-17, and TNF-α in serum	Liver necrosis	Unfolded protein response defects

MIA, maternal immune activation; poly (I:C), polyriboinosinic-polyribocytidylic acid; LPS, lipopolysaccharide, NE: not examined.

4.2. Immune Dysfunction Caused by Prenatal Exposure to LPS

LPS is used in MIA studies; however, these studies are less likely to be performed than studies using poly (I:C) as maternal inflammatory stimulation. The animal models of MIA induced by LPS are implicated in immune response modifications in offspring [70–80]. Previous studies have reported that cytokine levels at baseline were not changed by maternal LPS exposure in the prenatal period [70,72,75]. However, another study indicated high cytokine levels, including IL-1, IL-6, and IL-10, at baseline in offspring [71]. Exposure to maternal LPS in the prenatal period leads to different immune responses, such as immune overreaction or immune response failure, by the second attack of inflammation after birth (Figure 2) [70–72,74,75,79]. The animal model of immune overreaction shows high levels of cytokines, such as IL-1, IL-6, IL-17, and TNF-α, in serum after inflammatory stimuli. Contrarily, some reports also show that cytokine levels could not increase after inflammatory stimulation compared with control in offspring, and anti-inflammatory cytokines such as IL-10 showed a similar tendency [70,80] (Table 2). Immune response failure caused by exposure to MIA is implicated in suppressing MAPK p42/44 or delayed immune system maturation [70,75,80]. The reports on the mechanisms of immune dysfunction are scarce, and the mechanisms' details are still unclear. The immune overreaction might be associated with exposure to maternal LPS from the first to second trimester or low dose. The immune response failure might be associated with exposure to maternal LPS in the third trimester or high doses. The immune responses vary depending on the characteristics of maternal inflammatory stimulation, such as gestation period, the dose of prenatal inflammatory exposure, or the time of sample collection after the second attack of inflammation in offspring.

5. The Gestation Period, Inflammatory Magnitude, Inflammatory Type of MIA, and Immune Dysfunction Mechanism in Offspring

5.1. Alteration of the Immune System Affected by the Time of MIA

Prenatal development of the immune system in rodents is almost similar to that of humans. The prenatal immune system in rodents comprises cells originating from primitive hematopoiesis in York sac at 7.5 days' gestation. As the pregnancy progresses, the primary site of hematopoietic changes from the York sac to intraembryonic AGM, liver, bone marrow, thymus, and spleen. Diverse cell types in the immune system develop and mature at different gestational stages. Exposure to the maternal environment might significantly influence the fetal immune cells from the second to the third trimester because the critical period of immune system development in rodents is from 7.5 days' gestation to birth [81,82]. Recent studies support this hypothesis. In a meta-analysis investigating the association between MIA and immunological disorders [83,84], exposure to MIA at midgestation causes immune overreaction from the prenatal period to the preweaning stage, and the period of maternal inflammatory stimulation is one of the essential factors of immune dysfunction after birth [61]. The risk of schizophrenia is seven-fold in early pregnancy and three-fold in mid-pregnancy during the influenza pandemic [85]. Furthermore, microglia, the macrophages of the central nervous system, are derived from primitive myeloid progenitors of mouse embryos at 8 days' gestation and have been implicated in the pathogenesis of neurodevelopmental disorders [86]. The neurodevelopmental system is the most affected system at an early period of gestation. The effects of maternal infection on each organ and tissue might depend on the difference in the period when the inflammatory stimulation was received. Therefore, prenatal exposure to maternal infection is one of the essential factors of damage to organs and tissue, and a clinical phenotype is changed after birth.

5.2. Alteration of the Immune System Due to the Magnitude of Inflammatory Response or Type of Inflammatory Cytokines Present in the Prenatal Period

There are no reports about the importance of the magnitude or type of proinflammatory cytokines in abnormal immunity induced by MIA. Previous studies have shown an association between neurodevelopmental disorders and maternal influenza infection. Brown et al. examined the medical records of pregnant women and found an increased risk for schizophrenia caused by a maternal respiratory infection in offspring [81,85]. Neurodevelopmental disorders are possibly caused not only by influenza infection but also by other viral infections during gestation. These results indicate that the direct damage of the virus and immune regulatory components, such as cytokines or transcriptional factors, induced by MIA are crucial factors in organ injury or dysfunction after birth. Representative medicines, such as LPS or poly (I:C), used in MIA animal models activate different immune pathways. Their receptors include TLR-3 for poly (I:C) and TLR-4 for LPS. TLR-3 and TLR-4 activate NF-κB and AP-1 by the MyD88-dependent and Trif-dependent pathways, respectively, and result in the production of type I interferon and inflammatory cytokines [82,87]. Prenatal exposure to poly (I:C) or LPS leads to different neurodevelopmental or immune dysfunction disorders phenotypes.

Both poly (I:C) and LPS treatments cause anxiety-like behaviors in offspring. Poly (I:C) injection during gestation delays growth and sensorimotor development. LPS injection during gestation leads to reduced food intake and decreased body weight. IL-2, IL-5, and IL-6 serum levels in cases receiving poly (I:C) treatment are higher than in those receiving LPS treatment during gestation [88]. Moreover, the high concentrations of cytokines, such as IL-1β, IL-6, IL-8, IL-17, and IFN-γ, are linked to neurodevelopmental disorders in offspring [89–92]. Therefore, the difference in clinical features in neurodevelopmental disorders depends on the type of inflammatory molecules induced by the maternal inflammatory response in the fetus. In an animal model of schizophrenia, the increased cytokine level in maternal serum and fetal hippocampus induced by the injection of poly (I:C) was highly correlated with hippocampal neurogenesis impairment in offspring [93,94]. The magnitude of inflammatory response is strongly associated with the damaged tissue or organ phenotype. These results showed that the onset of neurodevelopmental disorders depends on the intensity of the inflammatory response and the kind of immunoregulatory molecules induced by inflammatory stimulation. Although an association between the mechanisms of immune dysfunction caused by MIA in offspring and the methods of inflammatory stimulation in pregnancy is partially elucidated, the whole picture of these mechanisms is still unclear. The elucidation of these findings is expected to contribute to the pathology of patients with immunological disorders, such as those with severe infections, autoinflammatory diseases, allergic diseases, and immunodeficiency diseases.

Table 2. Association between MIA using LPS and immune disorders caused by postnatal inflammatory stimuli.

Literature Authors (Year) (Ref#)	Species	Treatment of Pregnant Dam		Postnatal Treatment of Offspring				
		First Stimulation (μg/kg/dose)	Period (Gestational Day, GD)	Second Stimulation	Period (Postnatal Day, PD)	Findings	Histopathology	Assumed Pathogenesis
Lasaka et al. (2007) [83]	Rat	LPS (500)	Third trimester (GD 18)	LPS	PD 21	Decrease in IL-1, IL-6, and TNF-α in serum	NE	ND
Surriga et al. (2009) [73]	Rat	LPS (500)	Third trimester (GD 18)	LPS	PD 21	Decrease in IL6 mRNA expression in the liver	NE	Suppression of MAPK P42/44
Basta-Kaim et al. (2012) [77]	Rat	LPS (1000)	Second to third trimester (Every 2days from GD 7)	Concanavalin A	PD 30 and 90	Increase in IL-1β, IL-2, IL-6, and TNF-α in vitro	NE	Increased proliferative activity of splenocytes
Kirsten et al. (2013) [75]	Rat	LPS (100)	Second trimester (GD 9)	LPS	PD 60-67	Increase in IL-1β in serum	NE	Glucocorticoid dysregulation
Zager et al. (2013) [85]	Mouse	LPS (120)	Third trimester (GD 17)	LPS	PD 70	Increase in IL-12 in vitro	NE	Skewing of the cytokine balance towards Th1
Hsueh et al. (2017) [75]	Mouse	LPS (25, 25, 50)	Third trimester (GD 15, 16 and 17)	LPS	PD 56	Increase in IL-1, IL-6, IL-10, IL-12, IL-17, TNF-α, and IFN-γ in serum	NE	Increase in MCP-1 level
Adams et al. (2020) [82]	Mouse	LPS (10)	First to third trimester (GD 0, 7, 14)	LPS	PD 49	Increase in IL-1, IL-6, and IL-10 mRNA expression in the spleen	NE	Glucocorticoid dysregulation

MIA, maternal immune activation; LPS, lipopolysaccharide, NE: not examined, ND: not determined.

6. Epigenetic Changes in the Immune System

6.1. Importance of Epigenetic Alterations in Life

Epigenetic modifications, including DNA methylation, histone modification, and non-coding RNAs, often result in altered gene regulation without changing the DNA sequence and are associated with gene expression by changing the chromatin architecture [95,96]. Previous studies have reported that DNA methylation as well as hypomethylation can affect gene expression in various diseases and lead to schizophrenia by increasing transposon transfer [39,97]. Women in early pregnancy are more susceptible to these alterations [98–100], which could cause various diseases in offspring [101]. Moreover, prenatal exposure to famine could lead to epigenetic modifications, including low DNA methylation of the imprinted IGF2 gene; this epigenetic alteration persists six decades later in life [102,103]. Therefore, the epigenetic alterations due to exposure to adverse stimulations in fetuses affect them at birth and throughout their lifetime. The recent studies are focused on postnatal risk factors of each disease, which has slowly clarified the details of these factors. However, to understand the various diseases from the viewpoint implicated in the prenatal environment and epigenetic modifications, we can interpret the pathology of diseases more deeply. Research on the diagnosis and therapy by analyzing genes and the epigenome in the prenatal period is in progress. For example, several epigenetic abnormalities have been identified in patients with tumors, autoimmune diseases, diabetes mellitus, hematologic diseases, neurodevelopmental disorders, and infections [104].

6.2. Epigenetic Changes Induced by MIA in the Immune System

There are no reports on the direct relationship between epigenetic changes of immunological disorders in offspring and MIA; however, environmental factors other than MIA cause epigenetic changes in the immune system. Exposure to maternal farm environments increases the number of T regulatory cells in infants and decreases Th2 cytokine levels. These alterations are associated with demethylation at the forkhead box P3 promoter, which is one of the main transcription factors of Treg and is implicated in the immune response to inflammatory stimulation [105]. In animal models, immune molecules, such as cytokines and transcriptional factors, are transported from the dam to the pup through the placenta and change the activation of epigenetic modification enzymes. These modifications of epigenetic enzymes alter gene regulation of cytokine or transcriptional factors in the immune cells or signaling pathway [106–109]. IL-6 can enhance the activation of DNA methyltransferase 1 (DNMT1), suggesting the direct relationship between MIA and epigenetic alteration [107]. IL-17 may inhibit the histone deacetylase (HDAC) activity through the PI-3Kinase signaling pathway [108]. The main signaling pathways associated with the immune response, activated by cytokines, are JAK/STAT and MAPK/ERK signaling pathways. STAT proteins regulate histone acetylation at STAT-binding areas [106]. The MAPK/ERK signaling pathway is associated with epigenetic regulators involved in the histone acetyltransferase to chromatin [109]. HDAC induces an epigenetic modification of IL-10 expression [110]. H3K4 methylation suppresses NF-κB and results in decreased IL-6 expression [111]. Other studies show epigenetic modifications, such as DNA methylation, acetylation associated with polarization from naive T cells to Th1 and Th2, or cytokine production by a helper T cell [112–114]. Epigenetic alterations in the immune system cause various adverse effects on the host defense and may induce immune overreaction or immune response failure because of alterations in the gene expressions of inflammatory cytokine or transcriptional factors by changing the chromatin structure [115,116]. Further studies are required to investigate whether MIA directly interacts with epigenetic modifications of the immune system in offspring.

6.3. Prospects of Prevention and Treatment Using Epigenetic Therapy in the Prenatal Period

Prenatal diagnosis and treatment focus on preventing the onset of various diseases with genetic or epigenetic factors and reducing the medical costs for patients. Gene therapy for autoimmune disease in the postnatal period regulates the immune system, including the levels of proinflammatory cytokine or immune molecules or infiltration of lymphocytes. However, animal models of prenatal gene therapy for immunological disorders have yet to be reported. Gene therapy of an injection vector in the prenatal period can prevent hemophilia in offspring and is expected to be applied as a prenatal treatment for various diseases [117,118]. Epigenetic therapy in the postnatal period could treat diseases such as myelodysplastic syndrome, leukemia, cancer, heart failure, and diabetic retinopathy [104]; however, there are no reports about epigenetic therapy in the prenatal period. The application of epigenetic therapy during the prenatal period may suppress the onset of fatal diseases in the prenatal or neonatal period. However, this therapy has some disadvantages; it is not indicated for target cells, and activating gene expression in normal cells might lead to cancer [104]. We need to overcome many problems in the clinical field; however, significant benefits await epigenetic therapy's development. Thus, we need to evaluate the relationship between epigenetic alteration, maternal environments, and postnatal effect using an animal model.

7. Conclusions

The Association of Genetic Factors, Maternal Infection, and Postnatal Environmental Factors in Immune Dysfunction

Genetic factors are crucial to the onset of several human diseases, which are directly related to genetic diseases and are indirectly implicated in many diseases. In epidemiologic studies, exposure to a viral infection is the most critical factor that excessively activates the immune response in offspring. Maternal bacterial infection causes different immune responses in offspring, including immune overreaction or immune response failure. These clinical features in the immune system may depend on time, magnitude, and inflammatory type of MIA. In addition, postnatal environments are the ultimate determinants of immune overreaction or immune response failure. Immune overreaction leads to various diseases with immune hypersensitivity, including autoinflammatory, autoimmune and allergic diseases, and severe viral and bacterial infections. Immune response failure in offspring might cause immunodeficiency diseases and suppression of diseases with immune hypersensitivities, such as autoinflammatory, autoimmune, and allergic diseases and severe infections [119] (Figure 3).

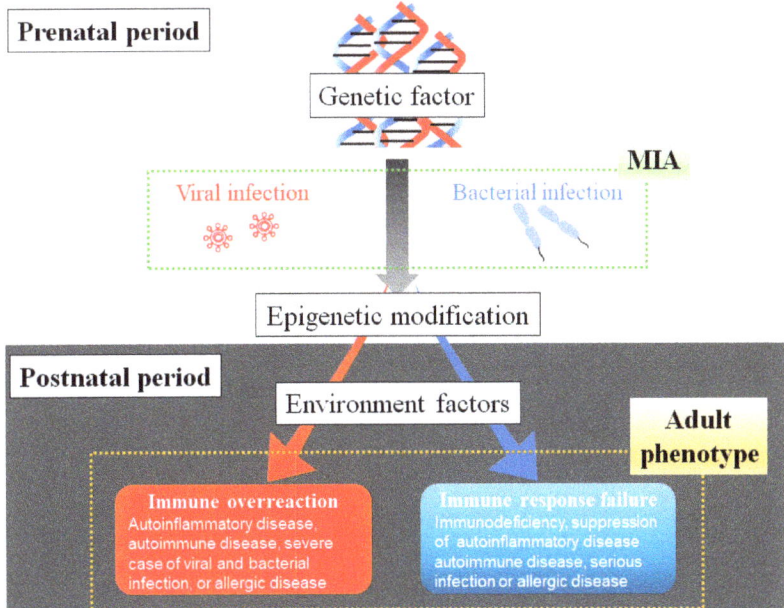

Figure 3. The association of genetic factors, maternal immune activation (MIA), and environmental factors in immune dysfunction after birth.

The goal of therapies was mainly to cure the disease or disorder after its onset until a few decades ago. Recently, treatments have been performed to prevent various contracting diseases. For instance, the treatment for hypertension, obesity, hyperlipidemia, and diabetes mellitus is aimed at preventing coronary artery disease or stroke in old age. Medical treatment is essential to prevent the crisis by removal of the risk factor. Additionally, the development of epigenetic alterations and genetic analysis at birth or shortly after birth may allow for the identification of individual disease susceptibility. In the future, the diagnosis and treatment of these diseases in the prenatal period may be achieved using an epigenetic analysis and suppression of various diseases associated with epigenetic modifications.

The determinants of the development of immune disorders, such as immune overreaction and immune response failure, in offspring depend on the characteristics of maternal inflammatory stimulation, including gestation period, the magnitude of maternal inflammation, and the kinds of immune molecules induced by MIA. The genetic factor and prenatal stimulations lead to the development of various diseases associated with immune system disorders. These constitutions are exacerbated by exposure to postnatal risk factors in offspring, leading to various diseases with abnormal immunity.

Author Contributions: All authors contributed significantly to this study, including the article's conception, drafting, revising, and critical reviewing. All authors approved the version of the manuscript and agreed on the journal to which the article has been submitted. The authors agree to be accountable for all aspects of the work. All authors have read and agreed to the published version of the manuscript.

Funding: This work was supported by JSPS KAKENHI (grant numbers 15K09713, 15K15405, 16H05364, 18K11659, 19K22696, 25293241, 24659512, 22390216, and 19390291).

Data Availability Statement: Not applicable.

Acknowledgments: We thank Mayumi Mitani and Tomoko Yasuda for their technical support.

Conflicts of Interest: The authors declare that the research was conducted without any commercial or financial relationships that could be construed as a potential conflict of interest.

References

1. Chen, T.; Liu, H.-X.; Yan, H.-Y.; Wu, D.-M.; Ping, J. Developmental origins of inflammatory and immune diseases. *Mol. Hum. Reprod.* **2016**, *22*, 858–865. [CrossRef]
2. Barker, D.J.; Osmond, C. Infant mortality, childhood nutrition, and ischaemic heart disease in England and Wales. *Lancet* **1986**, *1*, 1077–1081. [CrossRef]
3. Barker, D.J.; Winter, P.D.; Osmond, C.; Margetts, B.; Simmonds, S.J. Weight in infancy and death from ischaemic heart disease. *Lancet* **1989**, *2*, 577–580. [CrossRef]
4. Morea, M.; Miu, N.; Morea, V.F.; Cornean, R. Maternal obesity—A risk factor for metabolic syndrome in children. *Clujul Med* **2013**, *86*, 259–265.
5. Nilsen, F.M.; Ruiz, J.D.; Tulve, N.S. A Meta-Analysis of Stressors from the Total Environment Associated with Children's General Cognitive Ability. *Int. J. Environ. Res. Public Health* **2020**, *17*, 5451. [CrossRef]
6. Weijmans, M.; van der Graaf, Y.; Reitsma, J.; Visseren, F. Paternal or maternal history of cardiovascular disease and the risk of cardiovascular disease in offspring. A systematic review and meta-analysis. *Int. J. Cardiol.* **2015**, *179*, 409–416. [CrossRef]
7. Fuchs, O.; von Mutius, E. Prenatal and childhood infections: Implications for the development and treatment of childhood asthma. *Lancet Respir. Med.* **2013**, *1*, 743–754. [CrossRef]
8. Burke, H.; Leonardi-Bee, J.; Hashim, A.; Pine-Abata, H.; Chen, Y.; Cook, D.G.; Britton, J.R.; McKeever, T.M. Prenatal and Passive Smoke Exposure and Incidence of Asthma and Wheeze: Systematic Review and Meta-analysis. *Pediatrics* **2012**, *129*, 735–744. [CrossRef]
9. Gardener, H.; Spiegelman, D.; Buka, S.L. Prenatal risk factors for autism: Comprehensive meta-analysis. *Br. J. Psychiatry* **2009**, *195*, 7–14. [CrossRef]
10. Ashwood, P.; Krakowiak, P.; Hertz-Picciotto, I.; Hansen, R.; Pessah, I.N.; Van de Water, J. Associations of impaired behaviors with elevated plasma chemokines in autism spectrum disorders. *J. Neuroimmunol.* **2011**, *232*, 196–199. [CrossRef]
11. Terasaki, L.S.; Schwarz, J.M. Effects of Moderate Prenatal Alcohol Exposure during Early Gestation in Rats on Inflammation across the Maternal-Fetal-Immune Interface and Later-Life Immune Function in the Offspring. *J. Neuroimmune Pharmacol.* **2016**, *11*, 680–692. [CrossRef]
12. Shcherbitskaia, A.D.; Vasilev, D.S.; Milyutina, Y.P.; Tumanova, N.L.; Zalozniaia, I.V.; Kerkeshko, G.O.; Arutjunyan, A.V. Maternal Hyperhomocysteinemia Induces Neuroinflammation and Neuronal Death in the Rat Offspring Cortex. *Neurotox. Res.* **2020**, *38*, 408–420. [CrossRef]
13. Jain, S.; Baer, R.J.; McCulloch, C.E.; Rogers, E.; Rand, L.; Jelliffe-Pawlowski, L.; Piao, X. Association of Maternal Immune Activation during Pregnancy and Neurologic Outcomes in Offspring. *J. Pediatr.* **2021**, *238*, 87–93.e3. [CrossRef]
14. McKeever, T.M.; Lewis, S.A.; Smith, C.; Hubbard, R. The importance of prenatal exposures on the development of allergic disease: A birth cohort study using the West Midlands General Practice Database. *Am. J. Respir. Crit. Care Med.* **2002**, *166*, 827–832. [CrossRef]
15. Yue, Y.; Tang, Y.; Tang, J.; Shi, J.; Zhu, T.; Huang, J.; Qiu, X.; Zeng, Y.; Li, W.; Qu, Y.; et al. Maternal infection during pregnancy and type 1 diabetes mellitus in offspring: A systematic review and meta-analysis. *Epidemiology Infect.* **2018**, *146*, 2131–2138. [CrossRef]
16. Enstrom, A.M.; Onore, C.E.; Van de Water, J.A.; Ashwood, P. Differential monocyte responses to TLR ligands in children with autism spectrum disorders. *Brain. Behav. Immun.* **2010**, *24*, 64–71. [CrossRef]

17. Ashwood, P.; Krakowiak, P.; Hertz-Picciotto, I.; Hansen, R.; Pessah, I.; Van de Water, J. Elevated plasma cytokines in autism spectrum disorders provide evidence of immune dysfunction and are associated with impaired behavioral outcome. *Brain, Behav. Immun.* 2011, *25*, 40–45. [CrossRef]
18. Antoun, S.; Ellul, P.; Peyre, H.; Rosenzwajg, M.; Gressens, P.; Klatzmann, D.; Delorme, R. Fever during pregnancy as a risk factor for neurodevelopmental disorders: Results from a systematic review and meta-analysis. *Mol. Autism* 2021, *12*, 60. [CrossRef]
19. Han, V.X.; Patel, S.; Jones, H.F.; Nielsen, T.C.; Mohammad, S.S.; Hofer, M.J.; Gold, W.; Brilot, F.; Lain, S.J.; Nassar, N.; et al. Maternal acute and chronic inflammation in pregnancy is associated with common neurodevelopmental disorders: A systematic review. *Transl. Psychiatry* 2021, *11*, 71. [CrossRef]
20. Zinkernagel, R.M. Maternal antibodies, childhood infections, and autoimmune diseases. *N. Engl. J. Med.* 2001, *345*, 1331–1335. [CrossRef]
21. Hermann, E.; Truyens, C.; Alonso-Vega, C.; Even, J.; Rodriguez, P.; Berthe, A.; Gonzalez-Merino, E.; Torrico, F.; Carlier, Y. Human fetuses are able to mount an adultlike CD8 T-cell response. *Blood* 2002, *100*, 2153–2158. [CrossRef] [PubMed]
22. Douwes, J.; Cheng, S.; Travier, N.; Cohet, C.; Niesink, A.; McKenzie, J.; Cunningham, C.; Le Gros, G.; von Mutius, E.; Pearce, N. Farm exposure in utero may protect against asthma, hay fever and eczema. *Eur. Respir. J.* 2008, *32*, 603–611. [CrossRef]
23. Yu, J.; Liu, X.; Li, Y.; Meng, S.; Wu, F.; Yan, B.; Xue, Y.; Ma, T.; Yang, J.; Liu, J. Maternal exposure to farming environment protects offspring against allergic diseases by modulating the neonatal TLR-Tregs-Th axis. *Clin. Transl. Allergy* 2018, *8*, 34. [CrossRef] [PubMed]
24. Cai, L.; Wan, C.-L.; He, L.; Jong, S.; Chou, K.-C. Gestational Influenza Increases the Risk of Psychosis in Adults. *Med. Chem.* 2015, *11*, 676–682. [CrossRef] [PubMed]
25. Quagliato, L.A.; de Matos, U.; Nardi, A.E. Maternal immune activation generates anxiety in offspring: A translational meta-analysis. *Transl. Psychiatry* 2021, *11*, 245. [CrossRef]
26. Oncu-Oner, T.; Can, S. Meta-analysis of the relationship between Toxoplasma gondii and schizophrenia. *Ann. Parasitol.* 2022, *68*, 103–110.
27. Davies, C.; Segre, G.; Estradé, A.; Radua, J.; De Micheli, A.; Provenzani, U.; Oliver, D.; de Pablo, G.S.; Ramella-Cravaro, V.; Besozzi, M.; et al. Prenatal and perinatal risk and protective factors for psychosis: A systematic review and meta-analysis. *Lancet Psychiatry* 2020, *7*, 399–410. [CrossRef]
28. Selten, J.-P.; Termorshuizen, F. The serological evidence for maternal influenza as risk factor for psychosis in offspring is insufficient: Critical review and meta-analysis. *Schizophr. Res.* 2017, *183*, 2–9. [CrossRef]
29. Jiang, H.-Y.; Xu, L.-L.; Shao, L.; Xia, R.-M.; Yu, Z.-H.; Ling, Z.-X.; Yang, F.; Deng, M.; Ruan, B. Maternal infection during pregnancy and risk of autism spectrum disorders: A systematic review and meta-analysis. *Brain, Behav. Immun.* 2016, *58*, 165–172. [CrossRef]
30. Hu, C.-C.; Xu, X.; Xiong, G.-L.; Xu, Q.; Zhou, B.-R.; Li, C.-Y.; Qin, Q.; Liu, C.-X.; Li, H.-P.; Sun, Y.-J.; et al. Alterations in plasma cytokine levels in chinese children with autism spectrum disorder. *Autism Res.* 2018, *11*, 989–999. [CrossRef]
31. Eftekharian, M.M.; Ghafouri-Fard, S.; Noroozi, R.; Omrani, M.D.; Arsang-Jang, S.; Ganji, M.; Gharzi, V.; Noroozi, H.; Komaki, A.; Mazdeh, M.; et al. Cytokine profile in autistic patients. *Cytokine* 2018, *108*, 120–126. [CrossRef]
32. Molloy, C.; Morrow, A.; Meinzenderr, J.; Schleifer, K.; Dienger, K.; Manningcourtney, P.; Altaye, M.; Willskarp, M. Elevated cytokine levels in children with autism spectrum disorder. *J. Neuroimmunol.* 2006, *172*, 198–205. [CrossRef]
33. Guloksuz, S.A.; Abali, O.; Aktas Cetin, E.; Bilgic Gazioglu, S.; Deniz, G.; Yildirim, A.; Kawikova, I.; Guloksuz, S.; Leckman, J.F. Elevated plasma concentrations of S100 calcium-binding protein B and tumor necrosis factor alpha in children with autism spectrum disorders. *Braz. J. Psychiatry* 2017, *39*, 195–200. [CrossRef]
34. Xie, J.; Huang, L.; Li, X.; Li, H.; Zhou, Y.; Zhu, H.; Pan, T.; Kendrick, K.M.; Xu, W. Immunological cytokine profiling identifies TNF-α as a key molecule dysregulated in autistic children. *Oncotarget* 2017, *8*, 82390–82398. [CrossRef] [PubMed]
35. Jácome, M.C.I.; Chacòn, L.M.M.; Cuesta, H.V.; Rizo, C.M.; Santiesteban, M.W.; Hernandez, L.R.; García, E.N.; Fraguela, M.E.G.; Verdecia, C.I.F.; Hurtado, Y.V.; et al. Peripheral Inflammatory Markers Contributing to Comorbidities in Autism. *Behav. Sci.* 2016, *6*, 29. [CrossRef]
36. Suzuki, K.; Matsuzaki, H.; Iwata, K.; Kameno, Y.; Shimmura, C.; Kawai, S.; Yoshihara, Y.; Wakuda, T.; Takebayashi, K.; Takagai, S.; et al. Plasma Cytokine Profiles in Subjects with High-Functioning Autism Spectrum Disorders. *PLoS ONE* 2011, *6*, e20470. [CrossRef] [PubMed]
37. Al-Ayadhi, L.Y. Pro-inflammatory cytokines in autistic children in central Saudi Arabia. *Neurosciences* 2005, *10*, 155–158. [PubMed]
38. Han, V.X.; Jones, H.F.; Patel, S.; Mohammad, S.S.; Hofer, M.J.; Alshammery, S.; Maple-Brown, E.; Gold, W.; Brilot, F.; Dale, R.C. Emerging evidence of Toll-like receptors as a putative pathway linking maternal inflammation and neurodevelopmental disorders in human offspring: A systematic review. *Brain Behav. Immun.* 2022, *99*, 91–105. [CrossRef]
39. Bundo, M.; Toyoshima, M.; Okada, Y.; Akamatsu, W.; Ueda, J.; Nemoto-Miyauchi, T.; Sunaga, F.; Toritsuka, M.; Ikawa, D.; Kakita, A.; et al. Increased L1 Retrotransposition in the Neuronal Genome in Schizophrenia. *Neuron* 2014, *81*, 306–313. [CrossRef]
40. Zhu, N.; Zhang, D.; Wang, W.; Li, X.; Yang, B.; Song, J.; Zhao, X.; Huang, B.; Shi, W.; Lu, R.; et al. A Novel Coronavirus from Patients with Pneumonia in China, 2019. *N. Engl. J. Med.* 2020, *382*, 727–733. [CrossRef]
41. Wu, Z.; McGoogan, J.M. Characteristics of and Important Lessons From the Coronavirus Disease 2019 (COVID-19) Outbreak in China: Summary of a Report of 72 314 Cases From the Chinese Center for Disease Control and Prevention. *JAMA* 2020, *323*, 1239–1242. [CrossRef] [PubMed]

42. Fang, F.; Chen, Y.; Zhao, D.; Liu, T.; Huang, Y.; Qiu, L.; Hao, Y.; Hu, X.; Yin, W.; Liu, Z.; et al. Recommendations for the Diagnosis, Prevention, and Control of Coronavirus Disease-19 in Children-The Chinese Perspectives. *Front. Pediatr.* **2020**, *8*, 553394. [CrossRef] [PubMed]
43. Hu, J.; Wang, Y. The Clinical Characteristics and Risk Factors of Severe COVID-19. *Gerontology* **2021**, *67*, 255–266. [CrossRef] [PubMed]
44. Gold, M.S.; Sehayek, D.; Gabrielli, S.; Zhang, X.; McCusker, C.; Ben-Shoshan, M. COVID-19 and comorbidities: A systematic review and meta-analysis. *Postgrad. Med.* **2020**, *132*, 749–755. [CrossRef] [PubMed]
45. Parohan, M.; Yaghoubi, S.; Seraji, A.; Javanbakht, M.H.; Sarraf, P.; Djalali, M. Risk factors for mortality in patients with Coronavirus disease 2019 (COVID-19) infection: A systematic review and meta-analysis of observational studies. *Aging Male* **2020**, *23*, 1416–1424. [CrossRef]
46. Zheng, Z.; Peng, F.; Xu, B.; Zhao, J.; Liu, H.; Peng, J.; Li, Q.; Jiang, C.; Zhou, Y.; Liu, S.; et al. Risk factors of critical & mortal COVID-19 cases: A systematic literature review and meta-analysis. *J. Infect.* **2020**, *81*, e16–e25. [CrossRef]
47. Yildirim, Z.; Sahin, O.S.; Yazar, S.; Cetintas, V.B. Genetic and epigenetic factors associated with increased severity of Covid-19. *Cell Biol. Int.* **2021**, *45*, 1158–1174. [CrossRef]
48. Castro de Moura, M.; Davalos, V.; Planas-Serra, L.; Alvarez-Errico, D.; Arribas, C.; Ruiz, M.; Aguilera-Albesa, S.; Troya, J.; Valencia-Ramos, J.; Vélez-Santamaria, V.; et al. Epigenome-wide association study of COVID-19 severity with respiratory failure. *eBioMedicine* **2021**, *66*, 103339. [CrossRef]
49. Edlow, A.G.; Castro, V.M.; Shook, L.L.; Kaimal, A.J.; Perlis, R.H. Neurodevelopmental Outcomes at 1 Year in Infants of Mothers Who Tested Positive for SARS-CoV-2 During Pregnancy. *JAMA Netw. Open* **2022**, *5*, e2215787. [CrossRef]
50. Manti, S.; Leonardi, S.; Rezaee, F.; Harford, T.J.; Perez, M.K.; Piedimonte, G. Effects of Vertical Transmission of Respiratory Viruses to the Offspring. *Front. Immunol.* **2022**, *13*, 853009. [CrossRef]
51. Gee, S.; Chandiramani, M.; Seow, J.; Pollock, E.; Modestini, C.; Das, A.; Tree, T.; Doores, K.J.; Tribe, R.M.; Gibbons, D.L. The legacy of maternal SARS-CoV-2 infection on the immunology of the neonate. *Nat. Immunol.* **2021**, *22*, 1490–1502. [CrossRef] [PubMed]
52. Qin, Z.; Liu, F.; Blair, R.; Wang, C.; Yang, H.; Mudd, J.; Currey, J.M.; Iwanaga, N.; He, J.; Mi, R.; et al. Endothelial cell infection and dysfunction, immune activation in severe COVID-19. *Theranostics* **2021**, *11*, 8076–8091. [CrossRef] [PubMed]
53. Xu, S.-W.; Ilyas, I.; Weng, J.-P. Endothelial dysfunction in COVID-19: An overview of evidence, biomarkers, mechanisms and potential therapies. *Acta Pharmacol. Sin.* **2022**, *12*, 1–15. [CrossRef] [PubMed]
54. Sharps, M.C.; Hayes, D.J.; Lee, S.; Zou, Z.; Brady, C.A.; Almoghrabi, Y.; Kerby, A.; Tamber, K.K.; Jones, C.J.; Waldorf, K.M.A.; et al. A structured review of placental morphology and histopathological lesions associated with SARS-CoV-2 infection. *Placenta* **2020**, *101*, 13–29. [CrossRef] [PubMed]
55. Chmielewska, B.; Barratt, I.; Townsend, R.; Kalafat, E.; van der Meulen, J.; Gurol-Urganci, I.; O'Brien, P.; Morris, E.; Draycott, T.; Thangaratinam, S.; et al. Effects of the COVID-19 pandemic on maternal and perinatal outcomes: A systematic review and meta-analysis. *Lancet Glob. Health* **2021**, *9*, e759–e772. [CrossRef]
56. Wei, S.Q.; Bilodeau-Bertrand, M.; Liu, S.; Auger, N. The impact of COVID-19 on pregnancy outcomes: A systematic review and meta-analysis. *Can. Med Assoc. J.* **2021**, *193*, E540–E548. [CrossRef]
57. Lassi, Z.S.; Ana, A.; Das, J.K.; A Salam, R.; A Padhani, Z.; Irfan, O.; A Bhutta, Z. A systematic review and meta-analysis of data on pregnant women with confirmed COVID-19: Clinical presentation, and pregnancy and perinatal outcomes based on COVID-19 severity. *J. Glob. Health* **2021**, *11*, 05018. [CrossRef]
58. Shimizu, Y.; Tsukada, T.; Sakata-Haga, H.; Sakai, D.; Shoji, H.; Saikawa, Y.; Hatta, T. Exposure to Maternal Immune Activation Causes Congenital Unfolded Protein Response Defects and Increases the Susceptibility to Postnatal Inflammatory Stimulation in Offspring. *J. Inflamm. Res.* **2021**, *14*, 355–365. [CrossRef]
59. Rose, D.R.; Careaga, M.; Van de Water, J.; McAllister, K.; Bauman, M.D.; Ashwood, P. Long-term altered immune responses following fetal priming in a non-human primate model of maternal immune activation. *Brain, Behav. Immun.* **2017**, *63*, 60–70. [CrossRef]
60. Onore, C.E.; Schwartzer, J.J.; Careaga, M.; Berman, R.F.; Ashwood, P. Maternal immune activation leads to activated inflammatory macrophages in offspring. *Brain, Behav. Immun.* **2014**, *38*, 220–226. [CrossRef]
61. Hameete, B.C.; Fernández-Calleja, J.M.; de Groot, M.W.; Oppewal, T.R.; Tiemessen, M.M.; Hogenkamp, A.; de Vries, R.B.; Groenink, L. The poly(I:C)-induced maternal immune activation model; a systematic review and meta-analysis of cytokine levels in the offspring. *Brain, Behav. Immun. Health* **2021**, *11*, 100192. [CrossRef]
62. Tartaglione, A.M.; Villani, A.; Ajmone-Cat, M.A.; Minghetti, L.; Ricceri, L.; Pazienza, V.; De Simone, R.; Calamandrei, G. Maternal immune activation induces autism-like changes in behavior, neuroinflammatory profile and gut microbiota in mouse offspring of both sexes. *Transl. Psychiatry* **2022**, *12*, 1–10. [CrossRef]
63. Kim, S.; Kim, H.; Yim, Y.S.; Ha, S.; Atarashi, K.; Tan, T.G.; Longman, R.S.; Honda, K.; Littman, D.R.; Choi, G.B.; et al. Maternal gut bacteria promote neurodevelopmental abnormalities in mouse offspring. *Nature* **2017**, *549*, 528–532. [CrossRef]
64. Hsiao, E.Y.; McBride, S.W.; Chow, J.; Mazmanian, S.K.; Patterson, P.H. Modeling an autism risk factor in mice leads to permanent immune dysregulation. *Proc. Natl. Acad. Sci. USA* **2012**, *109*, 12776–12781. [CrossRef] [PubMed]
65. Committee on Infectious Diseases. Recommendations for Prevention and Control of Influenza in Children, 2018–2019. *Pediatrics* **2018**, *142*, e20182367. [CrossRef] [PubMed]

66. Ter Haar, N.; Oswald, M.; Jeyaratnam, J.; Anton, J.; Barron, K.; Brogan, P.; Cantarini, L.; Galeotti, C.; Grateau, G.; Hentgen, V.; et al. Recommendations for the management of autoinflammatory diseases. *Pediatr. Rheumatol.* **2015**, *13*, P133. [CrossRef]
67. Hidaka, F.; Matsuo, S.; Muta, T.; Takeshige, K.; Mizukami, T.; Nunoi, H. A missense mutation of the Toll-like receptor 3 gene in a patient with influenza-associated encephalopathy. *Clin. Immunol.* **2006**, *119*, 188–194. [CrossRef] [PubMed]
68. Kawashima, H.; Morichi, S.; Okumara, A.; Nakagawa, S.; Morishima, T.; the collaborating study group on influenza-associated encephalopathy in Japan. National survey of pandemic influenza A (H1N1) 2009-associated encephalopathy in Japanese children. *J. Med Virol.* **2012**, *84*, 1151–1156. [CrossRef] [PubMed]
69. Mori, S.-I.; Nagashima, M.; Sasaki, Y.; Mori, K.; Tabei, Y.; Yoshida, Y.; Yamazaki, K.; Hirata, I.; Sekine, H.; Ito, T.; et al. A novel amino acid substitution at the receptor-binding site on the hemagglutinin of H3N2 influenza A viruses isolated from 6 cases with acute encephalopathy during the 1997-1998 season in Tokyo. *Arch. Virol.* **1999**, *144*, 147–155. [CrossRef]
70. Surriga, O.; Ortega, A.; Jadeja, V.; Bellafronte, A.; Lasala, N.; Zhou, H. Altered hepatic inflammatory response in the offspring following prenatal LPS exposure. *Immunol Lett.* **2009**, *123*, 88–95. [CrossRef]
71. Hsueh, P.T.; Lin, H.H.; Wang, H.H.; Liu, C.L.; Ni, W.F.; Liu, J.K.; Chang, H.-H.; Sun, D.-S.; Chen, Y.-S.; Chen, Y.-L. Immune imbalance of global gene expression, and cytokine, chemokine and selectin levels in the brains of offspring with social deficits via maternal immune activation. *Genes Brain Behav.* **2018**, *17*, e12479. [CrossRef]
72. Kirsten, T.B.; Lippi, L.L.; Bevilacqua, E.; Bernardi, M.M. LPS exposure increases maternal corticosterone levels, causes placental injury and increases IL-1B levels in adult rat offspring: Relevance to autism. *PLoS ONE* **2013**, *8*, e82244. [CrossRef]
73. Cao, L.; Wang, J.; Zhu, Y.; Tseu, I.; Post, M. Maternal endotoxin exposure attenuates allergic airway disease in infant rats. *Am. J. Physiol. Lung Cell Mol. Physiol.* **2010**, *298*, 670–677. [CrossRef]
74. Basta-Kaim, A.; Szczęsny, E.; Leśkiewicz, M.; Głombik, K.; Ślusarczyk, J.; Budziszewska, B.; Regulska, M.; Kubera, M.; Nowak, W.; Wędzony, K.; et al. Maternal immune activation leads to age-related behavioral and immunological changes in male rat offspring—The effect of antipsychotic drugs. *Pharmacol Rep.* **2012**, *64*, 1400–1410. [CrossRef] [PubMed]
75. Hodyl, N.A.; Krivanek, K.M.; Lawrence, E.; Clifton, V.L.; Hodgson, D.M. Prenatal exposure to a pro-inflammatory stimulus causes delays in the development of the innate immune response to LPS in the offspring. *J. Neuroimmunol.* **2007**, *190*, 61–71. [CrossRef] [PubMed]
76. Gerhold, K.; Avagyan, A.; Seib, C.; Frei, R.; Steinle, J.; Ahrens, B.; Dittrich, A.M.; Blumchen, K.; Lauener, R.; Hamelmann, E. Prenatal initiation of endotoxin airway exposure prevents subsequent allergen-induced sensitization and airway inflammation in mice. *J. Allergy Clin. Immunol.* **2006**, *118*, 666–673. [CrossRef]
77. Blümer, N.; Herz, U.; Wegmann, M.; Renz, H. Prenatal lipopolysaccharide-exposure prevents allergic sensitization and airway inflammation, but not airway responsiveness in a murine model of experimental asthma. *Clin. Exp. Allergy* **2005**, *35*, 397–402. [CrossRef]
78. Kirsten, T.B.; De Oliveira, B.P.S.; De Oliveira, A.P.L.; Kieling, K.; De Lima, W.T.; Palermo-Neto, J.; Bernardi, M.M. Single early prenatal lipopolysaccharide exposure prevents subsequent airway inflammation response in an experimental model of asthma. *Life Sci.* **2011**, *89*, 15–19. [CrossRef] [PubMed]
79. Adams, R.C.M.; Smith, C. Exposure to Maternal Chronic Inflammation Transfers a Pro-Inflammatory Profile to Generation F2 via Sex-Specific Mechanisms. *Front Immunol.* **2020**, *11*, 48. [CrossRef]
80. Lasala, N.; Zhou, H. Effects of maternal exposure to LPS on the inflammatory response in the offspring. *J Neuroimmunol.* **2007**, *189*, 95–101. [CrossRef]
81. Brown, A.S. Prenatal Infection as a Risk Factor for Schizophrenia. *Schizophr. Bull.* **2006**, *32*, 200–202. [CrossRef]
82. Kawai, T.; Akira, S. TLR signaling. *Semin. Immunol.* **2007**, *19*, 24–32. [CrossRef]
83. Landreth, K.S. Critical windows in development of the rodent immune system. *Hum. Exp. Toxicol.* **2002**, *21*, 493–498. [CrossRef] [PubMed]
84. Park, J.E.; Jardine, L.; Gottgens, B.; Teichmann, S.A.; Haniffa, M. Prenatal development of human immunity. *Science* **2020**, *368*, 600–603. [CrossRef]
85. Brown, A.S.; Begg, M.D.; Gravenstein, S.; Schaefer, C.A.; Wyatt, R.J.; Bresnahan, M.; Babulas, V.P.; Susser, E.S. Serologic Evidence of Prenatal Influenza in the Etiology of Schizophrenia. *Arch. Gen. Psychiatry* **2004**, *61*, 774–780. [CrossRef] [PubMed]
86. Ginhoux, F.; Greter, M.; Leboeuf, M.; Nandi, S.; See, P.; Gokhan, S.; Mehler, M.F.; Conway, S.J.; Ng, L.G.; Stanley, E.R.; et al. Fate mapping analysis reveals that adult microglia derive from primitive macrophages. *Science* **2010**, *330*, 841–845. [CrossRef] [PubMed]
87. Kawasaki, T.; Kawai, T. Toll-like receptor signaling pathways. *Front. Immunol.* **2014**, *5*, 461. [CrossRef]
88. Arsenault, D.; St-Amour, I.; Cisbani, G.; Rousseau, L.-S.; Cicchetti, F. The different effects of LPS and poly I:C prenatal immune challenges on the behavior, development and inflammatory responses in pregnant mice and their offspring. *Brain Behav. Immun.* **2014**, *38*, 77–90. [CrossRef]
89. Masi, A.; Quintana, D.S.; Glozier, N.; Lloyd, A.R.; Hickie, I.B.; Guastella, A.J. Cytokine aberrations in autism spectrum disorder: A systematic review and meta-analysis. *Mol. Psychiatry* **2015**, *20*, 440–446. [CrossRef]
90. Goines, P.E.; Ashwood, P. Cytokine dysregulation in autism spectrum disorders (ASD): Possible role of the environment. *Neurotoxicology Teratol.* **2013**, *36*, 67–81. [CrossRef]
91. Smith, S.E.P.; Li, J.; Garbett, K.; Mirnics, K.; Patterson, P.H. Maternal Immune Activation Alters Fetal Brain Development through Interleukin-6. *J. Neurosci.* **2007**, *27*, 10695–10702. [CrossRef] [PubMed]

92. Choi, G.B.; Yim, Y.S.; Wong, H.; Kim, S.; Kim, H.; Kim, S.V.; Hoeffer, C.A.; Littman, D.R.; Huh, J.R. The maternal interleukin-17a pathway in mice promotes autism-like phenotypes in offspring. *Science* **2016**, *351*, 933–939. [CrossRef]
93. Zhao, Q.; Wang, Q.; Wang, J.; Tang, M.; Huang, S.; Peng, K.; Han, Y.; Zhang, J.; Liu, G.; Fang, Q.; et al. Maternal immune activation-induced PPARγ-dependent dysfunction of microglia associated with neurogenic impairment and aberrant postnatal behaviors in offspring. *Neurobiol. Dis.* **2019**, *125*, 1–13. [CrossRef]
94. Meyer, U.; Feldon, J.; Schedlowski, M.; Yee, B.K. Towards an immuno-precipitated neurodevelopmental animal model of schizophrenia. *Neurosci. Biobehav. Rev.* **2005**, *29*, 913–947. [CrossRef]
95. Quina, A.; Buschbeck, M.; Di Croce, L. Chromatin structure and epigenetics. *Biochem. Pharmacol.* **2006**, *72*, 1563–1569. [CrossRef] [PubMed]
96. Roadmap Epigenomics Consortium; Kundaje, A.; Meuleman, W.; Ernst, J.; Bilenky, M.; Yen, A.; Heravi-Moussavi, A.; Kheradpour, P.; Zhang, Z.; Wang, J. Integrative analysis of 111 reference human epigenomes. *Nature* **2015**, *518*, 317–330. [CrossRef]
97. Wilson, A.; Power, B.; Molloy, P.L. DNA hypomethylation and human diseases. *Biochim. Biophys. Acta (BBA) Rev. Cancer* **2007**, *1775*, 138–162. [CrossRef] [PubMed]
98. Tobi, E.W.; Slieker, R.C.; Stein, A.D.; Suchiman, H.E.D.; Slagboom, P.E.; Van Zwet, E.W.; Heijmans, B.T.; Lumey, L.H. Early gestation as the critical time-window for changes in the prenatal environment to affect the adult human blood methylome. *Int J Epidemiol.* **2015**, *44*, 1211–1223. [CrossRef]
99. Wang, S.; Tian, F.; Tang, Z.; Song, G.; Pan, Y.; He, B.; Bao, Q. Loss of imprinting of IGF2 correlates with hypomethylation of the H19 differentially methylated region in the tumor tissue of colorectal cancer patients. *Mol. Med. Rep.* **2012**, *5*, 1536–1540. [CrossRef]
100. Waterland, R.A.; Jirtle, R.L. Transposable Elements: Targets for Early Nutritional Effects on Epigenetic Gene Regulation. *Mol. Cell. Biol.* **2003**, *23*, 5293–5300. [CrossRef]
101. Zhang, L.; Lu, Q.; Chang, C. Epigenetics in Health and Disease. *Adv. Exp. Med. Biol.* **2020**, *1253*, 3–55. [CrossRef]
102. Heijmans, B.T.; Tobi, E.W.; Stein, A.D.; Putter, H.; Blauw, G.J.; Susser, E.S.; Slagboom, P.E.; Lumey, L.H. Persistent epigenetic differences associated with prenatal exposure to famine in humans. *Proc. Natl. Acad. Sci. USA* **2008**, *105*, 17046–17049. [CrossRef]
103. Vaiserman, A.; Lushchak, O. Prenatal famine exposure and adult health outcomes: An epigenetic link. *Environ. Epigenetics* **2021**, *7*, dvab013. [CrossRef] [PubMed]
104. Shamsi, M.B.; Firoz, A.S.; Imam, S.N.; Alzaman, N.; Samman, M.A. Epigenetics of human diseases and scope in future therapeutics. *J. Taibah Univ. Med Sci.* **2017**, *12*, 205–211. [CrossRef]
105. Schaub, B.; Liu, J.; Höppler, S.; Schleich, I.; Huehn, J.; Olek, S.; Wieczorek, G.; Illi, S.; von Mutius, E. Maternal farm exposure modulates neonatal immune mechanisms through regulatory T cells. *J. Allergy Clin. Immunol.* **2009**, *123*, 774–782.e5. [CrossRef]
106. Wei, L.; Vahedi, G.; Sun, H.-W.; Watford, W.T.; Takatori, H.; Ramos, H.L.; Takahashi, H.; Liang, J.; Gutierrez-Cruz, G.; Zang, C.; et al. Discrete Roles of STAT4 and STAT6 Transcription Factors in Tuning Epigenetic Modifications and Transcription during T Helper Cell Differentiation. *Immunity* **2010**, *32*, 840–851. [CrossRef] [PubMed]
107. Hodge, D.R.; Cho, E.; Copeland, T.D.; Guszczynski, T.; Yang, E.; Seth, A.K.; Farrar, W.L. IL-6 enhances the nuclear translocation of DNA cytosine-5-methyltransferase 1 (DNMT1) via phosphorylation of the nuclear localization sequence by the AKT kinase. *Cancer Genom. Proteom.* **2007**, *4*, 387–398.
108. Zijlstra, G.J.; Hacken, N.H.T.T.; Hoffmann, R.F.; van Oosterhout, A.J.M.; Heijink, I.H. Interleukin-17A induces glucocorticoid insensitivity in human bronchial epithelial cells. *Eur. Respir. J.* **2012**, *39*, 439–445. [CrossRef]
109. Ogryzko, V.V.; Schiltz, R.; Russanova, V.; Howard, B.H.; Nakatani, Y. The Transcriptional Coactivators p300 and CBP Are Histone Acetyltransferases. *Cell* **1996**, *87*, 953–959. [CrossRef]
110. Villagra, A.; Cheng, F.; Wang, H.-W.; Suarez, I.; Glozak, M.; Maurin, M.; Nguyen, D.; Wright, K.L.; Atadja, P.W.; Bhalla, K.; et al. The histone deacetylase HDAC11 regulates the expression of interleukin 10 and immune tolerance. *Nat. Immunol.* **2009**, *10*, 92–100, Erratum in *Nat. Immunol.* **2009**, *10*, 665. [CrossRef]
111. Xia, M.; Liu, J.; Wu, X.; Liu, S.; Li, G.; Han, C.; Song, L.; Li, Z.; Wang, Q.; Wang, J.; et al. Histone Methyltransferase Ash1l Suppresses Interleukin-6 Production and Inflammatory Autoimmune Diseases by Inducing the Ubiquitin-Editing Enzyme A20. *Immunity* **2013**, *39*, 470–481. [CrossRef]
112. Wilson, C.B.; Rowell, E.; Sekimata, M. Epigenetic control of T-helper-cell differentiation. *Nat. Rev. Immunol.* **2009**, *9*, 91–105. [CrossRef] [PubMed]
113. Ansel, K.M.; Lee, D.U.; Rao, A. An epigenetic view of helper T cell differentiation. *Nat. Immunol.* **2003**, *4*, 616–623. [CrossRef] [PubMed]
114. Lee, G.R.; Kim, S.T.; Spilianakis, C.; Fields, P.E.; Flavell, R.A. T Helper Cell Differentiation: Regulation by cis Elements and Epigenetics. *Immunity* **2006**, *24*, 369–379. [CrossRef] [PubMed]
115. Obata, Y.; Furusawa, Y.; Hase, K. Epigenetic modifications of the immune system in health and disease. *Immunol. Cell Biol.* **2015**, *93*, 226–232. [CrossRef]
116. Lee, C.-G.; Sahoo, A.; Im, S.-H. Epigenetic Regulation of Cytokine Gene Expression in T Lymphocytes. *Yonsei Med J.* **2009**, *50*, 322–330. [CrossRef]
117. David, A.L.; McIntosh, J.; Peebles, D.M.; Cook, T.; Waddington, S.; Weisz, B.; Wigley, V.; Abi-Nader, K.; Boyd, M.; Davidoff, A.M.; et al. Recombinant Adeno-Associated Virus-Mediated *In Utero* Gene Transfer Gives Therapeutic Transgene Expression in the Sheep. *Hum. Gene Ther.* **2011**, *22*, 419–426. [CrossRef]

118. Mattar, C.N.; Nathwani, A.C.; Waddington, S.N.; Dighe, N.; Kaeppel, C.; Nowrouzi, A.; Mcintosh, J.; Johana, N.B.; Ogden, B.; Fisk, N.M.; et al. Stable Human FIX Expression After 0.9G Intrauterine Gene Transfer of Self-complementary Adeno-associated Viral Vector 5 and 8 in Macaques. *Mol. Ther.* **2011**, *19*, 1950–1960. [CrossRef]
119. Piedimonte, G.; Harford, T. Effects of maternal–fetal transmission of viruses and other environmental agents on lung development. *Pediatr. Res.* **2020**, *87*, 420–426. [CrossRef]

Disclaimer/Publisher's Note: The statements, opinions and data contained in all publications are solely those of the individual author(s) and contributor(s) and not of MDPI and/or the editor(s). MDPI and/or the editor(s) disclaim responsibility for any injury to people or property resulting from any ideas, methods, instructions or products referred to in the content.

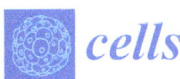

Article

Cannabinoid Mixture Affects the Fate and Functions of B Cells through the Modulation of the Caspase and MAP Kinase Pathways

Marie-Claude Lampron [1], Isabelle Paré [1], Mohammed Al-Zharani [2], Abdelhabib Semlali [3] and Lionel Loubaki [1,4,*]

[1] Héma-Québec, Medical Affairs and Innovation, 1070 Avenue des Sciences-de-la-Vie, Québec, QC G1V 5C3, Canada
[2] Department of Biology, College of Science, Imam Mohammad Ibn Saud Islamic University (IMSIU), Riyadh 11623, Saudi Arabia
[3] Groupe de Recherche en Écologie Buccale, Faculté de Médecine Dentaire, Université Laval, Québec, QC G1V 0A6, Canada
[4] Department of Biochemistry, Microbiology and Bioinformatics, Laval University, Québec, QC G1V 0A6, Canada
* Correspondence: lionel.loubaki@hema-quebec.qc.ca; Tel.: +1-418-780-4362

Abstract: Cannabis use is continuously increasing in Canada, raising concerns about its potential impact on immunity. The current study assessed the impact of a cannabinoid mixture (CM) on B cells and the mechanisms by which the CM exerts its potential anti-inflammatory properties. Peripheral blood mononuclear cells (PBMCs) were treated with different concentrations of the CM to evaluate cytotoxicity. In addition, flow cytometry was used to evaluate oxidative stress, antioxidant levels, mitochondrial membrane potential, apoptosis, caspase activation, and the activation of key signaling pathways (ERK1/2, NF-κB, STAT5, and p38). The number of IgM- and IgG-expressing cells was assessed using FluoroSpot, and the cytokine production profile of the B cells was explored using a cytokine array. Our results reveal that the CM induced B-cell cytotoxicity in a dose-dependent manner, which was mediated by apoptosis. The levels of ROS and those of the activated caspases, mitochondrial membrane potential, and DNA damage increased following exposure to the CM (3 µg/mL). In addition, the activation of MAP Kinase, STATs, and the NF-κB pathway and the number of IgM- and IgG-expressing cells were reduced following exposure to the CM. Furthermore, the exposure to the CM significantly altered the cytokine profile of the B cells. Our results suggest that cannabinoids have a detrimental effect on B cells, inducing caspase-mediated apoptosis.

Keywords: B cells; cannabinoids; apoptosis; caspase; oxidative stress

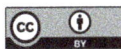

1. Introduction

Cannabis is the most widely used recreational drug in Canada. According to the Canadian Alcohol and Drugs Survey (CADS), the prevalence of cannabis use increased from 11% to 19% between 2017 and 2019 [1]. Cannabis is a complex plant containing ~500 phytochemicals, of which at least 60 belong to the phytocannabinoid class. These phytochemical compounds have shown therapeutic benefits as analgesics, anti-inflammatory agents, anti-emetics, and anticonvulsive agents, and they can improve muscle tone, mood state, cognition, and appetite [2,3].

Cannabinoids act through the endocannabinoid system (ECS), which includes the cannabinoid type 1 (CB1) and type 2 (CB2) receptors, their endogenous ligands (endocannabinoids), and the enzymes responsible for their synthesis and degradation [4]. Cannabinoids also modulate several non-cannabinoid receptors and ion channels, and they act through various receptor-independent pathways—for example, by delaying the reuptake of endocannabinoids and neurotransmitters (such as anandamide and adenosine) and by enhancing or inhibiting the binding of certain G-protein-coupled receptors to their ligands [4].

Cannabinoids affect various physiological processes, including the immune response. However, the effect of cannabinoids on immune cells is not well understood due to conflicting evidence. Cannabinoids have been shown to hinder the migration of leukocytes and the production of reactive oxygen species (ROS), and they have been shown to induce oxidative stress and the release of pro-inflammatory cytokines [5–9]. They can also limit the ability of macrophages to produce nitric oxide and IL-6 in response to lipopolysaccharides (LPSs), induce apoptosis in B and T cells, and reduce the cytolytic activity of natural killer (NK) cells [10–14]. However, cannabinoids have also been shown to stimulate the inflammatory response (mainly through their metabolites, which increase the secretion of some pro-inflammatory cytokines [15–18]) and promote the biosynthesis of eicosanoids, such as prostaglandins and leukotrienes (which are important mediators of inflammation) [19,20]. Of note, conflicting results have been reported regarding the effects of cannabinoids on B cells. El-Gohary et al. [21] reported that the oral ingestion of cannabis decreases the number of B cells, the serum levels of immunoglobulins (IgG and IgM), and the levels of the C3 and C4 complement proteins. By contrast, other studies have found no change in the number of B cells, an increase or decrease in IgE levels [22,23], a decrease in serum IgG levels, and an increase in IgD levels, with various impacts on IgA and IgM secretion [24,25]. Furthermore, one study reported that THC can cause a dose-dependent increase in B-cell proliferation [10,26], whereas other studies found that cannabinoids hinder B-cell proliferation in response to LPSs [26–29]. As we recently reported that a cannabinoid mixture (CM) can impair the quality of red blood cells (RBCs) and platelets by triggering RBC hemolysis and reducing platelet aggregation [30], we therefore wanted to assess the impact of exposure to a CM on B cells, as they produce antibodies, are involved in antigen presentation, and strongly express CB2 receptors (CB2Rs) [28], making them a cornerstone of the immune response.

2. Materials and Methods

2.1. Isolation and Storage of Peripheral Blood Mononuclear Cells

This study was approved by Héma-Québec's Research Ethics Committee (CER#2020-010), and all participants signed an informed consent form. Whole blood (450 mL) was collected using the Leukotrap® WB system (Haemonetics, Braintree, MA, USA) according to the manufacturer's instructions. Immediately after the blood donation, PBMCs were isolated using gradient centrifugation with a Ficoll-Paque solution (Cytiva, Vancouver, BC, Canada) and Leucosep tubes (Greiner Bio-One; Monroe, NC, USA) according to the manufacturer's instructions. PBMCs were collected and washed with DPBS (Thermo Fisher Scientific, Waltham, MA, USA) supplemented with 0.25% human albumin (CLS Behring, Ottawa, ON, Canada). The PBMCs were then suspended in a Plasma-Lyte solution (Baxter, Mississauga, ON, Canada) containing 5% human albumin and 18% CryoSure-Dex40 (WAK-Chemi medical, Steinbach, Germany), aliquoted, and frozen in liquid nitrogen for subsequent use.

2.2. Cell Culture and PBMC Exposure to a Cannabinoid Mixture

The PBMCs were thawed using the ThawSTAR™ system (BioLife Solutions, Bothell, WA, USA) and suspended in RPMI 1640 media (Thermo Fisher Scientific) supplemented with 20% fetal bovine serum (FBS; Thermo Fisher Scientific) and penicillin–streptomycin 1X (PEN/STREP; Sigma-Aldrich, St-Louis, MO, USA), and they were centrifuged for 10 min at $600 \times g$. The supernatant was discarded, and the cells were suspended in RPMI/20% FBS + PEN/STREP 1X at 1×10^6 cells/mL. The cells were then seeded in a 12-well plate (Sigma-Aldrich) and incubated for 3 hours at 37 °C/5% CO_2 to enable adherent cells to adhere. Then, different concentrations (ranging from 1 to 24 µg/mL) of the CM-8 components (#C-219, Cerilliant, Round Rock, TX, USA) or equivalent volume of methanol (MeOH; vehicle in which the CM is dissolved) were added to the required experimental conditions and incubated overnight at 37 °C/5% CO_2. This incubation time was based on the former blood donation deferral time after cannabis consumption that was used in our institution.

2.3. Cytotoxicity Assay

Following the cell culture and exposure to the CM, PBMC cytotoxicity was assessed through the quantification of lactate dehydrogenase (LDH) levels in the cell culture supernatant. Briefly, the PBMCs were suspended in RPMI/1% FBS + PEN/STREP 1X at 1×10^5 cells/mL and seeded in a 12-well plate (Sigma-Aldrich). The cells were then incubated for 3 hours at 37 °C/5% CO_2, before adding the CM or equivalent volume of MeOH, followed by an overnight incubation at 37 °C/5% CO_2. The cell supernatants were then collected for LDH quantification using a CyQUANT™ LDH Cytotoxicity Assay Kit (Cat#C20300, Fisher Scientific) according to the manufacturer instructions.

2.4. Apoptosis and CD45+/CD19+ Cell Count

In addition to cytotoxicity, PBMC apoptosis was assessed by using flow cytometry employing an Allophycocyanin (APC) conjugated-Annexin V Apoptosis Detection Kit (Cat# 640932; BioLegend, San Diego, CA, USA) according to the manufacturer's instructions. Furthermore, the number of CD45+/CD19+ cells was measured in each experimental condition of the dose-response assay. Briefly, following the overnight exposure to the CM, 50×10^3 cells were collected, washed in PBS, and stained with a fluorescein isothiocyanate (FITC)-conjugated anti-CD19 antibody (Clone HIB19; BD Biosciences, Franklin Lakes, NJ, USA) and an APC-conjugated anti-CD45 antibody (Clone HI20; BD Biosciences). Data were acquired using a BD Accuri™ C6 flow cytometer (BD Biosciences) and analyzed using FCS Express™ 6 software (De NovoSoftware, Los Angeles, CA, USA). Our gating strategy was as follows: first, all CD45+ cells were identified in a dot plot, and then CD19+ cells were identified in this population and the number of events enumerated. The acquisition volume was 200 µL.

2.5. Assessment of CB2R Expression

Along with the apoptosis assessment, the expression of CB2R was evaluated. Briefly, following the overnight exposure to the CM, 50×10^3 cells were collected, washed in PBS, and stained with a fluorescein isothiocyanate (FITC)-conjugated anti-CD19 antibody (Clone HIB19; BD Biosciences, Franklin Lakes, NJ, USA) and an Alexa Fluor® 647-conjugated Human Cannabinoid R2/CB2/CNR2 Antibody (Clone 352110R; R&D system). Data were acquired using the BD Accuri™ C6 flow cytometer (BD Biosciences) and analyzed using FCS Express™ 6 software (De NovoSoftware, Los Angeles, CA, USA). Our gating strategy was as follows: first, all CD19+ cells were identified in a dot plot, and then CB2R+ cells were identified in this population and the number of events enumerated.

2.6. Oxidative and Anti-Oxidative Stress Responses

To assess changes in the oxidative and anti-oxidative stress responses in B cells, PBMCs (with or without exposure to 3 µg/mL CM) were collected and stained with an APC-conjugated, anti-CD19 antibody (BD Biosciences) and exposed to CellROX™ Oxidative Stress Reagents (Cat# C10492, Thermo Fisher Scientific) according to the manufacturer's instructions. In addition, the anti-oxidative response was assessed by measuring the intracellular levels of glutathione (GSH) using an intracellular glutathione assay (Cat#9137, ImmunoChemistry, Davis, CA, USA) along with APC-conjugated, anti-CD19 antibody staining (BD Biosciences), according to the manufacturer's instructions. All data were acquired with the BD Accuri™ C6 flow cytometer (BD Biosciences) and analyzed using FCS Express™ 6 software (De Novo software). Our gating strategy was as follows: all cell populations were gated, and CD19+/ROS+ cells were identified in this population.

2.7. Mitochondrial Membrane Potential

To assess alterations in the mitochondrial membrane potential of B cells, PBMCs (with or without exposure to 3 μg/mL CM) were collected and stained using a MitoProbe™ DiOC2(3) Assay Kit (Cat# M34150, Thermo Fisher Scientific) along with an APC-conjugated, anti-CD19 antibody (BD Biosciences). All data were acquired with the BD Accuri™ C6 flow cytometer (BD Biosciences) and analyzed using FCS Express™ 6 software (De Novo software).

2.8. Apoptosis PCR Array

To investigate the differential expressions of apoptosis-related genes after exposure to the CM, real-time PCR was performed on purified B cells using an RT2 Profiler PCR Array for Human Apoptosis (cat#330231; PAHS-012ZD-6; Qiagen; Mississauga, ON, Canada). Briefly, PBMC (suspended in RPMI/20% FBS + PEN/STREP 1X at 1×10^6 cells/mL) were seeded in a 12-well plate (Sigma-Aldrich), incubated for 3 h at 37 °C/5% CO_2, and subsequently exposed to 3 μg/mL of the CM (Cerilliant) followed by an overnight incubation at 37 °C/5% CO_2. After the incubation, CD19+ cells were isolated using an EasySep™ Human B Cell Isolation Kit (cat#17954; Stemcell Technologies, Vancouver, BC, Canada) according to the manufacturer's instructions. Following isolation, the B cells from each experimental condition were transferred into a lysis buffer for total RNA extraction using a RiboPure™- Blood kit; (cat#AM1928; Thermo Fisher Scientific). The concentration and purity of the total RNA were assessed using a NanoDrop spectrophotometer (Thermo Fisher). The RNA was reverse-transcribed into cDNAs using a cDNA conversion kit (RT2 First Strand Kit; cat#330401; Qiagen), and a PCR array was performed using the SYBR Green master mix (cat#330504; Qiagen) along with an RT2 profiler plate. This plate was centrifuged for 1 min at $1000 \times g/25$ °C, and real-time PCR was carried out with a CFX-96 Real-Time PCR Detection System (Bio-Rad; Mississauga, ON, Canada) according to the manufacturer's instructions. The array measures the expressions of 84 key genes involved in apoptosis. Cycle threshold (CT) values were analyzed using the data analysis web portal at http://www.qiagen.com/geneglobe (accessed on 31 January 2023). The samples were assigned to control (untreated) and test groups (methanol and CM). The CT values were normalized based on a manual selection of reference genes. The data analysis web portal calculates the fold change/regulation using the delta-delta CT method, in which delta CT is calculated between a gene of interest and the average of several reference genes, followed by delta-delta CT calculations (Δ CT (Test Group)-Δ CT (Control Group)). The fold changes are then calculated as follows: $2^{(-\Delta\Delta CT)}$. The data analysis web portal also plots the heat map.

2.9. Assessment of Caspase Activation

To detect the activated caspases in the B cells, a Calbiochem® Caspase Detection Kit (FITC-VAD-FMK, cat#QIA90, Sigma-Aldrich) was used along with an APC-conjugated, anti-CD19 antibody (BD Biosciences). Briefly, PBMCs were cultured with or without 3 μg/mL CM as described above. Following the culture, the PBMCs were stained with the components of the detection kit and an anti-CD19 antibody (BD Biosciences). In addition, Z-VAD-FMK—a cell-permeable, irreversible pan-caspase inhibitor provided in the kit—was used to inhibit the caspase processing and apoptosis induced by the CM in the B cells. Data were acquired with the BD Accuri™ C6 flow cytometer (BD Biosciences). The gating strategy was as follows: first, all CD19+ cells were selected in a dot plot, and the activated caspases were identified in this CD19+ population.

2.10. Assessment of DNA Damage

Following the overnight exposure of the PBMCs to the CM (as described above), the PBMCs were collected and diluted at 5×10^5 cells/mL. Then, 50 μL of the cell suspension (25×10^3 cells) was transferred into flow cytometry tubes, DPBS + 2% FBS was added, and the cells were centrifuged for 5 min at $500 \times g$ at room temperature (RT). The cells were then fixed with a 1.5% paraformaldehyde solution (Sigma-Aldrich) for 20 min at RT, followed by a second wash with DPBS + 2% FBS. After the fixation step, the cells were permeabilized by exposing them to 90% methanol for 20 min at 4 °C. After another wash with DPBS + 2% FBS, the cells were stained with 5 µL of an Alexa Fluor® 488-conjugated, γH2AX antibody (Clone N1-431; BD Biosciences) and 20 µL of an APC-conjugated, CD19 antibody (BD Biosciences) for 20 min at RT. A final wash with DPBS + 2% FBS was performed before acquiring the data with the BD Accuri™ C6 flow cytometer (BD Biosciences). The gating strategy was as follows: first, all CD19+ cells were selected in a dot plot, and γH2AX+ cells were then identified in this CD19+ population.

2.11. Analysis of Cell Signaling Pathways

The signaling pathways involved in the development and functions of B cells were assessed using flow cytometry with the same protocol used to assess the DNA damage (described above). The only difference was the antibody used along with an FITC-conjugated, anti-CD19 antibody (BD Biosciences). For the assessment, 25×10^3 cells were stained using the following Alexa Fluor® 647 conjugated antibodies from BD Biosciences: phospho-NF-κB (Ser529; clone B33B4WP; Thermo Fisher Scientific), phospho-ERK1/2 (clone 20A), phospho-p38 (clone pT180/py182), and phospho-STAT5 (clone pY694). Data were acquired with the BD Accuri™ C6 flow cytometer. The gating strategy was as follows: cells were identified as CD19+ cells, and the cells positive for the aforementioned targets were identified in this CD19+ population. The data were analyzed using FCS Express™ 6 software (De Novo Software).

2.12. Detection and Enumeration of IgG-/IgM-Secreting B Cells

To evaluate the effect of the CM on B cells, a Human IgG/IgM Dual-Color B cell FluoroSpot kit (ELDB8079NL, R&D systems, Minneapolis, MN, USA) was used to quantify the IgG-/IgM-secreting cells according to the manufacturer's instructions. In total, 10^4 viable PBMCs (exposed or not exposed to the CM) were plated in each well of a 96-microplate provided in the kit. Images (6 pictures/well per condition) were acquired using an Olympus BX53 microscope equipped with a DP80 digital camera (Olympus, Shinjuku-ku, Tokyo, Japan) and they were analyzed using cellSens imaging software (Olympus).

2.13. Cytokine Expression Profiles of B Cells

Following exposure to the CM, the PBMCs were collected, and the B cells were isolated using an EasySep™ Human B Cell Isolation Kit (Stemcell Technologies) as described above. The B cells were then lysed in a cell lysis mix (Thermo Fisher Scientific), and the lysate was frozen for cytokine profiling. The amount of protein in each cell lysate was determined using a BCA Protein Assay (Thermo Fisher). The resulting data were used to normalize the results of the cytokine array, which was performed by Eve technologies Corp (Calgary, AB, Canada) using a Human Cytokine/Chemokine 71-Plex Discovery Assay® (HD71).

2.14. Statistical Analysis

All analyses were performed using GraphPad Prism 9.2.0 (GraphPad, San Diego, CA, USA). All values are reported as means ± standard errors of the mean, and statistical comparisons were carried out using a paired t-test, a Kruskal–Wallis test (i.e., a nonparametric ANOVA), a Wilcoxon matched-pairs signed-ranks test, or a Mann–Whitney test (where applicable). A p-value below 0.05 was considered statistically significant.

3. Results

3.1. Exposure to the Cannabinoid Mixture Favors B-Cell Apoptosis

Cannabinoids are detectable in the plasma within a few seconds after the first inhalation, and their bioavailability following inhalation varies widely (i.e., 2–56%), in part due to intra- and inter-subject variabilities in smoking dynamics causing some uncertainty in dose delivery [31,32]. Thus, doses were selected considering bioavailabilities of 2% (1 µg/mL),

6% (3 µg/mL), 12.5% (6 µg/mL), 25% (12 µg/mL), and 50% (24 µg/mL)—the equivalent of smoking 1 g of cannabis containing 24% of cannabinoids. This dose response revealed a dose-dependent increase in LDH levels, suggesting a significant cytotoxic effect of the CM on the PBMCs (Figure 1A). An Annexin V/PI analysis confirmed a dose-dependent increase in cell death in two specific PBMC subpopulations (P2 and P3) (Figure 1B,C), including B cells. The number of B cells was also significantly reduced at CM concentrations of at least 3 µg/mL (Figure 1D), which was associated with a significant decrease in the expression of CB2R (Figure 1E).

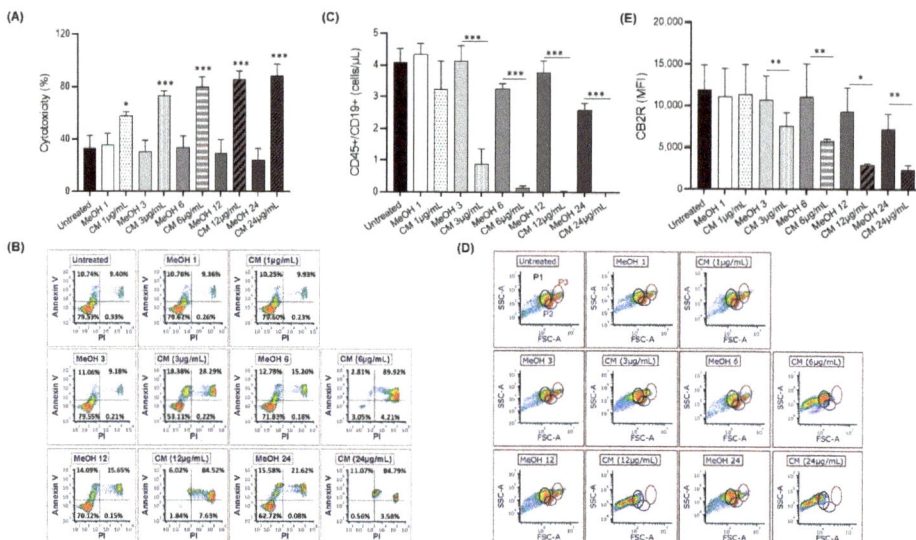

Figure 1. Cytotoxicity and Annexin V/PI expression after exposing PBMCs to a cannabinoid mixture. (**A**) PBMCs were exposed (or not) to different CM concentrations (1–24 µg/mL), and cytotoxicity was assessed using a lactate dehydrogenase assay. (**B**) Representative flow cytometry results of Annexin V/PI expression on PBMCs, which was measured to assess apoptosis following exposure to different doses of CM. (**C**) Representative flow cytometry results of the FSC/SSC profile of PBMCs following exposure to different CM concentrations. (**D**) Enumeration of B cells (CD45+/CD19+ cells) following exposure to different CM concentrations. (**E**) Expression of CB2R on B cells (CD19+/CB2R+ cells) following exposure to different CM concentrations. Data are presented as means and standard errors of the mean. * $p < 0.05$; ** $p < 0.001$; *** $p < 0.0001$. $n = 5$ experiments. CM = cannabinoid mixture; FSC = forward scatter; MeOH = methanol; SSC = side scatter. P1, P2, and P3 represent different populations of PBMCs.

3.2. Exposure to the Cannabinoid Mixture Significantly Reduces the Mitochondrial Membrane Potential of B Cells

We recently reported that a CM significantly increases the levels of ROS in oral cancer cells [33]. Therefore, we looked at ROS as a potential mechanism involved in the CM-induced death of B cells. From here on, we used the concentration of 3 µg/mL because, at this dose, we had a significant number of both living cells and cells undergoing apoptosis and not only dead cells. Thus, the cells were stained with an anti-CD19 antibody and a ROS marker. Exposure to 3 µg/mL CM significantly increased the intracellular levels of ROS in the CD19+ cells (Figure 2A), but it did not affect the anti-oxidative response (as measured via GSH levels) (Figure 2B).

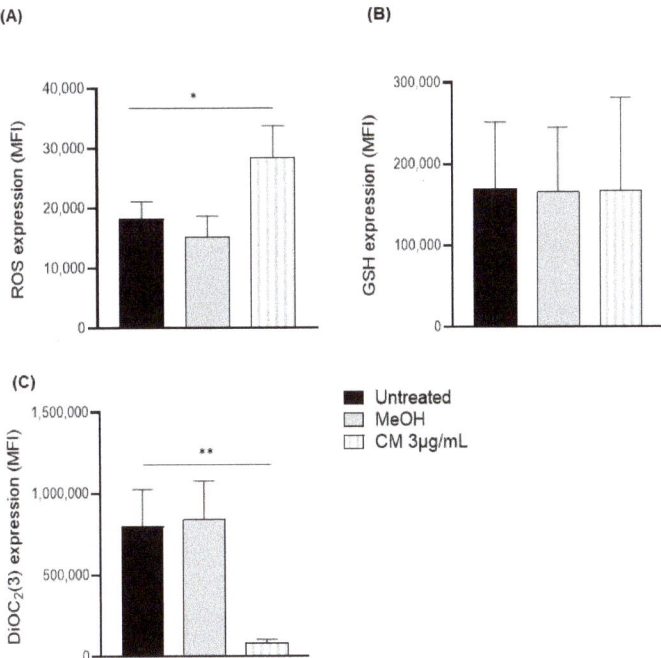

Figure 2. Response to oxidative and anti-oxidative stress, as well as mitochondrial membrane potential after exposing PBMCs to a cannabinoid mixture. PBMCs were exposed (or not) to 3 µg/mL of CM and stained with an APC-conjugated, anti-CD19 antibody and (**A**) treated with CellROX™ Oxidative Stress Reagents to measure ROS levels or (**B**) exposed to intracellular glutathione assay components to measure the anti-oxidative response via flow cytometry. (**C**) The mitochondrial membrane potential of CD19+ cells was also assessed via flow cytometry using a MitoProbe™ DiOC$_2$(3) Assay Kit. Data are presented as means and standard errors of the mean. * $p < 0.05$; ** $p < 0.001$. $n = 5$ experiments. CM = cannabinoid mixture; GSH = glutathione; MeOH = methanol; MFI = median fluorescence unit; ROS = reactive oxygen species.

Increased levels of ROS have been associated with mitochondrial damage [34]. Thus, using a MitoProbe™ DiOC$_2$(3) Assay Kit, we measured the mitochondrial membrane potential of the B cells (CD19+ cells). The CM also reduced the median fluorescence intensity (MFI) of the B cells by 10-fold (untreated: 797,704.9 ± 228,317.31; methanol: 839,641.2 ± 237,704.82 MFI; CM-treated: 79,188.6 ± 25,246.65 MFI) (Figure 2C).

3.3. The Cannabinoid Mixture Induces B-Cell Apoptosis through the Caspase Pathway

To identify the pathways involved in the CM-induced apoptosis of the B cells, we analyzed the expressions of 84 genes involved in apoptosis using a PCR array. The PBMCs were exposed to 3 µg/mL of the CM overnight, the B cells were isolated using an EasySep™ Human B Cell Isolation Kit, and their RNA was extracted. cDNAs were generated, and a real-time PCR was performed according to the manufacturer's instructions. Among the 84 genes analyzed, 3 were upregulated by ≥3-fold after exposure to the vehicle: LTBR (3.55-fold), TNFRSF1A (3.15-fold), and TNFRSF25 (4.34-fold). By contrast, after exposure to the CM, 27 were significantly upregulated compared with the untreated B cells: BAG1 (3.63-fold), BCL2L10 (7.07-fold), BIK (7.07-fold), BIRC5 (7.07-fold), CD40LG (5.63-fold), CIDEA (7.07-fold), CRADD (7.07-fold), CYCS (3.17-fold), DAPK1 (7.07-fold), FADD (3.20-fold), FASLG (7.07-fold), GADD45A (4.38-fold), HRK (3.60-fold), IL10 (3.10-fold), LTA (4.48-fold), LTBR (3.85-fold), NOL3 (7.07-fold), TNF (5.85-fold), TNFRSF11B (7.07-fold),

TNFRSF21 (13.11-fold), TNFRSF25 (8.95-fold), TNFSF8 (3.74-fold), TP73 (7.07-fold), TRADD (7.07-fold), TRAF3 (3.00-fold), and both CASP14 (7.07-fold) and CASP5 (7.07-fold) (Figure 3A).

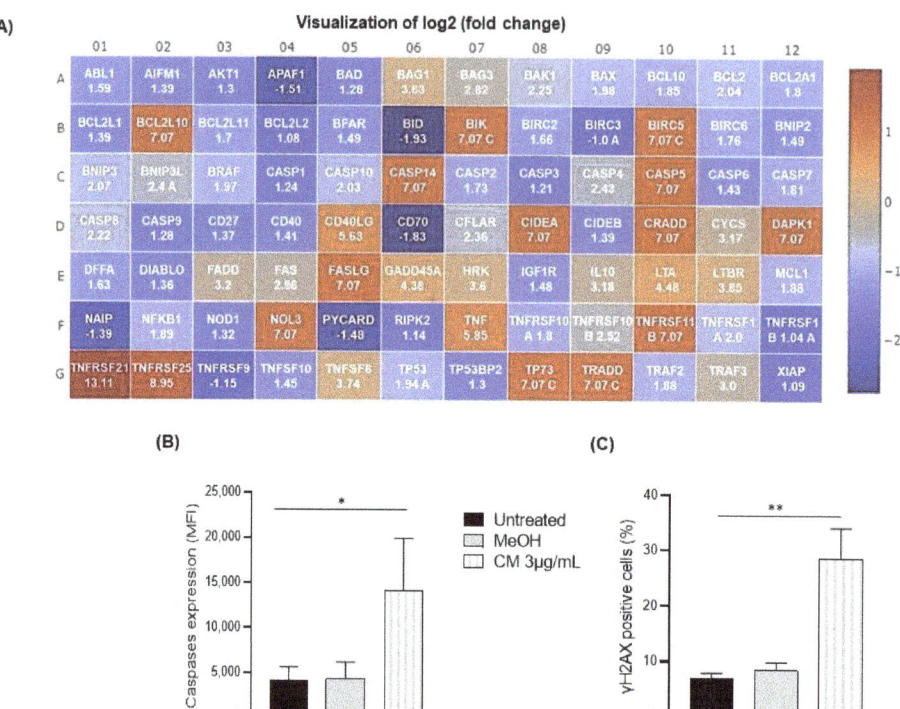

Figure 3. Apoptosis and DNA damage after exposing PBMCs to a cannabinoid mixture. PBMCs were exposed (or not) to 3 µg/mL of the CM, and B cells were isolated using an EasySep™ Human B Cell Isolation Kit. (A) Heatmap of CM compared to the untreated condition. (B) Activated caspase levels in CD19+ cells were assessed via flow cytometry using a Caspase Detection Kit. (C) DNA damage, as measured by the expression of γH2AX, was assessed via flow cytometry. Data are presented as means and standard errors of the mean. *: $p < 0.05$, **: $p < 0.001$. $n = 5$ experiments. CM = cannabinoid mixture; MeOH = methanol; MFI = median fluorescence unit.

Based on this finding, we explored the caspase pathway given its role in the initiation and execution of cell death [35]. A flow cytometry analysis of the activated caspases revealed a 4-fold increase in the level of activated caspase in the CM-treated B cells (22,068.7 ± 4433.30 MFI) compared to the untreated (5211.3 ± 1119.55 MFI) or vehicle-treated B cells (6424.3 ± 1900.61 MFI) (Figure 3B). In addition, we found that the CM potently increased the expression of the DNA damage marker γH2AX in the B cells by ~4-fold (untreated: 6.9 ± 0.95% of positive cells; methanol: 8.4 ± 1.42; CM: 28.7 ± 5.43% of positive cells; Figure 3C).

To confirm that caspase activation is involved in the CM-induced apoptosis of the B cells, PBMCs were treated with the pan caspase inhibitor Z-VAD-FMK and exposed to the CM. CM-induced B-cell death was significantly abrogated by the caspase inhibitor (untreated: 63.0 ± 10% of living cells; methanol: 63.2 ± 10.48% of living cells; CM: 19.4 ± 5.65; Z-VAD-FMK+ CM: 44.6 ± 11.63% of living cells, Figure 4A–C).

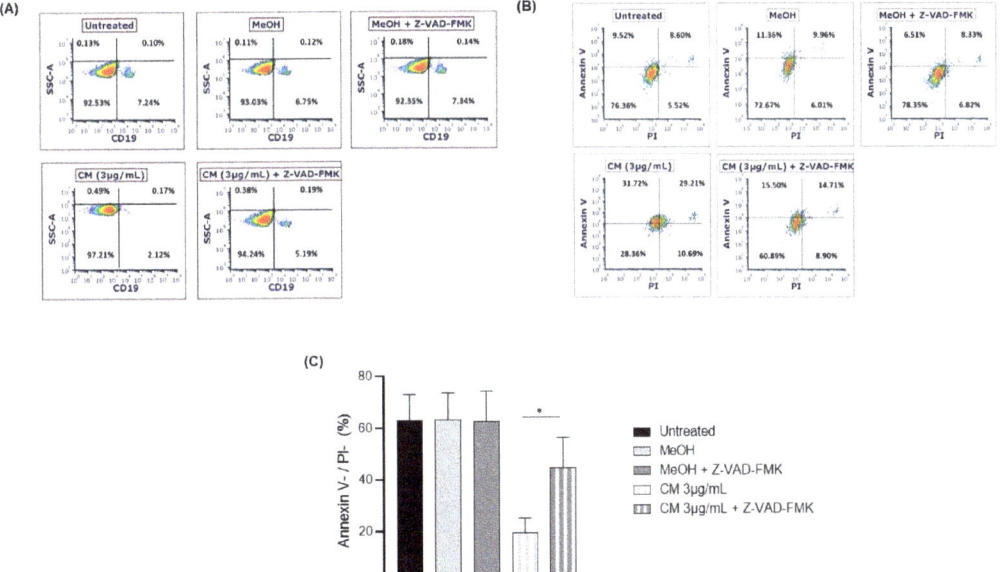

Figure 4. Death of B cells after co-treatment with the caspase inhibitor Z-VAD-FMK and the cannabinoid mixture. PBMCs were exposed (or not) to the caspase inhibitor Z-VAD-FMK and subsequently exposed (or not) to 3 µg/mL of the CM. After exposure to the CM, PBMCs were stained with an anti-CD19 antibody and (**A**) the persistence of the B-cell population, and (**B,C**) the levels of non-apoptotic cells (i.e., Annexin V/PI levels) were measured. Data are presented as means and standard errors of the mean. *: $p < 0.05$. $n = 5$ experiments. CM = cannabinoid mixture; FSC = forward scatter; MeOH = methanol; SSC = side scatter.

3.4. The Cannabinoid Mixture Affects B-Cell Signaling Pathways and Function

ERK, NF-κB, STAT5, and p38 have been shown to play important roles in B-cell proliferation, differentiation, survival, and immunoglobulin production [36–39]. Thus, we explored the phosphorylation of these key signaling molecules. The CM reduced the phosphorylation of ERK1/2 (untreated: 61% ± 6.96% of positive cells; methanol: 58.45% ± 5.75; CM: 18.7% ± 9.03% of positive cells); of NF-κB (untreated: 68.8% ± 3.60% of positive cells; methanol: 67.6% ± 5.31; CM: 18.1% ± 3.22% of positive cells); of STAT5 (untreated: 63.1% ± 5.34% of positive cells; methanol: 53.4% ± 2.95; CM: 7.5% ± 1.8% of positive cells); and of p38 (untreated: 32.4% ± 4.75% of positive cells; methanol: 37.7% ± 5.83%; CM: 8% ± 2.65% of positive cells; Figure 5A), which was associated with a significant reduction in the number of IgM- and IgG-expressing B cells (Figure 5B–D).

3.5. The Cannabinoid Mixture Affects the Cytokine Secretion Profile of B Cells

Using a Human Cytokine/Chemokine 71-Plex Discovery Assay® (HD71), we analyzed how the CM affects the cytokine secretion profile of B cells. Our results reveal that twenty-one (21) cytokines, including IL-6 and TNF-α, were not detected. Eighteen (17) cytokines were not modulated ($n = 17$), while thirteen cytokines (13), including RANTES and IL-27, were downregulated. Finally, eight (8) cytokines, including IFN-α2 and CXCL9, were upregulated ($n = 5$) (Figure 6).

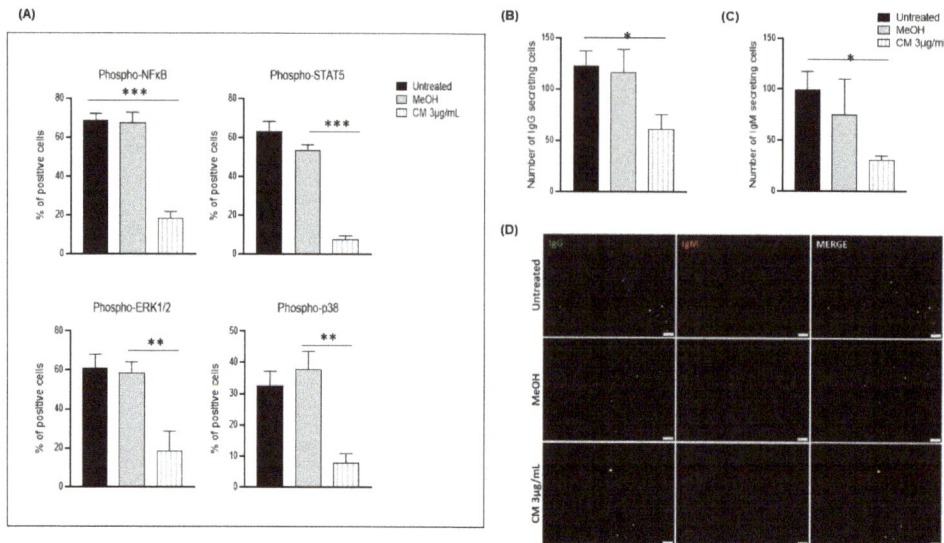

Figure 5. MAP Kinase, NF-κB, and STAT signaling pathways after exposing PBMCs to the cannabinoid mixture. PBMCs were exposed (or not) to 3 μg/mL of the CM and co-stained with an APC-conjugated, anti-CD19 antibody coupled with Alexa Fluor® 647-conjugated phospho-NF-κB, phospho-ERK1/2, phospho-p38, or phospho-STAT5 antibodies. (**A**) Representative histograms of the expressions of the aforementioned proteins with and without CM exposure. Number of (**B**) IgG-secreting cells and (**C**) number of IgM-secreting cells were quantified using FluoroSpot. (**D**) Representative fluorescence microscopy image of IgG- and IgM-secreting cells. Data are presented as means and standard errors of the mean. *: $p < 0.05$. ** $p < 0.001$; *** $p < 0.0001$. $n = 5$ experiments. CM = cannabinoid mixture; MeOH = methanol; UT = untreated.

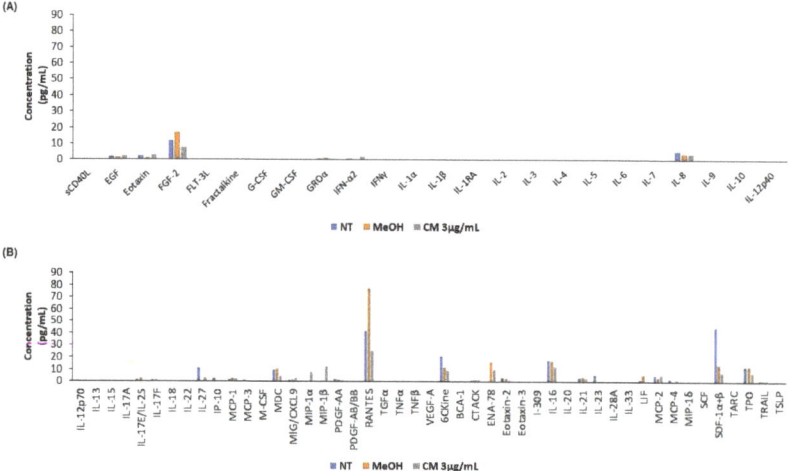

Figure 6. Cytokine profile after exposing B cells to the cannabinoid mixture. PBMCs were exposed (or not) to 3 μg/mL of CM, and B cells were isolated using an EasySep™ Human B Cell Isolation Kit. B cells were then lysed, and a cytokine array was performed. (**A**,**B**) Representative histograms of the expression of the 71 proteins tested by the cytokine array.

4. Discussion

We recently reported that a CM impairs the quality of RBCs and platelets by triggering RBC hemolysis and reducing platelet aggregation [30]. However, to the best of our knowledge, the effects of a CM on B-cell cytotoxicity and the pathways driving cell death have not been investigated. Here, we showed that exposing PBMCs to various concentrations of a CM (1–24 µg/mL) caused significant cytotoxicity to B cells and limited their ability to produce immunoglobulins.

Cannabinoids are detectable in the plasma within a few seconds after the first inhalation, and their concentration peaks within 3-10 minutes [40,41]. They are quickly eliminated by pyrolysis, and their bioavailability following inhalation varies widely (i.e., 2−56%) [31,32,42]. For example, it has been found that, six minutes after the inhalation of 13 mg of THC (i.e., 2.5×10^{19} THC molecules), only 2.8% of this THC (1.4×10^{14} molecules/mL) is detectable in the plasma [31]. Moreover, it has also been found that, one minute after intravenously administering a single bolus of 5 mg of THC (i.e., 9.55×10^{18} molecules), the plasma concentration of THC is 4.28×10^{14} molecules/mL [43], suggesting the rapid elimination of cannabinoids and, more importantly, a large difference between the administered dose and that measured in the blood.

Given this evidence, we selected concentrations corresponding to bioavailabilities of 2% (1 µg/mL), 6% (3 µg/mL), 12.5% (6 µg/mL), 24% (12 µg/mL), and 50% (24 µg/mL), which equate to inhaling a joint containing 1 g of cannabis with 24% of cannabinoids. Using this range of concentrations, the CM induced cytotoxicity in a dose-dependent manner in the PBMCs, particularly in the B cells. Indeed, we observed that the CM significantly reduced the number of B cells, which is consistent with a previous study conducted by El-Gohary et al. [21], who reported that cannabis users have lower PBMC, T-cell, B-cell, and NK-cell counts than non-users. This cytotoxicity may be explained by the expressions of the cannabinoid receptors on immune cells, particularly that of CB2R, which is known to mediate most of the immunosuppressive effects of the ECS [20,44] and is highly expressed on the surface of B cells [28]. This hypothesis is further supported by the significant reduction in the expression of CB2R following the exposure to the CM, suggesting that its activation occurs through an internalization mechanism, as reported by Atwood et al. [45].

Based on the dose response of the CM, we decided to continue all our experiments with the concentration of 3 µg/mL because this allowed us to have both living cells and cells undergoing apoptosis, which is in line with our goal of documenting the mechanism involved in CM-induced B-cell death. Thus, to explore the mechanisms involved in CM-induced B-cell death, we assessed the production of ROS, since cannabinoids have been shown to induce apoptosis in human monocytes through an increased production of ROS and the disruption of mitochondrial integrity [46]. Thus, as expected, the CM significantly reduced the mitochondrial membrane potential, which resulted in a mitochondrial free radical leak and, thus, explains the increase in the levels of intracellular ROS. Of interest, a similar increase in oxidative stress has been reported in synthetic cannabinoid users [47]. In addition to the increase in the production of ROS, no modulation of the anti-oxidative response (GSH) was observed, which suggests that an imbalance in redox homeostasis is a mechanism involved in the B-cell apoptosis observed herein. Indeed, the expressions of 27 genes involved in apoptosis were significantly altered after exposure to the CM, including those of caspases, which we further explored given their roles in the initiation and execution of cell death [35,48]. As expected, the CM significantly increased the levels of activated caspases. Further, apoptosis was abrogated when the PBMCs were co-treated with the pan caspase inhibitor Z-VAD-FMK, thus confirming the roles of caspases in the CM-induced apoptosis of the B cells. However, this inhibition was not complete, which suggests the involvement of other mechanisms in addition to caspases. This hypothesis is supported by the findings obtained by McKallip et al. [14], who reported that the exposure of mice (in vivo) to a pan caspase inhibitor prior to THC administration partially blocked the apoptotic effects of THC, which also suggests the involvement of mechanisms other than caspases, as well as supporting the findings of our apoptosis gene array.

The study of the intracellular signaling pathways in the B cells, carried out to characterize the molecular events responsible for the functional modifications that are elicited in these cells following exposure to the CM, revealed a reduction in the levels of phosphorylated ERK1/2, NF-κB, STAT5, and p38, which are involved in B-cell proliferation, differentiation, survival, and immunoglobulin production [36–39]. More specifically, ERK1/2 phosphorylation is one of the signaling events that canonically occurs following CB2R stimulation by an agonist; it may be considered a biomarker to verify CB2R activation, and it also plays a key role in the efficient generation of IgG-bearing B cells by promoting their survival [36,49]. In addition, the phosphorylation of NF-κB, which is important for B-cell maturation and activation, mediated through the B-cell receptor (BCR) [39,50], was reduced by exposure to the CM, thus suggesting the potential ability of cannabinoids to impair B-cell activation. Furthermore, the phosphorylation of STAT5 and p38, which have been reported to regulate B-cell proliferation and survival, was also reduced following exposure to the CM [37,38]. Together, these data could explain the significantly reduced number of IgG- and IgM-expressing cells reported herein, which was associated with the downregulated levels of cytokines that are involved in B-cell immunoglobulin production, such as RANTES and IL-27 [51,52], while some cytokines, such as IFN-α2, which lower the threshold for B-cell activation, were upregulated, probably as a compensatory mechanism [53]. We can also talk about another potential compensatory mechanism which is the increase in the expression of CXCL9 with the aim to maintain the expression of its receptor CXCR3 given its role in the differentiation of B cells [54].

Taken together, these results suggest that cannabinoids exert negative impacts on key aspects of B-cell fate and the immune response in general. They also raise concerns about the ability of cannabis users to effectively fight certain infections. Indeed, cannabis users have been reported to have a higher risk of fungal exposure (as cannabis may contain inhalable Aspergillus organisms) and infection associated with an increased variety of immunologic lung disorders [55–57]. Furthermore, these detrimental effects were observed following exposure to a concentration as low as 3 μg/mL, which suggests, as also observed by Melèn et al. [58], that even occasional cannabis users might exhibit (transitory) B-cell death.

5. Conclusions

To the best of our knowledge, this study provides the first evidence that a brief (in vitro) exposure of PBMCs to a CM impairs their survival and function. Specifically, the CM triggered B-cell death in a dose-dependent manner, despite being rapidly eliminated. Although our in vitro model likely reproduces several features of cannabis use, further studies conducted in cannabis users are required to confirm and better understand the impact of cannabis use on the immune system.

Author Contributions: Conceptualization, L.L. and A.S.; methodology, L.L., M.A.-Z. and A.S.; formal analysis, M.-C.L. and L.L.; investigation, M.-C.L. and L.L.; resources, L.L. and A.S.; data curation, M.-C.L. and I.P.; writing—original draft preparation, L.L. and M.-C.L.; writing—review and editing, M.-C.L., L.L., A.S. and M.A.-Z.; project administration, L.L. All authors have read and agreed to the published version of the manuscript.

Funding: This project was funded by Héma-Québec (AMI-33424) and by the Deanship of Scientific Research at Imam Mohammed Ibn Saoud Islamic University (IMSIU) through Research Partnership Program no. RP-21-09-87.

Institutional Review Board Statement: The study was conducted in accordance with the Declaration of Helsinki and approved by the Institutional Review Board (or Ethics Committee) of Héma-Québec (protocol code CER#2020-010, approved on 02-03-2020).

Informed Consent Statement: Informed consent was obtained from all subjects involved in the study.

Data Availability Statement: Not applicable.

Acknowledgments: We acknowledge Tony Tremblay for cannabinoid quantification and Samuel Rochette for discussion on the manuscript and English editing. The authors extend their appreciation to the Deanship of Scientific Research at Imam Mohammed IBN Saud Islamic University (IMSIU) for funding and supporting this work through Research Partnership Program no. RP-21-09-87.

Conflicts of Interest: The authors declare no conflict of interest.

References

1. Canadian Alcohol and Drugs Survey (CADS): Summary of Results for 2019. Available online: https://www.canada.ca/en/health-canada/services/canadian-alcohol-drugs-survey/2019summary.html (accessed on 25 November 2022).
2. Henshaw, F.R.; Dewsbury, L.S.; Lim, C.K.; Steiner, G.Z. The Effects of Cannabinoids on Pro- and Anti-Inflammatory Cytokines: A Systematic Review of *In Vivo* Studies. *Cannabis Cannabinoid Res.* **2021**, *6*, 177–195. [CrossRef] [PubMed]
3. Andre, C.M.; Hausman, J.-F.; Guerriero, G. Cannabis Sativa: The Plant of the Thousand and One Molecules. *Front. Plant Sci.* **2016**, *7*, 19. [CrossRef]
4. Argenziano, M.; Tortora, C.; Bellini, G.; Di Paola, A.; Punzo, F.; Rossi, F. The Endocannabinoid System in Pediatric Inflammatory and Immune Diseases. *Int. J. Mol. Sci.* **2019**, *20*, 5875, Erratum in *IJMS* **2020**, *21*, 2757. [CrossRef]
5. Begg, M.; Pacher, P.; Batkai, S.; Oseihyiaman, D.; Offertaler, L.; Mo, F.; Liu, J.; Kunos, G. Evidence for Novel Cannabinoid Receptors. *Pharmacol. Ther.* **2005**, *106*, 133–145. [CrossRef] [PubMed]
6. Cencioni, M.T.; Chiurchiù, V.; Catanzaro, G.; Borsellino, G.; Bernardi, G.; Battistini, L.; Maccarrone, M. Anandamide Suppresses Proliferation and Cytokine Release from Primary Human T-Lymphocytes Mainly via CB_2 Receptors. *PLoS ONE* **2010**, *5*, e8688. [CrossRef]
7. Coopman, K.; Smith, L.D.; Wright, K.L.; Ward, S.G. Temporal Variation in CB2R Levels Following T Lymphocyte Activation: Evidence That Cannabinoids Modulate CXCL12-Induced Chemotaxis. *Int. Immunopharmacol.* **2007**, *7*, 360–371. [CrossRef] [PubMed]
8. McHugh, D.; Tanner, C.; Mechoulam, R.; Pertwee, R.G.; Ross, R.A. Inhibition of Human Neutrophil Chemotaxis by Endogenous Cannabinoids and Phytocannabinoids: Evidence for a Site Distinct from CB_1 and CB_2. *Mol. Pharm.* **2008**, *73*, 441–450. [CrossRef] [PubMed]
9. Ortega-Gutiérrez, S.; Molina-Holgado, E.; Guaza, C. Effect of Anandamide Uptake Inhibition in the Production of Nitric Oxide and in the Release of Cytokines in Astrocyte Cultures. *Glia* **2005**, *52*, 163–168. [CrossRef]
10. Carayon, P.; Marchand, J.; Dussossoy, D.; Derocq, J.M.; Jbilo, O.; Bord, A.; Bouaboula, M.; Galiègue, S.; Mondière, P.; Pénarier, G.; et al. Modulation and Functional Involvement of CB2 Peripheral Cannabinoid Receptors during B-Cell Differentiation. *Blood* **1998**, *92*, 3605–3615. [CrossRef]
11. Schatz, A.R.; Lee, M.; Condie, R.B.; Pulaski, J.T.; Kaminski, N.E. Cannabinoid Receptors CB1 and CB2: A Characterization of Expression and Adenylate Cyclase Modulation within the Immune System. *Toxicol. Appl. Pharm.* **1997**, *142*, 278–287. [CrossRef]
12. Chang, Y.H.; Lee, S.T.; Lin, W.W. Effects of Cannabinoids on LPS-Stimulated Inflammatory Mediator Release from Macrophages: Involvement of Eicosanoids. *J. Cell Biochem.* **2001**, *81*, 715–723. [CrossRef] [PubMed]
13. Nagarkatti, P.; Pandey, R.; Rieder, S.A.; Hegde, V.L.; Nagarkatti, M. Cannabinoids as Novel Anti-Inflammatory Drugs. *Future Med. Chem.* **2009**, *1*, 1333–1349. [CrossRef] [PubMed]
14. McKallip, R.J.; Lombard, C.; Martin, B.R.; Nagarkatti, M.; Nagarkatti, P.S. Δ^9-Tetrahydrocannabinol-Induced Apoptosis in the Thymus and Spleen as a Mechanism of Immunosuppression In Vitro and In Vivo. *J. Pharm. Exp.* **2002**, *302*, 451–465. [CrossRef] [PubMed]
15. Krishnan, G.; Chatterjee, N. Endocannabinoids Alleviate Proinflammatory Conditions by Modulating Innate Immune Response in Muller Glia during Inflammation. *Glia* **2012**, *60*, 1629–1645. [CrossRef] [PubMed]
16. Berdyshev, E.V.; Boichot, E.; Germain, N.; Allain, N.; Anger, J.-P.; Lagente, V. Influence of Fatty Acid Ethanolamides and Δ9-Tetrahydrocannabinol on Cytokine and Arachidonate Release by Mononuclear Cells. *Eur. J. Pharmacol.* **1997**, *330*, 231–240. [CrossRef]
17. Mukhopadhyay, P.; Pan, H.; Rajesh, M.; Bátkai, S.; Patel, V.; Harvey-White, J.; Mukhopadhyay, B.; Haskó, G.; Gao, B.; Mackie, K.; et al. CB_1 Cannabinoid Receptors Promote Oxidative/Nitrosative Stress, Inflammation and Cell Death in a Murine Nephropathy Model: CB_1 Antagonists for Nephropathy. *Br. J. Pharmacol.* **2010**, *160*, 657–668. [CrossRef] [PubMed]
18. Khoury, M.; Cohen, I.; Bar-Sela, G. "The Two Sides of the Same Coin"—Medical Cannabis, Cannabinoids and Immunity: Pros and Cons Explained. *Pharmaceutics* **2022**, *14*, 389. [CrossRef]
19. Ricciotti, E.; FitzGerald, G.A. Prostaglandins and Inflammation. *ATVB* **2011**, *31*, 986–1000. [CrossRef]
20. Turcotte, C.; Chouinard, F.; Lefebvre, J.S.; Flamand, N. Regulation of Inflammation by Cannabinoids, the Endocannabinoids 2-Arachidonoyl-Glycerol and Arachidonyl-Ethanolamide, and Their Metabolites. *J. Leukoc. Biol.* **2015**, *97*, 1049–1070. [CrossRef]
21. El-Gohary, M.; Eid, M.A. Effect of Cannabinoid Ingestion (in the Form of Bhang) on the Immune System of High School and University Students. *Hum. Exp. Toxicol.* **2004**, *23*, 149–156. [CrossRef]
22. Rachelefsky, G.S.; Opelz, G.; Mickey, M.R.; Lessin, P.; Kiuchi, M.; Silverstein, M.J.; Stiehm, E.R. Intact Humoral and Cell-Mediated Immunity in Chronic Marijuana Smoking. *J. Allergy Clin. Immunol.* **1976**, *58*, 483–490. [CrossRef] [PubMed]

23. Newton, C.A.; Klein, T.W. Cannabinoid 2 (CB2) Receptor Involvement in the down-Regulation but Not up-Regulation of Serum IgE Levels in Immunized Mice. *J. Neuroimmune Pharm.* **2012**, *7*, 591–598. [CrossRef]
24. Nahas, G.G.; Osserman, E.F. Altered Serum Immunoglobulin Concentration in Chronic Marijuana Smokers. In *Drugs of Abuse, Immunity, and Immunodeficiency*; Friedman, H., Specter, S., Klein, T.W., Eds.; Advances in Experimental Medicine and Biology; Springer: Boston, MA, USA, 1991; Volume 288, pp. 25–32. ISBN 978-1-4684-5927-2.
25. Ngaotepprutaram, T.; Kaplan, B.L.F.; Carney, S.; Crawford, R.; Kaminski, N.E. Suppression by Δ9-Tetrahydrocannabinol of the Primary Immunoglobulin M Response by Human Peripheral Blood B Cells Is Associated with Impaired STAT3 Activation. *Toxicology* **2013**, *310*, 84–91. [CrossRef]
26. Derocq, J.M.; Ségui, M.; Marchand, J.; Le Fur, G.; Casellas, P. Cannabinoids Enhance Human B-Cell Growth at Low Nanomolar Concentrations. *FEBS Lett.* **1995**, *369*, 177–182. [CrossRef]
27. Klein, T.W.; Newton, C.A.; Widen, R.; Friedman, H. The Effect of Delta-9-Tetrahydrocannabinol and 11-Hydroxy-Delta-9-Tetrahydrocannabinol on T-Lymphocyte and B-Lymphocyte Mitogen Responses. *J. Immunopharmacol.* **1985**, *7*, 451–466. [CrossRef]
28. Croxford, J.L.; Yamamura, T. Cannabinoids and the Immune System: Potential for the Treatment of Inflammatory Diseases? *J. Neuroimmunol.* **2005**, *166*, 3–18. [CrossRef] [PubMed]
29. Tanasescu, R.; Constantinescu, C.S. Cannabinoids and the Immune System: An Overview. *Immunobiology* **2010**, *215*, 588–597. [CrossRef] [PubMed]
30. Lampron, M.-C.; Desbiens-Tremblay, C.; Loubaki, L. In Vitro Exposure of Whole Blood to a Cannabinoid Mixture Impairs the Quality of Red Blood Cells and Platelets. *Blood Transfus.* **2022**. [CrossRef]
31. Nahas, G.G. The Pharmacokinetics of THC in Fat and Brain: Resulting Functional Responses to Marihuana Smoking. *Hum. Psychopharmacol. Clin. Exp.* **2001**, *16*, 247–255. [CrossRef]
32. Huestis, M.A. Human Cannabinoid Pharmacokinetics. *Chem. Biodivers.* **2007**, *4*, 1770–1804. [CrossRef]
33. Loubaki, L.; Rouabhia, M.; Zahrani, M.A.; Amri, A.A.; Semlali, A. Oxidative Stress and Autophagy Mediate Anti-Cancer Properties of Cannabis Derivatives in Human Oral Cancer Cells. *Cancers* **2022**, *14*, 4924. [CrossRef] [PubMed]
34. Li, X.; Fang, P.; Mai, J.; Choi, E.T.; Wang, H.; Yang, X. Targeting Mitochondrial Reactive Oxygen Species as Novel Therapy for Inflammatory Diseases and Cancers. *J. Hematol. Oncol.* **2013**, *6*, 19. [CrossRef] [PubMed]
35. Lopez, K.E.; Bouchier-Hayes, L. Lethal and Non-Lethal Functions of Caspases in the DNA Damage Response. *Cells* **2022**, *11*, 1887. [CrossRef] [PubMed]
36. Sanjo, H.; Hikida, M.; Aiba, Y.; Mori, Y.; Hatano, N.; Ogata, M.; Kurosaki, T. Extracellular Signal-Regulated Protein Kinase 2 Is Required for Efficient Generation of B Cells Bearing Antigen-Specific Immunoglobulin G. *Mol. Cell Biol.* **2007**, *27*, 1236–1246. [CrossRef] [PubMed]
37. Heltemes-Harris, L.M.; Farrar, M.A. The Role of STAT5 in Lymphocyte Development and Transformation. *Curr. Opin. Immunol.* **2012**, *24*, 146–152. [CrossRef] [PubMed]
38. Khiem, D.; Cyster, J.G.; Schwarz, J.J.; Black, B.L. A P38 MAPK-MEF2C Pathway Regulates B-Cell Proliferation. *Proc. Natl. Acad. Sci. USA* **2008**, *105*, 17067–17072. [CrossRef]
39. Sasaki, Y.; Iwai, K. Roles of the NF-кB Pathway in B-Lymphocyte Biology. In *B Cell Receptor Signaling*; Kurosaki, T., Wienands, J., Eds.; Current Topics in Microbiology and Immunology; Springer International Publishing: Cham, Germany, 2015; Volume 393, pp. 177–209. ISBN 978-3-319-26131-7.
40. Owens, S.M.; McBay, A.J.; Reisner, H.M.; Perez-Reyes, M. 125I Radioimmunoassay of Delta-9-Tetrahydrocannabinol in Blood and Plasma with a Solid-Phase Second-Antibody Separation Method. *Clin. Chem.* **1981**, *27*, 619–624. [CrossRef]
41. Vandevenne, M.; Vandenbussche, H.; Verstraete, A. Detection Time of Drugs of Abuse in Urine. *Acta Clin. Belg.* **2000**, *55*, 323–333. [CrossRef]
42. Vandrey, R.; Herrmann, E.S.; Mitchell, J.M.; Bigelow, G.E.; Flegel, R.; LoDico, C.; Cone, E.J. Pharmacokinetic Profile of Oral Cannabis in Humans: Blood and Oral Fluid Disposition and Relation to Pharmacodynamic Outcomes. *J. Anal. Toxicol.* **2017**, *41*, 83–99. [CrossRef]
43. Agurell, S.; Halldin, M.; Lindgren, J.E.; Ohlsson, A.; Widman, M.; Gillespie, H.; Hollister, L. Pharmacokinetics and Metabolism of Delta 1-Tetrahydrocannabinol and Other Cannabinoids with Emphasis on Man. *Pharm. Rev.* **1986**, *38*, 21–43.
44. Capozzi, A.; Caissutti, D.; Mattei, V.; Gado, F.; Martellucci, S.; Longo, A.; Recalchi, S.; Manganelli, V.; Riitano, G.; Garofalo, T.; et al. Anti-Inflammatory Activity of a CB2 Selective Cannabinoid Receptor Agonist: Signaling and Cytokines Release in Blood Mononuclear Cells. *Molecules* **2021**, *27*, 64. [CrossRef]
45. Atwood, B.K.; Wager-Miller, J.; Haskins, C.; Straiker, A.; Mackie, K. Functional Selectivity in CB_2 Cannabinoid Receptor Signaling and Regulation: Implications for the Therapeutic Potential of CB_2 Ligands. *Mol. Pharm.* **2012**, *81*, 250–263. [CrossRef]
46. Wu, H.-Y.; Huang, C.-H.; Lin, Y.-H.; Wang, C.-C.; Jan, T.-R. Cannabidiol Induced Apoptosis in Human Monocytes through Mitochondrial Permeability Transition Pore-Mediated ROS Production. *Free Radic. Biol. Med.* **2018**, *124*, 311–318. [CrossRef] [PubMed]
47. Guler, E.; Bektay, M.; Akyildiz, A.; Sisman, B.; Izzettin, F.; Kocyigit, A. Investigation of DNA Damage, Oxidative Stress, and Inflammation in Synthetic Cannabinoid Users. *Hum. Exp. Toxicol.* **2020**, *39*, 1454–1462. [CrossRef] [PubMed]
48. Lombard, C.; Nagarkatti, M.; Nagarkatti, P. CB2 Cannabinoid Receptor Agonist, JWH-015, Triggers Apoptosis in Immune Cells: Potential Role for CB2-Selective Ligands as Immunosuppressive Agents. *Clin. Immunol.* **2007**, *122*, 259–270. [CrossRef]

49. Wang, J.; Xu, J.; Peng, Y.; Xiao, Y.; Zhu, H.; Ding, Z.-M.; Hua, H. Phosphorylation of Extracellular Signal-Regulated Kinase as a Biomarker for Cannabinoid Receptor 2 Activation. *Heliyon* **2018**, *4*, e00909. [CrossRef] [PubMed]
50. Barnabei, L.; Laplantine, E.; Mbongo, W.; Rieux-Laucat, F.; Weil, R. NF-KB: At the Borders of Autoimmunity and Inflammation. *Front. Immunol.* **2021**, *12*, 716469. [CrossRef] [PubMed]
51. Kimata, H.; Yoshida, A.; Ishioka, C.; Fujimoto, M.; Lindley, I.; Furusho, K. RANTES and Macrophage Inflammatory Protein 1 Alpha Selectively Enhance Immunoglobulin (IgE) and IgG4 Production by Human B Cells. *J. Exp. Med.* **1996**, *183*, 2397–2402. [CrossRef]
52. Morita, Y.; Masters, E.A.; Schwarz, E.M.; Muthukrishnan, G. Interleukin-27 and Its Diverse Effects on Bacterial Infections. *Front. Immunol.* **2021**, *12*, 678515. [CrossRef] [PubMed]
53. Braun, D.; Caramalho, I.; Demengeot, J. IFN-α/β Enhances BCR-dependent B Cell Responses. *Int. Immunol.* **2002**, *14*, 411–419. [CrossRef]
54. Muehlinghaus, G.; Cigliano, L.; Huehn, S.; Peddinghaus, A.; Leyendeckers, H.; Hauser, A.E.; Hiepe, F.; Radbruch, A.; Arce, S.; Manz, R.A. Regulation of CXCR3 and CXCR4 Expression during Terminal Differentiation of Memory B Cells into Plasma Cells. *Blood* **2005**, *105*, 3965–3971. [CrossRef] [PubMed]
55. Kagen, S.; Kurup, V.; Sohnle, P.; Fink, J. Marijuana Smoking and Fungal Sensitization. *J. Allergy Clin. Immunol.* **1983**, *71*, 389–393. [CrossRef] [PubMed]
56. Bailey, K.L.; Wyatt, T.A.; Katafiasz, D.M.; Taylor, K.W.; Heires, A.J.; Sisson, J.H.; Romberger, D.J.; Burnham, E.L. Alcohol and Cannabis Use Alter Pulmonary Innate Immunity. *Alcohol* **2019**, *80*, 131–138. [CrossRef] [PubMed]
57. Caiaffa, W.T.; Vlahov, D.; Graham, N.M.; Astemborski, J.; Solomon, L.; Nelson, K.E.; Muñoz, A. Drug Smoking, Pneumocystis Carinii Pneumonia, and Immunosuppression Increase Risk of Bacterial Pneumonia in Human Immunodeficiency Virus-Seropositive Injection Drug Users. *Am. J. Respir. Crit. Care Med.* **1994**, *150*, 1493–1498. [CrossRef] [PubMed]
58. Melén, C.M.; Merrien, M.; Wasik, A.M.; Panagiotidis, G.; Beck, O.; Sonnevi, K.; Junlén, H.-R.; Christensson, B.; Sander, B.; Wahlin, B.E. Clinical Effects of a Single Dose of Cannabinoids to Patients with Chronic Lymphocytic Leukemia. *Leuk. Lymphoma* **2022**, *63*, 1387–1397. [CrossRef]

Disclaimer/Publisher's Note: The statements, opinions and data contained in all publications are solely those of the individual author(s) and contributor(s) and not of MDPI and/or the editor(s). MDPI and/or the editor(s) disclaim responsibility for any injury to people or property resulting from any ideas, methods, instructions or products referred to in the content.

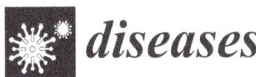

Article

Comparative Study on MNVT of OPV Type I and III Reference Products in Different Periods

Xiyan Wang [†], Ruirui Ren [†], Bo Ma, Jing Xie, Yan Ma, Hong Luo, Yu Guo, Ling Ding, Liang Zhang, Mengyuan Zhang, Tianlang Wang, Zhichao Shuang and Xiujuan Zhu *

Beijing Institute of Biological Products Co., Ltd., Beijing 100176, China
* Correspondence: zhuxiujuan1@sinopharm.com
† These authors contributed equally to this work and should be regarded as co-first authors.

Abstract: Widespread vaccination using the oral live attenuated polio vaccine (OPV) and Sabin strain inactivated vaccine (sIPV) have greatly reduced the incidence of polio worldwide. In the period post-polio, the virulence of reversion of the Sabin strain makes the use of OPV gradually becoming one of the major safety hazards. The verification and release of OPV has become the top priority. The monkey neurovirulence test (MNVT) is the gold standard for detecting whether OPV meets the criteria, which are recommended by the WHO and Chinese Pharmacopoeia. Therefore, we statistically analyzed the MNVT results of type I and III OPV at different stages: 1996–2002 and 2016–2022. The results show that the upper and lower limits and C value of the qualification standard of type I reference products in 2016–2022 have decreased compared with the corresponding scores in the 1996–2002 period. The upper and lower limit and C value of the qualified standard of type III reference products were basically the same as the corresponding scores in the 1996–2002. We also found significant differences in the pathogenicity of the type I and III in the cervical spine and brain, with the decreasing trend in the diffusion index of the type I and type III in the cervical spine and brain. Finally, two evaluation criteria were used to judge the OPV test vaccines from 2016 to 2022. The vaccines all met the test requirements under the evaluation criteria of the above two stages. Based on the characteristics of OPV, data monitoring was one of the most intuitive methods to judge changes in virulence.

Keywords: OPV; MNVT; neurovirulence; reference product; vaccine

1. Introduction

Poliomyelitis is an acute infectious disease caused by poliovirus (PV), which seriously endangers children's health [1,2]. The virus causes motor neuron cell damage by invading the central nervous system, mostly affecting motor neurons in the anterior horn of the spinal cord, leading to acute flaccid paralysis (AFP) with muscle atrophy. Its wide spread in the world has led to paralysis, or even death, of countless children, or life-long affliction with post-polio syndrome (PPS) [3–6].

There are three serotypes of poliovirus: poliovirus type I, poliovirus type II and poliovirus type III. In 2015, the WHO announced that wild-type poliovirus type II was completely eradicated and type I and III strains became a priority for prevention [7]. Therefore, mass vaccination with vaccines became an important means of preventing poliomyelitis. The data evaluation model shows that after widespread vaccination, 5 million additional cases of paralytic poliomyelitis were prevented during 1960–1987, and 24 million cases were prevented globally during 1988–2021 [8].

Inactivated poliovirus vaccine (IPV) and live attenuated oral poliovirus vaccine (OPV) are the important methods to prevent poliomyelitis from happening. The intestinal immune effect induced by OPV can better prevent the transmission of wild virus compared with IPV, but at the same time, it is accompanied by a virulence of regression phenomenon higher than IPV [9]. To better prevent the spread of the poliovirus, comprehensive vaccination has become a necessary method. However, large-scale vaccination means that manufacturers need to strictly enforce quality control for vaccines to reduce the incidence of clinically adverse reactions.

In the process of vaccine production, we need to complete a large number of experiments to provide data support for the verification of vaccine safety and effectiveness. MNVT is used to detect the virulence of seed virus strains and OPV stock solution, and then determine whether the vaccine virulence is qualified. This test is crucial in the vaccine inspection process. In this paper, MNVT experiment results of OPV production process at the Beijing Institute of Biological Products Co., ltd. (Beijing Companies, Beijing, China) were statistically compared to provide a basis for vaccine quality control.

MNVT has high repeatability and sensitivity in virulence testing with a half-century history of application, which is an essential step in evaluating the safety of live attenuated polio vaccine [10]. In accordance with the WHO and the Chinese Pharmacopoeia, the animals were infected with virus by intraspinal injection or intracerebral injection, the glia in the central nervous system (CNS) was activated, and the peripheral immune cells infiltrated and spread to the whole CNS. The semi quantitative score was made by observing the pathological changes to evaluate the batch release of live attenuated vaccines [11].

In the 1980s, fixed upper and lower limits and C values were set as criteria for determining whether the MNVT was acceptable. In the past, we have completed the statistics of MNVT data for three types of reference products from 1996 to 2002, and verified the differences between the experimental batch's MNVT results and those from before the 1980s [12]. Each laboratory should establish its own judgment standard, recommended by the WHO, after completing experiments with the continuous accumulation of experimental data. Therefore, after 2013, the M value of the first ten experiments and the C value calculated were used by combining the standard deviations as the evaluation criteria for vaccine eligibility.

In this paper, the MNVT results of type I and type III were counted using references from 2016–2022 and compared with the results of 1996–2002. With respect to pathological test results, the mean fraction of lesions at neutrophilic sites and C values were determined. Furthermore, there were certain differences in the criteria for determining MNVT in different time periods, which was used to further improve the OPV MNVT test results and provide a certain database for subsequent experiments.

2. Materials and Methods

2.1. Animals

According to the requirements of the Chinese Pharmacopoeia and WHO regulations, we selected Macaca mulatta (over 1.5 kg) as the test animal, which were provided by the Beijing Institute of Xieerxin Biology Resource (Beijing, China) and Xiangcheng Longrui Experimental Animal Co., Ltd. (Henan, China). We selected monkeys before the test and isolated them for 6 weeks. After blood sampling and testing, we ensured that the monkeys did not carry tuberculosis, B virus, foam virus (FV) or other acute infectious diseases, and there were no neutralizing antibodies against poliovirus in serum. Type I and type III were immunized in 14 and 22 heads of monkeys, respectively, to ensure that the effective number of monkeys after the test was not less than 11 and 18.

All animals were housed in a room maintained at 16–26 °C with an alternating 12 h light/dark cycle (AM. 7:00–PM. 19:00). Food and water were autoclaved. The operation process of animal experiment conforms to the national Regulations on the Administration of Experimental Animals and has been reviewed by the Ethics Committee of Experimental Animal Welfare of Beijing Company. The manufacturers of experimental animals have obtained the production license of experimental animals approved by the Beijing Municipal Science Committee and the domestication and breeding license of wild animals approved by the Beijing Landscaping Bureau.

All efforts were made to minimize animal pain and suffering and the number of animals used during the experiments.

2.2. Materials

The reference product of type I and type III provided by the WHO (I—1981, III—1981), the monovalent virus stock solution of OPV was provided by Beijing companies.

2.3. Methods

MNVT is widely used in the detection of attenuated live vaccines. As an important standard for judging neurovirulence, this method has been used in vaccine quality control in the pharmaceutical industry for more than 50 years. Since 1996, all the experimental steps were carried out in accordance with the requirements of the WHO Regulations for the Manufacture and Testing of Live Attenuated Oral Polio Vaccine and the Pharmacopoeia of the People's Republic of China (current edition).

The experiment was divided into a vaccine group to be tested and a reference vaccine group. The number of effective monkeys in each group of type I should be more than 11, and the number of effective monkeys of type III should be more than 18. The group of reference and vaccine to be tested should be carried out in parallel. All animals were injected between the first and second lumbar vertebrae, and each monkey was injected with 0.1 mL of sample (the virus content should be 6.5~7.5 LgCCID50/mL).

Spinal cord injection can make the virus directly invade the central nervous system (CNS) tissue. After vaccination, it is observed for 17–22 consecutive days, and the daily feed intake (normal; feed intake 1/2; feed intake 1/3; feed intake waste), fecal conditions (fecal formation; fecal beach; fecal porridge) and motor status (normal climbing; hind limbs unable to move; limbs unable to move) were recorded. If an animal dies during clinical observation, the animal shall be dissected to further confirm the cause of death, and the number of animals killed during observation shall not exceed one quarter before the experiment can be established.

At the end of observation period, sections of the CNS of monkeys were taken for histological examination, and the thickness of the sections was 10–15 μm. Five pathological sections were prepared from each animal, resulting in a total of 29 tissues: 10 tissues from the cervical enlargement, 12 tissues from the lumbar enlargement, 1 from the cerebellum, 1 from the pons, 2 from the medulla oblongata, 2 from the midbrain, 2 from the cortex, and 2 from the thalamus. The specific distribution is as follows:

Slice 1: Swollen neck, 10 slices.
Slice 2: Waist puffed, 12 slices.
Slice 3: 1 section of cerebellum and pontine and 2 sections of medulla oblongata.
Slice 4: Midbrain and cortex, 3 slices.
Slice 5: Thalamus, 1 slice.

After fixation, staining and depigmentation, the pathological sections were prepared, and the lesions in each monkey were observed by microscopic examination and counted using a 4-level scoring method. The scoring process was performed independently by the same experimenter and criteria were as follows:

Score 1: Only cellular invasion like perivascular cufflike leukocyte aggregates; Low, moderate or high cellular invasion by non-neural lesions (which alone would not be sufficient to indicate a positive monkey).
Score 2: Cellular infiltration and little neuronal damage.
Score 3: Cell invasion and extensive neuronal damage.
Score 4: Massive neuronal damage with or without cell invasion.

Of concern is that monkeys with neuronal damage in slices, but without a needle track should be considered valid monkeys. Trauma-induced damage in sections without specific pathological changes was not considered valid. Sections could not be included in the scoring if the damage on the sections was a result of trauma and not specific viral damage. Pathological sections were scored by scoring method to determine the activity of virus-induced neuropathy. When the mean value of the reference vaccine was between the upper and lower limits, the vaccine to be tested can be judged to be qualified based on the respective standard values. If the mean value of the vaccine to be tested exceeds the upper and lower limits, the experimental result does not hold.

The mean value of the reference lesion, the total within test error (s2) and combined sample standard deviation (s) were calculated using the sampling error of the statistical mean. The upper limit of type I was calculated as M+s, the lower limit was calculated as M-s, the upper limit of type III was calculated in the same way as type I, and the lower limit comes from M-s/2.

The acceptability constant (C value) was the difference between the average lesion score of the vaccine to be tested and the average lesion score of the reference vaccine. The calculation method is as follows: $C_1 = 2.3\sqrt{2S^2/N_1}$, $C_2 = 2.6\sqrt{2S^2/N_1}$, $C_3 = 1.6\sqrt{2S^2/N_2}$. The results were judged as follows: the average lesion score ($\bar{x}_{test}$) of the vaccine to be tested was compared with the average lesion score ($\bar{x}_{ref}$) of the reference product, if $\bar{x}_{test} - \bar{x}_{ref} < C_1$, the vaccine was qualified, otherwise it is unqualified; $C_1 < \bar{x}_{test} - \bar{x}_{ref} < C_2$ requires it to be retested and recalculated after the retest. If $\bar{x}_{(test1+test2)} - \bar{x}_{(ref1+ref2)}/2 > C_3$, it will be judged unqualified.

3. Results

3.1. Statistics of Pathological Test Results of Type I MNVT

The results of 19 tests were counted using references from 2016 to 2022 and it was found that the pathological score of the reference products fluctuated greatly, the upper and lower limits gradually narrowed (Figure 1); there were three consecutive batches of results approaching the lower limit, which further narrows the upper and lower limits. Compared with 1996–2002, it could be more intuitively found that the mean value of the 19 tests (0.383) decreased by 0.222, the upper limit (0.591) decreased by 0.392 and the lower limit (0.231) decreased by 0.166; the value has a relative increase of 0.018, with no significant change (Table 1).

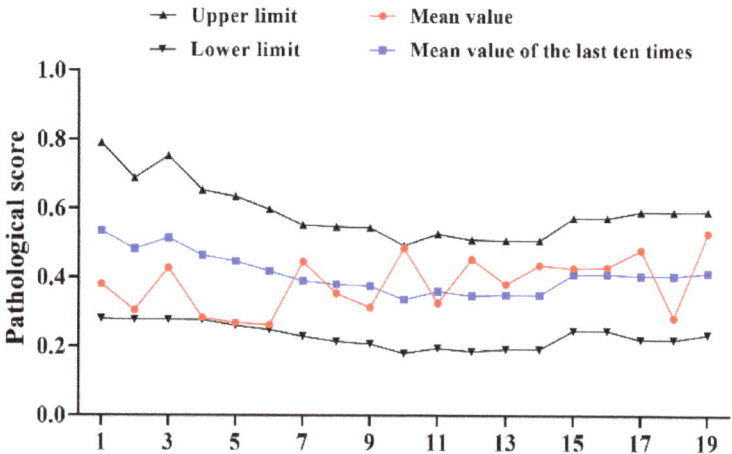

Figure 1. Statistical of pathological score of type I reference product in 2016–2022. N = 19 times.

Table 1. Statistics for two stage of type I.

Stage	1996–2002	2016–2022	Increase	Decrease
Mean value	0.605	0.383	-	0.222
Combined sample standard deviation (s)	0.161	0.179	0.018	-
upper limit	0.591	0.938	0.347	-
lower limit	0.397	0.231	-	0.166

3.2. Statistics of Pathological Test Results of Type III MNVT

A total of 12 trials of type III reference products were completed from 2016–2022. The results demonstrated that the pathological score of the reference product fluctuated from 2016 to 2022, the upper and lower limits gradually narrowed down (Figure 2). Different from the changes of type I, the pathological data of type III references have decreased to varying degrees compared with the past. The average mean value of the 12 experiments (0.538) was decreased by 0.194, the upper limit (0.940) was 0.211 lower than the past average (1.151) and just the lower limit (0.440) was improved by 0.131 compared to the past (0.309) (Table 2). Although all were within the qualified range, the results still require our close attention.

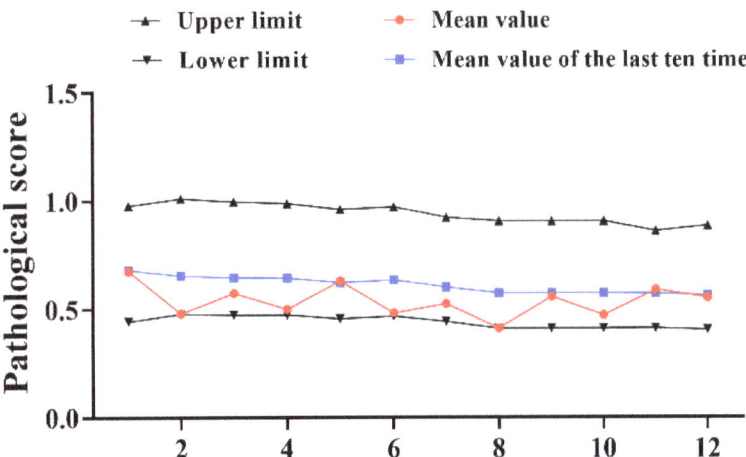

Figure 2. Statistical of pathological score of type III reference product in 2016–2022. N = 12 times.

Table 2. Statistics for two stage of type III.

Stage	1996–2002	2016–2022	Increase	Decrease
Mean value	0.732	0.538	-	0.194
Combined sample standard deviation (s)	0.423	0.331	-	0.092
upper limit	1.151	0.940	-	0.211
lower limit	0.309	0.440	0.131	-

3.3. Comparison of Lesion Scores in Different Neurotropic Sites of Type I and Type III

The pathological scores of three parts of all reference products from 2016 to 2022 were counted. As the results displayed (Figure 3), the degree of lesions in the enlarged lumbar region was still significantly higher than that in the cervical spine and brain. There was no significant difference between type III and type I lumbar lesions ($p > 0.05$), although the cervical spine and brain lesions index was significantly higher than type I ($p < 0.001$). As before, we compared the statistical data from 1996 to 2002 (Table 3), and the overall lesion score decreased. The coefficient of variation (CV) was calculated based on the standard deviation value of the previous ten times. Compared with the 1996–2002 period, we found that the coefficient of variation of type I has increased, and that of type III decreased, indicating that the degree of dispersion of pathological scores of the two reference products was inconsistent.

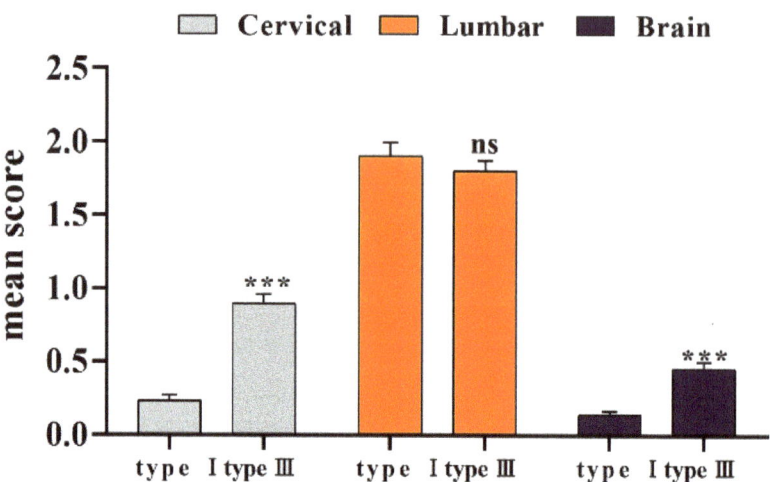

Figure 3. Statistical of pathological lesion tissue of type I and type III. *** $p < 0.01$ compared with type I group.

Table 3. Statistics of the average lesion scores in different central nervous systems from 1996–2002 and 2016–2022.

CNS	Type I		Type III	
	1996–2002	2016–2022	1996–2002	2016–2022
Cervical	0.276	0.118	0.532	0.449
Lumbar	1.404	0.953	1.187	0.900
Brain	0.127	0.070	0.473	0.229
Coefficient of variation (cv)	0.346	0.437	0.851	0.543
Extramedullary diffusion index	0.223	0.167	0.459	0.429

The average pathological scores of the lumbar spine, neck and brain marrow of the reference article are the same as the previous ones.

The statistical data from 1996 to 2002 was compared (Table 3), and the overall pathological score decreased. The coefficient of variation (CV) value was calculated based on the standard deviation of ten/the average M value of ten. Compared with 1996–2002, we found that the coefficient of variation of type I increased, and type III decreased, so it was reflected that the dispersion degree of the two references were inconsistent. At the same time, the extramedullary diffusion index in the two periods were compared. The lumbar spinal cord was the part inoculated in the MNVT, and the motor neurons in the anterior horn were also the most concentrated, the lesions of the lumbar spine were the most serious compared with the cervical spine and the brain. Although the diffusion index of the two to the neck and brain was not much different between the two periods, there was still a slight downward trend now compared with the past. It was also consistent with the change trend of the pathological mean.

3.4. C Value Statistic

The C value (C1, C2, C3) represents the acceptable range of the difference between the vaccine test and the reference lesion score, and the change of the C value directly affects whether the vaccine was qualified or not. We counted the changes of C value in the above two stages. The data illustrated that (Table 4) the C value of type I and type III decreased. The results displayed that although the virulence of vaccines has declined in recent years, the qualification limit of the test vaccines has gradually become stricter, the pass rate of the vaccines has decreased and the difficulty has increased.

Table 4. 1996–2002 and 2016–2022 C value statistics.

C Value	1996–2002	2016–2021	Increase	Decrease
Type I C1	0.224	0.160	-	−0.064
Type I C2	0.253	0.180	-	−0.073
Type I C3	0.110	0.081	-	−0.029
Type III C1	0.282	0.243	-	−0.039
Type III C2	0.318	0.274	-	−0.044
Type III C3	0.139	0.123	-	−0.016

3.5. MNVT Results of Test Vaccines in 2016–2022

The MNVT results of type I (Table 5) and III (Table 6) OPV stock solution tested were collected by all Beijing companies from 2016 to 2022 and calculated based on the results of the same batch of reference products. The virulence of all the test vaccines were all within the qualified range. In addition, we also compared with the fixed C1 value at the past stage and found that the results of the test vaccines were still qualified under different reference values, which further verifies the reliability of the calculation method at this stage.

Table 5. The mean value of type I OPV stock solution between 2016 and 2022 and the MNVT qualification under different judgment standards.

NO.	Positive Monkeys	$Mean_{test}$	$Mean_{ref}$	$Mean_{test} - Mean_{ref}$	2016–2022	1996–2002 (0.224)
1	13	0.461	0.381	0.08	qualified	qualified
2	13	0.279	0.306	−0.027	qualified	qualified
3	14	0.449	0.428	0.021	qualified	qualified
4	14	0.407	0.284	0.123	qualified	qualified
5	14	0.273	0.270	0.003	qualified	qualified
6	14	0.266	0.263	0.003	qualified	qualified
7	14	0.360	0.446	−0.086	qualified	qualified
8	14	0.476	0.355	0.121	qualified	qualified
9	14	0.268	0.314	−0.046	qualified	qualified
10	14	0.449	0.486	−0.037	qualified	qualified
11	13	0.286	0.327	−0.041	qualified	qualified
12	13	0.417	0.453	−0.036	qualified	qualified
13	14	0.381	0.381	0	qualified	qualified
14	14	0.491	0.436	0.055	qualified	qualified
15	14	0.444	0.428	0.016	qualified	qualified
16	12	0.398	0.43	−0.032	qualified	qualified
17	13	0.552	0.48	0.072	qualified	qualified
18	13	0.399	0.285	0.114	qualified	qualified
19	14	0.429	0.529	−0.1	qualified	qualified

Table 6. The mean value of type III OPV stock solution between 2016 and 2022 and the MNVT qualification under different judgment standards.

NO.	Positive Monkeys	Mean$_{test}$	Mean$_{ref}$	Mean$_{test}$−Mean$_{ref}$	2016–2022	1996–2002 (0.282)
1	22	0.712	0.676	0.036	qualified	qualified
2	21	0.531	0.481	0.05	qualified	qualified
3	21	0.544	0.575	−0.031	qualified	qualified
4	20	0.382	0.500	−0.118	qualified	qualified
5	20	0.468	0.630	−0.162	qualified	qualified
6	22	0.536	0.482	0.054	qualified	qualified
7	21	0.542	0.525	0.017	qualified	qualified
8	22	0.582	0.413	0.169	qualified	qualified
9	21	0.478	0.558	−0.08	qualified	qualified
10	22	0.647	0.472	0.175	qualified	qualified
11	21	0.619	0.590	0.029	qualified	qualified
12	21	0.524	0.553	−0.029	qualified	qualified

4. Discussions

Although the Global Polio Eradication Initiative (GPEI) promised to eradicate polio by 2000, the disease has remained endemic in some countries for the past 20 years [13]. However, the incidence of poliomyelitis in the world has been greatly reduced, the crucial reason for this is vaccination.

OPV are one of the most successful methods for controlling PV infections, the intestinal mucosal immunity and systemic immunity caused by OPV make the immune effect much higher than that of IPV, which could more effectively prevent the spread of wild poliovirus (WPV). However, because of outbreaks associated with circulating vaccine-derived poliovirus (cVDPVs) [14–16], most people have recognized that the risk of OPV reversion of virulence is significantly higher than that of IPV. Based on the difference in immune efficacy between the OPV and IPV, complete cessation of OPV use is still not possible. Instead, because of the continued emergence of cVDPVs, OPV production and use potentially needs to increase progressively. In 2016, the WHO recommended at least one dose of IPV preceding routine immunization with OPV vaccination to reduce vaccine-associated paralytic polio (VAPPs) and VDPVs until PV could be eradicated [17–19]. We have completed the transformation from tOPV to bOPV before and have been using it until now, making great contributions to the world's prevention of poliomyelitis, which also means that we have greater responsibility. The significance of our comparison and analysis of the MNVT results for the reference product in the above two stages is to further ensure whether the virulence of OPV is continuously applicable.

Although MNVT is the gold standard for detecting vaccine neurotoxicity, it cannot explain many potential neurotoxicity mechanisms and lacks reproducibility [20,21]. The WHO also recommended detection methods other than MNVT. We found that the detection of spontaneous neurotoxic response of OPV by PCR and restriction endonuclease cleavage (MAPREC) is highly sensitive and reliable. This method can predict the experimental results of MNVT [22,23]. We also completed the quantitative analysis of viruses in OPV through MAPREC, further ensuring the full tracking of virulence [24], which is used for the safety and consistency control of OPV together with MNVT. Although the application of MNVT and MAPREC is mature enough, new alternative methods are still crucial for considering the 3Rs (Replacement, Reduction and Refinement) and methods optimization.

A correlativity study showed that transgenic mice maybe are one of the best alternative models. PVR-Tg21 transgenic animals developed by Japanese scholars in 1990 indicated the same virus sensitivity as MNVT [25–27]. We are currently doing more work to try to determine the feasibility and sensitivity of transgenic mouse models. In addition to in vivo methods, new in vitro molecular diagnosis is still the focus of attention in the future, we need most effort to further ensure the absolute safety and effectiveness of each vaccine.

5. Conclusions

To further ensure whether the virulence of OPV vaccine is continuously applicable, the results of MNVT experiments over the past decades were counted, compared and analyzed. The statistical results illustrated that the average lesion score of type I was on a downward trend, which was different from that in the 1996–2002 period. Compared with the same trend, the C value has also decreased, which suggests that the qualification rate of our vaccine may be affected. However, compared with the changes of type I, type III maintained relatively stable virulence in the above two stages. The reason of decreasingly pathological value of type I also needs to be further investigated.

In addition to the reference products, we have counted the MNVT results of OPV vaccine stock solution from 2016 to 2022. The data showed that the results met the test requirements under different evaluation criteria in 1996–2002 and 2016–2022. Nevertheless, we also need to constantly monitor the virulence changes of reference products to strictly control the qualification rate of vaccines.

Author Contributions: Conceptualization, data collection, investigation, writing and review—X.W. and R.R.; Supervision—X.Z.; Data contribution—X.W., R.R., B.M., J.X., Y.M., H.L., Y.G., L.D., L.Z., M.Z., T.W. and Z.S. All authors have read and agreed to the published version of the manuscript.

Funding: This research received no external funding.

Institutional Review Board Statement: All experiments have passed the review of the Ethics Committee of Laboratory Animal Welfare of Beijing Institute of Biological Products Co., Ltd. (The first approval date was 1 July 2014, before which there were no welfare ethics approval requirements for animal experiments in China).

Informed Consent Statement: Not applicable.

Data Availability Statement: Not applicable.

Acknowledgments: The authors would like to acknowledge the following collaborators for assistance in developing this review: Beijing company QC laboratory.

Conflicts of Interest: The authors declare no conflict of interest.

References

1. Kidd, D.; Williams, A.J.; Howard, R.S. Poliomyelitis. *Postgrad. Med. J.* **1996**, *72*, 641–647. [PubMed]
2. Cabrerizo, M. Grupo Para El Estudio de Las Infecciones Por Enterovirus Y Parechovirus GPEELIPEYP. Importancia de los enterovirus en neuropediatria: De los poliovirus a otros enterovirus [Importance of enteroviruses in neuropaediatrics: From polioviruses to other enteroviruses]. *Rev. Neurol.* **2017**, *64*, S35–S38. [PubMed]
3. Howard, R.S. Poliomyelitis and the postpolio syndrome. *BMJ* **2005**, *330*, 1314–1318. [CrossRef]
4. Tiffreau, V.; Rapin, A.; Serafi, R.; Percebois-Macadré, L.; Supper, C.; Jolly, D.; Boyer, F.-C. Post-polio syndrome and rehabilitation. *Ann. Phys. Rehabil. Med.* **2010**, *53*, 42–50. [CrossRef] [PubMed]
5. Gerloff, N.; Mandelbaum, M.; Pang, H.; Collins, N.; Brown, B.; Sun, H.; Harrington, C.; Hecker, J.; Agha, C.; Burns, C.C.; et al. Direct detection of polioviruses using a recombinant poliovirus receptor. *PLoS ONE* **2021**, *16*, e0259099. [CrossRef] [PubMed]
6. Shapiro, L.T.; Sherman, A.L. Medical Comorbidities and Complications Associated with Poliomyelitis and Its Sequelae. *Phys. Med. Rehabil. Clin. N. Am.* **2021**, *32*, 591–600. [CrossRef] [PubMed]
7. Previsani, N.; Tangermann, R.H.; Tallis, G.; Jafari, H.S. World Health Organization Guidelines for Containment of Poliovirus Following Type-Specific Polio Eradication—Worldwide, 2015. *MMWR Morb. Mortal. Wkly. Rep.* **2015**, *64*, 913–917. [CrossRef] [PubMed]
8. Badizadegan, K.; Kalkowska, D.A.; Thompson, K.M. Polio by the Numbers—A Global Perspective. *J. Infect. Dis.* **2022**, *226*, 1309–1318. [CrossRef]
9. Bandyopadhyay, A.S.; Garon, J.; Seib, K.; Orenstein, W.A. Polio vaccination: Past, present and future. *Future Microbiol.* **2015**, *10*, 791–808. [CrossRef]
10. Contreras, G.; Furesz, J.; Karpinski, K.; Grinwich, K.; Gardell, C. Experience in Canada with the new revised monkey neurovirulence test for oral poliovirus vaccine. *J. Biol. Stand.* **1988**, *16*, 195–205.
11. Levenbook, I.S.; Pelleu, L.J.; Elisberg, B.L. The monkey safety test for neurovirulence of yellow fever vaccines: The utility of quantitative clinical evaluation and histological examination. *J. Biol. Stand.* **1987**, *15*, 305–313. [CrossRef] [PubMed]
12. Yang, J.Y.; Wang, H.Y.; Ke, W.H.; Ma, J.M. Statistical analysis of the standard of reference viruses for monkey neurovirulence test in oral poliomyelitis vaccine(OPV). *Prog. Microbiol. Immunol.* **2005**, 7–12. [CrossRef]

13. World Health Assembly Global Eradication of Poliomyelitis by the Year 2000 (Resolution 41.28). 1988. Available online: http://www.who.int/csr/ihr/polioresolution4128en.pdf (accessed on 4 June 2019).
14. Kew, O.; Morris-Glasgow, V.; Landaverde, M.; Burns, C.; Shaw, J.; Garib, Z.; André, J.; Blackman, E.; Freeman, C.J.; Jorba, J. Outbreak of Poliomyelitis in Hispaniola Associated with Circulating Type 1 Vaccine-Derived Poliovirus. *Science* **2002**, *296*, 356. [CrossRef] [PubMed]
15. Ekaterina, K.; Majid, L.; Tatiana, Z.; Svetlana, P.; Elvira, R.; Elena, C.; Anatoly, G.; Olga, I.; Tatyana, E.; Galina, L. Pressure for Pattern-Specific Intertypic Recombination between Sabin Polioviruses: Evolutionary Implications. *Viruses* **2017**, *9*, 353.
16. Burns, C.C.; Diop, O.M.; Sutter, R.W.; Kew, O.M. Vaccine-derived polioviruses. *J. Infect. Dis.* **2014**, *210* (Suppl. 1), S283–S293. [CrossRef] [PubMed]
17. Ciapponi, A.; Bardach, A.; Ares, L.R.; Glujovsky, D.; Cafferata, M.L.; Cesaroni, S.; Bhatti, A. Sequential inactivated (IPV) and live oral (OPV) poliovirus vaccines for preventing poliomyelitis. *Cochrane Database Syst. Rev.* **2019**, *12*, CD011260. [CrossRef]
18. Falleiros-Arlant, L.H.; Ayala, S.E.G.; Domingues, C.; Brea, J.; Colsa-Ranero, A. Current status of poliomyelitis in Latin America. *Estado Actual Polio. Latinoamérica. Rev. Chil. Infectol.* **2020**, *37*, 701–709. [CrossRef]
19. Shimizu, H. Poliovirus vaccine. *Uirusu* **2012**, *62*, 57–65. [CrossRef]
20. May Fulton, C.; Bailey, W.J. Live Viral Vaccine Neurovirulence Screening: Current and Future Models. *Vaccines* **2021**, *9*, 710. [CrossRef]
21. Rubin, S.A.; Afzal, M.A. Neurovirulence safety testing of mumps vaccines–historical perspective and current status. *Vaccine* **2011**, *29*, 2850–2855. [CrossRef]
22. Sarcey, E.; Serres, A.; Tindy, F.; Chareyre, A.; Ng, S.; Nicolas, M.; Vetter, E.; Bonnevay, T.; Abachin, E.; Mallet, L. Quantifying low-frequency revertants in oral poliovirus vaccine using next generation sequencing. *J. Virol. Methods* **2017**, *246*, 75–80. [CrossRef] [PubMed]
23. Bidzhieva, B.; Laassri, M.; Chumakov, K. MAPREC assay for quantitation of mutants in a recombinant flavivirus vaccine strain using near-infrared fluorescent dyes. *J. Virol. Methods* **2011**, *175*, 14–19. [PubMed]
24. Li, N.; Ding, L.; Ma, M.; Sun, Q.Y.; Wang, H.Y.; Li, T. Evaluation of the neurovirulence of type III Sabin strain poliovirus through MAPREC and MNVT. *Chin. Med. Biotechnol.* **2019**, *6*, 494–499.
25. Ren, R.; Costantini, F.; Gorgacz, E.J.; Lee, J.J.; Racaniello, V.R. Transgenic mice expressing a human poliovirus receptor: A new model for poliomyelitis. *Cell* **1990**, *63*, 353–362. [PubMed]
26. Abe, S.; Ota, Y.; Doi, Y.; Nomoto, A.; Nomura, T.; Chumakov, K.M.; Hashizume, S. Studies on neurovirulence in poliovirus-sensitive transgenic mice and cynomolgus monkeys for the different temperature-sensitive viruses derived from the Sabin type 3 virus. *Virology* **1995**, *210*, 160–166. [CrossRef]
27. Koike, S.; Taya, C.; Aoki, J.; Matsuda, Y.; Ise, I.; Takeda, H.; Matsuzaki, T.; Amanuma, H.; Yonekawa, H.; Nomoto, A. Characterization of three different transgenic mouse lines that carry human poliovirus receptor gene—Influence of the transgene expression on pathogenesis. *Arch. Virol.* **1994**, *139*, 351–363. [CrossRef]

Disclaimer/Publisher's Note: The statements, opinions and data contained in all publications are solely those of the individual author(s) and contributor(s) and not of MDPI and/or the editor(s). MDPI and/or the editor(s) disclaim responsibility for any injury to people or property resulting from any ideas, methods, instructions or products referred to in the content.

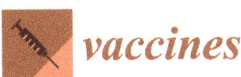

Review

Neutrophil Extracellular Traps and NLRP3 Inflammasome: A Disturbing Duo in Atherosclerosis, Inflammation and Atherothrombosis

Puneetpal Singh [1,*], Nitin Kumar [1], Monica Singh [1], Manminder Kaur [2], Gurjinderpal Singh [3], Amit Narang [4], Abhinav Kanwal [5], Kirti Sharma [1], Baani Singh [1], Mario Di Napoli [6] and Sarabjit Mastana [7]

1. Division of Molecular Genetics, Department of Human Genetics, Punjabi University, Patiala 147002, India
2. Department of Neurology, MK Neuro Centre, Patiala 147002, India
3. Department of Neurology, Bhatia Hospital Neuro and Multispecialty, Patiala 147002, India
4. Department of Neurosurgery, All India Institute of Medical Sciences (AIIMS), Bathinda 151005, India
5. Department of Pharmacology, All India Institute of Medical Sciences (AIIMS), Bathinda 151005, India
6. Department of Neurological Service, Annunziata Hospital, Sulmona, 67039 L'Aquila, Italy
7. Human Genomics Laboratory, School of Sport, Exercise and Health Sciences, Loughborough University, Loughborough LE11 3TU, UK
* Correspondence: puneetpalsingh@pbi.ac.in

Abstract: Atherosclerosis is the formation of plaque within arteries due to overt assemblage of fats, cholesterol and fibrous material causing a blockage of the free flow of blood leading to ischemia. It is harshly impinging on health statistics worldwide because of being principal cause of high morbidity and mortality for several diseases including rheumatological, heart and brain disorders. Atherosclerosis is perpetuated by pro-inflammatory and exacerbated by pro-coagulatory mediators. Besides several other pathways, the formation of neutrophil extracellular traps (NETs) and the activation of the NOD-like receptor family pyrin domain containing 3 (NLRP3) inflammasome contribute significantly to the initiation and propagation of atherosclerotic plaque for its worst outcomes. The present review highlights the contribution of these two disturbing processes in atherosclerosis, inflammation and atherothrombosis in their individual as well as collaborative manner.

Keywords: atherosclerosis; inflammation; atherothrombosis; neutrophils; monocytes; macrophages; neutrophil extracellular traps; NLRP3 inflammasome

1. Introduction

Atherosclerosis is the development of plaque within the walls of arteries due to the accumulation of low density lipoproteins (LDLs), calcium, fats and cholesterol [1]. This plaque may progress to a larger size due to the involvement of immune cells causing an obstruction to the free flow of blood, which is rich in oxygen and nutrients to be delivered to different parts of the body. Other factors contributing to atherosclerosis are hypertension, tobacco smoking, diabetes, obesity and sedentary life style [2]. If the plaque remains inflamed and untreated, it causes ischemia and may rupture causing thrombus formation [3]. Generally, atherosclerosis is considered to be a problem related to heart diseases only, although it can upset any middle or large-sized artery supplying blood to any organ. Atherosclerosis is the reason for substantial morbidity and mortality for several disorders including myocardial infarction, coronary artery disease, chronic kidney disease, peripheral artery disease and stroke [1].

Thorough investigation of the signaling pathways of oxidative stress, proprotein convertase subtilisin/kexin type 9 (PCSK9), Notch signaling, Wnt signaling, mitochondrial dysfunction, pathways of cellular death, cellular excitotoxicity, dysregulated efferocytosis and many more have uncovered the pathogenesis of atherosclerosis to a large extent [1,4].

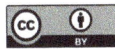

Besides these, two important cellular signaling pathways, namely the formation of neutrophil extracellular traps (NETs) and the activation of the NOD-like receptor family pyrin domain containing 3 (NLRP3) inflammasome, have started unraveling a significant contribution in the inflammatory trajectory from atherosclerosis to ischemia and to infarction and post-infarction phase.

Atherosclerosis, Inflammation and Atherothrombosis

Atherosclerosis is the primary culprit in several diseases, and is perpetuated by inflammation to cause atherothrombosis, leading to ischemia and infarction [1–3]. Atherosclerosis is triggered by the accumulation and circulation of LDL particles in the blood which are rich in cholesterol, packed with phospholipids and coated with apolipoproteins [5]. These LDL enter intima from endothelium either through leaky junctions in the glycocalyx created by dying or dividing cells under the effect of transmural pressure [5] or by the process of transcytosis [6]. LDLs in intima are oxidized due to the availability of free radicals there or the catalysis of metal ions by the Fenton reaction. The endothelial layer comprises tightly placed cells that separate the blood from the vessel wall. These tight junctions may leak due to disturbed blood flow promoting the uptake of LDLs and lipoproteins. Endothelial cells are activated owing to oxidation of these LDLs and lipoproteins resulting in pronounced activation of intracellular adhesion molecule 1 (ICAM1), vascular cell adhesion molecule 1 (VCAM1) and selectins (P and E) [7]. These mediators augment the adhesion of monocytes, leukocytes and chemokine receptors such as C-C Chemokine Receptor type 2 (CCR2) and type 5 (CCR5) [8]. Chemokines help in the migration of monocyte-adhesion molecules into intima. Here, these monocytes mature into macrophages due to local macrophage colony stimulating factors (M-CSF). These macrophages exhibit scavenger receptors that bind with lipoproteins to cause foaming of LDLs (lipid laden cells). In early lesions, these macrophages are recruited; however, in the advanced form of lesions, they proliferate. These foam cells play a role in the efflux of the cholesterol or undergo apoptosis/necrosis supplementing the necrotic core with cholesterol esters. These lipid-rich macrophages incite the inflammatory cycle and provide neo-epitopes further inviting humoral and adaptive immune functions [5,6]. The dysregulated transendothelial flux of LDL causes enlargement and inflammation of intima commencing atherosclerosis [1] (Figure 1A).

The atherosclerotic plaque is propagated by the incessant accrual of lipids and oxidized LDLs. The resident smooth muscle cells (SMC) migrate from media to intima thereby thickening the plaque [1]. The inflammatory leukocytes reach the plaque site which is supplemented by extracellular components of interstitial collagen, proteoglycans, elastin and glycosaminoglycans. Components of plaque denuded from the lesion reach adjoining lymph nodes and present themselves as antigens for T and B cells [2]. T cells start localizing on plaque and Th1 cells invoke interferon gamma (IFNγ) which impairs the ability of SMCs to synthesize interstitial collagen and repair the fibrous cap over the necrotic core, further complicating the atherosclerotic plaque, whereas Th1 cells regress the lesion by producing anti-inflammatory cytokines (IL-2, IL-3 and IL-10). Macrophages and SMCs undergo necrosis and their impaired clearance (dysregulated efferocytosis) from the necrotic core makes a lipid-rich core of the atheroma [1,3] (Figure 1B). Slowly and steadily plaque is calcified by the accumulation of calcium over it, making it more vulnerable to rupture. Atherosclerotic plaques with a large lipid core and thin fibrous cap are more susceptible to rupture and incite thrombosis, whereas lesser lipid cores with a thick fibrous cap are stable [3,4]. In the case of stable plaques, another thrombotic event may emerge from lesions, called plaque erosion. This eroded lesion has been observed to have matrix components with a thin fibrous cap, less lipids and few leukocytes. It has been observed that innate immune participation through pattern recognition receptors (PRR) and polymorphonuclear leukocytes (PMLCs) amplifies the thrombotic events [1,8,9].

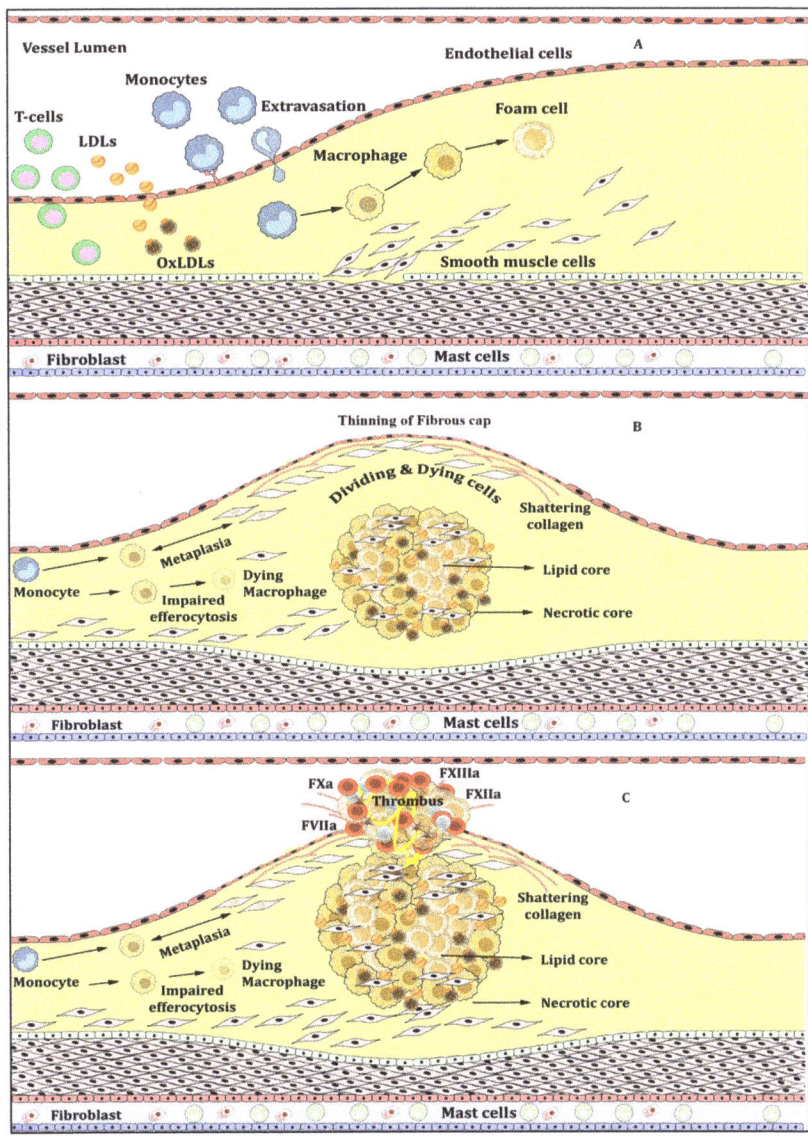

Figure 1. Initiation of atherosclerosis (**A**), progression (**B**) and rupture of atherosclerotic plaque (**C**).

Generally, dysregulated extracellular matrix turnover, inflammation and coagulation along with local systemic factors progress the plaque to rupture. The components of the extracellular matrix overlay the fibrous cap over the plaque [1,10]. Tissue growth factor-beta (TGF-β) induces the synthesis of interstitial collagen. The entry of inflammatory mediators such as macrophages and T cell lymphocytes; leukocyte adhesion molecules such as ICAM-1, VCAM, selectin P and selectin E; chemokines such as monocyte chemoattractant protein-1 (MCP-1), CCR-2 and CCR-5; interleukins including interleukin-1 beta (IL-1β), interleukin-6 (IL-6), interleukin-18 (IL-18), tumor necrosis factor–alpha (TNF-α), IFNγ and cluster of differentiation 40 (CD40); cytokines such as granulocyte macrophage colony-stimulating factor (GMS-CF) and acute phase reactant; C-reactive protein (CRP) along with mediators of fibrosis such as matrix metalloproteinases (MMP), cathepsins, cystatin

C and tissue inhibitor of MMPs (TIMP) render the plaque skeleton unable to sustain the pressure and the plaque ruptures [2,3,10,11]. The internal components of plaques are then exposed to the blood which invites thrombogenic molecules such as prothrombin produced by macrophages (Figure 1C). SMCs trigger thrombus formation which is the most formidable complication of atherosclerosis [6,12]. This dysfunctional endothelium and persistent thrombi generate an ischemic insult causing ischemia. These fibrin-rich thrombi activate the process of clot formation which is observed to be rich in fibrin strands, platelet clumps and NETs [12,13].

Several strategies to identify vulnerable individuals based on their immunophenotyping and surrogate end points have been suggested to alleviate the risk of atherosclerosis-driven diseases [14].Some studies have suggested that targeting epigenetic stimulators of inflammation with inhibition of Bromodomain and extraterminal motifs (BETs) can drastically reduce the expression of the worst outcomes of atherosclerosis. Studies have also suggested that therapeutic vaccination such as epitopes binding to apoB100 may reduce lesion formation. Moreover, the induction of T regulatory cells (Tregs) inhibits LDL-triggered activation of macrophages [15]. All these methods of blocking or inhibiting atherosclerotic propagation can be helpful in formulating personalized medicine for several diseases.

2. NETs, NETosis and Atherosclerosis

Serving as immune sentinels, neutrophils are the first to react against infectious agents and the first to reach the site of injury to catch and kill pathogens by phagocytosis to resolve inflammation (clearing pro-inflammatory stimuli) and repair tissue (promote angiogenesis) [8]. A few years ago, a new anti-pathogen strategy of neutrophils was discovered whereby on meeting a pathogen, neutrophils make a mesh-like structure called a neutrophil extracellular trap (NET) that ensnares and neutralizes pathogens [11]. NETs are web-like structures formed via decondensation of their chromatin by citrullination of arginine by peptidyl arginine deiminase 4 (PAD4) [13]. This loose chromatin becomes embedded with azurophilic granules and cytosolic proteins. The components of decondensed chromatin include predominantly positively charged proteins along with cell-free DNA and RNA. Although 70% of the proteins are histones, the rest belongs to the cytoplasm, metabolic pathways and cytoskeleton. Almost 20 proteins have been identified in the NET proteome (NETome) that participate in NET formation. These include neutrophil elastase (NE), proteinase-3 (PR3), myeloperoxidase (MPO), Cathepsin G, Keratinocyte transglutaminase, factor XIIIa, alpha-defensins and citrullinated histones (ctH) [16].

When neutrophils fail to resolve inflammation by phagocytosis and pro-inflammatory stimuli are non-subsiding and incessant then NETs are formed and thrown on the microbes (pro-inflammatory stimulus) either by breaking the plasma membrane with the pore-forming protein Gasdermin D (GSDMD) causing the death of the neutrophil (suicidal NETosis) or by transporting these NETs by membrane blebbing or vesicular exocytosis (vital NETosis) [10,13]. NETosis is the process by which the neutrophil expels its nuclear material outside the cell; however this term was earlier used for neutrophil death (Figure 2).

NET formation or NETosis is initiated by several triggers; otherwise, resting neutrophils are non-inflammatory and do not undergo NETosis [8]. Vital NETosis is observed mostly during infection rather than sterile injury, whereas suicidal NETosis is associated with sterile and noninfectious complications [13]. Several stimuli have been observed to initiate the formation of NETs such as phorbol-12-myristate-13-acetate (PMA) [17], bacterial toxin; ionomycin, lipopolysaccharides (LPS) [10], some cytokines such as IL-1β, TNFα and IL-8 [11], microbe size [18], activated platelets [19], reactive oxygen species (ROS) burst [20], histone acetylation [21], etc.

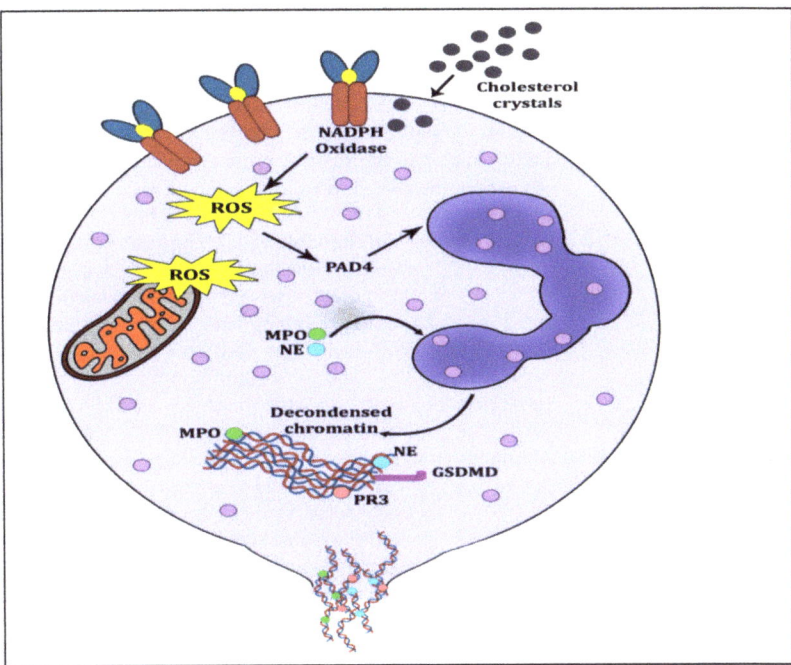

Figure 2. Overview of suicidal NETosis. Cholesterol crystals interact with free radicals and generate NADPH-oxidase-induced reactive oxygen species (ROS). ROS stimulate peptidyl arginine deiminase 4 (PADI4) to citrullinate arginine resulting in loosening of chromatin from histone. Myeloperoxidase (MPO) and neutrophil elastase (NE) migrate to the nuclear membrane for its rupturing by further decondensation of the chromatin. This decondensed chromatin exhibits a mesh-like structure called neutrophil extracellular trap (NET), which is ejected into the cytoplasm, where it is embedded with azurophilic granules and cytosolic proteins. Finally, this NET is ejected through the membrane rupturing of the neutrophil and causing its death.

Atherosclerosis is considered to be the chief culprit in the pathology of several complex disorders, and is propelled by vascular inflammation [1]. The inflammatory trigger by lipid-rich foam cells in atherosclerosis is considered to be the central event when these accumulate in the subendothelial area of an injured artery [1,3,5]. In order to clarify whether NETs are formed during and contribute to atherosclerosis, earlier studies have shown that neutrophils were either present with condensed nuclei or were luminar rather than lesional, suggesting that neutrophils are less likely to participate in atherosclerosis development [22,23]. In essential hypertension patients, abundant NET formation was observed but when they were treated with angiotensin II (AngII), NETs were substantially reduced [24]. It has been observed that a mouse knockout for *ApoE-/-* expresses heightened NET formation and interferon-alpha (IFN-α) expression in atherosclerotic arteries. When these mice were injected daily with Cl-amidine, which is an inhibitor of the PAD4 enzyme, recruitment of neutrophils and macrophages into intima was significantly reduced, hence mitigating NET formation and reducing atherosclerotic load by delaying carotid thrombosis [22]. This suggests that PAD4 is a paramount enzyme for histone citrullination and recruitment of NETs during atherosclerosis. Another study demonstrated that NETs are not formed in mice with NE blocked in *Klebsiella pneumoniae* infection suggesting NE is vital for NET formation [20]. They observed that during an ROS burst, NE sheds off from azurophilic granules and moves to the nucleus for chromatin decondensation. It has also been observed that MPO significantly induces NET formation in *Candida albicans* infection as neutrophils from MPO-deficient patients fail to form NETs [25]. Most of these studies have been carried out on murine models, and thus PAD4-driven NETosis has been shown to occur in experimental mouse models only; however, in humans it does not influence fatty streak formation or increasing plaque size [26]. However, the same study also observed that it participates in the atherothrombotic advancement of intimal lesions prone to plaque erosion. Plaque erosion is a complication where flowing blood within arteries does not disrupt the cap of the atherosclerotic plaque but an acute thrombus is eroded from intima, where endothelial cells are damaged (endothelial denudation). Another study examined NET formation and its contribution to atherogenesis using a myeloid-specific deletion of PAD4 in *ApoE-/-* knockout mice [27]. The authors proposed strongly that NETs promote atherosclerosis in both murines and humans and this NET-driven atherogenesis is governed by PAD4, because in their experiment of PAD4 deletion in myeloid cells, a reduced NET formation and attenuated inflammatory response were observed [27].

NETs and NETosis not only participate in atherosclerosis but also contribute to thrombus formation. NETs induce a scaffold of DNA that exhibits a red blood cell (RBC)-rich thrombus along with von Willebrand factor (vWF), fibronectin and fibrinogen in experimental deep venous thrombus in baboons [12]. This inference is corroborated by a study in humans showing that activated platelets interact with neutrophils to generate tissue factors that provoke neutrophils to induce thrombogenic signals promoting atherogenesis in ST-segment elevation acute myocardial infarction (STEMI) [28]. NETs participate significantly in prothrombotic signaling by triggering the oxidation of LDLs, generating ROS, endothelial dysfunction, apoptosis, fibrin-formation-induced platelet aggregation, accumulation of vWF and fibrinogen [29]. NETs are observed to interact with inflammatory platelets to promote thrombosis via immune-related GTPase family M protein (IRGM) and its orthologs [30]. Carriers of the homozygote TT genotype of the R262W polymorphism within the Src homology 2B (SH2B) protein 3 (LNK/SH2B3) gene show augmented platelet–neutrophil aggregation leading to heightened atherosclerosis and atherothrombosis in an oxidized phospholipid (oxPL)-dependent manner [31]. Alluding to contradictions and confusions, a remarkable piece of research has answered three important queries related to the role and relevance of NETs and NETosis in an experimental murine model of atherosclerosis [32]. First, they incubated neutrophils with cholesterol crystals and observed that cholesterol crystals prompt neutrophils to synthesize NETs and undergo suicidal NETosis. Second, to investigate whether NETosis participates in atherosclerosis, NETs were observed abundantly within atherosclerotic lesions of aortic roots in mice lacking ApoE (*ApoE-/-*) who were nurtured with high-fat diets (HFD) for 8 continuous weeks. ApoE is the master player of reverse cholesterol transport, whereby it carries and transfers a larger volume of LDLs to the liver, and then these LDLs are transported to bile [33]. Therefore, its absence (*ApoE-/-*) caused hypercholesterolemia which led to an accumulation of leukocytes and plaque formation. This suggests that during hypercholesterolemia, neutrophils make NETs abundantly contiguous to cholesterol crystals. Third, to understand whether NETosis contributes to atherogenesis, they developed triple-knockout mice for ApoE and two important components of the nuclear material expelled by NETs, i.e., NE and PR3 (*ApoE$^{-/-}$/NE$^{-/-}$/PR3$^{-/-}$*), and compared these with *ApoE-/-* mice. It was observed that the aortic roots of triple-knockout mice had no NET formation, reduced levels of IL-1β and fewer lesional T cells which produce cytokine IL-17. IL-17 is observed to perpetuate inflammation by inviting other pro-inflammatory cytokines such as TNF-α, IL-1β and IFN-γ [34]. This demonstrates that components of NETs, namely, NE and PR3, are required for inflammation in atherosclerosis that propels atherogenesis. To corroborate this finding, they further injected *ApoE-/-* mice with DNase, an enzyme that neutralizes DNA material, and observed that the lesion size was significantly reduced (by approximately three times), whereas lesion size was unaffected after injecting DNase into *ApoE$^{-/-}$/NE$^{-/-}$/PR3$^{-/-}$* mice, who had no NET formation. It suggested that even during hypercholesterolemia caused by *ApoE$^{-/-}$* absence, no NETs were formed because NE and PR3 were neutralized by the DNase, proving that these two are paramount for NET formation. Furthermore, this study clarified that cholesterol crystals invoke neutrophils to form NETs and exercise NETosis, components of which prime macrophages to initiate NLRP3 inflammasome activation, finally converting immature forms of IL-1β (pro-IL-1β) and IL-18 (Pro-IL-18) to mature forms and release them with the help of pore-forming Gasdermin D into the extracellular space [13].

3. NLRP3 Inflammasome Activation and Atherosclerosis

NLRP3 is present in the cytoplasm as an inactive protein but is activated on sensing danger from several cellular triggers [9,35]. NLRP3 inflammasome activation has been observed to play a central role in initiating the inflammatory cascade in several diseases [36]. It is a multiprotein complex that contains an adapter (ASC or PYCARD), a receptor (NLRP3) and an effector (pro-caspase-1) along with domains such as telomerase-associated protein 1 (TP1 or NACHT), neuronal apoptosis inhibitory protein (NAIP), N-terminal pyrin domain (PYD) and leucine-rich repeat (LRR). On sensing damage or danger signals by NACHT, it triggers signaling where ASC forms speck-like clusters and pro-caspase 1 (Pro-CASP1) is recruited to the ASC speck clusters. ASC and Pro-CASP1 cleave proteolytically the active caspase-1 (CASP-1), which matures pro-IL1β to IL-1β and pro-IL18 to IL-18. During this maturation, CASP-1 induces pyroptosis, which is a form of lytic cell death triggered by the formation of plasma membrane pores by gasdermin D, leading to a flux of ions (K^+ and Ca^{2+}) and releasing mature IL-1β and IL-18 into the extracellular space [37] (Figure 3).

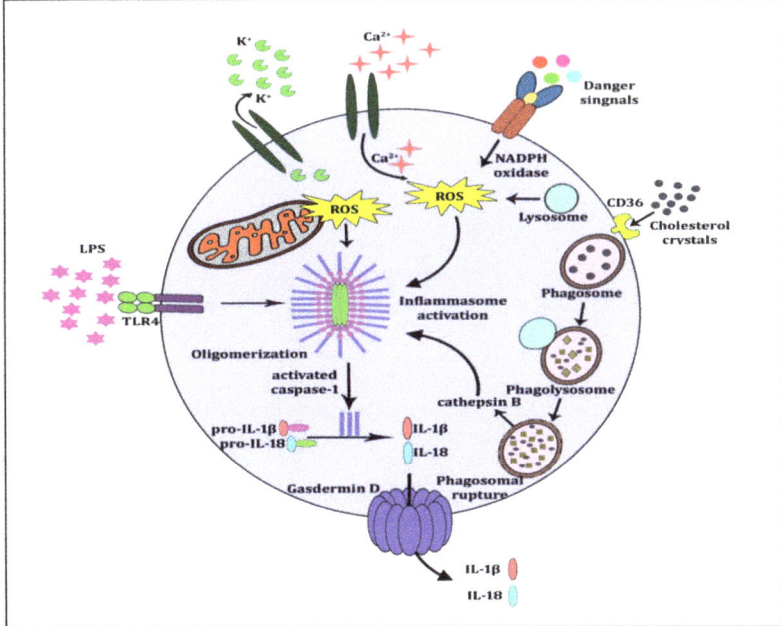

Figure 3. NLRP3 inflammasome activation. Cholesterol crystals are internalized by CD36 and taken by phagosomes for phagocytosis. Cholesterol crystals are broken down and lysosomes attach to phagosomes to form phagolysosomes. Because of the size and chemistry of the cholesterol crystals, the phagolysosome ruptures and undegraded crystals along with cathepsin B are exposed in cytoplasm. This is the priming signal for NLRP3 inflammasome activation. Other signals such as K^+ efflux, Ca^{2+} influx and lipopolysaccharide (LPS) may also trigger the NLRP3 inflammasome. Immature forms of IL-1β and IL-18 (pro-IL-1β and pro-Il-18) are proteolytically cleaved by activated caspase-1. These mature cytokines IL-1β and IL-18 are released into the extra cellular space by pore-forming Gasdermin D.

It is well known now that for the activation of the NLRP3 inflammasome, two molecular signals are required. First, a nuclear factor kappa B (NF-κB)-dependent priming signal promotes the upregulation of IL-1β and NLRP3, and then a second signal triggers the oligomerization or activation of the NLRP3 inflammasome [38]. During atherosclerosis, cholesterol crystals evoke NETs to provide the first priming signal for macrophages, whereas the production of pro-IL-1β provides the second signal for the activation of the NLRP3 inflammasome and the release of mature cytokines. The NLRP3 inflammasome is triggered by different danger signals such as cholesterol crystals in atherosclerosis [39], uric acid crystals in gout [40] and amyloid-beta in Alzheimer's [41]. It is also activated in response to other triggers such as a reduced K^+ concentration in the cytoplasm resulting in P2X purinoceptor 4 (P2X4) receptor-mediated K^+ efflux [42]. Necrotic cells of the ischemic core discharge Ca^{2+} which increases in extracellular spaces prompting an increased influx and decreased efflux of Ca^{2+} [43]. Extensive Ca^{2+} influx induces cytochrome C dislocation which impairs the mitochondrial function of ATP production leading to ROS generation [44], which triggers NLRP3 inflammasome activation [45].

A pioneer work by Duewell et al. [39] revealed that cholesterol crystals are taken up by macrophages, whereby they are degraded in phagosomes and transferred to lysosomes. These undegraded cholesterol crystals (undegraded because of their size and chemistry) invoke rupture of the phagolysosomal membrane releasing lysosomal cysteine protease cathepsin B, which is taken up as a danger signal for the priming and activation of the NLRP3 inflammasome and release of mature IL-1β. Another study showed that complement component 5a (CC5a) along with TNF-α invokes a signal for cholesterol-crystal-induced NLRP3 inflammasome activation [46]. Undegraded cholesterol crystals released after phagolysosomal membrane breach trigger the priming signal for the NLRP3 inflammasome to produce a premature form of IL-1β (pro-IL-1β) which is considered to be the activation signal for the oligomerization of the NLRP3 inflammasome to release mature IL-1β [32]. Basic calcium phosphate crystals (BCPC) are considered to be present with inflammatory macrophages in developing atherosclerotic plaque, and are internalized by macrophages [47] and initiate signals for the activation of the NLRP3 inflammasome [48]. Fatty acid palmitate promotes neointima formation by upregulation of inflammatory pathways and exerts a pro-inflammatory effect on vascular smooth muscle cells by stimulating the expression of C-reactive protein (CRP), TNF-α and inducible nitric oxide (iNOS) [49]. This palmitate prompts NLRP3 inflammasome activation through mitochondrial ROS production and lysosomal degradation [50]. Expounding on several triggers of NLRP3 inflammasome activation, two things are equivocally believed. First, NLRP3 is required as a general sensing receptor for all sorts of cellular debris. Second, many stimuli (K^+ efflux, Ca^{2+} influx, cathepsin B and ROS formation) are generated due to the breakdown of cellular organelles.

Almost 20 years ago, the NLRP1 inflammasome was discovered, which was considered to be present in leukocytes and activated by PYCARD to release mature caspase1 and 5 [51]. Later several inflammasomes such as the NLR Family CARD Domain Containing 4 (NLRC4), Interferon-inducible protein 2 (AIM2), Pyrin and Interferon inducible protein 16 (IFI16) were discovered [52]. Earlier, when research on NOD-like receptors (NLRs) was in its infancy, it was believed that NOD-like receptor proteins (NLRPs) create inflammasomes only through caspase-1 activation, which was termed the "canonical inflammasome". Then later, it was observed that inflammasomes can be formed by NLRPs through other methods such as with alternate caspases (caspase-11), which sense intracellular lipopolysaccharide (LPS) as a danger signal [53]. This was termed the "non-canonical inflammasome". NLRP3 can trigger both types of inflammasome activation.

The role of NLRP3 inflammasome activation in atherosclerosis and atherogenesis can be understood by the role of two terrible cytokines produced by it, i.e., IL-1β and IL-18. Inflammation itself does not initiate atherogenesis; rather it invites several intermediaries, especially cytokines, which mediate both inflammation and immune signaling. IL-1β plays both of these roles as a key messenger for propelling inflammatory signaling to atherothrombosis [54].

A study investigated the role of IL-1β in the progression of atherosclerosis by engineering double-knockout mice ($ApoE^{-/-}/IL-1β^{-/-}$) [55]. The study revealed that the area and size of the lesion at the aortic sinus decreased by 30% in $ApoE^{-/-}/IL-1β^{-/-}$ mice of 12 to 24 weeks of age when compared with $ApoE^{-/-}/IL-1β^{+/+}$ mice. Similarly, a significant reduction in VCAM-1 and MCP-1 mRNA levels was evident in $ApoE^{-/-}/IL-1β^{-/-}$ mice. The results suggested that *IL-1β* plays a significant role in the progression of atherosclerosis by downregulating VCAM-1 and MCP-1 expression in an injured aorta. Lately, it has been revealed that IL-1β helps in leukocyte accumulation and recruitment into atherosclerotic aortas, suggesting its role in speeding up atherosclerosis [56]. Moreover, IL-1β expression drives vascular calcification, angiotensin II (AngII)-induced hypertension and vascular remodeling [57]. Therefore, strategies for blocking IL-1β through inhibitors and agonists have proved to be very beneficial for atherosclerosis-driven diseases [58]. Similarly, IL-18, another proinflammatory cytokine produced by the activation of the NLRP3 inflammasome, is expressed in macrophages and plays a significant role in inflammatory and immune signaling by the synthesis of T cells, natural killer cells and IFNγ [59]. A study has revealed that it is rampantly present in atherosclerotic plaques and influences plaque destabilization [60]. Another study comprising knockout mice for $ApoE^{-/-}$ and $IL18^{-/-}$ revealed that this double knockout had reduced lesion size and lesser lesion composition [61]. It suggests that even in hypercholesterolemia, the absence of IL-18 attenuates lesion size and its concomitants. Another study explained its role in plaque destabilization by setting up an inflammatory hyper-response after binding to interleukin-18 receptor alpha chain (IL-18Ra) through NF-kB [62]. The CANTOS (Canakinumab Anti-inflammatory Thrombosis Outcome Study) research has substantiated the clinical relevance of blocking IL-1β and IL-18 for curtailing atherothrombosis in post-acute myocardial ischemia [63]. Nevertheless, a proposition that in advanced lesions, especially in the fibrous cap, IL-1β is atheroprotective for outward vessel remodeling and stabilizing the plaque by maintaining the thickness of fibrous cap and collagen content, cannot be ignored [64].

4. NETosis-NLRP3 Inflammasome Activation Link: A Maleficent Crosstalk

Clinical research on the signaling pathways leading to atherosclerosis has suggested that components of NETosis evoke NLRP3 inflammasome activation, which releases the proinflammatory cytokines IL-1β and IL-18. Both of these cytokines are very harmful for stimulating the atherosclerotic plaque to atherothrombosis and its rupture leading to ischemia. A study has revealed that monocyte-derived macrophages generate strong signals for inflammasome activation when they are incubated with NETs and then with cholesterol crystals [32]. This shows that NETs prime macrophages to produce pro-IL-1β and cholesterol crystals induce phagolysosomal damage due to internalization by binding to CD36 (a glycoprotein on the plasma membrane of macrophages). When macrophages ingest cholesterol crystals as cellular debris, they destroy them into phagosomes; these phagosomes deliver the degraded contents to lysosomes (phagolysosomes) where they are further degraded by acid hydrolases. These hydrolyzed contents of cholesterol crystals may cause the rupture of the phagolysosome membrane and the release of its contents into the cytoplasm which otherwise are exported outside the cell by membrane transporters [39,65]. These undegraded cholesterol crystals released into the cytoplasm due to phagolysosomal membrane rupture, are taken as danger signals which are sensed by PRRs, termed danger-associated molecular patterns (DAMPs) and pathogen-associated molecular patterns (PAMPs). NLRP3 is a significant member of the innate immune system which is a PRR and is activated in response to these danger signals. During NLRP3 inflammasome activation, it transposes ASC and regulates caspase-1 (CASP1) stimulation, which further proteolytically cleaves the mature forms of the proinflammatory cytokines IL-1β from pro-IL-1β and IL-18 from pro-IL-18. Present abundantly in atheromatous lesions, both IL-1β and IL-18 help in plaque development and its progression to ischemic stroke [66].

The consequent release of undegraded cholesterol crystals into the cytoplasm sets the wheel of inflammatory cascade (activating NLRP3 inflammasome) in motion through cycles of internalization of cholesterol crystals and continued phagolysosome rupturing (Figure 4). During acute inflammation, resolvins and selectins induce neutrophil apoptosis; they are engulfed and phagocytosed by macrophages in an effort to resolve inflammation and improve healing [67]. Hence, it is worthwhile to infer from the experimental evidence that cholesterol crystals incite both neutrophils and macrophages to initiate pronounced inflammation (NETosis and NLRP3 inflammasome activation) and destroy the neutrophil–macrophage amity which is otherwise anti-inflammatory, pro-healing and pro-repair [67].

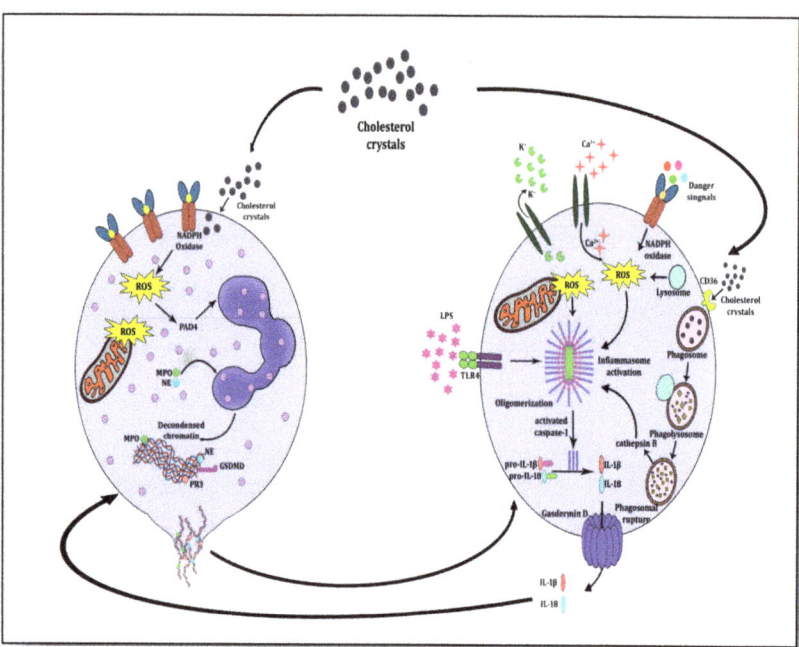

Figure 4. Neutrophil-macrophage crosstalk for mutually inciting atherosclerosis and igniting inflammation. Components of NETs (dead mitochondria and cfDNA) prime macrophages and components of NLRP3 inflammasome activation (IL-1β and IL-18) induce neutrophils to form NETs. Cholesterol crystals evoke signals for both neutrophils and macrophages for the development of NETs and prime NLRP3 inflammasome by interacting with reactive oxygen species (ROS) and CD36-mediated internalization, respectively.

To understand whether the NLRP3 inflammasome promotes NET formation during atherosclerosis, mice deficient with Abca1/g1 in myeloid cells were engineered with Nlrp3/caspase1/caspase11 deletion and bone marrow cells of these mice were transported to $Ldlr^{-/-}$ mice, which were fed with Western-type diet (WTD) [68]. They observed that lesion size significantly decreased in myeloid Abca1/g1-deficient $Ldlr^{-/-}$ mice due to Nlrp3/caspase1/caspase11 deficiency. Abca1/g1-deficient myeloid cells enhanced the cleavage of caspase 1 in splenic monocytes and macrophages and also in neutrophils to induce NET formation in atherosclerotic plaques. This indicates a cycle of heightened inflammation whereby the amassed cholesterol induces NLRP3 inflammasome activation which further promotes NET formation and NETosis in atherosclerotic plaques [68]. Another study has substantiated this inference and demonstrated that the canonical NLRP3 inflammasome plays a significant role in NETosis in sterile conditions [69]. This study has three important findings: first, PAD4, which is required for histone citrullination and decondensation of chromatin during NETosis, is required for NLRP3 oligomerization by mediating protein levels of ASC and NLRP3 post-transcriptionally. Second, genetic ablation of NLRP3 results in impaired signaling; hence, it significantly reduces NET formation in mouse neutrophils suggesting that NLRP3 components help in nuclear and plasma membrane rupture. Third, NLRP3 inhibition with a pharmacological antagonist attenuates NETosis in both mouse and human neutrophils. This study has shown that NLRP3 insufficiency leads to lesser NET formation in the thrombi of an experimental mouse model of deep venous thrombosis.

All of this suggests that PAD4 is required for NLRP3 inflammasome activation which propels NETosis both in vivo and in vitro under non-sterile conditions. Interestingly, IL-1β, a final product of NLRP3 inflammasome activation, is observed to play a significant role in NET formation and induces NETosis in systemic inflammatory response syndrome (SIRS) and abdominal aortic aneurysms (AAA) [11,70]. Moreover, cytokine IL-18 enhances the influx of Ca^{2+} into neutrophils which generates mitochondrial ROS and induces NET formation [71]. It has been demonstrated that similar processes are evident in NLRP3 inflammasome activation and in the generation of NETs [72]. Inflammasome activation proceeds to osmotic swelling of the cells, cell necrosis and finally the release of proinflammatory IL-1β, IL-18 and some DAMPs such as interleukin 1 alpha (IL-1α), high mobility group box 1 (HMGB1) proteins and ATPs. During this process, activated CASP1/11 cleaves GSDMD which neutralizes the membrane via pore formation and eventually cause pyroptosis, an inflammation-stimulated type of cell death. A similar process is evident in neutrophils where the NLRP3 inflammasome activation triggers the cleavage of GSDMD which helps in the degradation of the granular membrane, decondensation of chromatin, dissolution of the plasma membrane and expulsion of the components of NETs [72].

On the other hand, NET components including cfDNA stimulate NLRP3 inflammasome in macrophages [73]. Three significant inferences are evident from the analysis of these previously mentioned research reports. First, PAD4 is the hallmark for NET generation, and it also stimulates NLRP3 inflammasome activation. Second, cholesterol crystals trigger priming and activating signals for NLRP3 inflammasome activation and also initiate NET formation and prompt NETosis. Third, components of NETs (dead mitochondria and cfDNA) prime NLRP3 to activate the inflammasome, whereas IL-1β and IL-18 stimulate neutrophils for NET formation. Although it was known that NLRP3 inflammasome activation in macrophages is responsible for delayed wound healing in diabetic mice, it has been revealed that NET production in diabetic wounds triggers NLRP3 inflammasome activation and releases IL-1β in macrophages causing a sustained inflammatory response and prolonging wound healing [74]. Furthermore, NETs elicit signals for ROS generation triggering thioredoxin interacting protein (TXNIP) activation and both of these induce NLRP3 inflammasome activation. On summing up, one may reason to believe that both NLRP3 inflammasome activation and NETosis are triggered simultaneously, primarily by cholesterol crystals, and together these processes not only participate in triggering atherosclerosis but also perpetuate it with inflammation and exacerbate it with atherogenesis, finally leading to ischemia and infarction.

5. Future Directions

It is beyond doubt that our understanding of mediators that propel inflammation on atherosclerosis has improved considerably over last few years but translating this knowledge from bench to bedside still needs to be enhanced. The complex etiology coupled with several phases of atherosclerotic lesion and more so their different responses to inflammation-resolving drug targets have complicated its utility for improving anti-atherosclerosis strategies. Future studies based on multiomics platforms should weigh the collaborative contribution of these inflammatory perpetrators against trained immunity (de facto innate immune memory) and should develop some quantifiable measure stratified with risk severity so that their genetic or pharmacological inhibition may prove beneficial for specific stages of atherosclerotic lesions showing recuperative dose response. Gene expression studies along with clinical data sets in atherosclerosis may jointly be used to develop polygenic risk scores which can offer risk-stratified quantitative measures for specific immunophenotypes. Such strategies for harnessing gene-immune signatures may be the future of personalized medicine, whereby a formidable impact of the NETs–NLRP3 inflammasome nexus on atherosclerosis and its affiliated worst outcomes can be curtailed.

Author Contributions: P.S., M.S. and N.K. conceived the idea and set the focus and outline of the manuscript. M.K., G.S., A.K., A.N., S.M. and M.D.N. contributed their opinions and text especially for the mechanism of atherosclerosis. P.S., M.S. and N.K. wrote the manuscript. N.K., M.S., K.S. and B.S. reviewed the literature and assembled together all the ideas contributed by the authors in the manuscript. P.S., M.S. and S.M. looked after the assimilation of ideas and putting them together. P.S., M.S., A.K., N.K., A.N., M.D.N. and S.M. edited and enriched the manuscript. P.S. and N.K. drew the figures. All authors have read and agreed to the published version of the manuscript.

Funding: This research was funded from the Senior Research Fellowship awarded to Nitin Kumar by the Human Resource Development Group (HRDG) of the Council of Scientific and Industrial Research (CSIR), New Delhi (09/140(0174)/2018-EMR-1).

Institutional Review Board Statement: Not applicable.

Informed Consent Statement: Not applicable.

Data Availability Statement: Data collected from different research papers for writing this review paper are available from the corresponding author, and can be shared on request.

Acknowledgments: Senior Research Fellowship awarded to Nitin Kumar by Human Resource Development Group (HRDG) of Council of Scientific and Industrial Research (CSIR), New Delhi (09/140(0174)/2018-EMR-1).

Conflicts of Interest: The authors declare no conflict of interest. The funding agency has no role in the design of the study; in the collection, analyses or interpretation of data; in the writing of the manuscript; or in the decision to publish the results.

References

1. Libby, P.; Buring, J.E.; Badimon, L.; Hansson, G.K.; Deanfield, J.; Bittencourt, M.S.; Tokgözoğlu, L.; Lewis, E.F. Atherosclerosis. *Nat. Rev. Dis. Primers* **2019**, *5*, 56. [CrossRef] [PubMed]
2. Lechner, K.; von Schacky, C.; McKenzie, A.L.; Worm, N.; Nixdorff, U.; Lechner, B.; Kränkel, N.; Halle, M.; Krauss, R.M.; Scherr, J. Lifestyle factors and high-risk atherosclerosis: Pathways and mechanisms beyond traditional risk factors. *Eur. J. Prev. Cardiol.* **2020**, *27*, 394–406. [CrossRef] [PubMed]
3. Tabas, I.; García-Cardeña, G.; Owens, G.K. Recent insights into the cellular biology of atherosclerosis. *J. Cell. Biol.* **2015**, *209*, 13–22. [CrossRef]
4. Kong, P.; Cui, Z.-Y.; Huang, X.-F.; Zhang, D.-D.; Guo, R.-J.; Han, M. Inflammation and atherosclerosis: Signaling pathways and therapeutic intervention. *Signal Transduct. Target. Ther.* **2022**, *7*, 131. [CrossRef] [PubMed]
5. Dabagh, M.; Jalali, P.; Tarbell, J.M. The transport of LDL across the deformable arterial wall: The effect of endothelial cell turnover and intimal deformation under hypertension. *Am. J. Physiol. Heart Circ. Physiol.* **2009**, *297*, H983–H996. [CrossRef]
6. Noble, M.I.M.; Drake-Holland, A.J.; Vink, H. Hypothesis: Arterial glycocalyx dysfunction is the first step in the atherothrombotic process. *QJM* **2008**, *101*, 513–518. [CrossRef]
7. Björkegren, J.L.M.; Lusis, A.J. Atherosclerosis: Recent developments. *Cell* **2022**, *185*, 1630–1645. [CrossRef]
8. Bonaventura, A.; Vecchié, A.; Abbate, A.; Montecucco, F. Neutrophil Extracellular Traps and Cardiovascular Diseases: An Update. *Cells* **2020**, *9*, 231. [CrossRef]
9. Tschopp, J.; Schroder, K. NLRP3 inflammasome activation: The convergence of multiple signalling pathways on ROS production? *Nat. Rev. Immunol.* **2010**, *10*, 210–215. [CrossRef]
10. Thiam, H.R.; Wong, S.L.; Qiu, R.; Kittisopikul, M.; Vahabikashi, A.; Goldman, A.E.; Goldman, R.D.; Wagner, D.D.; Waterman, C.M. NETosis proceeds by cytoskeleton and endomembrane disassembly and PAD4-mediated chromatin decondensation and nuclear envelope rupture. *Proc. Natl. Acad. Sci. USA* **2020**, *117*, 7326–7337. [CrossRef] [PubMed]
11. Keshari, R.S.; Jyoti, A.; Dubey, M.; Kothari, N.; Kohli, M.; Bogra, J.; Barthwal, M.K.; Dikshit, M. Cytokines induced neutrophil extracellular traps formation: Implication for the inflammatory disease condition. *PLoS ONE* **2012**, *7*, e48111. [CrossRef] [PubMed]
12. Fuchs, T.A.; Brill, A.; Duerschmied, D.; Schatzberg, D.; Monestier, M.; Myers, D.D.; Wrobleski, S.K.; Wakefield, T.W.; Hartwig, J.H.; Wagner, D.D. Extracellular DNA traps promote thrombosis. *Proc. Natl. Acad. Sci. USA* **2010**, *107*, 15880–15885. [CrossRef] [PubMed]
13. Jorch, S.K.; Kubes, P. An emerging role for neutrophil extracellular traps in noninfectious disease. *Nat. Med.* **2017**, *23*, 279–287. [CrossRef] [PubMed]

14. Engelen, S.E.; Robinson, A.J.B.; Zurke, Y.-X.; Monaco, C. Therapeutic strategies targeting inflammation and immunity in atherosclerosis: How to proceed? *Nat. Rev. Cardiol.* **2022**, *19*, 522–542. [CrossRef]
15. Tabas, I.; Lichtman, A.H. Monocyte-Macrophages and T Cells in Atherosclerosis. *Immunity* **2017**, *47*, 621–634. [CrossRef]
16. Döring, Y.; Soehnlein, O.; Weber, C. Neutrophil Extracellular Traps in Atherosclerosis and Atherothrombosis. *Circ. Res.* **2017**, *120*, 736–743. [CrossRef]
17. Damascena, H.L.; Silveira, W.A.A.; Castro, M.S.; Fontes, W. Neutrophil Activated by the Famous and Potent PMA (Phorbol Myristate Acetate). *Cells* **2022**, *11*, 2889. [CrossRef] [PubMed]
18. Branzk, N.; Lubojemska, A.; Hardison, S.E.; Wang, Q.; Gutierrez, M.G.; Brown, G.D.; Papayannopoulos, V. Neutrophils sense microbe size and selectively release neutrophil extracellular traps in response to large pathogens. *Nat. Immunol.* **2014**, *15*, 1017–1025. [CrossRef]
19. Clark, S.R.; Ma, A.C.; Tavener, S.A.; McDonald, B.; Goodarzi, Z.; Kelly, M.M.; Patel, K.D.; Chakrabarti, S.; McAvoy, E.; Sinclair, G.D.; et al. Platelet TLR4 activates neutrophil extracellular traps to ensnare bacteria in septic blood. *Nat. Med.* **2007**, *13*, 463–469. [CrossRef]
20. Papayannopoulos, V.; Metzler, K.D.; Hakkim, A.; Zychlinsky, A. Neutrophil elastase and myeloperoxidase regulate the formation of neutrophil extracellular traps. *J. Cell. Biol.* **2010**, *191*, 677–691. [CrossRef]
21. Hamam, H.J.; Khan, M.A.; Palaniyar, N. Histone Acetylation Promotes Neutrophil Extracellular Trap Formation. *Biomolecules* **2019**, *9*, 32. [CrossRef]
22. Knight, J.S.; Luo, W.; O'Dell, A.A.; Yalavarthi, S.; Zhao, W.; Subramanian, V.; Guo, C.; Grenn, R.C.; Thompson, P.R.; Eitzman, D.T.; et al. Peptidylarginine deiminase inhibition reduces vascular damage and modulates innate immune responses in murine models of atherosclerosis. *Circ. Res.* **2014**, *114*, 947–956. [CrossRef]
23. Megens, R.T.A.; Vijayan, S.; Lievens, D.; Döring, Y.; van Zandvoort, M.A.M.J.; Grommes, J.; Weber, C.; Soehnlein, O. Presence of luminal neutrophil extracellular traps in atherosclerosis. *Thromb. Haemost.* **2012**, *107*, 597–598. [CrossRef] [PubMed]
24. Chrysanthopoulou, A.; Gkaliagkousi, E.; Lazaridis, A.; Arelaki, S.; Pateinakis, P.; Ntinopoulou, M.; Mitsios, A.; Antoniadou, C.; Argyriou, C.; Georgiadis, G.S.; et al. Angiotensin II triggers release of neutrophil extracellular traps, linking thromboinflammation with essential hypertension. *JCI Insight* **2021**, *6*, e148668. [CrossRef] [PubMed]
25. Metzler, K.D.; Fuchs, T.A.; Nauseef, W.M.; Reumaux, D.; Roesler, J.; Schulze, I.; Wahn, V.; Papayannopoulos, V.; Zychlinsky, A. Myeloperoxidase is required for neutrophil extracellular trap formation: Implications for innate immunity. *Blood* **2011**, *117*, 953–959. [CrossRef] [PubMed]
26. Franck, G.; Mawson, T.L.; Folco, E.J.; Molinaro, R.; Ruvkun, V.; Engelbertsen, D.; Liu, X.; Tesmenitsky, Y.; Shvartz, E.; Sukhova, G.K.; et al. Roles of PAD4 and NETosis in Experimental Atherosclerosis and Arterial Injury: Implications for Superficial Erosion. *Circ. Res.* **2018**, *123*, 33–42. [CrossRef]
27. Liu, Y.; Carmona-Rivera, C.; Moore, E.; Seto, N.L.; Knight, J.S.; Pryor, M.; Yang, Z.-H.; Hemmers, S.; Remaley, A.T.; Mowen, K.A.; et al. Myeloid-Specific Deletion of Peptidylarginine Deiminase 4 Mitigates Atherosclerosis. *Front. Immunol.* **2018**, *9*, 1680. [CrossRef]
28. Stakos, D.A.; Kambas, K.; Konstantinidis, T.; Mitroulis, I.; Apostolidou, E.; Arelaki, S.; Tsironidou, V.; Giatromanolaki, A.; Skendros, P.; Konstantinides, S.; et al. Expression of functional tissue factor by neutrophil extracellular traps in culprit artery of acute myocardial infarction. *Eur. Heart J.* **2015**, *36*, 1405–1414. [CrossRef] [PubMed]
29. Moschonas, I.C.; Tselepis, A.D. The pathway of neutrophil extracellular traps towards atherosclerosis and thrombosis. *Atherosclerosis* **2019**, *288*, 9–16. [CrossRef] [PubMed]
30. Sun, S.; Zou, X.; Wang, D.; Liu, Y.; Zhang, Z.; Guo, J.; Lu, R.; Huang, W.; Wang, S.; Li, Z.; et al. IRGM/Irgm1 deficiency inhibits neutrophil-platelet interactions and thrombosis in experimental atherosclerosis and arterial injury. *Biomed. Pharmacother.* **2023**, *158*, 114152. [CrossRef]
31. Dou, H.; Kotini, A.; Liu, W.; Fidler, T.; Endo-Umeda, K.; Sun, X.; Olszewska, M.; Xiao, T.; Abramowicz, S.; Yalcinkaya, M.; et al. Oxidized Phospholipids Promote NETosis and Arterial Thrombosis in LNK(SH2B3) Deficiency. *Circulation* **2021**, *144*, 1940–1954. [CrossRef]
32. Warnatsch, A.; Ioannou, M.; Wang, Q.; Papayannopoulos, V. Inflammation. Neutrophil extracellular traps license macrophages for cytokine production in atherosclerosis. *Science* **2015**, *349*, 316–320. [CrossRef]
33. Mahley, R.W.; Huang, Y.; Weisgraber, K.H. Putting cholesterol in its place: ApoE and reverse cholesterol transport. *J. Clin. Invest.* **2006**, *116*, 1226–1229. [CrossRef]
34. Allam, G.; Abdel-Moneim, A.; Gaber, A.M. The pleiotropic role of interleukin-17 in atherosclerosis. *Biomed. Pharmacother.* **2018**, *106*, 1412–1418. [CrossRef]
35. Dostert, C.; Pétrilli, V.; Van Bruggen, R.; Steele, C.; Mossman, B.T.; Tschopp, J. Innate immune activation through Nalp3 inflammasome sensing of asbestos and silica. *Science* **2008**, *320*, 674–677. [CrossRef] [PubMed]
36. Wang, Z.; Zhang, S.; Xiao, Y.; Zhang, W.; Wu, S.; Qin, T.; Yue, Y.; Qian, W.; Li, L. NLRP3 Inflammasome and Inflammatory Diseases. *Oxid. Med. Cell. Longev.* **2020**, *2020*, 4063562. [CrossRef] [PubMed]
37. Bergsbaken, T.; Fink, S.L.; Cookson, B.T. Pyroptosis: Host cell death and inflammation. *Nat. Rev. Microbiol.* **2009**, *7*, 99–109. [CrossRef] [PubMed]
38. He, Y.; Hara, H.; Núñez, G. Mechanism and Regulation of NLRP3 Inflammasome Activation. *Trends Biochem. Sci.* **2016**, *41*, 1012–1021. [CrossRef]

39. Duewell, P.; Kono, H.; Rayner, K.J.; Sirois, C.M.; Vladimer, G.; Bauernfeind, F.G.; Abela, G.S.; Franchi, L.; Nuñez, G.; Schnurr, M.; et al. NLRP3 inflammasomes are required for atherogenesis and activated by cholesterol crystals. *Nature* **2010**, *464*, 1357–1361. [CrossRef]
40. Martinon, F.; Pétrilli, V.; Mayor, A.; Tardivel, A.; Tschopp, J. Gout-associated uric acid crystals activate the NALP3 inflammasome. *Nature* **2006**, *440*, 237–241. [CrossRef]
41. Ising, C.; Venegas, C.; Zhang, S.; Scheiblich, H.; Schmidt, S.V.; Vieira-Saecker, A.; Schwartz, S.; Albasset, S.; McManus, R.M.; Tejera, D.; et al. NLRP3 inflammasome activation drives tau pathology. *Nature* **2019**, *575*, 669–673. [CrossRef]
42. Muñoz-Planillo, R.; Kuffa, P.; Martínez-Colón, G.; Smith, B.L.; Rajendiran, T.M.; Núñez, G. K$^+$ efflux is the common trigger of NLRP3 inflammasome activation by bacterial toxins and particulate matter. *Immunity* **2013**, *38*, 1142–1153. [CrossRef] [PubMed]
43. Murakami, T.; Ockinger, J.; Yu, J.; Byles, V.; McColl, A.; Hofer, A.M.; Horng, T. Critical role for calcium mobilization in activation of the NLRP3 inflammasome. *Proc. Natl. Acad. Sci. USA* **2012**, *109*, 11282–11287. [CrossRef]
44. Feng, G.; Yang, X.; Li, Y.; Wang, X.; Tan, S.; Chen, F. LPS enhances platelets aggregation via TLR4, which is related to mitochondria damage caused by intracellular ROS, but not extracellular ROS. *Cell. Immunol.* **2018**, *328*, 86–92. [CrossRef]
45. Shimada, K.; Crother, T.R.; Karlin, J.; Dagvadorj, J.; Chiba, N.; Chen, S.; Ramanujan, V.K.; Wolf, A.J.; Vergnes, L.; Ojcius, D.M.; et al. Oxidized mitochondrial DNA activates the NLRP3 inflammasome during apoptosis. *Immunity* **2012**, *36*, 401–414. [CrossRef] [PubMed]
46. Samstad, E.O.; Niyonzima, N.; Nymo, S.; Aune, M.H.; Ryan, L.; Bakke, S.S.; Lappegård, K.T.; Brekke, O.-L.; Lambris, J.D.; Damås, J.K.; et al. Cholesterol crystals induce complement-dependent inflammasome activation and cytokine release. *J. Immunol.* **2014**, *192*, 2837–2845. [CrossRef]
47. Nadra, I.; Mason, J.C.; Philippidis, P.; Florey, O.; Smythe, C.D.W.; McCarthy, G.M.; Landis, R.C.; Haskard, D.O. Proinflammatory activation of macrophages by basic calcium phosphate crystals via protein kinase C and MAP kinase pathways: A vicious cycle of inflammation and arterial calcification? *Circ. Res.* **2005**, *96*, 1248–1256. [CrossRef]
48. Pazár, B.; Ea, H.-K.; Narayan, S.; Kolly, L.; Bagnoud, N.; Chobaz, V.; Roger, T.; Lioté, F.; So, A.; Busso, N. Basic calcium phosphate crystals induce monocyte/macrophage IL-1β secretion through the NLRP3 inflammasome in vitro. *J. Immunol.* **2011**, *186*, 2495–2502. [CrossRef] [PubMed]
49. Wu, D.; Liu, J.; Pang, X.; Wang, S.; Zhao, J.; Zhang, X.; Feng, L. Palmitic acid exerts pro-inflammatory effects on vascular smooth muscle cells by inducing the expression of C-reactive protein, inducible nitric oxide synthase and tumor necrosis factor-α. *Int. J. Mol. Med.* **2014**, *34*, 1706–1712. [CrossRef]
50. Wen, H.; Gris, D.; Lei, Y.; Jha, S.; Zhang, L.; Huang, M.T.-H.; Brickey, W.J.; Ting, J.P.-Y. Fatty acid-induced NLRP3-ASC inflammasome activation interferes with insulin signaling. *Nat. Immunol.* **2011**, *12*, 408–415. [CrossRef]
51. Martinon, F.; Burns, K.; Tschopp, J. The inflammasome: A molecular platform triggering activation of inflammatory caspases and processing of proIL-beta. *Mol. Cell.* **2002**, *10*, 417–426. [CrossRef]
52. Broz, P.; Dixit, V.M. Inflammasomes: Mechanism of assembly, regulation and signalling. *Nat. Rev. Immunol.* **2016**, *16*, 407–420. [CrossRef] [PubMed]
53. Yi, Y.-S. Caspase-11 non-canonical inflammasome: A critical sensor of intracellular lipopolysaccharide in macrophage-mediated inflammatory responses. *Immunology* **2017**, *152*, 207–217. [CrossRef]
54. Lim, G.B. IL-1 signalling in atherosclerosis. *Nat. Rev. Cardiol.* **2019**, *16*, 200. [CrossRef] [PubMed]
55. Kirii, H.; Niwa, T.; Yamada, Y.; Wada, H.; Saito, K.; Iwakura, Y.; Asano, M.; Moriwaki, H.; Seishima, M. Lack of interleukin-1beta decreases the severity of atherosclerosis in ApoE-deficient mice. *Arterioscler. Thromb. Vasc. Biol.* **2003**, *23*, 656–660. [CrossRef]
56. Hettwer, J.; Hinterdobler, J.; Miritsch, B.; Deutsch, M.-A.; Li, X.; Mauersberger, C.; Moggio, A.; Braster, Q.; Gram, H.; Robertson, A.A.B.; et al. Interleukin-1β suppression dampens inflammatory leucocyte production and uptake in atherosclerosis. *Cardiovasc. Res.* **2022**, *118*, 2778–2791. [CrossRef]
57. Ren, X.-S.; Tong, Y.; Ling, L.; Chen, D.; Sun, H.-J.; Zhou, H.; Qi, X.-H.; Chen, Q.; Li, Y.-H.; Kang, Y.-M.; et al. NLRP3 Gene Deletion Attenuates Angiotensin II-Induced Phenotypic Transformation of Vascular Smooth Muscle Cells and Vascular Remodeling. *Cell. Physiol. Biochem.* **2017**, *44*, 2269–2280. [CrossRef]
58. Libby, P. Interleukin-1 Beta as a Target for Atherosclerosis Therapy: Biological Basis of CANTOS and Beyond. *J. Am. Coll. Cardiol.* **2017**, *70*, 2278–2289. [CrossRef] [PubMed]
59. Badimon, L. Interleukin-18: A potent pro-inflammatory cytokine in atherosclerosis. *Cardiovasc. Res.* **2012**, *96*, 172–175; discussion 176–180. [CrossRef] [PubMed]
60. Mallat, Z.; Corbaz, A.; Scoazec, A.; Besnard, S.; Lesèche, G.; Chvatchko, Y.; Tedgui, A. Expression of interleukin-18 in human atherosclerotic plaques and relation to plaque instability. *Circulation* **2001**, *104*, 1598–1603. [CrossRef]
61. Elhage, R.; Jawien, J.; Rudling, M.; Ljunggren, H.-G.; Takeda, K.; Akira, S.; Bayard, F.; Hansson, G.K. Reduced atherosclerosis in interleukin-18 deficient apolipoprotein E-knockout mice. *Cardiovasc. Res.* **2003**, *59*, 234–240. [CrossRef]
62. Bhat, O.M.; Kumar, P.U.; Giridharan, N.V.; Kaul, D.; Kumar, M.J.M.; Dhawan, V. Interleukin-18-induced atherosclerosis involves CD36 and NF-κB crosstalk in Apo E-/- mice. *J. Cardiol.* **2015**, *66*, 28–35. [CrossRef]
63. Ridker, P.M.; MacFadyen, J.G.; Thuren, T.; Libby, P. Residual inflammatory risk associated with interleukin-18 and interleukin-6 after successful interleukin-1β inhibition with canakinumab: Further rationale for the development of targeted anti-cytokine therapies for the treatment of atherothrombosis. *Eur. Heart J.* **2020**, *41*, 2153–2163. [CrossRef] [PubMed]

64. Gomez, D.; Baylis, R.A.; Durgin, B.G.; Newman, A.A.C.; Alencar, G.F.; Mahan, S.; St Hilaire, C.; Müller, W.; Waisman, A.; Francis, S.E.; et al. Interleukin-1β has atheroprotective effects in advanced atherosclerotic lesions of mice. *Nat. Med.* **2018**, *24*, 1418–1429. [CrossRef]
65. Ogura, Y.; Sutterwala, F.S.; Flavell, R.A. The inflammasome: First line of the immune response to cell stress. *Cell* **2006**, *126*, 659–662. [CrossRef]
66. Paramel Varghese, G.; Folkersen, L.; Strawbridge, R.J.; Halvorsen, B.; Yndestad, A.; Ranheim, T.; Krohg-Sørensen, K.; Skjelland, M.; Espevik, T.; Aukrust, P.; et al. NLRP3 Inflammasome Expression and Activation in Human Atherosclerosis. *J. Am. Heart Assoc.* **2016**, *5*, e003031. [CrossRef]
67. Serhan, C.N.; Savill, J. Resolution of inflammation: The beginning programs the end. *Nat. Immunol.* **2005**, *6*, 1191–1197. [CrossRef] [PubMed]
68. Westerterp, M.; Fotakis, P.; Ouimet, M.; Bochem, A.E.; Zhang, H.; Molusky, M.M.; Wang, W.; Abramowicz, S.; la Bastide-van Gemert, S.; Wang, N.; et al. Cholesterol Efflux Pathways Suppress Inflammasome Activation, NETosis, and Atherogenesis. *Circulation* **2018**, *138*, 898–912. [CrossRef] [PubMed]
69. Münzer, P.; Negro, R.; Fukui, S.; di Meglio, L.; Aymonnier, K.; Chu, L.; Cherpokova, D.; Gutch, S.; Sorvillo, N.; Shi, L.; et al. NLRP3 Inflammasome Assembly in Neutrophils Is Supported by PAD4 and Promotes NETosis Under Sterile Conditions. *Front. Immunol.* **2021**, *12*, 683803. [CrossRef]
70. Meher, A.K.; Spinosa, M.; Davis, J.P.; Pope, N.; Laubach, V.E.; Su, G.; Serbulea, V.; Leitinger, N.; Ailawadi, G.; Upchurch, G.R. Novel Role of IL (Interleukin)-1β in Neutrophil Extracellular Trap Formation and Abdominal Aortic Aneurysms. *Arterioscler. Thromb. Vasc. Biol.* **2018**, *38*, 843–853. [CrossRef] [PubMed]
71. Liao, T.-L.; Chen, Y.-M.; Tang, K.-T.; Chen, P.-K.; Liu, H.-J.; Chen, D.-Y. MicroRNA-223 inhibits neutrophil extracellular traps formation through regulating calcium influx and small extracellular vesicles transmission. *Sci. Rep.* **2021**, *11*, 15676. [CrossRef] [PubMed]
72. Sollberger, G.; Choidas, A.; Burn, G.L.; Habenberger, P.; Di Lucrezia, R.; Kordes, S.; Menninger, S.; Eickhoff, J.; Nussbaumer, P.; Klebl, B.; et al. Gasdermin D plays a vital role in the generation of neutrophil extracellular traps. *Sci. Immunol.* **2018**, *3*, eaar6689. [CrossRef] [PubMed]
73. Hu, Q.; Shi, H.; Zeng, T.; Liu, H.; Su, Y.; Cheng, X.; Ye, J.; Yin, Y.; Liu, M.; Zheng, H.; et al. Increased neutrophil extracellular traps activate NLRP3 and inflammatory macrophages in adult-onset Still's disease. *Arthritis Res. Ther.* **2019**, *21*, 9. [CrossRef] [PubMed]
74. Liu, D.; Yang, P.; Gao, M.; Yu, T.; Shi, Y.; Zhang, M.; Yao, M.; Liu, Y.; Zhang, X. NLRP3 activation induced by neutrophil extracellular traps sustains inflammatory response in the diabetic wound. *Clin. Sci.* **2019**, *133*, 565–582. [CrossRef] [PubMed]

Disclaimer/Publisher's Note: The statements, opinions and data contained in all publications are solely those of the individual author(s) and contributor(s) and not of MDPI and/or the editor(s). MDPI and/or the editor(s) disclaim responsibility for any injury to people or property resulting from any ideas, methods, instructions or products referred to in the content.

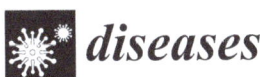

Article

Demographic and Social Patterns of the Mean Values of Inflammatory Markers in U.S. Adults: A 2009–2016 NHANES Analysis

Rose Calixte [1], Zachary Ye [2], Raisa Haq [3], Salwa Aladhamy [4] and Marlene Camacho-Rivera [1,*]

1. School of Public Health, SUNY Downstate Health Sciences University, Brooklyn, NY 11203, USA
2. College of Medicine, SUNY Downstate Health Sciences University, Brooklyn, NY 11203, USA
3. School of Medicine, City University of New York, New York, NY 10031, USA
4. College of Optometry, Pennsylvania State University, State College, PA 16802, USA
* Correspondence: marlene.camacho-rivera@downstate.edu; Tel.: +1-718-270-4386

Abstract: Several studies have reported on the negative implications of elevated neutrophil-to-lymphocyte ratio (NLR) and elevated platelet-to-lymphocyte ratio (PLR) levels associated with outcomes in many surgical and medical conditions, including cancer. In order to use the inflammatory markers NLR and PLR as prognostic factors in disease, a normal value in disease-free individuals must be identified first. This study aims (1) to establish mean values of various inflammatory markers using a healthy and nationally representative U.S. adult population and (2) to explore heterogeneity in the mean values by sociodemographic and behavioral risk factors to better specify cutoff points accordingly. The National Health and Nutrition Examination Survey (NHANES) of aggregated cross-sectional data collected from 2009 to 2016 was analyzed; data extracted included markers of systemic inflammation and demographic variables. We excluded participants who were under 20 years old or had a history of an inflammatory disease such as arthritis or gout. Adjusted linear regression models were used to examine the associations between demographic/behavioral characteristics and neutrophil counts, platelet counts, lymphocyte counts, as well as NLR and PLR values. The national weighted average NLR value is 2.16 and the national weighted average PLR value is 121.31. The national weighted average PLR value for non-Hispanic Whites is 123.12 (121.13–125.11), for non-Hispanic Blacks it is 119.77 (117.49–122.06), for Hispanic people it is 116.33 (114.69–117.97), and for participants of other races it is 119.84 (116.88–122.81). Non-Hispanic Blacks and Blacks have significantly lower mean NLR values (1.78, 95% CI 1.74–1.83 and 2.10, 95% CI 2.04–2.16, respectively) as compared with that of non-Hispanic Whites (2.27, 95% CI 2.22–2.30, $p < 0.0001$). Subjects who reported a non-smoking history had significantly lower NLR values than subjects who reported any smoking history and higher PLR values than current smokers. This study provides preliminary data for demographic and behavioral effects on markers of inflammation, i.e., NLR and PLR, that have been associated with several chronic disease outcomes, suggesting that different cutoff points should be set according to social factors.

Keywords: inflammation; cancer; biomarkers; neutrophil; platelet; lymphocyte; smoking

Citation: Calixte, R.; Ye, Z.; Haq, R.; Aladhamy, S.; Camacho-Rivera, M. Demographic and Social Patterns of the Mean Values of Inflammatory Markers in U.S. Adults: A 2009–2016 NHANES Analysis. *Diseases* **2023**, *11*, 14. https://doi.org/10.3390/diseases11010014

Academic Editor: Omar Cauli

Received: 28 September 2022
Revised: 28 December 2022
Accepted: 16 January 2023
Published: 20 January 2023

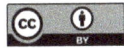

Copyright: © 2023 by the authors. Licensee MDPI, Basel, Switzerland. This article is an open access article distributed under the terms and conditions of the Creative Commons Attribution (CC BY) license (https://creativecommons.org/licenses/by/4.0/).

1. Introduction

Inflammatory cells have been found to play roles in a variety of chronic conditions, such as cardiovascular disease [1], chronic kidney disease [2], and cancer [3–7]. Hematological components of the systemic inflammatory response (SIR), also known as SIR biomarkers, are increasingly becoming potential prognostic factors of various diseases [8]. Two such inflammatory response markers that have been widely used are the neutrophil-to-lymphocyte ratio (NLR) and the platelet-to-lymphocyte ratio (PLR).

NLR is the ratio of circulating neutrophils to lymphocytes and can be calculated from a complete blood count [9]. An elevated NLR value has been associated with shorter survival in lung [3], pancreatic [4], and colorectal [5] cancers and serves as a marker of infectious pathologies and post-operative complications [6,10]. However, there is no current standard value that is considered to be a normal vs. abnormal NLR value. Current studies have defined NLR cutoff points contingent to their respective methodologies and populations. Some studies have reported NLR values organized into intervals [11,12], while other studies have chosen to define a cutoff point based on the median value calculated from the sample (NLR > 3.5) [2], and other studies have defined an elevated NLR based on poor survival in their sample (NLR > 5) [5].

Another inflammatory marker that has potential prognostic value for disease is the PLR, which is the ratio of circulating platelets to lymphocytes. An elevated PLR has been shown to be an independent prognostic factor for cardiovascular diseases, especially heart failure. It has been found that heart failure patients have both higher PLR values and higher NLR values [13]. PLR has also been associated with a worse prognosis or poorer oncological outcomes such as poorer overall survival and more advanced staging in a variety of malignancies, including gastric [14], colorectal [15], and pancreatic [16] cancers. The standard reference range for PLR is also uncertain, as this value appears to vary depending on a variety of factors [17].

It has been established that elevated NLR and PLR values are generally prognostic factors of mortality and morbidity in the diseases they are associated with. While current studies have looked at the significance of NLR and PLR in diseased populations, not much is known about the NLR and PLR values in normal, healthy populations. Having universal reference values based on a large and healthy population will allow for better use of these markers, which can lead to potential clinical significance in determining if a patient is in good health. One study tried to determine the limits of the values of NLR that were observable in an adult, non-geriatric population and identified them as 0.78–3.53 [18]. However, NLR and PLR values have been shown to differ based on demographic factors [17,19]. There has also been an association found between smoking status and NLR and PLR levels. Smoking appears to increase NLR [20] and decrease PLR [20,21]. As such, this study aims (1) to establish mean values of various inflammatory markers using a healthy and nationally representative U.S. adult population and (2) to explore heterogeneity in the mean values by sociodemographic and behavioral risk factors to better specify cutoff points accordingly.

2. Materials and Methods

The National Health and Nutrition Examination Survey (NHANES), a population-based survey that is designed to assess the health and nutritional status of non-institutionalized adults and children in the United States, was used for analysis. The NHANES uses a complex, multistage, probability sampling design to produce a nationally representative sample. In this study, we aggregated cross-sectional data collected from 2009 to 2016 and extracted various, validated measures of general inflammation (lymphocyte, monocyte, segmented neutrophil, eosinophil, basophil, platelet count, NLR, and PLR), demographic characteristics (age, sex, race, and body mass index), and social factors (education level, nativity to USA, smoking status, and alcohol usage).

Consenting participants complete a detailed in-person interview that is conducted by a trained professional on topics encompassing their demographic, socioeconomic, dietary, and health-related information. Measures of age, sex, race, education, nativity to USA, smoking status, and alcohol usage are obtained at that time. After an in-home interview, participants are scheduled an appointment at a Mobile Examination Center (MEC) where medical, physiologic, and laboratory tests are administered by trained medical staff [22]. At this time, body mass index is measured using bioelectrical impedance. Hematology testing is performed on blood specimens collected from participants and evaluated for neutrophil (1000 cells/μL), monocyte (1000 cells/μL), segmented neutrophil (1000 cells/μL), eosinophil (1000 cells/μL), basophil (1000 cells/μL), and platelet (1000 cells/μL) counts. Cell counts are determined using the Coulter MAXMs method (Beckman Coulter, Miami, FL, USA).

We excluded participants who were under 20 years old or had a history of inflammatory disease such as arthritis or gout. The final sample consisted of 16,849 subjects across all of the survey waves. We categorized age into four categories (20–29, 30–59, 60–79, and ≥80) to balance across sample sizes and because the NHANES has stopped reporting the actual age of anyone over 80 years old and uses 80 as a ceiling for age. We categorized BMI into four clinically important categories (underweight, normal weight, overweight, and obese).

We summarized all variables of interest using appropriate descriptive statistics such as unweighted mean (95% confidence interval) or unweighted frequency (percent) and weighted mean (95% CI) or weighted proportion (95% CI). We tested for bivariate association between demographic and behavioral characteristics on general inflammatory markers using linear regression models for each outcome. We tested for independent predictors of inflammatory markers using multiple linear regressions. We preprocessed the data using the SAS 9.4® software and analyzed the data using the Stata/SE version 16 software, with appropriate complex survey design methodology to provide nationally representative estimates. Results with p-value ≤ 0.05 are significant.

3. Results

3.1. Mean Inflammatory Marker Values in U.S. Adults

We present summary statistics of the study population with 95% confidence intervals in Table 1. The weighted study population is 62.5% non-White Hispanics, 11.6% non-Hispanic Black, and 16.7 % Hispanics. The proportions of males and females in the population are equally distributed. Over 82% of the study population are between 20 years old and 59 years old. Over 66% of the included participants are either overweight or obese. About 32% have a college degree or more. Moreover, close to 79% of the population are U.S. born citizens. About 60% of the included participants are non-smokers and just under 12% of the participants are non-drinkers. In the weighted population, the national mean for lymphocytes (1000 cells/μL) is 2.14 (95% CI = 2.11–2.16), the national mean for monocytes (1000 cells/μL) is 0.56 (95% CI = 0.55–0.56), the national mean for neutrophils (1000 cells/μL) is 4.28 (95% CI = 4.23–4.34), the national mean for eosinophils (1000 cells/μL) is 0.20 (95% CI = 0.19–0.20), the national mean for basophils (1000 cells/μL) is 0.05 (95% CI = 0.04–0.05), the national mean for platelet count (1000 cells/μL) is 238.89 (95% CI = 237.26–240.53), the national mean NLR value is 2.16 (95% CI = 2.13–2.19), And the national mean PLR value is 121.31 (95% CI = 102.01–122.61). The national weighted average (95% CI) numbers for the inflammatory markers are within the normal range for healthy people.

Table 1. Sociodemographic and clinical characteristics of the NHANES sample: 2009–2016.

Characteristics of Interest [1]		Unweighted Sample	Weighted Population
Race	Non-Hispanic White	6177 (36.7)	62.46 (58.54–66.22)
	Non-Hispanic Black	3493 (20.7)	11.65 (9.949–13.6)
	Hispanic	4615 (27.4)	16.7 (13.99–19.8)
	Other	2564 (15.2)	9.2 (8.01–10.53)
Sex	Male	8550 (50.7)	50.47 (49.86–51.26)
	Female	8299 (49.3)	49.53 (48.74–50.32)
Age (years)	20–29	3822 (22.7)	24.63 (23.1–26.23)
	30–59	9366 (55.6)	58.86 (57.41–60.29)
	60–79	3025 (18.0)	14.02 (13.15–14.94)
	80+	636 (3.8)	2.49 (2.2–2.8)
Education	<High School	3902 (23.2)	15.62 (14.1–17.27)
	High School/General Educational Development	3636 (21.6)	20.81 (19.62–22.06)
	Some College, or Associate of Arts	4997 (29.7)	31.72 (30.29–33.18)
	>College Graduate	4291 (25.5)	31.85 (29.52–34.28)
Nativity	United States born	11,042 (65.5)	78.83 (76.49–80.99)
	Non-United States born	5797 (34.4)	21.17 (19.01–23.51)

Table 1. Cont.

Characteristics of Interest [1]		Unweighted Sample	Weighted Population
Body mass index (Kg/m^2)	Underweight (<18.5)	291 (1.7)	1.791(1.527–2.098)
	Normal weight (18.5–24.9)	4999 (29.7)	31.43 (29.89–33.01)
	Overweight (25.0–29.9)	5369 (31.9)	33.75 (32.68–34.83)
	Obese (>30)	5404 (32.1)	33.03 (31.7–34.39)
Smoking status	Non-smoker	10,107 (60.0)	59.63 (58.06–61.18)
	Current smoker	3454 (20.5)	19.74 (18.73–20.78)
	Former smoker	3272 (19.4)	20.63 (19.36–21.96)
Alcohol usage	Non-drinker	2133 (12.7)	11.61 (10.29–13.07)
	Moderate drinker	4807 (28.5)	32.83 (31.5–34.19)
	Heavy drinker	7406 (44.0)	55.56 (54.14–56.97)
Lymphocytes (1000 cells/μL)		2.17 (2.15–2.19)	2.14 (2.11–2.16)
Monocytes (1000 cells/μL)		0.55 (0.54–0.55)	0.56 (0.55–0.56)
Segmented neutrophils (1000 cells/μL)		4.23 (4.2–4.27)	4.28 (4.23–4.34)
Eosinophils (1000 cells/μL)		0.2 (0.2–0.2)	0.20 (0.19–0.20)
Basophils number (1000 cells/μL)		0.05 (0.04–0.05)	0.05 (0.04–0.05)
Platelet count (1000 cells/μL)		239.46 (238.45–240.47)	238.89 (237.26–240.53)
Neutrophil/lymphocyte ratio (NLR)		2.12 (2.10–2.14)	2.16 (2.13–2.19)
Platelet/lymphocyte ratio (PLR)		120.19 (119.48–120.91)	121.31 (120.01–122.61)

[1] We summarized the data using unweighted mean (95% CI), unweighted count (percent), weighted mean (95% CI), and weighted proportion (95% CI).

3.2. Univariate Associations of Demographic Factors and Inflammatory Markers

We present the results of the univariate regression model for inflammatory markers in Table 2. On average, non-Hispanic Black adults have higher lymphocyte counts, higher platelet counts, lower monocyte counts, lower neutrophil counts, lower eosinophil counts, lower basophil counts, and lower NLR values than non-Hispanic Whites. However, the mean inflammatory marker counts for within racial categories are within a normal range. A gender difference was also observed within the inflammatory markers, with adult males having lower mean lymphocyte counts, lower mean neutrophil counts, lower mean platelet counts, and lower mean PLR values as compared with those of female adults. However, on average, adult males had higher NLR values, higher eosinophil counts, and higher monocyte counts than adult females in the U.S. population. The mean values for inflammatory markers were different for U.S.-born participants vs. non-U.S.-born participants. As compared with non-U.S.-born adults, U.S.-born adults had lower mean lymphocyte counts, higher mean monocyte counts, higher mean neutrophil counts, higher mean platelet counts, and higher mean NLR values. However, foreign born adults had higher PLR values as compared with U.S.-born adults. Participants with normal BMI values had the lowest mean values for lymphocyte counts and neutrophil counts, but the highest mean value for PLR. Comparing across demographic and clinical categories, the mean values for all inflammatory markers are within the normal range.

3.3. Multivariable Regression Results for Inflammatory Markers

We present the results of the multivariable regression model for inflammatory markers in Table 3. The results of the multivariable model reveal that, on average, lymphocyte count data are significantly higher in non-Hispanic Blacks and Hispanics as compared with non-Hispanic Whites. On average, lymphocyte counts are significantly higher for females as compared with males. Participants who were 30–79 years old had significantly lower mean lymphocyte counts vs. participants who were between 20 and 29 years old. Non-U.S.-born participants in the NHANES also have significantly higher mean lymphocyte counts vs. U.S.-born participants. Overweight and obese participants have significantly higher mean lymphocyte counts as compared with normal weight participants. Current smokers also have significantly higher mean lymphocyte counts as compared with those who had never smoked.

Table 2. Univariate associations of sociodemographic characteristics with clinical inflammatory markers: NHANES 2009–2016.

Sociodemographic Characteristics [2]		Lymphocytes (1000 Cells/μL)	Monocytes (1000 Cells/μL)	Segmented Neutrophils (1000 Cells/μL)
Race	Non-Hispanic White	2.09 (2.05–2.12)	0.57 (0.56–0.58)	4.37 (4.30–4.44)
	Non-Hispanic Black	2.24 (2.20–2.27)	0.52 (0.51–0.53)	3.66 (3.58–3.74)
	Hispanic	2.26 (2.20–2.29)	0.55 (0.54–0.56)	4.44 (4.36–4.53)
	Other	2.15 (2.12–2.19)	0.52 (0.51–0.53)	4.13 (4.03–4.23)
Sex	Male	2.09 (2.06–2.13)	0.58 (0.57–0.59)	3.95 (3.92–3.97)
	Female	2.18 (2.16–2.21)	0.54 (0.54–0.55)	4.11 (4.08–4.14)
Age (years)	20–29	2.27 (2.23–2.30)	0.56 (0.55–0.57)	4.38 (4.28–4.47)
	30–59	2.14 (2.11–2.17)	0.55 (0.54–0.55)	4.27 (4.22–4.33)
	60–79	1.94 (1.90–1.99)	0.57 (0.55–0.59)	4.13 (4.04–4.21)
	80+	1.94 (1.69–2.19)	0.62 (0.60–0.64)	4.36 (4.17–4.55)
Education	<High School	2.23 (2.20–2.27)	0.56 (0.55–0.58)	4.46 (4.36–4.56)
	High School/General Educational Development	2.20 (2.16–2.25)	0.57 (0.56–0.59)	4.45 (4.37–4.52)
	Some College, or Associate of Arts	2.17 (2.14–2.20)	0.56 (0.55–0.58)	4.35 (4.28–4.43)
	>College Graduate	2.02 (1.20–2.05)	0.53 (0.52–0.54)	4.01 (3.94–4.09)
Nativity	United States born	2.12 (2.10–2.15)	0.56 (0.55–0.57)	4.34 (4.28–4.40)
	Non-United States born	2.19 (2.17–2.21)	0.53 (0.52–0.54)	4.08 (4.01–4.14)
Body mass index (Kg/m²)	Underweight (<18.5)	2.09 (1.99–2.19)	0.52 (0.49–0.54)	4.06 (3.77–4.33)
	Normal weight (18.5–24.9)	2.01 (1.99–2.02)	0.53 (0.52–0.53)	3.40 (3.92–3.07)
	Overweight (25.0–29.9)	2.12 (2.08–2.15)	0.56 (0.55–0.56)	4.18 (4.10–4.25)
	Obese (>30)	2.28 (2.25–2.31)	0.58 (0.57–0.59)	4.66 (4.59–4.72)
Smoking status	Non-smoker	2.09 (2.07–2.11)	0.54 (0.53–0.54)	4.09 (4.04–4.15)
	Current smoker	2.36 (2.32–2.42)	0.60 (0.59–0.60)	4.87 (4.77–4.97)
	Former smoker	2.04 (2.01–2.07)	0.57 (0.56–0.57)	4.26 (4.17–4.36)
Alcohol usage	Non-drinker	2.16 (2.10–2.22)	0.54 (0.53–0.56)	4.17 (4.07–4.27)
	Moderate drinker	2.08 (2.04–2.12)	0.54 (0.53–0.55)	4.19 (4.12–4.27)
	Heavy drinker	2.16 (2.13–2.18)	0.57 (0.56–0.58)	4.34 (4.28–4.41)

Sociodemographic Characteristics		Eosinophils (1000 Cells/μL)	Basophils (1000 Cells/μL)	Platelet/Lymphocyte Ratio
Race	Non-Hispanic White	0.20 (0.19–0.20)	0.05 (0.45–0.05)	123.12 (121.13–125.11)
	Non-Hispanic Black	0.18 (0.17–0.19)	0.04 (0.04–0.05)	119.77 (117.49–122.06)
	Hispanic	0.20 (0.20–0.21)	0.04 (0.04–0.05)	116.33 (114.69–117.97)
	Other	0.21 (0.20–0.22)	0.04 (0.04–0.05)	119.84 (116.88–122.81)
Sex	Male	0.24 (0.24–0.24)	0.04 (0.04–0.05)	117.75 (116.25–119.26)
	Female	0.20 (0.20–0.20)	0.04 (0.04–0.05)	124.94 (123.28–126.61)

Table 2. Cont.

Sociodemographic Characteristics		Eosinophils (1000 Cells/μL)	Basophils (1000 Cells/μL)	Platelet/Lymphocyte Ratio
Age (years)	20–29	0.19 (0.19–0.20)	0.04 (0.04–0.05)	114.92 (113.02–116.83)
	30–59	0.19 (0.19–0.20)	0.05 (0.04–0.05)	121.67 (120.17–123.18)
	60–79	0.21 (0.20–0.22)	0.05 (0.05–0.05)	128.62 (125.83–131.42)
	80+	0.22 (0.20–0.23)	0.05 (0.04–0.05)	133.78 (127.83–139.73)
Education	<High School	0.21 (0.20–0.22)	0.05 (0.04–0.05)	115.05 (112.75–117.35)
	High School/General Educational Development	0.20 (0.19–0.21)	0.05 (0.05–0.05)	118.93 (116.61–121.24)
	Some College, or Associate of Arts	0.19 (0.19–0.20)	0.05 (0.05–0.05)	121.08 (119.24–122.91)
	>College Graduate	0.18 (0.18–0.19)	0.04 (0.04–0.04)	126.11 (124.03–128.19)
Nativity	United States born	0.19 (0.19–0.20)	0.05 (0.05–0.05)	122.78 (121.22–124.33)
	Non-United States born	0.20 (0.20–0.21)	0.04 (0.04–0.04)	115.85 (114.17–117.52)
Body mass index (Kg/m^2)	Underweight (<18.5)	0.17 (0.15–0.19)	0.05 (0.04–0.06)	124.61 (118.82–130.40)
	Normal weight (18.5–24.9)	0.18 (0.17–0.18)	0.04 (0.04–0.04)	125.01 (122.93–127.09)
	Overweight (25.0–29.9)	0.20 (0.19–0.20)	0.04 (0.04–0.05)	120.21 (118.34–122.08)
	Obese (>30)	0.21 (0.21–0.22)	0.05 (0.05–0.05)	118.56 (116.79–120.32)
Smoking status	Non-smoker	0.18 (0.18–0.19)	0.04 (0.04–0.04)	123.51 (122.08–124.94)
	Current smoker	0.22 (0.22–0.23)	0.06 (0.05–0.06)	111.02 (108.89–113.16)
	Former smoker	0.20 (0.20–0.21)	0.05 (0.04–0.05)	124.77 (122.55–127.00)
Alcohol usage	Non-drinker	0.19 (0.18–0.20)	0.04 (0.38–0.05)	122.41 (119.53–125.29)
	Moderate drinker	0.19 (0.18–0.20)	0.04 (0.04–0.05)	124.21 (122.17–126.25)
	Heavy drinker	0.20 (0.20–0.21)	0.05 (0.05–0.05)	119.87 (118.14–121.60)

Sociodemographic Characteristics		Platelet Count (1000 Cells/μL)	Neutrophil/Lymphocyte Ratio
Race	Non-Hispanic White	235.64 (233.72–237.56)	2.27 (2.22–2.31)
	Non-Hispanic Black	243.92 (240.75–247.09)	1.78 (1.74–1.83)
	Hispanic	245.18 (242.85–247.50)	2.10 (2.04–2.16)
	Other	240.52 (236.65–244.39)	2.03 (1.98–2.08)
Sex	Male	243.37 (242.34–244.40)	2.19 (2.15–2.23)
	Female	263.52 (262.50–264.54)	2.14 (2.10–2.17)
Age (years)	20–29	242.92 (240.37–245.46)	2.06 (2.01–2.11)
	30–59	240.68 (238.76–242.60)	2.13 (2.1–2.17)
	60–79	227.22 (223.46–230.98)	2.35 (2.29–2.41)
	80+	211.45 (206.22–216.68)	2.81 (2.64–2.97)

Table 2. Cont.

Sociodemographic Characteristics		Platelet Count (1000 Cells/μL)	Neutrophil/Lymphocyte Ratio
Education	<High School	238.89 (235.65–242.13)	2.16 (2.09–2.22)
	High School/General Educational Development	239.56 (236.47–242.65)	2.19 (2.14–2.24)
	Some College, or Associate of Arts	241.24 (239.15–243.33)	2.17 (2.12–2.21)
	>College Graduate	235.18 (232.56–237.81)	2.15 (2.09–2.20)
Nativity	United States born	239.20 (237.44–240.94)	2.21 (2.17–2.25)
	Non-United States born	236.40 (233.73–239.07)	1.98 (1.95–2.02)
Body mass index (Kg/m²)	Underweight (<18.5)	237.38 (227.95–246.81)	2.13 (1.95–2.31)
	Normal weight (18.5–24.9)	232.19 (230.01–234.37)	2.14 (2.09–2.20)
	Overweight (25.0–29.9)	233.71 (231.61–235.80)	2.14 (2.10–2.18)
	Obese (>30)	249.83 (247.43–252.24)	2.19 (2.15–2.23)
Smoking status	Non-smoker	239.27 (237.45–241.08)	2.1 (2.07–2.13)
	Current smoker	241.36 (238.94–243.78)	2.22 (2.17–2.28)
	Former smoker	234.08 (231.28–236.87)	2.28 (2.23–2.34)
Alcohol usage	Non-drinker	242.17 (238.08–246.26)	2.1 (2.03–2.15)
	Moderate drinker	237.01 (234.20–239.81)	2.2 (2.15–2.25)
	Heavy drinker	238.37 (236.25–240.5)	2.17 (2.13–2.20)

[2] We present group means (95% CI) of inflammatory markers for each level of the predictors of interest.

Table 3. Multivariable analyses of inflammatory markers of the U.S. population: NHANES 2009–2016.

Sociodemographic Characteristics		Lymphocytes (1000 Cells/μL)	Monocytes (1000 Cells/μL)	Segmented Neutrophils (1000 Cells/μL)
		Estimate (95% CI)	Estimate (95% CI)	Estimate (95% CI)
Race	Non-Hispanic White	REF	REF	REF
	Non-Hispanic Black	0.058 (0.014–0.102) *	−0.055 (−0.066—−0.044) ***	−0.852 (−0.960—−0.745) ***
	Hispanic	0.0683 (0.017–0.120) *	−0.012 (−0.027—−0.002)	0.080 (−0.051–0.213)
	Other	0.060 (−0.005–0.125)	−0.023 (−0.039—−0.007) **	0.053 (−0.084–0.190)
Sex	Male	REF	REF	REF
	Female	0.116 (0.080–0.153) ***	−0.047 (−0.056—−0.037) ***	0.053 (0.165–0.318) ***
Age (years)	20–29	REF	REF	REF
	30–59	−0.145 (−0.188—−0.103) *	−0.016 (−0.028—−0.005) **	−0.123 (−0.211—−0.344) **
	60–79	−0.312 (−0.370—−0.253) *	0.002 (−0.018–0.023)	−0.252 (−0.353—−0.150) ***
	80+	−0.228 (−0.514–0.058)	0.062 (0.370–0.087) ***	0.062 (−0.157–0.281)

Table 3. Cont.

Sociodemographic Characteristics		Lymphocytes (1000 Cells/μL)	Monocytes (1000 Cells/μL)	Segmented Neutrophils (1000 Cells/μL)
		Estimate (95% CI)	Estimate (95% CI)	Estimate (95% CI)
Education	<High School	REF	REF	REF
	High School/General Educational Development	0.002 (−0.046–0.050)	0.001 (−0.141–0.016)	−0.816 (−0.203–0.040)
	Some College, or Associate of Arts	−0.242 (−0.783–0.030)	0.001 (−0.012–0.140)	−0.159 (−0.289—0.029) *
	>College Graduate	−0.095 (−0.147—0.043) ***	−0.027 (−0.038—0.007) **	−0.331 (−0.454—0.209) ***
Nativity	United States born	REF	REF	REF
	Non-United States born	0.063 (0.023–0.104) **	−0.016 (−0.029—0.003) **	−0.234 (−0.341—0.127) ***
Body mass index (Kg/m²)	Underweight (<18.5)	−0.012 (−0.117–0.093)	−0.004 (−0.029–0.021)	−0.034 (−0.334–0.267)
	Normal weight (18.5–24.9)	REF	REF	REF
	Overweight (25.0–29.9)	0.139 (0.096–0181) ***	0.025 (0.015–0.034) ***	0.237 (0.145–0.329) ***
	Obese (>30)	0.286 (0.241–0.330) ***	0.055 (0.044–0.066) ***	0.720 (0.632–0.809) ***
Smoking status	Non-smoker	REF	REF	REF
	Current smoker	0.282 (0.231–0.333) ***	0.054 (0.043–0.065) ***	0.756 (0.662–0.850) ***
	Former smoker	0.005 (−0.038–0.049)	0.016 (0.003–0.029) **	0.100 (0.008–0.191) *
Alcohol usage	Non-drinker	REF	REF	REF
	Moderate drinker	−0.011 (−0.093–0.070)	−0.015 (−0.031–0.001)	0.025 (−0.075–0.013)
	Heavy drinker	−0.200 (−0.091–0.051)	−0.003 (−0.17–0.012)	0.015 (−0.072–0.103)

Sociodemographic Characteristics		Eosinophils (1000 Cells/μL)	Basophils (1000 Cells/μL)	
		Estimate (95% CI)		Estimate (95% CI)
Race	Non-Hispanic White	REF		REF
	Non-Hispanic Black	−0.018 (−0.027—0.010) ***		−0.005 (−0.009—0.002) **
	Hispanic	−0.003 (−0.0130–0.007)		−0.002 (−0.007–0.002)
	Other	0.016 (0.002–0.030) *		−0.001 (−0.005–0.004)
Sex	Male	REF		REF
	Female	−0.020 (−0.028—0.012) ***		0.002 (−0.001–0.005)
Age (years)	20–29	REF		REF
	30–59	−0.001 (−0.010–0.008)		0.004 (0.001–0.006) *
	60–79	0.011 (−0.002–0.024)		0.007 (0.002–0.011) **
	80+	0.032 (0.012–0.053) **		0.010 (0.003–0.017) **
Education	<High School	REF		REF
	High School/General Educational Development	−0.007 (−0.021–0.007)		−0.001 (−0.004–0.003)
	Some College, or Associate of Arts	−0.009 (−0.020–0.003)		−0.001 (−0.005–0.003)
	>College Graduate	−0.011 (−0.023–0.001)		−0.002 (−0.005—0.001) *

Table 3. Cont.

Sociodemographic Characteristics		Eosinophils (1000 Cells/µL)	Basophils (1000 Cells/µL)
		Estimate (95% CI)	Estimate (95% CI)
Nativity	United States born	REF	REF
	Non-United States born	0.010 (0.001–0.020) **	−0.002 (−0.005–0.001)
Body mass index (Kg/m²)	Underweight (<18.5)	−0.003 (−0.027–0.020)	0.003 (−0.006–0.127)
	Normal weight (18.5–24.9)	REF	REF
	Overweight (25.0–29.9)	0.018 (0.009–0.027) ***	0.003 (−0.001–0.006)
	Obese (>30)	0.036 (0.027–0.046) ***	0.011 (0.008–0.015) ***
Smoking status	Non-smoker	REF	REF
	Current smoker	0.039 (0.029–0.049) ***	0.034 (0.010–0.018) ***
	Former smoker	0.012 (0.001–0.022) *	0.002 (−0.002–0.005)
Alcohol usage	Non-drinker	REF	REF
	Moderate drinker	−0.002 (−0.013–0.009)	0.002 (−0.003–0.006)
	Heavy drinker	0.030 (−0.008–0.014)	0.004 (−0.001–0.009)

Sociodemographic Characteristics		Platelet Count	Neutrophil/Lymphocyte Ratio
		Estimate (95% CI)	Estimate (95% CI)
Race	Non-Hispanic White	REF	REF
	Non-Hispanic Black	3.404 (−0.383–7.190)	−0.445 (−0.517–−0.372) ***
	Hispanic	10.682 (7.000–14.370) ***	−0.030 (−0.0136–0.076)
	Other	11.102 (5.512–16.690) ***	−0.0653 (−0.0156–0.025)
Sex	Male	REF	REF
	Female	27.174 (25.060–29.289) ***	−0.029 (−0.074–0.0153)
Age (years)	20–29	REF	REF
	30–59	−2.709 (−3.215–4.968)	0.090 (0.031–0.150) **
	60–79	−15.183 (−19.935–−10.429) ***	0.278 (0.204–0.351) ***
	80+	−25.420 (−31.748–−19.094) ***	0.707 (−0.162–0.038) ***
Education	<High School	REF	REF
	High School/General Educational Development	0.876 (−3.215–4.968)	−0.034 (−0.0121–0.052)
	Some College, or Associate of Arts	−0.157 (−4.287–3.972)	−0.0470 (−0.0133–0.049)
	>College Graduate	−2.177 (−6.894–2.540)	−0.062 (−0.016–0.038)
Nativity	United States born	REF	REF
	Non-United States born	−7.830 (−11.931–−3.729) ***	−0.186 (−0.258–−0.113) ***
Body mass index (Kg/m²)	Underweight (<18.5)	−2.310 (−12.510–7.888)	−0.0262 (−0.0232–0.179)
	Normal weight (18.5–24.9)	REF	REF
	Overweight (25.0–29.9)	5.643 (2.840–8.446) ***	−0.110 (−0.171–−0.049) ***
	Obese (>30)	18.059 (14.911–21.207) ***	−0.034 (−0.099–0.031)

Table 3. Cont.

Sociodemographic Characteristics		Platelet Count	Neutrophil/Lymphocyte Ratio
		Estimate (95% CI)	Estimate (95% CI)
Smoking status	Non-smoker	REF	REF
	Current smoker	3.908 (0.739–7.077) *	0.11 (0.05–0.171) ***
	Former smoker	0.600 (−2.494–3.634)	0.076 (0.018–134) *
Alcohol usage	Non-drinker	REF	REF
	Moderate drinker	−1.433 (−6.490–3.624)	
	Heavy drinker	0.847 (−3.783–5.477) ***	2.27 (2.038–2.508) ***

* $p < 0.05$, ** $p < 0.01$, *** $p < 0.001$; REF refers to referent group.

On average, monocyte counts are significantly lower in non-Hispanic Blacks as compared with those in non-Hispanic Whites. Additionally, females have a lower mean monocyte count vs. that of males. Non-U.S.-born NHANES participants have significantly lower monocyte counts. However, the mean monocyte counts for overweight and obese members of the U.S. adult population are significantly higher than the mean monocyte count for normal weight participants. Current and former smokers both have significantly higher mean monocyte counts vs. those who have never smoked.

On average, non-Hispanic Blacks have significantly lower neutrophil counts vs. non-Hispanic Whites. Females, on average, have significantly higher neutrophil counts vs. males. Participants aged 30–79, on average, have significantly lower neutrophil counts vs. participants aged 20–29. Neutrophil counts are significantly lower for non-U.S.-born participants. Neutrophil counts are significantly higher for overweight and obese NHANES participants. Former and current smokers both have significantly higher mean neutrophil counts vs. those who had never smoked.

Eosinophil counts are significantly lower in non-Hispanic Blacks vs. non-Hispanic Whites. On average, females also have significantly lower eosinophil counts as compared with males and those born outside of the USA have significantly higher eosinophil counts as compared with participants declaring themselves as U.S. born. Additionally, overweight and obese NHANES participants have significantly higher mean eosinophil counts vs. normal weight participants. Likewise, former and current smokers have significantly higher mean eosinophil counts vs. never smokers.

Basophil counts, on average, are significantly lower in non-Hispanic Blacks vs. non-Hispanic Whites. Participants aged 20–29 have a significantly lower mean basophil count vs. those of participants in the age groups 30–59, 60–79, and 80 and older. Mean basophils counts are significantly higher in obese NHANES participants as compared to normal-weight NHANES participants. Additionally, current smokers have significantly higher basophil counts vs. those who had never smoked.

On average, platelet counts are significantly higher in Hispanics and others as compared with non-Hispanic Whites. Females also have significantly higher platelet counts than males. Participants aged 20–29 have a significantly higher mean platelet count vs. those of participants in the age groups 30–59, 60–79, and 80 and older. Participants who are overweight and obese have significantly higher mean platelet counts as compared with participants with normal weight. Current smokers also have a significantly higher mean platelet count as compared with those who had never smoked. However, participants born outside of the United States have a significantly lower mean platelet count as compared with U.S.-born participants.

The mean NLR value for non-Hispanic Blacks is significantly lower as compared with non-Hispanic Whites. On average, NLR values are also significantly lower in non-U.S.-born participants as compared with U.S.-born participants. Participants aged 20–29 have a significantly higher mean NLR value vs. those of participants in the age groups 30–59, 60–79, and 80 and older. Additionally, current smokers and former smokers have significantly higher mean NLR values as compared with that of those who had never smoked.

The mean PLR value for non-Hispanic Blacks is significantly lower as compared with non-Hispanic Whites. Participants aged 20–29 have a significantly lower mean PLR value vs. that of participants in the age groups 30–59, 60–79, and 80 and older. Additionally, current smokers have a significantly higher mean PLR value as compared with those who had never smoked. Participants in the obese category also had a higher mean PLR value as compared with normal weight participants.

4. Discussion

NLR and PLR values have been used as predictors of mortality in patients with various types of cancers, acute coronary syndrome, and other chronic inflammatory states [1–6]. These markers have also been reported to predict mortality rates of patients affected by the novel coronavirus [23,24]. While there is a growing body of research on the prognostic power of NLR, PLR, and associated white blood cell counts in regard to disease progression and outcomes, not much is known about contributors of blood cellular variations in the general, healthy population. There are some studies that have tried to define a range of normal values but were only investigated with a small study cohort and, moreover, were not looked at across various demographic and behavioral factors. The present study analyzed a large U.S. dataset of over 16,000 participants and reported the mean values of lymphocyte count, monocyte count, segmented neutrophil count, eosinophil count, basophil count, platelet count, NLR, and PLR for the general, healthy population and stratified values by various demographic and behavioral factors. NLR and PLR values were found to vary significantly with race, age, and smoking status. The mean NLR value in the non-Hispanic White population is 2.27, while the non-Hispanic Black population has a mean NLR value of 1.78. The national weighted average PLR value in the non-Hispanic White population is 123.12, while the non-Hispanic Black population has a national weighted average PLR value of 119.77. Participants born outside of the USA were also found to have significantly lower NLR values than U.S.-born participants. These findings have been replicated in other epidemiological studies that have examined inflammatory markers among Latinos, and have been partially explained by differences in behavioral risk factors and acculturative stress [25,26]. Participants aged 20–29 had a mean NLR value of 2.06, while the age groups 30–59, 60–79, and over 80 had mean NLR values of 2.13, 2.35, and 2.81, respectively. Participants aged 20–29 had a mean PLR value of 114.92, while the age groups 30–59, 60–79, and over 80 had mean PLR values of 121.67, 128.62, and 133.78, respectively. Smoking status endorsed a significant difference in mean NLR values in which non-smokers had a mean NLR value of 2.1, current smokers had a mean NLR value of 2.22, and former smokers had a mean NLR value of 2.28. Smoking status also endorsed a significant difference in mean PLR values in which non-smokers had a mean PLR value of 123.51, current smokers had a mean PLR value of 111.02, and former smokers had a mean PLR value of 124.77.

Generally, a higher NLR value and a higher PLR value have been correlated with high mortality and poor prognosis in non-healthy populations [27–30]. However, in the general, healthy population there are not yet standardized values for a normal range of NLR and PLR values that consider various modifiable and nonmodifiable factors. In this study, it was found that the mean NLR and PLR values differed by factors such as race, age, and smoking status. The results showed that non-Hispanic Blacks had the lowest mean NLR value of all racial groups, which was consistent with previous studies [19]. A higher prevalence of benign ethnic neutropenia in populations of African descent may explain the lower mean NLR value in non-Hispanic Blacks but further investigation is needed [31,32].

Participants aged 20–29, on average, had lower NLR and PLR values than participants older than age 30. Higher NLR and PLR values in older populations may be attributed to multiple causes. One such cause is the complex process of immunosenescence, i.e., the age-related decline of the immune system. Immunosenescence can cause decreased production of white blood cells such as lymphocytes, neutrophils, monocytes, and regulatory B and T cells as reflected by age-related response to inflammation, including increased susceptibility to infections, varied responses to vaccines and immunomodulators, and increased prevalence of chronic inflammatory states or conditions [33]. Altered levels of white blood cell production would directly affect NLR and PLR values, thus, explaining the higher range of NLR and PLR values for older age groups.

Smoking status was found to be significantly associated with NLR values, in which non-smokers were found to have the lowest NLR levels as compared with current and former smokers. Smoking status was also found to be significantly associated with PLR values, in which current smokers were found to have the lowest PLR levels as compared with non-smokers and former smokers. These findings are consistent with previous studies, that establish NLR increases with increasing pack-years [34] and PLR decreases with increasing pack-years [21]. Increased NLR values in current and former smokers can possibly be explained by the changes in white blood cell counts that are caused by gaseous and particulate cigarette smoke. Decreased PLR values in current smokers are also due mostly to cigarette smoke causing changes in white blood cell counts, since current smoking is known to be correlated with thrombogenic effects, likely related to increased platelet counts and enhanced platelet function [35]. Direct activation of epithelial and immune cells in the oral and conducting airways induces the secretion of proinflammatory factors such as IL-8 and TNF-alpha and recruitment of white blood cells such as neutrophils that can potentially modulate NLR and PLR levels and cause chronic inflammation [36].

In general, inflammation has been implicated as a causative factor or major contributor to morbidity in an increasing number of chronic conditions. Aging and smoking, as discussed above, are two common causes of increased inflammation. COVID-19 also causes an acute hyperinflammatory state, which, if prolonged, can cause widespread damage to multiple organ systems [24], contributing to the increasingly recognized long COVID syndrome. However, one of the most recognized causes of inflammation is malignancy. Tumors can release systemic cytokines that predispose the body to developing many inflammatory sequelae, including atherosclerosis, thrombosis, and paraneoplastic manifestations [23]. These inflammatory phenomena are associated with worse prognosis in cancer patients and can also lead to eventual increased risk for cardiovascular and cerebrovascular disease [29]. Indeed, the inflammatory marker high sensitivity C-reactive protein is already used to screen for coronary disease predisposed by chronic low-level inflammation. The NLR and PLR, as other markers of inflammation, can serve as adjunctive markers to guide clinicians and their patients about the treatment, prognosis, and counseling in the course of cancer.

The current study has several strengths and limitations. One major strength is the use of a large, nationally representative non-institutionalized sample of US residents. This comprehensive dataset allows examination of natural contributors of blood cellular variations across various factors to be able to derive statistically significant differences in NLR and PLR values in different groups of people. Some limitations include the exclusion of patients with any chronic inflammatory conditions and as a result may have caused an underestimation of inflammatory marker levels in the general population. Another limitation, and possible area of further research, is the correlation of NLR and PLR values with other well-known markers of inflammation, such as C-Reactive protein, which may give further insight into how overall inflammation is modulated by demographic and behavioral factors.

5. Conclusions

In conclusion, the present analysis of a large U.S. dataset of over 16,000 subjects reports the mean values of neutrophil-to-lymphocyte and platelet-to-lymphocyte ratios in a healthy, general population, using various demographic and behavioral factors. The NLR and PLR values significantly varied with race, age, nativity, and smoking status. It was found that non-Hispanic Blacks, older people, people born in the USA, and people who have a current or past smoking history had higher NLR values. The differences in inflammatory markers by nativity highlight the need to better uncover the biobehavioral mechanisms and pathways linking acculturation with health outcomes. These findings have important clinical implications because they indicate the need to set different cutoff points by race, age, and sex for predictive markers using in risk assessment of various illnesses.

Author Contributions: Conceptualization, M.C.-R. and R.C.; methodology, M.C.-R. and R.C.; software, R.C.; validation, R.C.; formal analysis, R.C.; investigation, M.C.-R., Z.Y., R.H., S.A. and R.C.; resources, M.C.-R., Z.Y. and Z.Y.; data curation, M.C.-R. and R.C.; writing—original draft preparation—M.C.-R., Z.Y., R.H., S.A. and R.C.; writing—review and editing, M.C.-R., Z.Y., R.H., S.A. and R.C.; visualization, M.C.-R., Z.Y., R.H., S.A. and R.C.; supervision, M.C.-R. and R.C.; project administration, M.C.-R. All authors have read and agreed to the published version of the manuscript.

Funding: This research received no external funding.

Institutional Review Board Statement: As the analytic sample of the NHANES was derived from de-identified publicly available data, Institutional Review Board approval was not required for this study.

Informed Consent Statement: Not applicable.

Data Availability Statement: Data supporting these results are from the publicly available National Health and Nutrition Examination Survey. Datasets, questionnaires, and related documentation can be found at https://wwwn.cdc.gov/nchs/nhanes (accessed on 1 August 2022).

Conflicts of Interest: The authors declare no conflict of interest.

References

1. Bhat, T.; Teli, S.; Rijal, J.; Bhat, H.; Raza, M.; Khoueiry, G.; Meghani, M.; Akhtar, M. Neutrophil to lymphocyte ratio and cardiovascular diseases: A review. *Expert Rev. Cardiovasc. Ther.* **2013**, *11*, 55–59. [CrossRef] [PubMed]
2. Turkmen, K.; Guney, I.; Yerlikaya, F.H.; Tonbul, H.Z. The relationship between neutrophil-to-lymphocyte ratio and inflammation in end-stage renal disease patients. *Ren. Fail.* **2012**, *34*, 155–159. [CrossRef] [PubMed]
3. Cedrés, S.; Torrejon, D.; Martínez, A.; Martinez, P.; Navarro, A.; Zamora, E.; Mulet-Margalef, N. Neutrophil to lymphocyte ratio (NLR) as an indicator of poor prognosis in stage IV non-small cell lung cancer. *Clin. Transl. Oncol.* **2012**, *14*, 864–869. [CrossRef] [PubMed]
4. An, X.; Ding, P.R.; Li, Y.H.; Wang, F.-H.; Shi, Y.-X.; Wang, Z.-Q.; He, Y.-J.; Xu, R.-H. Elevated neutrophil to lymphocyte ratio predicts survival in advanced pancreatic cancer. *Biomarkers* **2010**, *15*, 516–522. [CrossRef] [PubMed]
5. Walsh, S.R.; Cook, E.J.; Goulder, F.; Justin, T.A.; Keeling, N.J. Neutrophil-lymphocyte ratio as a prognostic factor in colorectal cancer. *J. Surg. Oncol.* **2005**, *91*, 181–184. [CrossRef]
6. Cho, H.; Hur, H.W.; Kim, S.W.; Kim, S.H.; Kim, J.H.; Kim, Y.T.; Lee, K. Pre-treatment neutrophil to lymphocyte ratio is elevated in epithelial ovarian cancer and predicts survival after treatment. *Cancer Immunol. Immunother.* **2009**, *58*, 15–23. [CrossRef]
7. Sun, X.; Xue, Z.; Yasin, A.; He, Y.; Chai, Y.; Li, J.; Zhang, K. Colorectal Cancer and Adjacent Normal Mucosa Differ in Apoptotic and Inflammatory Protein Expression. *Eng. Regen.* **2022**, *2*, 279–287. [CrossRef]
8. Guthrie, G.J.; Charles, K.A.; Roxburgh, C.S.; Horgan, P.G.; McMillan, D.C.; Clarke, S.J. The systemic inflammation-based neutrophil-lymphocyte ratio: Experience in patients with cancer. *Crit. Rev. Oncol. Hematol.* **2013**, *88*, 218–230. [CrossRef]
9. Proctor, M.J.; Morrison, D.S.; Talwar, D.; Balmer, S.M.; Fletcher, C.D.; O'Reilly, D.S.J.; Foulis, A.K.; Horgan, P.G.; McMillan, D.C. A comparison of inflammation-based prognostic scores in patients with cancer. A Glasgow Inflammation Outcome Study. *Eur. J. Cancer* **2011**, *47*, 2633–2641. [CrossRef]
10. Farah, R.; Ibrahim, R.; Nassar, M.; Najib, D.; Zivony, Y.; Eshel, E. The neutrophil/lymphocyte ratio is a better addition to C-reactive protein than CD64 index as a marker for infection in COPD. *Panminerva Med.* **2017**, *59*, 203–209. [CrossRef]
11. Azab, B.; Bhatt, V.R.; Phookan, J.; Murukutla, S.; Kohn, N.; Terjanian, T.; Widmann, W.D. Usefulness of the neutrophil-to-lymphocyte ratio in predicting short- and long-term mortality in breast cancer patients. *Ann. Surg. Oncol.* **2012**, *19*, 217–224. [CrossRef] [PubMed]
12. Núñez, J.; Núñez, E.; Bodí, V.; Sanchis, J.; Miñana, G.; Mainar, L.; Santas, E.; Merlos, P.; Rumiz, E.; Darmofal, H.; et al. Usefulness of the neutrophil to lymphocyte ratio in predicting long-term mortality in ST segment elevation myocardial infarction. *Am. J. Cardiol.* **2008**, *101*, 747–752. [CrossRef] [PubMed]
13. Durmus, E.; Kivrak, T.; Gerin, F.; Sunbul, M.; Sari, I.; Erdogan, O. Neutrophil-to-Lymphocyte Ratio and Platelet-to-Lymphocyte Ratio are Predictors of Heart Failure. *Arq. Bras. Cardiol.* **2015**, *105*, 606–613. [CrossRef] [PubMed]
14. Xu, Z.; Xu, W.; Cheng, H.; Shen, W.; Ying, J.; Cheng, F.; Xu, W. The Prognostic Role of the Platelet-Lymphocytes Ratio in Gastric Cancer: A Meta-Analysis. *PLoS ONE* **2016**, *11*, e0163719. [CrossRef] [PubMed]
15. Gu, X.; Gao, X.S.; Qin, S.; Li, X.; Qi, X.; Ma, M.; Yu, H.; Sun, S.; Zhou, D.; Wang, W.; et al. Elevated Platelet to Lymphocyte Ratio Is Associated with Poor Survival Outcomes in Patients with Colorectal Cancer. *PLoS ONE* **2016**, *11*, e0163523. [CrossRef] [PubMed]
16. Song, W.; Tian, C.; Wang, K.; Zhang, R.J.; Zou, S.B. Preoperative platelet lymphocyte ratio as independent predictors of prognosis in pancreatic cancer: A systematic review and meta-analysis. *PLoS ONE* **2017**, *12*, e0178762. [CrossRef]
17. Wu, L.; Zou, S.; Wang, C.; Tan, X.; Yu, M. Neutrophil-to-lymphocyte and platelet-to-lymphocyte ratio in Chinese Han population from Chaoshan region in South China. *BMC Cardiovasc. Disord.* **2019**, *19*, 125. [CrossRef]
18. Forget, P.; Khalifa, C.; Defour, J.P.; Latinne, D.; Van Pel, M.C.; De Kock, M. What is the normal value of the neutrophil-to-lymphocyte ratio? *BMC Res. Notes* **2017**, *10*, 12. [CrossRef]
19. Azab, B.; Camacho-Rivera, M.; Taioli, E. Average values and racial differences of neutrophil lymphocyte ratio among a nationally representative sample of United States subjects. *PLoS ONE* **2014**, *9*, e112361. [CrossRef]
20. Gumus, F.; Solak, I.; Eryilmaz, M.A. The effects of smoking on neutrophil/lymphocyte, platelet/ /lymphocyte ratios. *Bratisl. Lek. Listy.* **2018**, *119*, 116–119. [CrossRef]
21. Pujani, M.; Chauhan, V.; Singh, K.; Rastogi, S.; Agarwal, C.; Gera, K. The effect and correlation of smoking with platelet indices, neutrophil lymphocyte ratio and platelet lymphocyte ratio. *Hematol. Transfus Cell Ther.* **2021**, *43*, 424–429. [CrossRef] [PubMed]

22. Ahluwalia, N.; Dwyer, J.; Terry, A.; Moshfegh, A.; Johnson, C. Update on NHANES Dietary Data: Focus on Collection, Release, Analytical Considerations, and Uses to Inform Public Policy. *Adv. Nutr.* **2016**, *7*, 121–134. [CrossRef] [PubMed]
23. Lin, C.; Arevalo, Y.A.; Nanavati, H.D.; Lin, D.M. Racial differences and an increased systemic inflammatory response are seen in patients with COVID-19 and ischemic stroke. *Brain Behav. Immun. Health* **2020**, *8*, 100137. [CrossRef] [PubMed]
24. Sarkar, S.; Kannan, S.; Khanna, P.; Singh, A.K. Role of platelet-to-lymphocyte count ratio (PLR), as a prognostic indicator in COVID-19: A systematic review and meta-analysis. *J. Med. Virol.* **2022**, *94*, 211–221. [CrossRef] [PubMed]
25. Torres, J.M.; Epel, E.S.; To, T.M.; Lee, A.; Aiello, A.E.; Haan, M.N. Cross-border ties, nativity, and inflammatory markers in a population-based prospective study of Latino adults. *Soc. Sci. Med.* **2018**, *211*, 21–30. [CrossRef] [PubMed]
26. Scholaske, L.; Wadhwa, P.D.; Entringer, S. Acculturation and biological stress markers: A systematic review. *Psychoneuroendocrinology* **2021**, *132*, 105349. [CrossRef]
27. Xie, X.; Fu, X.; Zhang, Y.; Huang, W.; Huang, L.; Deng, Y.; Yan, D.; Yao, R. U-shaped relationship between platelet-lymphocyte ratio and postoperative in-hospital mortality in patients with type A acute aortic dissection. *BMC Cardiovasc. Disord.* **2021**, *21*, 569. [CrossRef]
28. Shen, Y.; Huang, X.; Zhang, W. Platelet-to-lymphocyte ratio as a prognostic predictor of mortality for sepsis: Interaction effect with disease severity-a retrospective study. *BMJ Open* **2019**, *9*, e022896. [CrossRef]
29. Zhai, G.; Wang, J.; Liu, Y.; Zhou, Y. Platelet-lymphocyte ratio as a new predictor of in-hospital mortality in cardiac intensive care unit patients. *Sci. Rep.* **2021**, *11*, 23578. [CrossRef]
30. Kumar, P.; Law, S.; Sriram, K.B. Evaluation of platelet lymphocyte ratio and 90-day mortality in patients with acute exacerbation of chronic obstructive pulmonary disease. *J. Thorac. Dis.* **2017**, *9*, 1509–1516. [CrossRef]
31. Howard, R.; Scheiner, A.; Kanetsky, P.A.; Egan, K.M. Sociodemographic and lifestyle factors associated with the neutrophil-to-lymphocyte ratio. *Ann. Epidemiol.* **2019**, *38*, 11–21. [CrossRef] [PubMed]
32. Hsieh, M.; Chin, K.; Link, B.; Stroncek, D.; Wang, E.; Everhart, J.; Tisdale, J.F.; Rodgers, G. Benign Ethnic Neutropenia in Individuals of African Descent: Incidence, Granulocyte Mobilization, and Gene Expression Profiling. *Blood* **2005**, *106*, 3069. [CrossRef]
33. Castelo-Branco, C.; Soveral, I. The immune system and aging: A review. *Gynecol. Endocrinol.* **2014**, *30*, 16–22. [CrossRef] [PubMed]
34. Tulgar, Y.K.; Cakar, S.; Tulgar, S.; Dalkilic, O.; Cakiroglu, B.; Uyanik, B.S. The effect of smoking on neutrophil/lymphocyte and platelet/lymphocyte ratio and platelet indices: A retrospective study. *Eur. Rev. Med. Pharmacol. Sci.* **2016**, *20*, 3112–3118.
35. Ghahremanfard, F.; Semnani, V.; Ghorbani, R.; Malek, F.; Behzadfar, A.; Zahmatkesh, M. Effects of cigarette smoking on morphological features of platelets in healthy men. *Saudi Med. J.* **2015**, *36*, 847–850. [CrossRef]
36. Lee, J.; Taneja, V.; Vassallo, R. Cigarette smoking and inflammation: Cellular and molecular mechanisms. *J. Dent. Res.* **2012**, *91*, 142–149. [CrossRef]

Disclaimer/Publisher's Note: The statements, opinions and data contained in all publications are solely those of the individual author(s) and contributor(s) and not of MDPI and/or the editor(s). MDPI and/or the editor(s) disclaim responsibility for any injury to people or property resulting from any ideas, methods, instructions or products referred to in the content.

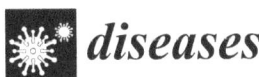

Article

Are Drugs Associated with Microscopic Colitis? A Systematic Review and Meta-Analysis

Zahid Ijaz Tarar [1], Umer Farooq [2], Mustafa Gandhi [1], Faisal Kamal [3], Moosa Feroze Tarar [4], Veysel Tahan [5], Harleen Kaur Chela [6] and Ebubekir Daglilar [6,*]

[1] Department of Medicine, University of Missouri, Columbia, MO 65212, USA
[2] Department of Medicine, Rochester General Hospital, Rochester, NY 14621, USA
[3] Division of Gastroenterology, University of California, San Francisco, CA 94143, USA
[4] Department of Medicine, Services Institute of Medical Sciences, Lahore 54000, Pakistan
[5] Division of Gastroenterology and Hepatology, University of Missouri, Columbia, MO 65212, USA
[6] Division of Gastroenterology and Hepatology, Charleston Area Medical Center, West Virginia University School of Medicine, Charleston, WV 25303, USA
* Correspondence: ebubekir.daglilar@hsc.wvu.edu

Citation: Tarar, Z.I.; Farooq, U.; Gandhi, M.; Kamal, F.; Tarar, M.F.; Tahan, V.; Chela, H.K.; Daglilar, E. Are Drugs Associated with Microscopic Colitis? A Systematic Review and Meta-Analysis. *Diseases* 2023, *11*, 6. https://doi.org/ 10.3390/diseases11010006

Academic Editors: Vasso Apostolopoulos, Jack Feehan and Vivek P. Chavda

Received: 19 November 2022
Revised: 19 December 2022
Accepted: 23 December 2022
Published: 29 December 2022

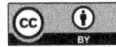

Copyright: © 2022 by the authors. Licensee MDPI, Basel, Switzerland. This article is an open access article distributed under the terms and conditions of the Creative Commons Attribution (CC BY) license (https:// creativecommons.org/licenses/by/ 4.0/).

Abstract: There is growing evidence of the association of Microscopic Colitis (MC) with the use of specific medications such as proton pump inhibitors (PPIs), Selective serotonin reuptake inhibitors (SSRIs), Non-Steroidal anti-inflammatory drugs (NSAIDs), Statins and H2-receptor antagonists (H2RA). In our study, we calculated the pooled odds of MC in patients using these drugs. We performed a detailed search of major databases, including PubMed/Medline, Scopus, web of science, and Embase, to include the studies in which odds of MC were reported after using above mentioned drugs. A random-effects model was used to pool the estimates. Thirteen studies were included in our analysis consisting of 304,482 patients (34,194 cases and 270,018 controls). In eight studies, the control group consisted of a random population selected based on age, gender and same birth year, whereas 3 studies recruited patients who presented with diarrhea and underwent colonoscopy and biopsy to rule out MC. Two studies reported odds of MC for both diarrhea and random control groups. Patients taking PPIs were more likely to develop MC, AOR 2.65 (95% CI 1.81–3.50, I^2 98.13%). Similarly, higher odds of association were found in patients taking SSRIs (OR 2.12, 95% CI 1.27–2.96, I^2 96.46%), NSAIDs (OR 2.02, 95% CI 1.33–2.70, I^2 92.70%) and Statins (OR 1.74, 95% CI 1.19–2.30, I^2 96.36%). No difference in odds of developing MC was seen in patients using H2RA compared to the control group (OR 2.70, 95% CI 0.32–5.08, I^2 98.67%). We performed a subgroup analysis based on the control group and found higher odds of MC in patients on PPIs compared to the random control group (OR 4.55, 95% CI 2.90–6.19, I^2 98.13%). Similarly, higher odds of MC were noted for SSRI (OR 3.23, 95% CI 1.54–4.92, I^2 98.31%), NSAIDs (OR 3.27, 95% CI 2.06–4.48, I^2 95.38%), and Statins (OR 2.23, 95% CI 1.41–3.06, I^2 98.11%) compared to the random control group. Contrary lower odds of MC were seen in the PPI and H2RA group compared to the diarrhea control group (OR 0.68, 95% CI 0.48–0.88, I^2 7.26%), (OR 0.46, 95% CI 0.14–0.78, I^2 0%) respectively. We found no difference in odds of MC in patients on SSRIs (OR 0.96, 95% CI 0.49–1.42, I^2 37.89%), NSAIDs (OR 1.13, 95% CI 0.49–1.76, I^2 59.37%) Statins (OR 0.91, 95% 0.66–1.17, I^2 0%) and H2RA (OR 3.48, 95% CI −0.41–7.36, I^2 98.89%) compared to the diarrhea control group. We also analyzed the association use of PPIs and NSAIDs with the development of collagenous colitis (CC) and lymphocytic colitis. Only the use of NSAIDs was associated with increased odds of developing collagenous colitis (OR 1.61, 95% CI 1.50–1.72, I^2 0%). No increased odds of CC and LC were seen in PPI users. PPIs, NSAIDs, SSRIs, and Statins are associated with an increased risk of MC compared to the random control group. On the contrary, the use of PPIs, NSAIDs, SSRIs, and Statins is not associated with an increased risk of MC when compared to the diarrhea control group.

Keywords: microscopic colitis; drug use; PPIs; NSAIDs; SSRIs; statins

1. Introduction

Microscopic colitis (MC) is a chronic inflammatory disease of the large intestine, consistent with two histological subtypes, lymphocytic colitis (LC) and collagenous colitis (CC). The most common presentation of MC is chronic watery diarrhea associated with abdominal pain, fecal urgency, and incontinence [1,2]. Microscopic colitis was considered a disease of old age, but now the incidence is rising in the younger population. The updated incidence and prevalence of MC are 25.8 cases/per 100,000 and 246.2/per 100,000, as reported by Tome et al. in an epidemiological study performed in Olmsted County, MN, USA [3,4]. The possible explanation for the increasing incidence of MC is better awareness and understanding of the disease and better and readily available diagnostic modalities such as endoscopy and biopsy [5].

The inflammation of the colon in response to luminal antigen exposure is suggested to underlie the mechanism of MC, but the exact pathogenesis is still unclear [6]. Endoscopic examination in MC usually reveals normal mucosa. Diagnosis is often established with a microscopic examination, which shows increased intraepithelial lymphocytes, inflamed lamina propria, and damage to the epithelial surface in both LC and CC [7,8]. The histological presence of collagenous bands allows for the differentiation between the two subtypes of MC and is only seen in CC [1,9].

Female sex and increasing age are the established risk factors associated with MC [3]. There is growing evidence that MC is related to other autoimmune diseases such as celiac disease, thyroid disorders, and rheumatic diseases, and the use of certain medications such as proton pump inhibitors (PPIs), Selective serotonin reuptake inhibitors (SSRIs), Non-steroidal anti-inflammatory drugs (NSAIDs), and Statins [2,10–13].

In our meta-analysis, we aimed to study the association of PPIs, SSRIs, NSAIDs, Statins, and H2RA with microscopic colitis. We further examined the association of PPIs and NSAIDs with subtypes of MC, including subgroup analysis for LC and CC. This is the first systematic review and meta-analysis on this topic to the best of our knowledge.

2. Methods

2.1. Data Search and Screening

We designed and performed an electronic literature search of Medline/PubMed, Embase Ovid, Cochrane Central Register for controlled trials, Scopus, and web of science from inception to 30 September 2022. We followed the preferred reporting items for the systematic review and meta-analysis (PRISMA) statement. Zahid Tarar (ZT) and Umer Farooq (UF) designed the search strategy, which was approved by Ebubekir Daglilar (ED). Both ZT and UF independently searched the databases mentioned above and registers. We designed three questions for our analysis. (1) Is there an association between medication use and microscopic colitis? (2) what are the odds of developing microscopic colitis in patients taking certain medications, including PPIs, SSRIs, NSAIDs, Statins, and H2RA? (3) what are the odds of developing collagenous and lymphocytic colitis in patients taking PPIs and NSAIDs? We included medical subject headings [Mesh] and free-text terms in our search. Following free text terms were used in different combinations: "(Microscopic colitis) AND (Drugs) OR (Medications) AND (Proton pump inhibitors) AND (PPIs OR SSRIs OR Statins OR H2RA OR NSAIDs) AND (Collagenous Colitis) AND/OR (Lymphocytic Colitis)". All search fields were used in all databases and registers except in Scopus, where the "Article title, keywords, and abstract" field was used. We also hand-searched the reference list of included studies.

2.2. Eligibility Criteria and Study Selection

We included the studies which meet the following criteria. (1) Reported odds of microscopic colitis in patients taking PPIs, SSRIs, NSAIDs, Statins, or H2RA; (2) Defined a control group; (3) Age above 18; (4): Reported odds of developing LC and CC while on PPIs or NSAIDs.

The following exclusion criteria were used (1) Studies in which odds ratios were not provided, or just *p*-value was provided; (2) Case reports or case series; (3) Abstracts or conference articles; (4) Letter to editors, Review articles and editorials; (5) Studies in which outcome data were missing; (6) Studies in a foreign language. Two investigators (ZT and UF) independently screened the abstracts, titles, and complete reports to identify the eligible studies based on pre-defined inclusion criteria. Any conflict or disagreement between the reviewers was resolved through discussion or by a third reviewer (MG). All references were downloaded in Endnote 11, and duplicate studies were removed manually and automatically.

2.3. Data Extraction

Data were extracted into Microsoft excel by two reviewers (ZT and MT). They independently pulled the information about study design, first author, year of publication, country of study, study cohort characteristics (age, sex, sample size), duration of the study, period of medication use, percentage of patients taking medications in both cases and control group, odds of developing MC in patients taking drugs, odds of developing CC and LC in patients taking PPIs or NSAIDs. We did not conduct an analysis on the odds of LC and CC for stains, SSRIs, and H2RA due to a lack of data availability. Once data was extracted, a third reviewer (ED) independently reviewed the extracted data sheet, and the final data sheet was prepared after discussion.

2.4. Statistical Analysis

We calculated the pooled odds ratio from each study's reported adjusted odds ratios. A random-effects model was used to calculate the pooled Odds ratio with 95% CI, and *p*-value < 0.05 was considered statistically significant. Cochrane chi-square test and I^2 statistics were used to test heterogeneity. Heterogeneity of 0, 25%, 50% and 75% were interpreted as absent, low, moderate and high, as described by the Cochrane Handbook for Systematic review [14]. Forest plots were created to report the results. The funnel plot and nonparametric trim and fill analysis for asymmetry were used to assess the publication bias. We used STATA software 17 to conduct the meta-analysis.

3. Results

3.1. Search Results and Study Characteristics

Figure 1 outlines the summary of the selection process. On the initial search of electronic databases and registers, we identified 3181 reports (1107 from PubMed/Medline, 1187 from Scopus, 568 from web of science, 221 from Embase, and 98 from Registers). After removing 1423 duplicate records, 1758 articles were screened, and finally, 45 reports were considered for eligibility. Of these 45 articles, 13 studies fulfilled the selection criteria and were included in the final analysis. Eight studies [11,13,15–20] used random control adjusted for age, sex, GP practice, or birth year.

In contrast, three studies [8,9,12] used diarrhea controls in which colonoscopy and biopsy were performed to rule out microscopic colitis. Masclee et al. [21] and Pascua et al. [22] reported the odds of MC in both random community controls and diarrhea controls. In five studies [9,11,15,16,20], odds of collagenous and lymphocytic colitis were calculated in patients on either PPIs or NSAIDs. Supplementary Table S1 details the characteristics of included studies.

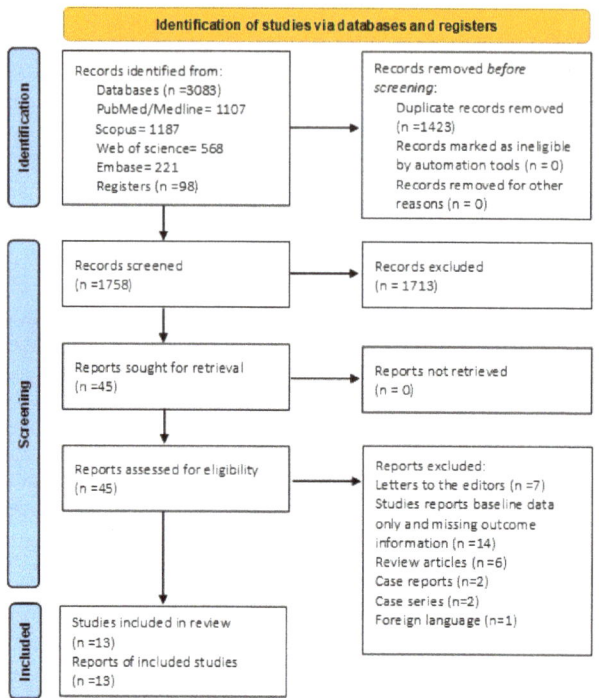

Figure 1. Prisma flow diagram for search and selection process of meta-analysis.

3.2. Pooled Odds of MC in Patients Taking PPIs and Subgroup Analysis Based on Control Groups

Nine studies [8,9,12,13,17–19,21,22] reported the odds of microscopic colitis in patients using proton pump inhibitors. Studies by Masclee et al. [21] and Pascua et al. [22] reported two different Odds ratios based on the control groups (Community random and diarrhea controls). Pooled Odds of MC in patients taking PPIs were 2.65 (95% CI 1.81–3.50, I^2 98.13%). On subgroup analysis, lower odds of MC (OR 0.68, 95% CI 0.48–0.88, I^2 7.26%) were found compared to the diarrhea control group, while greater odds were seen compared to the random control group (OR 4.55, 95% CI 2.90–6.19, I^2 98.13%). A statistically significant difference was seen between the groups ($p < 0.0001$) (Figure 2).

3.3. Pooled Odds of MC in Patients Taking SSRIs and Subgroup Analysis Based on Control Groups

Higher pooled odds of MC were observed in patients taking SSRI (OR 2.12(95% CI 1.27–2.96, I^2 96.46%). We included nine different odds ratios from 8 studies [8,9,12,17–19,21,22] to calculate the pooled odds ratio because Pascua et al. [22] provided two ratios based on two different control groups. Greater odds of MC were seen in patients taking SSRIs when compared to random health controls (OR 3.23, 95% CI 1.54–4.92, I^2 98.31%), whereas on the contrary, no difference in odds of MC was noted in comparison to the diarrhea control group (OR 0.96, 95% CI 0.49–1.42, I^2 37.89%) (Figure 3).

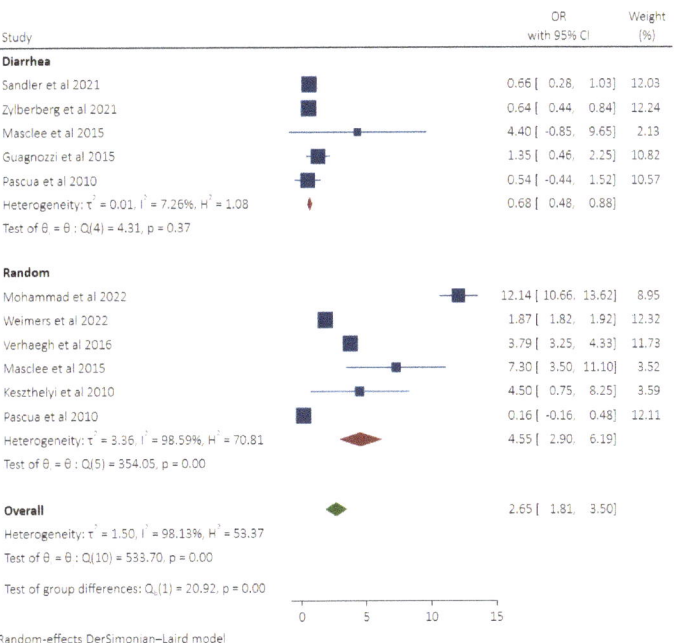

Figure 2. Pooled odds of MC in PPI users with subgroup analysis based on control groups (Diarrhea vs. Random Control) [8,9,12,13,17–19,21,22].

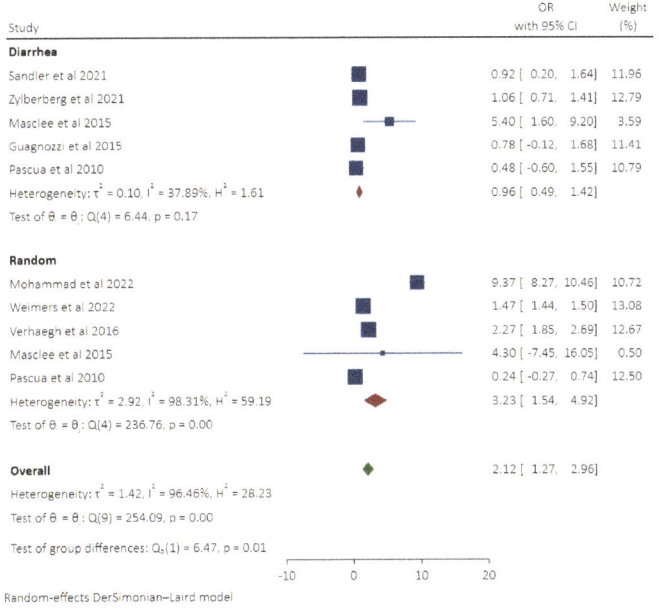

Figure 3. Pooled odds of MC in SSRI users with subgroup analysis based on control groups (Diarrhea vs. Random Control) [8,9,12,17–19,21,22].

3.4. Pooled Odds of MC in Patients Taking NSAIDs and Subgroup Analysis Based on Control Groups

Eight studies [8,9,12,13,17–19,21] provided the adjusted odds of MC in patients who were currently taking NSAIDs or were on them in the past. Patients taking NSAIDs had greater odds of developing MC (OR 2.02, 95% CI 1.33–2.70, I^2 92.70%). On subgroup analysis based on the control group, we found higher odds of MC in patients taking NSAIDs in comparison to the random control group (OR 3.27, 95% CI 2.06–4.48, I^2 95.38%), whereas no difference in odds of MC was noted when compared to the diarrhea control patient group (OR 1.13, 95% CI 0.49–1.76, I^2 59.37%). A statistically significant difference was noted between these two groups p (0.001) (Figure 4).

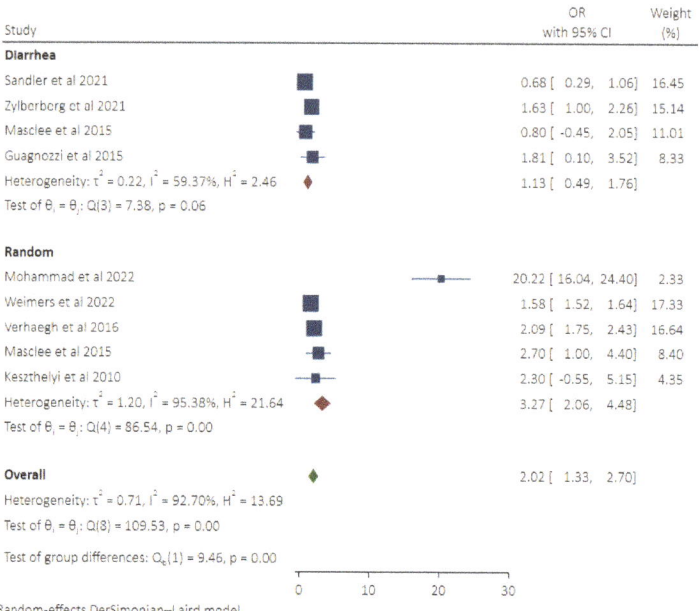

Figure 4. Pooled odds of MC in NSAIDs users with subgroup analysis based on control groups (Diarrhea vs. Random Control) [8,9,12,13,17–19,21].

3.5. Pooled Odds of MC in Patients Taking Statins with Subgroup Analysis of Diarrhea versus Random Controls

Pooled odds of MC in statin users were 1.74 (95% CI 1.19–2.30, I^2 96.36%) calculated from 9 adjusted odd ratios obtained from 7 studies [8,9,17–19,21,22]. Higher odds of MC were seen in patients taking statins compared to the healthy random control group (OR 2.23, 95% CI 1.41–3.06, I^2 98.11%). No significant difference in odds of MC was found in statin users compared to the diarrhea control group (OR 0.91, 95% CI 0.66–1.17, I^2 0%) (Figure 5).

3.6. Pooled Odds of MC in Patients Taking H2RA and Subgroup Analysis Based on Control Groups

H2 receptor antagonist use was not associated with increased odds of MC (OR 2.70, 95% CI −0.32–5.08, I^2 98.67%) based on the data provided in four studies [9,17–19]. Lower odds of MC were seen in patients using H2RA compared to the diarrhea control group (OR 0.46, 95% CI 0.14–0.78, I^2 0%). Similar odds of MC were seen compared to the community control patient population (OR 3.48, 95% CI −0.41–7.36, I^2 98.89%). No significant difference was seen between the groups (p 0.13) (Figure 6).

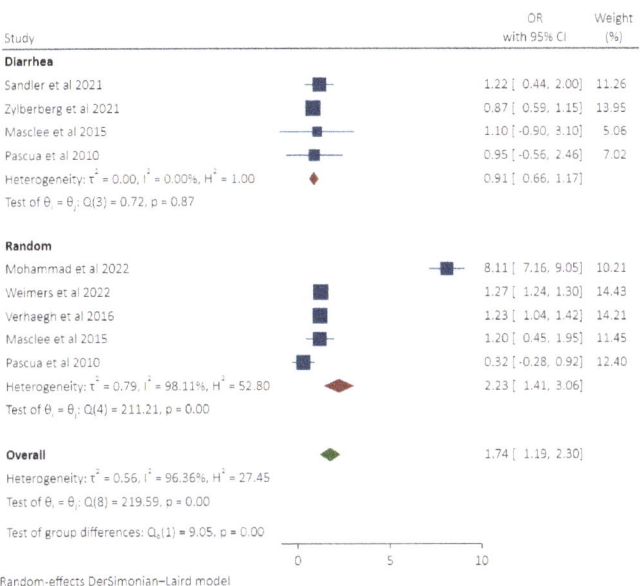

Figure 5. Pooled odds of MC in Statin users with subgroup analysis based on control groups (Diarrhea vs. Random Control) [8,9,17–19,21,22].

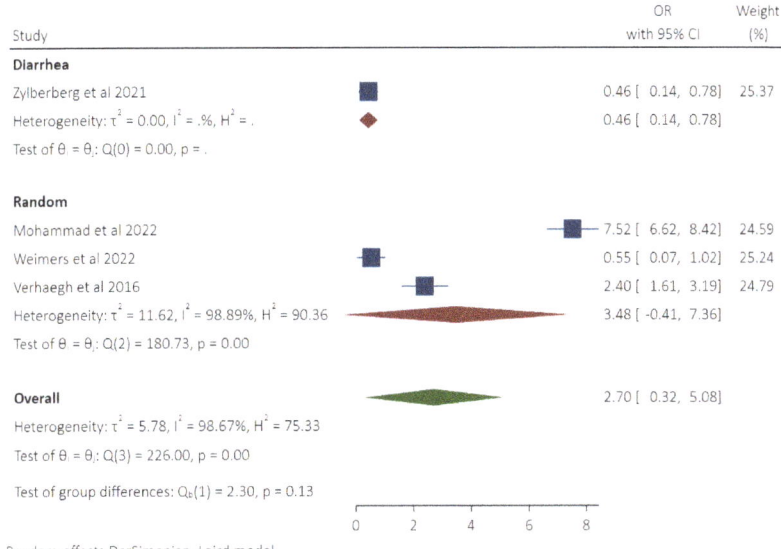

Figure 6. Pooled odds of MC in H2RA users with subgroup analysis based on control groups (Diarrhea vs. Random Control) [9,17–19].

3.7. Subgroup Analysis on the Association of LC and CC with the Use of PPIs and NSAIDs

We performed a subgroup analysis to determine the risk of developing collagenous colitis or lymphocytic colitis in patients taking proton pump inhibitors or NSAIDs. Similar odds of CC and LC (3.97, 95% CI 0.35–7.59, I^2 99.28%), (2.33, 95% CI 0.64–4.01, I^2 98.64%) respectively were seen in patients taking PPIs compared to control group. No statistically significant difference was seen between both groups (p 0.42). Odds of CC (OR 1.61, 95% CI

1.50–1.72, I^2 0%) were significantly higher in patients on NSAIDs, whereas similar odds of LC were found in NSAIDs users (OR 1.18, 95% CI 0.43–1.92, I^2 84.26%) compared to the control group. No significant difference between the CC and LC groups was seen (p 0.25) (Figure 7A,B).

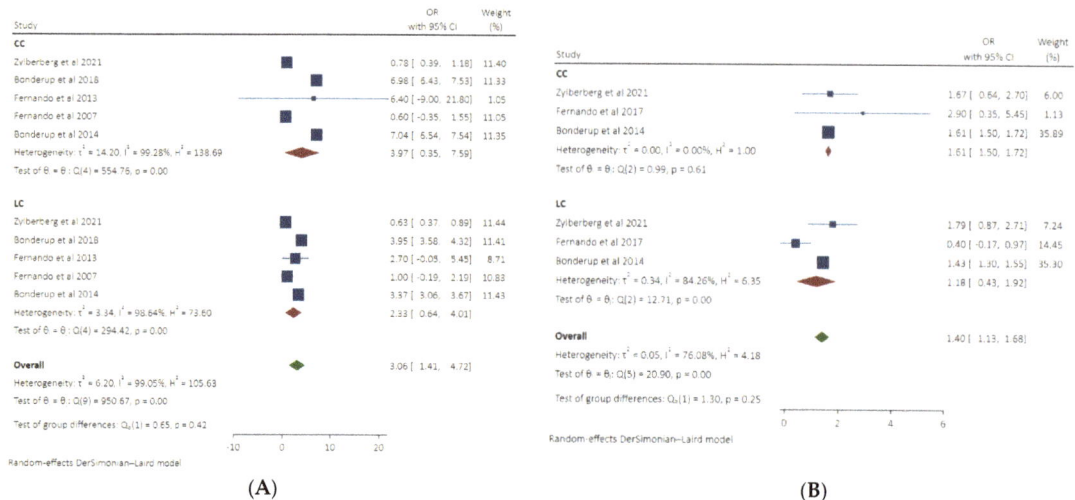

Figure 7. (**A**): Pooled odds of Lymphocytic and collagenous colitis in PPI users. (**B**): Pooled odds of Lymphocytic and collagenous colitis in NSAIDs users [8,9,12,13,17–19,21,22].

4. Quality Assessment

We evaluated the quality of included studies using the Methodological Index for Nonrandomized Studies (MINORS) criteria [23]. MINORS criteria score such studies on twelve items. Individual items are scored from 0 to 2 (2 when reported and adequate; 1 when inadequately reported; 0 if not reported). Scores from each item were summed up. The quality of studies was classified as high quality ($\geq$11), fair (score 6–10), or poor (score $\leq$ 5). Two authors (UF and ZT) conducted the quality assessment separately, and any disagreement was resolved by consensus with a third reviewer (FK). The quality assessment of studies is summarized in Supplementary Table S2.

5. Publication Bias

Visible asymmetry was noted on funnel plots, but the nonparametric trim and fill test was negative for any publication bias (Supplementary Figure S1a–e).

6. Discussion

In our analysis, we reported the effect of medication use on the development of microscopic colitis. We demonstrated that certain medications such as proton pump inhibitors, SSRIs, NSAIDs, and Statins are associated with an increased risk of MC, but H2RA use was not associated with an increased risk of MC when compared to random control groups. This is the first meta-analysis on this topic to the best of our knowledge, and the results of our analysis are significant.

Our results showed that using PPIs is associated with significantly higher odds of MC, in accordance with the results of the previous studies [12,18,19,21]. It is postulated that changes in gut flora, electrolyte imbalance due to acid suppression, and intestinal dysbiosis caused by PPIs are the possible underlying mechanism of MC development [24–26]. The noteworthy result in our analysis is that when MC cases were compared with diarrhea controls, the use of PPI was associated with decreased pooled odds of MC, while in studies in which random controls were selected, the risk of MC in PPI users was high. These results raise a question about the association of MC with PPI use because patients who suffer from gastrointestinal symptoms are more likely to get a PPI prescription compared to the healthy control group, and a similar observation has been made by Law et al. [27]. On subgroup analysis, it was found that the use of PPI was not associated with a greater likelihood of CC or LC. Lower odds of MC compared to diarrhea control and higher odds with random control warrant further prospective trials to establish or negate the association of MC with PPIs.

Data on the association of MC with the use of H2RA is conflicting. As the effect of H2RA on acid secretion is like PPIs, it is thought that they can cause intestinal dysbiosis, leading to MC. Our analysis did not find increased odds of MC in patients taking H2RA. A recent study by Zylberberg et al. [9] reported lower odds of MC in patients taking H2RA. In another study by Mohammad et al. [17], significantly higher odds of MC in association with H2RA were reported. The noteworthy fact is that Zylberberg et al. [9] recruited a diarrhea control group as a comparison, while Mohammad et al. [17] conducted a population-based study.

The NSAIDs inhibit prostaglandin synthesis, which results in increased gut permeability and impairs the integrity of the mucosal barrier resulting in an influx of bacteria and toxins into the intestinal lumen. The reaction to these luminal antigens is considered an underlying pathogenetic factor for the development of MC in NSAID users [17,28]. We reported significantly higher odds of MC in patients taking NSAIDs, and these results reinforce the results of previously conducted studies [9,12,13,17,19,21,29]. We also found that the odds of developing CC are higher in NSAID users, though no significantly higher risk of LC was seen in patients taking NSAIDs. On subgroup analysis based on the control group, we demonstrated that when MC cases using NSAIDs were compared to the diarrhea control group, no difference in risk of MC was seen, while when MC cases were compared to a healthy random control group, significantly greater odds of MC were noted. This discrepancy in results based on the control group in PPI and NSAIDs group warrants us to be careful about interpreting these results.

We demonstrated greater odds of MC in statin users, which is consistent with the results reported in the studies performed earlier [8,17–19]. In subgroup comparison to diarrhea and random control groups, no difference in odds of MC was seen. The underlying mechanism involved in MC development in statin users is not precise; however, inflammatory effects resulting from the downregulation of anti-tumor necrosis factor and upregulation of pro-inflammatory cytokines such as IL-8 by statin can contribute [17,30,31].

The effect of SSRI on the causation of MC is not well studied, although a few factors which have been considered potential contributors and reported in the literature are the following. First, it is said that serotonin possesses inflammatory characteristics, as seen in cases of colitis [32]. Moreover, a higher number of enterochromaffin cells are seen in MC patients, which secrete more serotonin. This results in the upregulation of immune-mediated markers by activating the nervous system, enhancing chloride secretion and gut motility [33,34]. We demonstrated that patients on SSRI are associated with greater odds of developing MC, which is consistent with the finding in most of the studies we included in our analysis. We did not find any difference in the odds of MC compared to diarrhea or random healthy controls.

Our study has several strengths. We conducted a detailed literature search of all the major database engines and a manual search of the bibliography of included studies. Two investigators searched and screened the databases separately, and a third reviewer approved the final studies included in the analysis. We emailed the primary and corresponding authors to get any missing information and avoid duplication of results. We performed a subgroup analysis based on control groups to prevent overestimating the effects from reports where healthy controls were recruited. We used a random-effect model to provide a more conservative and generalized pooled odds of MC in patients on different medications. We also did a sensitivity analysis to minimize the effect of any study affecting the results. Moreover, this is the first meta-study analyzing the association of MC with a particular medication.

There are a few limitations of our meta-analysis. The first few studies used random healthy controls as a comparison. In contrast, in other studies, diarrhea controls were recruited, leading to an overestimation of results due to differences in medication exposure between both control groups. Second, drug dosage was not provided in most of the included reports. Furthermore, it was not clearly stated if a patient was taking two medications which can result in MC at the time of the study. Moreover, only a few studies separately provided LC and CC odds. In addition, many reported medications are available over the counter in many countries where these studies are performed, so noted exposure can be overestimated or even underestimated.

Supplementary Materials: The following supporting information can be downloaded at: https://www.mdpi.com/article/10.3390/diseases11010006/s1.

Author Contributions: Conceptualization, Z.I.T. and E.D.; methodology, Z.I.T. and U.F.; software, Z.I.T. and U.F.; validation, Z.I.T., U.F., V.T. and E.D.; formal analysis, Z.I.T.; investigation, Z.I.T. and M.F.T.; resources, Z.I.T.; data curation, M.G., Z.I.T. and U.F., writing—original draft preparation, Z.I.T., M.G. and F.K.; writing—review and editing, H.K.C., V.T. and E.D.; visualization, H.K.C.; supervision, V.T. and E.D.; project administration, Z.I.T. and E.D.; funding acquisition, No funding. All authors have read and agreed to the published version of the manuscript.

Funding: This research received no external funding.

Institutional Review Board Statement: It is a systematic review and meta-analysis performed on retrospective data; IRB approval is not required/waived.

Informed Consent Statement: This analysis is performed on retrospective study data; informed consent is not required.

Data Availability Statement: This analysis is performed on publicly available data, which can be shared on request.

Conflicts of Interest: The authors declared no potential conflict of interest for this article's research, authorship, and publication.

References

1. Miehlke, S.; Verhaegh, B.; Tontini, G.E.; Madisch, A.; Langner, C.; Munch, A. Microscopic colitis: Pathophysiology and clinical management. *Lancet Gastroenterol. Hepatol.* **2019**, *4*, 305–314. [CrossRef]
2. Miehlke, S.; Guagnozzi, D.; Zabana, Y.; Tontini, G.E.; Kanstrup Fiehn, A.M.; Wildt, S.; Bohr, J.; Bonderup, O.; Bouma, G.; D'Amato, M.; et al. European guidelines on microscopic colitis: United European Gastroenterology and European Microscopic Colitis Group statements and recommendations. *United Eur. Gastroenterol. J.* **2021**, *9*, 13–37. [CrossRef]
3. Tome, J.; Sehgal, K.; Kamboj, A.K.; Harmsen, W.S.; Kammer, P.P.; Loftus, E.V., Jr.; Tremaine, W.J.; Khanna, S.; Pardi, D.S. The Epidemiology of Microscopic Colitis in Olmsted County, Minnesota: Population-Based Study from 2011 to 2019. *Clin. Gastroenterol. Hepatol.* **2022**, *20*, 1085–1094. [CrossRef]
4. Gentile, N.M.; Khanna, S.; Loftus, E.V., Jr.; Smyrk, T.C.; Tremaine, W.J.; Harmsen, W.S.; Zinsmeister, A.R.; Kammer, P.P.; Pardi, D.S. The epidemiology of microscopic colitis in Olmsted County from 2002 to 2010: A population-based study. *Clin. Gastroenterol. Hepatol.* **2014**, *12*, 838–842. [CrossRef]
5. Andrews, C.N.; Beck, P.L.; Wilsack, L.; Urbanski, S.J.; Storr, M. Evaluation of endoscopist and pathologist factors affecting the incidence of microscopic colitis. *Can. J. Gastroenterol.* **2012**, *26*, 515–520. [CrossRef]
6. Pardi, D.S. Diagnosis and Management of Microscopic Colitis. *Am. J. Gastroenterol.* **2017**, *112*, 78–85. [CrossRef]
7. Rasmussen, M.A.; Munck, L.K. Systematic review: Are lymphocytic colitis and collagenous colitis two subtypes of the same disease-microscopic colitis? *Aliment. Pharmacol. Ther.* **2012**, *36*, 79–90. [CrossRef]
8. Sandler, R.S.; Keku, T.O.; Woosley, J.T.; Galanko, J.A.; Peery, A.F. Medication use and microscopic colitis. *Aliment. Pharmacol. Ther.* **2021**, *54*, 1193–1201. [CrossRef]
9. Zylberberg, H.M.; Kamboj, A.K.; De Cuir, N.; Lane, C.M.; Khanna, S.; Pardi, D.S.; Lebwohl, B. Medication use and microscopic colitis: A multicentre retrospective cohort study. *Aliment. Pharmacol. Ther.* **2021**, *53*, 1209–1215. [CrossRef]
10. Bohr, J.; Wickbom, A.; Hegedus, A.; Nyhlin, N.; Hultgren Hornquist, E.; Tysk, C. Diagnosis and management of microscopic colitis: Current perspectives. *Clin. Exp. Gastroenterol.* **2014**, *7*, 273–284.

11. Fernandez-Banares, F.; Esteve, M.; Espinos, J.C.; Rosinach, M.; Forne, M.; Salas, A.; Viver, J.M. Drug consumption and the risk of microscopic colitis. *Am. J. Gastroenterol.* **2007**, *102*, 324–330. [CrossRef]
12. Guagnozzi, D.; Lucendo, A.J.; Angueira, T.; Gonzalez-Castillo, S.; Tenias, J.M. Drug consumption and additional risk factors associated with microscopic colitis: Case-control study. *Rev. Esp. Enferm. Dig.* **2015**, *107*, 347–353.
13. Keszthelyi, D.; Jansen, S.V.; Schouten, G.A.; de Kort, S.; Scholtes, B.; Engels, L.G.; Masclee, A.A. Proton pump inhibitor use is associated with an increased risk for microscopic colitis: A case-control study. *Aliment. Pharmacol. Ther.* **2010**, *32*, 1124–1128. [CrossRef]
14. Page, M.J.; Moher, D.; Bossuyt, P.M.; Boutron, I.; Hoffmann, T.C.; Mulrow, C.D.; Shamseer, L.; Tetzlaff, J.M.; Akl, E.A.; Brennan, S.E.; et al. PRISMA 2020 explanation and elaboration: Updated guidance and exemplars for reporting systematic reviews. *BMJ* **2021**, *372*, n160. [CrossRef]
15. Fernandez-Banares, F.; de Sousa, M.R.; Salas, A.; Beltran, B.; Piqueras, M.; Iglesias, E.; Gisbert, J.P.; Lobo, B.; Puig-Divi, V.; Garcia-Planella, E.; et al. Epidemiological risk factors in microscopic colitis: A prospective case-control study. *Inflamm. Bowel Dis.* **2013**, *19*, 411–417.
16. Bonderup, O.K.; Fenger-Gron, M.; Wigh, T.; Pedersen, L.; Nielsen, G.L. Drug exposure and risk of microscopic colitis: A nationwide Danish case-control study with 5751 cases. *Inflamm. Bowel Dis.* **2014**, *20*, 1702–1707. [CrossRef]
17. Mohammed, A.; Ghoneim, S.; Paranji, N.; Waghray, N. Quantifying risk factors for microscopic colitis: A nationwide, retrospective cohort study. *Indian J. Gastroenterol.* **2022**, *41*, 181–189. [CrossRef]
18. Verhaegh, B.P.; de Vries, F.; Masclee, A.A.; Keshavarzian, A.; de Boer, A.; Souverein, P.C.; Pierik, M.J.; Jonkers, D.M. High risk of drug-induced microscopic colitis with concomitant use of NSAIDs and proton pump inhibitors. *Aliment. Pharmacol. Ther.* **2016**, *43*, 1004–1013. [CrossRef]
19. Weimers, P.; Vedel Ankersen, D.; Lophaven, S.N.; Bonderup, O.K.; Munch, A.; Lynge, E.; Lokkegaard, E.C.L.; Munkholm, P.; Burisch, J. Microscopic Colitis in Denmark: Regional Variations in Risk Factors and Frequency of Endoscopic Procedures. *J. Crohns Colitis* **2022**, *16*, 49–56. [CrossRef]
20. Bonderup, O.K.; Nielsen, G.L.; Dall, M.; Pottegard, A.; Hallas, J. Significant association between the use of different proton pump inhibitors and microscopic colitis: A nationwide Danish case-control study. *Aliment. Pharmacol. Ther.* **2018**, *48*, 618–625. [CrossRef]
21. Masclee, G.M.; Coloma, P.M.; Kuipers, E.J.; Sturkenboom, M.C. Increased risk of microscopic colitis with use of proton pump inhibitors and non-steroidal anti-inflammatory drugs. *Am. J. Gastroenterol.* **2015**, *110*, 749–759. [CrossRef]
22. Pascua, M.F.; Kedia, P.; Weiner, M.G.; Holmes, J.; Ellenberg, J.; Lewis, J.D. Microscopic colitis and Medication Use. *Clin. Med. Insights Gastroenterol.* **2010**, *2010*, 11–19. [CrossRef]
23. Slim, K.; Nini, E.; Forestier, D.; Kwiatkowski, F.; Panis, Y.; Chipponi, J. Methodological index for non-randomized studies (minors): Development and validation of a new instrument. *ANZ J. Surg.* **2003**, *73*, 712–716. [CrossRef]
24. Imhann, F.; Bonder, M.J.; Vich Vila, A.; Fu, J.; Mujagic, Z.; Vork, L.; Tigchelaar, E.F.; Jankipersadsing, S.A.; Cenit, M.C.; Harmsen, H.J.; et al. Proton pump inhibitors affect the gut microbiome. *Gut* **2016**, *65*, 740–748. [CrossRef]
25. Lewis, S.J.; Franco, S.; Young, G.; O'Keefe, S.J. Altered bowel function and duodenal bacterial overgrowth in patients treated with omeprazole. *Aliment. Pharmacol. Ther.* **1996**, *10*, 557–561. [CrossRef]
26. Mullin, J.M.; Gabello, M.; Murray, L.J.; Farrell, C.P.; Bellows, J.; Wolov, K.R.; Kearney, K.R.; Rudolph, D.; Thornton, J.J. Proton pump inhibitors: Actions and reactions. *Drug Discov. Today* **2009**, *14*, 647–660. [CrossRef]
27. Law, E.H.; Badowski, M.; Hung, Y.T.; Weems, K.; Sanchez, A.; Lee, T.A. Association Between Proton Pump Inhibitors and Microscopic Colitis. *Ann. Pharmacother.* **2017**, *51*, 253–263. [CrossRef]
28. Gleeson, M.H.; Davis, A.J. Non-steroidal anti-inflammatory drugs, aspirin and newly diagnosed colitis: A case-control study. *Aliment. Pharmacol. Ther.* **2003**, *17*, 817–825. [CrossRef]
29. Keszthelyi, D.; Penders, J.; Masclee, A.A.; Pierik, M. Is microscopic colitis a drug-induced disease? *J. Clin. Gastroenterol.* **2012**, *46*, 811–822. [CrossRef]
30. Aktunc, E.; Kayhan, B.; Arasli, M.; Gun, B.D.; Barut, F. The effect of atorvastatin and its role on systemic cytokine network in treatment of acute experimental colitis. *Immunopharmacol. Immunotoxicol.* **2011**, *33*, 667–675. [CrossRef]
31. Guimbaud, R.; Bertrand, V.; Chauvelot-Moachon, L.; Quartier, G.; Vidon, N.; Giroud, J.P.; Couturier, D.; Chaussade, S. Network of inflammatory cytokines and correlation with disease activity in ulcerative colitis. *Am. J. Gastroenterol.* **1998**, *93*, 2397–2404. [CrossRef] [PubMed]
32. El-Salhy, M.; Gundersen, D.; Hatlebakk, J.G.; Hausken, T. High densities of serotonin and peptide YY cells in the colon of patients with lymphocytic colitis. *World J. Gastroenterol.* **2012**, *18*, 6070–6075. [CrossRef] [PubMed]
33. Kim, D.Y.; Camilleri, M. Serotonin: A mediator of the brain-gut connection. *Am. J. Gastroenterol.* **2000**, *95*, 2698–2709. [CrossRef]
34. Khan, W.I.; Ghia, J.E. Gut hormones: Emerging role in immune activation and inflammation. *Clin. Exp. Immunol.* **2010**, *161*, 19–27. [CrossRef]

Disclaimer/Publisher's Note: The statements, opinions and data contained in all publications are solely those of the individual author(s) and contributor(s) and not of MDPI and/or the editor(s). MDPI and/or the editor(s) disclaim responsibility for any injury to people or property resulting from any ideas, methods, instructions or products referred to in the content.

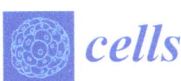

Article

Hepatic Peroxisome Proliferator-Activated Receptor Alpha Dysfunction in Porcine Septic Shock

Jolien Vandewalle [1,2,*], Bruno Garcia [3,4], Steven Timmermans [1,2], Tineke Vanderhaeghen [1,2], Lise Van Wyngene [1,2], Melanie Eggermont [1,2], Hester Dufoor [1,2], Céline Van Dender [1,2], Fëllanza Halimi [5], Siska Croubels [5], Antoine Herpain [3,6,7] and Claude Libert [1,2,*]

1. VIB Center for Inflammation Research, VIB, 9052 Ghent, Belgium
2. Department for Biomedical Molecular Biology, Faculty of Sciences, Ghent University, 9052 Ghent, Belgium
3. Experimental Laboratory of Intensive Care, Université Libre de Bruxelles, 1050 Brussels, Belgium
4. Department of Intensive Care, Centre Hospitalier Universitaire de Lille, 59000 Lille, France
5. Department of Pathobiology, Pharmacology and Zoological Medicine, Faculty of Veterinary Medicine, Ghent University, 9820 Merelbeke, Belgium
6. Department of Intensive Care, Erasme University Hospital—HUB, Université Libre de Bruxelles, 1050 Brussels, Belgium
7. Department of Intensive Care, St.-Pierre University Hospital, Université Libre de Bruxelles, 1050 Brussels, Belgium
* Correspondence: jolien.vandewalle@irc.vib-ugent.be (J.V.); claude.libert@irc.vib-ugent.be (C.L.)

Abstract: Despite decades of research, sepsis remains one of the most urgent unmet medical needs. Mechanistic investigations into sepsis have mainly focused on targeting inflammatory pathways; however, recent data indicate that sepsis should also be seen as a metabolic disease. Targeting metabolic dysregulations that take place in sepsis might uncover novel therapeutic opportunities. The role of peroxisome proliferator-activated receptor alpha (PPARα) in liver dysfunction during sepsis has recently been described, and restoring PPARα signaling has proven to be successful in mouse polymicrobial sepsis. To confirm that such therapy might be translated to septic patients, we analyzed metabolic perturbations in the liver of a porcine fecal peritonitis model. Resuscitation with fluids, vasopressor, antimicrobial therapy and abdominal lavage were applied to the pigs in order to mimic human clinical care. By using RNA-seq, we detected downregulated PPARα signaling in the livers of septic pigs and that reduced PPARα levels correlated well with disease severity. As PPARα regulates the expression of many genes involved in fatty acid oxidation, the reduced expression of these target genes, concomitant with increased free fatty acids in plasma and ectopic lipid deposition in the liver, was observed. The results obtained with pigs are in agreement with earlier observations seen in mice and support the potential of targeting defective PPARα signaling in clinical research.

Keywords: sepsis; swine; metabolism; PPARα; free fatty acids

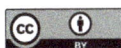

1. Introduction

Sepsis 3.0 defines sepsis as a life-threatening organ dysfunction caused by a dysregulated host response to infection [1]. Sepsis is the most important cause of morbidity and mortality in human patients admitted to intensive care units (ICU), with a significant cost impact in health care worldwide. Recent estimates suggest a yearly burden of 48.9 million sepsis cases and 11 million deaths worldwide [2]. After five decades of research, no innovative drugs addressing mechanistic pathways have become available to treat septic patients. Sepsis is classically considered as an overreaction of the immune system. However, anti-inflammatory drugs have failed in clinical trials [3]. Current management of sepsis is supportive rather than curative and essentially relies on antibiotics to eradicate the bacterial infection, fluid resuscitation with a vasopressor to maintain an adequate tissular perfusion and mechanical support for organs at risk of failing [4,5]. Recent studies have described the possible role of metabolic changes that take place in the liver during sepsis, and targeting these alterations holds much interest for the management of sepsis [4,6].

One of the promising targets is peroxisome proliferator-activated receptor alpha (PPARα) signaling. PPARα is a 52 kDa protein highly expressed in metabolic tissues and activated by free fatty acids (FFAs) and other lipid derivatives. As a member of the nuclear receptor family, PPARα has a conserved modular structure consisting of an N-terminal domain, important for transcriptional activation, a DNA-binding domain that contains zinc fingers, a short hinge region and the C-terminal ligand-binding domain [7,8]. Upon activation, PPARα regulates gene transcription by forming a heterodimer with retinoid X receptor and binding to specific DNA sequences referred to as PPARα response elements (PPRE). PPARα regulates a wide variety of genes, of which most are involved in diverse aspects of lipid metabolism, including FFA transport, oxidation of FFAs and ketogenesis (for example *ACOX1, HMGCS2, CPT1* and *CPT2*). In this way, PPARα orchestrates metabolic homeostasis during energy deprivation, the latter leading to the release of FFAs from white adipose tissue [7,8].

Sepsis is typically associated with the induction of a starvation response due to an increased energy need on the one hand, and anorexia (defined by a lack of food intake and/or appetite) on the other [6,9,10]. Despite the essential role of PPARα to cope with starvation, recent studies in murine sepsis have found that PPARα expression dramatically declines and hence loses function in the liver [11,12]. This results in impaired lipid metabolism, coinciding with ectopic lipid accumulation, lipotoxicity and increased mortality. Preventing PPARα dysfunction reduces sepsis mortality, making this pathway an interesting target to evaluate in clinical research [11,12]. The above-mentioned studies were performed on mice, but it remains to be confirmed whether these observations also occur in human sepsis.

Rodents are used in 94% of all sepsis studies because of their low cost, well-characterized genome and the opportunity to generate and use transgenic strains [13]. However, mice are less suitable as a model for sepsis due to their high resilience to infection, different pathophysiology to humans and technical constraints for performing a goal-orientated resuscitation and source control [14]. Therefore, validation of mice preclinical findings in a larger mammalian animal model enhances the translational potential towards human sepsis drastically [13]. Pigs are appropriate animal models to close the gap between rodent and human studies given their homology in size, physiology and pathophysiology, especially when studying metabolic and infectious diseases [15,16].

In this current study, we report that sepsis-induced changes in the liver, as observed in mice, are actually also relevant in a porcine peritonitis model. Based on bulk RNA sequencing (RNA-seq), we found PPARα dysfunction and concomitant lipid accumulation in the blood and liver of septic pigs in direct relation to the degree of hemodynamic alterations in the animals. Our results strengthen the potential validity of poor PPARα signaling as a new therapeutic target for human sepsis patients.

2. Materials and Methods

2.1. Experimental Procedure

Fecal peritonitis resulting in septic shock was introduced in nine pigs (*Sus scrofa domesticus*, RA-SE Genetics, Belgium, weighing ± 50 kg) (5 ♂ and 4 ♀) by intraperitoneal instillation of 3 g/kg of autologous feces previously collected from the animal's enclosure and diluted in 300 mL of 5% glucose solution. As a control, three sham pigs (2 ♂ and 1 ♀), consisting of anesthesia and surgical preparation but without sepsis induction, were applied. Animals were fasted for 18 h prior to the start of the experiment, with free access to water. All the septic animals developed shock (mean arterial pressure (MAP) ≤ 50 mmHg)—within 5.9 ± 1.4 h after the onset of sepsis—and were then left untreated for 1 h to consolidate multi-organ dysfunction. Resuscitation fluids, norepinephrine (NE), antibiotics treatment and abdominal lavage were applied during the following 8 h to mimic human clinical cares, after which the animals were euthanized for organ isolation (liver and plasma). The study protocol for the pigs followed the EU Directive (2010/63/EU) for animal experiments and was approved by the local animal ethics committee (Comité Ethique du Bien-Être Animal; protocol number 724N) from the Université Libre de Bruxelles (ULB) in Brussels (Belgium). Pig experiments were performed in the Experimental Laboratory of Intensive Care of the ULB (LA1230406) and under the ARRIVE guidelines and MQTiPSS recommendations. Analysis of the samples was performed in the Inflammation Research Center (IRC) in Zwijnaarde. A detailed description of the experimental procedure to induce septic shock in the pigs is provided in [17]. Samples were isolated from the NE group at the end of the experiment (vasopressor 2 timepoint). Note, we isolated one extra pig that was used for a pilot experiment.

2.2. Biological Samples

Systemic blood samples for FFA analysis were collected from the femoral artery at the end of the experiment and immediately centrifuged, and plasma was frozen at −20 °C until further processing. FFAs were determined via colorimetric assays according to the manufacturer's instructions (KA1667, Abnova, Taipei City, Taiwan).

2.3. Liver Transcriptomic Analysis

Liver biopsies taken from the fourth segment were isolated and stored in RNALater (AM7021, Invitrogen, Waltham, MA, USA). RNA was isolated using the Aurum total RNA mini kit (732-6820, Biorad, Temse, Belgium). RNA quality was checked with the Agilent RNA 6000 Pico Kit (Agilent Technologies, Santa Clara, CA, USA). The RNA was used for creating an Illumina sequencing library using the Illumina TruSeqLT stranded RNA-seq library protocol (VIB Nucleomics Core, Belgium) and paired-end sequencing (2 × 150 bp) was done on an Illumina Novaseq 6000. The obtained reads were mapped to the pig (*Sus scrofa*, Sscrofa11.1) reference transcriptome/genome with hisat v2.0.4 [18]. Gene-level read counts were obtained with the feature Counts software (part of the subread package) [19]. Multimapping reads were excluded from the assignment. Differential gene expression was assessed with the DESeq2 package [20], with the FDR set at 5%. Motif finding for multiple motifs, or de novo motif finding, was performed using the HOMER software [21]. We used the promoter region (start offset: −500 bp, end offset: 50 bp downstream of transcription start site TSS) to search for known motif enrichment and de novo motifs. Gene ontology (GO) term enrichment on selected groups of genes was performed via the Enrichr tool [22].

2.4. LipidTOX Staining

Liver pieces (~1 cm^3) were isolated and stored in cold antigenfix for 1–2 h. Then, the liver was washed twice in cold PBS and put in 34% sucrose at 4 °C while constantly agitating for at least 10 h and up to 24 h. The next day, liver pieces were stored in NEC50 and frozen at −80 °C until further processing. Cryostat sections of 20 μm thickness were rehydrated in PBS for 5 min after which the sections were blocked in blocking buffer (2% BSA, 1% fetal calf serum, 1% goat serum, in 0.5% saponin) for 30 min at RT. The antibody mix (LipidTOX Deep Red (1:400, Life Technologies Europe B.V., Merelbeke, Belgium); Acti-stain 488 Phalloidin (1:150, PHDG1, Cytoskeleton Inc., St. Denver, CO, USA)) was added and incubated for 2 h at RT. After washing with PBS for 5 min, nuclear staining (Hoechst (1:1.000, Sigma-Aldrich N.V., Hoeilaart, Belgium)) was added for 5 min at RT. Slides were washed in PBS for 5 min, quickly rinsed in water to remove residual salt and mounted. For each cryosection, eight Z-stacks of 3 areas per coupe were imaged with a spinning disk confocal microscope (Zeiss, White Plains, NY, USA), using a 40× Plan-Apochromat objective lens (1.4 Oil DIC (UV) VIS-IR M27, Zeiss)) at a pixel size of 0.167 μm and at optimal Z-resolution (240 mm). Z-stacks were processed in Volocity (PerkinElmer, Waltham, MA, USA) and the amount of lipid droplets was calculated. We had two biological samples per group (sham vs. sepsis). Two liver pieces from each pig were isolated and 3 areas per liver piece were analyzed for technical variance. The average was taken of the six technical repeats per animal and the biological data was used for analyses.

2.5. Datasets and Databases

RNA-seq data of the pigs are deposited at the National Center for Biotechnology Information (NCBI) Gene Expression Omnibus public database (http://www.ncbi.nlm.nih.gov/geo/) under accession number GSE218636 (accessed on 23 November 2022). PPARα responsive genes are retrieved from the publicly available dataset deposited at the NCBI under accession number GSE139484 (accessed on 23 November 2019). PPARα responsive genes are considered as those responsive to the PPARα agonist GW7647 in sham condition. Genes involved in FA oxidation are retrieved from MGI (http://www.informatics.jax.org/vocab/gene_ontology/) with GO:0019395 (accessed on 18 October 2022). 121 genes are involved in this pathway of which 87 are found in pigs.

2.6. Statistics

Figures are generated in Graphpad prism 9. When comparing sham versus sepsis data, a Student's *t*-test was used in an unpaired two-tailed fashion. Mean ± SEM is shown in bar graphs. Violin plots were analyzed with a Wilcoxon signed-rank test.

3. Results

3.1. Hepatic PPARα Dysfunction in Porcine Septic Shock

3.1.1. Inflammation and Metabolic Dysregulation in Liver upon Septic Shock

All the septic animals developed shock (mean arterial pressure (MAP) ≤ 50 mmHg)—within 5.9 ± 1.4 h after the onset of sepsis—with severe tissular hypoperfusion (Figure 1). Septic shock induced an hyperdynamic cardiovascular response, restored by the introduction of fluid expansion and subsequent NE infusion, which normalized tissular perfusion for the entire period of septic shock resuscitation. Multiple organ failure was observed, with respiratory and renal dysfunction, on top of circulatory failure and severe capillary leakage. Clinical parameters measured at the timepoint just before euthanizing are summarized in Table 1. A more comprehensive description of the model severity and the response to resuscitation care can be found in the princeps study publication [17].

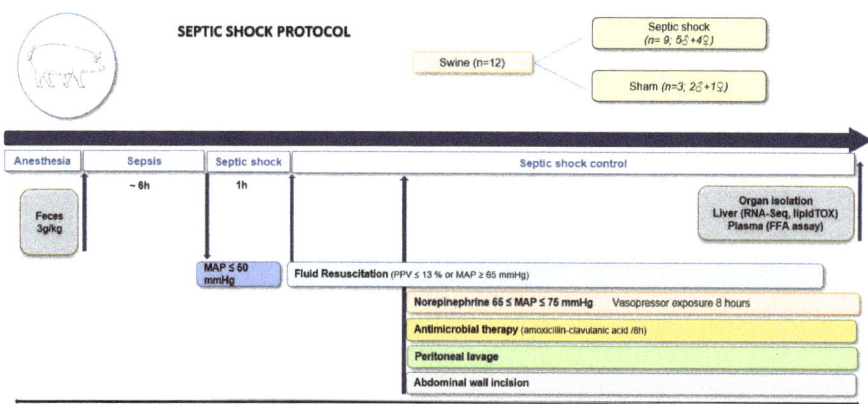

Figure 1. Protocol timeline. Animals were allowed to develop sepsis until a severe hypotension with mean arterial pressure (MAP) ≤ 50 mmHg was obtained. Severe hypotension (MAP between 45 and 50 mmHg) was allowed for one hour. Thereafter, full resuscitation was started, aiming to restore the pulse pressure variation (PPV) to ≤13% or MAP ≥ 65 mmHg. After achieving this objective, antibiotics and abdominal lavage were applied to control the infection. Norepinephrine was added to the infusion to maintain a MAP of 65–75 mmHg for 8 h. After this timepoint, the animals were euthanized to collect liver and plasma for subsequent analysis (i.e., ~18 h after the start of the experiment).

Table 1. Clinical parameters determined in pigs just before euthanizing.

		Sham	Septic Shock	p-Value
Hemodynamic parameters	MAP (mmHg)	68 ± 2	68 ± 3	0.85
	HR (/min)	87 ± 3	155 ± 21	0.03
	CO (L/min)	6 ± 1	9 ± 2	0.03
	NE (µg/kg/min)	0 ± 0	1 ± 0.84	0.08
	SvO_2 (%)	64 ± 3	73 ± 5	0.02
	PCO_2 gap (mmHg)	5 ± 1	5 ± 5	0.98
Respiratory function	RR (/min)	17 ± 3	20 ± 3	0.10
	Tidal Volume (mL)	375 ± 35	385 ± 50	0.76
	$PaCO_2$ (mm Hg)	52 ± 1	47 ± 5	0.15
	PaO_2/FiO_2 ratio	330 ± 58	253 ± 58	0.07
Metabolism	T°	38.8 ± 0.8	38.8 ± 0.4	0.80
	Glucose (mg/dL	107 ± 10	115 ± 23	0.61
	Lactate (mmol/L)	0.9 ± 0.00	2 ± 1.1	0.12
	pH	7.46 ± 0.01	7.42 ± 0.06	0.26
	Base excess (mmol/L)	12 ± 1	5 ± 5	0.03

MAP: mean arterial pressure, HR: heart rate, CO: cardiac output, NE: norepinephrine requirement, SvO_2: mixed venous oxygen saturation, pCO_2 gap: veno-arterial difference in CO_2 partial pressure, RR: respiratory rate, $PaCO_2$: partial pressure of carbon dioxide, PaO_2/FiO_2: ratio of arterial oxygen partial pressure to fractional inspired oxygen.

Relative differences in transcriptional changes observed in the liver upon septic shock were visualized with principal component analysis (PCA) and a clear separation of sham versus sepsis samples was observed (Figure 2A). Sepsis induced significant upregulation of 1892 genes and downregulation of 2043 genes in the liver of the pigs ($p < 0.05$) compared to sham animals (Figure 2B). A list of differentially expressed genes and their expression level is included in the supplementals (Table S1). To obtain information on the processes that were specifically induced or inhibited in the septic pigs by these upregulated and downregulated genes, they were analyzed via gene set enrichment against various libraries using Enrichr. Genes upregulated in the liver upon sepsis were associated with the immune system, innate immune system and neutrophil degranulation (Figure 2C). These are typical pathways activated upon inflammation. The downregulated genes were associated with metabolism, more specifically metabolism of lipids and FFAs, as well as amino acids and steroids (Figure 2D). As targeting the inflammatory pathway in sepsis trials did not result in successful therapeutic targets [3] and based on our previous studies in murine sepsis [12], we focused on the pathways that are predicted to be downregulated upon sepsis. Restoring downregulated pathways that normally have a protective function could provide novel therapeutic opportunities.

3.1.2. PPARα Dysfunction

Analysis of the downregulated genes with Wiki pathway analysis identified PPARα signaling as most affected pathway during sepsis (Figure 3A). Motif analysis by HOMER of the downregulated genes ($p < 0.05$ and with a mouse orthologue) upon sepsis revealed a PPARα motif in the top 5 of the known motifs (Figure 3B). The mean log fold change (LFC) upon sepsis of the 293 downregulated genes that contain a PPRE identified by HOMER was −1.8 (Table S2). This PPARα motif was not retrieved in the motifs of the upregulated genes ($p < 0.05$ and with a mouse orthologue), the top motifs of which were generally associated with the inflammatory response (Figure 3B), e.g., the NF-κB DNA binding motif. To study the effect of PPARα loss of function genome wide, we plotted the LFC upon sepsis of all PPARα-induced genes (Appendix A). The median LFC of these genes was −0.27 and significantly differed from the baseline LFC 0 (Figure 3C), which confirms that PPARα appears significantly less active as a transcription factor in sepsis than sham pigs. As PPARα is involved in FFA oxidation, the LFC of all genes involved in FFA oxidation based on gene ontology analysis (GO:0019395), and which depend on PPARα for their expression, were compared between sham and sepsis samples. The median LFC of these genes was −1.07 (Figure 3D) (Table S3). As an illustration, we plotted the expression level of PPARα and several PPARα targets involved in β-oxidation and ketogenesis to compare the expression in septic livers to those in sham condition (Figure 3E). The mRNA expression of PPARα in septic animals was only 36% of that in sham animals. Likewise, genes involved in the FFA β-oxidation pathway were reduced by more than half upon sepsis. Interestingly, PPARα levels in the liver correlated negatively with the NE requirement of the septic pigs (Figure 3F). This correlation implies that pigs with lower PPARα levels have a higher need for NE infusion to maintain their blood pressure, which is indicative of a more severe sepsis. Together, these data support the notion that PPARα signaling is dysfunctional in the liver of septic pigs and correlates with sepsis severity.

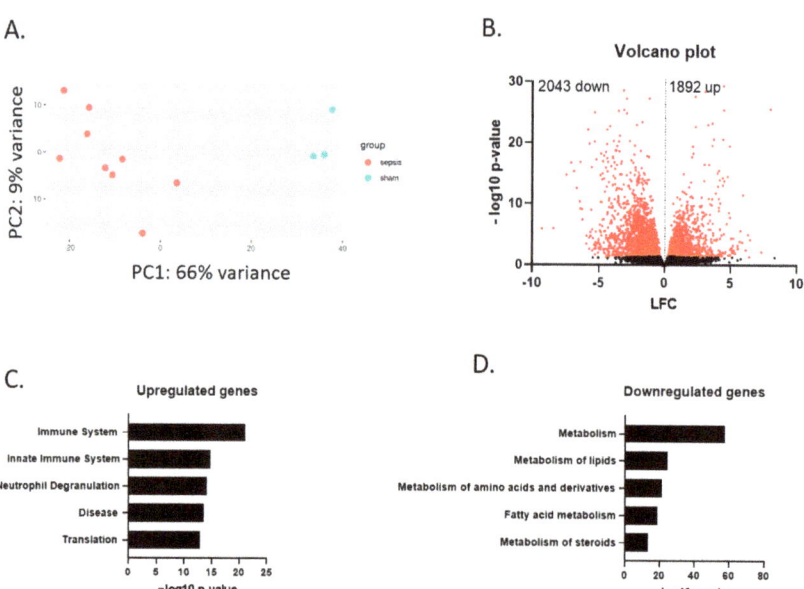

Figure 2. Metabolic dysregulation in livers of porcine sepsis. (**A**) PCA plot of overall gene expression in liver samples from sham and sepsis pigs. PCA plot clarifies the variance within samples per condition. (**B**) Volcano plot with differential expression of genes affected by sepsis compared to sham, as measured by bulk RNA sequencing. Genes significantly affected are indicated with red dots ($p < 0.05$). Genes with $-\log 10$ p-value above 30 are omitted for clarity of the plot. (**C**) Top five enriched gene ontology (GO) terms for genes that are upregulated upon sepsis ($p < 0.05$). (**D**) Top five enriched GO terms for genes that are downregulated upon sepsis ($p < 0.05$). Analyses of (**C**,**D**) was performed with the Enrichr tool.

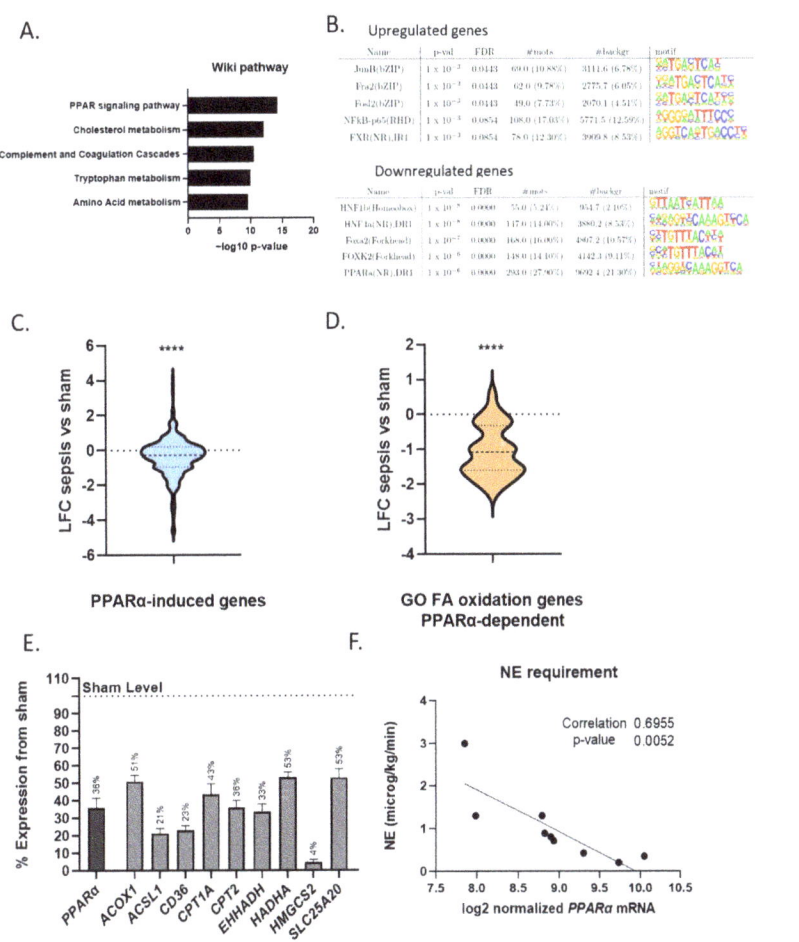

Figure 3. PPARα dysfunction in livers of porcine sepsis. (**A**) Top five enriched gene ontology (GO) terms for genes that are downregulated upon sepsis ($p < 0.05$). Analysis was performed with the Wiki pathway tool. (**B**) Homer motif analysis to detect DNA binding motifs in the 500 base pairs upstream of the transcription start site of up- and down regulated genes upon sepsis ($p < 0.05$ and for genes with a mouse orthologue). Top five motifs ranked according to p-value is shown. (**C**) Violin plot showing LFC upon sepsis of genes that are known to be induced by the PPARα agonist GW7647 in murine sepsis ($p < 0.05$). LFC of the porcine genes with a mouse orthologue upon sepsis is displayed (389 genes). Median and upper and lower quartiles are shown with a horizontal dotted line in the violin plot. Median is significantly different from baseline LFC 0. **** $p < 0.0001$. (**D**) Violin plot showing LFC upon sepsis of genes involved in FA oxidation (GO00193951, 121 genes) that are known to be induced by the PPARα agonist GW7647 (34/121) in murine sepsis ($p < 0.05$). LFC of the porcine genes with a mouse orthologue upon sepsis is displayed (29 genes). Median and upper and lower quartiles are shown with a horizontal dotted line in the violin plot. Median is significantly different from baseline LFC 0. **** $p < 0.0001$. (**E**) Expression level of PPARα and genes involved in β-oxidation of FFAs and ketogenesis is displayed. The expression level of sham pigs is set as 100% and compared to the level in sepsis pigs. (**F**) Correlation curve plotting the norepinephrine (NE) requirement of each septic pig to their PPARα mRNA level in the liver (RNA-seq counts are log2 normalized). Data is analyzed with a simple linear regression. R^2 depicts correlation of 0.6955. The slope is significantly different from zero. N = 9.

3.1.3. Increased FFA in Blood and Ectopic Lipid Accumulation in Liver

Since PPARα is the major transcription factor involved in β-oxidation of FFAs, and since we observe significant problems with the expression of PPARα and genes involved in FFA β-oxidation, we hypothesized that FFAs will accumulate in the blood due to processing problems. Indeed, total FFAs were increased significantly in the pig's blood upon sepsis (Figure 4A). When FFAs are high in circulation, the liver sequestrates them in lipid droplets [12]. To investigate whether ectopic lipid accumulation is occurring in the liver of septic pigs, cryosections of liver were stained with LipidTOX, a fluorescent dye with high affinity for neutral lipids. Extensive lipid droplet accumulation was observed in the livers of septic animals, whereas this was only minimal in sham samples (Figure 4B,C), indicating more lipid accumulation in the liver of septic subjects.

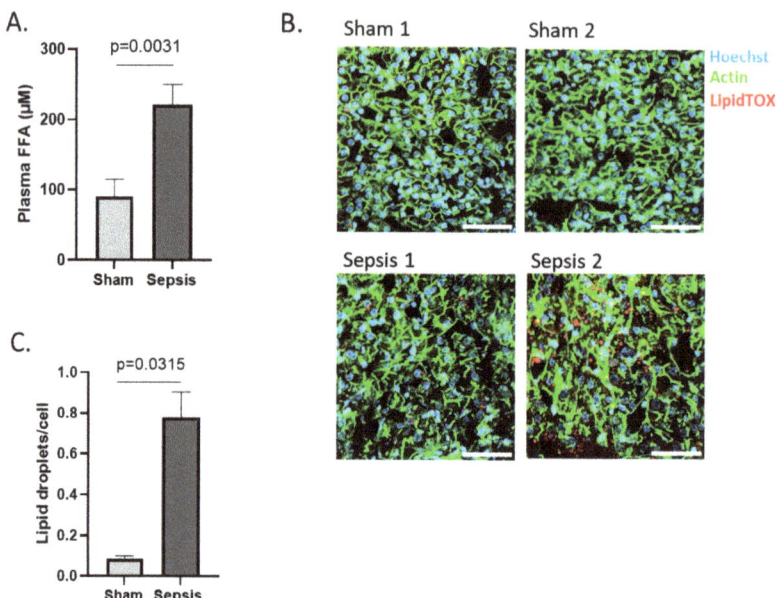

Figure 4. Metabolic disease parameters in blood and liver of porcine sepsis. (**A**) Concentration FFA in plasma of sham (n = 3) and sepsis (n = 9) pigs. (**B**) Immunofluorescent images of porcine liver after sham or sepsis. Cryosections were stained with Hoechst (blue), acti-stain (green) and lipidTOX (red). Z-stacks (8/region) were generated in 3 areas scattered across the entire tissue section. White scale bar = 50 μm. One representative picture of each biological repeat is shown. (**C**) The amount of lipid droplets (LDs)/cell were calculated for each Z-stack. Averages of the amount of the LDs were converged for each subject and biological replicates (n = 2) are used in the figure.

4. Discussion

In contrast to the Sepsis 2.0 definition, the latest definition of sepsis no longer refers to inflammation as an essential pathway [1]. One of the reasons for this adjustment is that clinical trials targeting the inflammatory pathway have failed to provide significant survival benefits [3]. Potential clarifications for this failure might be the use of inappropriate animals as preclinical models. Given the complex nature of sepsis, it is unlikely that findings based on one species will be able to mimic all aspects of the clinical and biological complexity observed in human sepsis. Therefore, it is advisable to confirm key findings in other mammals, such as pigs [23].

Next, it has become increasingly clear that other pathways, such as certain metabolic pathways, are playing a crucial role in the pathogenesis of sepsis [4]. A large proteomic and metabolic screen on the plasma of human sepsis patients identified glucose metabolism and FFA β-oxidation pathways as being significantly different between sepsis survivors and non-survivors [24]. Moreover, these pathways differed consistently among several sets of patients, and diverged more as death approached [24]. FFA β-oxidation is a multistep process that breaks down FFAs in the mitochondria to produce energy. In times of starvation, lipolysis liberates FFAs from adipose tissue to foresee in energy [25]. In septic subjects, lipolysis is observed as a way to cope with the negative energy balance that is the result of an increased energy need and a decreased food intake during sepsis [9,10,26]. However, we recently observed that the transformation of FFAs to acetyl-CoA and ketones fails due to defects in PPARα signaling, leading to an accumulation of these substrates. Indeed, already 6 h after the onset, FFAs increase in the blood of septic mice [12]. Similarly, FFAs increase in the blood of septic patients and these levels correlate well with the clinical severity [12]. Mice with a deletion of PPARα in their hepatocytes display an increased mortality upon sepsis [27]. Preventing PPARα dysfunction with pemafibrate, however, reduces sepsis mortality. Pemafibrate is a novel selective PPARα modulator (SPPARMα) that restores PPARα expression, thereby decreasing FFA plasma levels and lipid accumulation in the liver [12]. Together these data reveal PPARα as an interesting new target for sepsis.

The role of PPARα in human sepsis patients has already been investigated. In the blood of septic children, the decreased expression of PPARα responsive genes was observed, with lower levels being associated with a more severe disease status [28]. Nevertheless, the major FFA-metabolizing organ which depends on PPARα is the liver. Determination of hepatic PPARα levels and function in human sepsis patients is, however, challenging, primarily due to the coagulation problems in sepsis patients. Post-mortem liver biopsies could identify lower PPARα levels in non-surviving critically ill patients [27]; however, these results should be interpreted with caution as RNA quality rapidly declines after death [29].

We studied the liver of septic pigs in order to minimize the gap between mouse and human research. In the current study, we analyzed the liver of septic pigs, since the liver plays a key role in metabolic rearrangements. In accordance with the literature [30], upregulated genes in porcine livers upon sepsis are generally associated with inflammatory pathways, whereas downregulated genes are linked to metabolic pathways. Interestingly, the pathway affected with the highest probability is PPARα signaling. PPARα targets related to FFA β-oxidation are especially reduced in the livers of sepsis pigs, which might explain the increased FFA levels in plasma and lipid accumulation in their livers. In murine sepsis, reduced mRNA expression of PPARα and its targets involved in FFA β-oxidation could indeed be linked to a reduced capability of liver explants to metabolize palmitic acid ex vivo, as measured with the Seahorse technology [12].

The strength of this current study is the use of an advanced ICU animal model that follows the MQTiPSS recommendations (including abdominal lavage, antimicrobial therapy and early vasopressor introduction) with the aim of improving the clinical translatability of experimental findings. A downside of doing this type of research, especially when using pigs, is the high cost in comparison to research using rodents as the animal model. This downside can be countered by performing interdisciplinary or multicenter studies involving the isolation of several tissues and organs simultaneously. The collaborative study reported here is an example. Liver biopsies and plasma were isolated from septic shock pigs that were also used in a study on the myocardial effects of vasopressors [17]. Due to logistical reasons, we were, however, not able to quantify FFA β-oxidation ex vivo in the pig samples, so conclusive proof of the link between PPARα resistance on the one hand and FFA increase and lipotoxicity on the other is lacking in pigs. Moreover, a determination of mitochondrial number might be interesting, as the number of mitochondria can also influence FFA β-oxidation capacity in cells. Lastly, the effect of the PPARα agonist pemafibrate on hepatic PPARα function, lipotoxicity and survival still needs to be determined to solidify the proposed hypotheses.

Collectively, these data suggest that problems with PPARα expression and activity in the liver might contribute to problems with β-oxidation of FFAs. This in turn leads to deposition of lipid storages in the liver upon sepsis. The data obtained in porcine septic subjects thus confirm the results obtained in murine sepsis and support the potential of targeting defective PPARα signaling in the clinic. Elucidation of the upstream signal(s) causing PPARα dysfunction might uncover novel therapeutic opportunities in sepsis. Moreover, clinical trials are warranted to validate the therapeutic applicability of this axis (i.e., PPARα resistance–FFA increase–lipotoxicity) in human individuals with sepsis.

Supplementary Materials: The following supporting information can be downloaded at https://www.mdpi.com/article/10.3390/cells11244080/s1, Table S1: differentially expressed genes (up and down) in liver upon septic shock, Table S2: mean log fold change (LFC) upon sepsis of the 293 downregulated genes that contain a PPRE motif, Table S3: LFC of all genes involved in FFA oxidation and which depend on PPARα for their expression.

Author Contributions: Conceptualization, J.V. and C.L.; in vivo work, B.G. and A.H.; processing samples, J.V., T.V., L.V.W., M.E., H.D. and C.V.D.; RNA-seq analysis, S.T.; writing—original draft preparation, J.V.; writing—review and editing, J.V., F.H., S.C., A.H. and C.L.; supervision, C.L. All authors have read and agreed to the published version of the manuscript.

Funding: An FWO grant (11Z2718N) to J.V. supported this work. Funding of this work was further provided by the Special Research Fund of Ghent University (GOA and Methusalem Program (BOF.MET.2021.0001.0)).

Institutional Review Board Statement: The study protocol for the pigs followed the EU Directive (2010/63/EU) for animal experiments and was approved by the local animal ethics committee (Comité Ethique du Bien-Être Animal; protocol number 724N) from the Université Libre de Bruxelles (ULB) in Brussels (Belgium).

Informed Consent Statement: Not applicable.

Data Availability Statement: RNA-seq data of the pigs are deposited at the National Center for Biotechnology Information (NCBI) Gene Expression Omnibus public database (http://www.ncbi.nlm.nih.gov/geo/) under accession number GSE218636 (accessed on 23 November 2022). PPARα responsive genes are retrieved from the publicly available dataset deposited at the NCBI under accession number GSE139484 (accessed on 23 November 2019). PPARα responsive genes are considered as those responsive to the PPARα agonist GW7647 in sham condition. Genes involved in FA oxidation are retrieved from MGI (http://www.informatics.jax.org/vocab/gene_ontology/) with GO:0019395 (accessed on 18 October 2022). 121 genes are involved in this pathway of which 87 genes were found in pig.

Acknowledgments: We acknowledge the VIB Nucleomics Core for sequencing analysis, the VIB Bioimaging core Ghent for imaging support and Fuhong Su, Jacques Creteur and Fabio Taccone for support with the pig experiments.

Conflicts of Interest: The authors declare no conflict of interest.

Appendix A

PPARα-induced genes are selected based on their response to the PPARα agonist GW7647 in mice livers (i.e., significantly upregulated by GW7647 ($p < 0.05$) [12]) and with a pig orthologue.

References

1. Singer, M.; Deutschman, C.S.; Seymour, C.; Shankar-Har, M.; Annane, D.; Angus, D.C. The Third International Consensus Definitions for Sepsis and Septic Shock (Sepsis-3). *JAMA* **2016**, *315*, 801–810. [CrossRef] [PubMed]
2. Rudd, K.E.; Johnson, S.C.; Agesa, K.M.; Shackelford, K.A.; Tsoi, D.; Kievlan, D.R.; Colombara, D.v.; Ikuta, K.S.; Kissoon, N.; Finfer, S.; et al. Global, Regional, and National Sepsis Incidence and Mortality, 1990–2017: Analysis for the Global Burden of Disease Study. *Lancet* **2020**, *395*, 200–211. [CrossRef] [PubMed]
3. Cavaillon, J.; Singer, M.; Skirecki, T. Sepsis Therapies: Learning from 30 Years of Failure of Translational Research to Propose New Leads. *EMBO Mol. Med.* **2020**, *12*, e10128. [CrossRef] [PubMed]
4. van Wyngene, L.; Vandewalle, J.; Libert, C. Reprogramming of Basic Metabolic Pathways in Microbial Sepsis: Therapeutic Targets at Last? *EMBO Mol. Med.* **2018**, *10*, e8712. [CrossRef] [PubMed]

5. Evans, L.; Rhodes, A.; Alhazzani, W.; Antonelli, M.; Coopersmith, C.M.; French, C.; Machado, F.R.; Mcintyre, L.; Ostermann, M.; Prescott, H.C.; et al. Surviving Sepsis Campaign: International Guidelines for Management of Sepsis and Septic Shock 2021. *Intensive Care Med.* **2021**, *47*, 1181–1247. [CrossRef]
6. Vandewalle, J.; Libert, C. Sepsis: A Failing Starvation Response. *Trends Endocrinol. Metab.* **2022**, *33*, 292–304. [CrossRef]
7. Goldstein, I.; Baek, S.; Presman, D.M.; Paakinaho, V.; Swinstead, E.E.; Hager, G.L. Transcription Factor Assisted Loading and Enhancer Dynamics Dictate the Hepatic Fasting Response. *Genome Res.* **2017**, *27*, 427–439. [CrossRef]
8. Kersten, S.; Stienstra, R. The Role and Regulation of the Peroxisome Proliferator Activated Receptor Alpha in Human Liver. *Biochimie* **2017**, *136*, 75–84. [CrossRef]
9. Wang, A.; Huen, S.C.; Luan, H.H.; Yu, S.; Zhang, C.; Gallezot, J.-D.D.; Booth, C.J.; Medzhitov, R. Opposing Effects of Fasting Metabolism on Tissue Tolerance in Bacterial and Viral Inflammation. *Cell* **2016**, *166*, 1512–1525.e12. [CrossRef]
10. Peterson, S.J.; Tsai, A.A.; Scala, C.M.; Sowa, D.C.; Sheean, P.M.; Braunschweig, C.L. Adequacy of Oral Intake in Critically Ill Patients 1 Week after Extubation. *J. Am. Diet. Assoc.* **2010**, *110*, 427–433. [CrossRef]
11. Colaço, H.; Barros, A.; Neves-Costa, A.; Seixas, E.; Pedroso, D.; Velho, T.; Willmann, K.; Yi, H.-S.; Shong, M.; Benes, V.; et al. Host-Dependent Induction of Disease Tolerance to Infection by Tetracycline Antibiotics. *Immunity* **2020**, *12*, 53–67. [CrossRef]
12. van Wyngene, L.; Vanderhaeghen, T.; Timmermans, S.; Vandewalle, J.; van Looveren, K.; Souffriau, J.; Wallacys, C.; Eggermont, M.; Ernst, S.; van Hamme, E.; et al. Hepatic PPARα Function and Lipid Metabolic Pathways Are Dysregulated in Polymicrobial Sepsis. *EMBO Mol. Med.* **2020**, *12*, e11319. [CrossRef] [PubMed]
13. Zingarelli, B.; Coopersmith, C.M.; Drechsler, S.; Efron, P.; Marshall, J.C.; Moldawer, L.; Wiersinga, W.J.; Xiao, X.; Osuchowski, M.F.; Thiemermann, C. Part I: Minimum Quality Threshold in Preclinical Sepsis Studies (MQTiPSS) for Study Design and Humane Modeling Endpoints. *Shock* **2019**, *51*, 10. [CrossRef] [PubMed]
14. Guillon, A.; Preau, S.; Aboab, J.; Azabou, E.; Jung, B.; Silva, S.; Textoris, J.; Uhel, F.; Vodovar, D.; Zafrani, L.; et al. Preclinical Septic Shock Research: Why We Need an Animal ICU. *Ann. Intensive Care* **2019**, *9*, 66. [CrossRef]
15. Bassols, A.; Costa, C.; Eckersall, P.D.; Osada, J.; Sabrià, J.; Tibau, J. The Pig as an Animal Model for Human Pathologies: A Proteomics Perspective. *Proteom. Clin. Appl.* **2014**, *8*, 715–731. [CrossRef]
16. Meurens, F.; Summerfield, A.; Nauwynck, H.; Saif, L.; Gerdts, V. The Pig: A Model for Human Infectious Diseases. *Trends Microbiol.* **2012**, *20*, 50–57. [CrossRef]
17. Garcia, B.; Su, F.; Dewachter, L.; Favory, R.; Khaldi, A.; Moiroux-Sahraoui, A.; Annoni, F.; Vasques-Nóvoa, F.; Rocha-Oliveira, E.; Roncon-Albuquerque, R.; et al. Myocardial Effects of Angiotensin II Compared to Norepinephrine in an Animal Model of Septic Shock. *Crit. Care* **2022**, *26*, 281. [CrossRef]
18. Kim, D.; Paggi, J.M.; Park, C.; Bennett, C.; Salzberg, S.L. Graph-Based Genome Alignment and Genotyping with HISAT2 and HISAT-Genotype. *Nat. Biotechnol.* **2019**, *37*, 907–915. [CrossRef]
19. Liao, Y.; Smyth, G.K.; Shi, W. FeatureCounts: An Efficient General Purpose Program for Assigning Sequence Reads to Genomic Features. *Bioinformatics* **2014**, *30*, 923–930. [CrossRef]
20. Love, M.I.; Huber, W.; Anders, S. Moderated Estimation of Fold Change and Dispersion for RNA-Seq Data with DESeq2. *Genome Biol.* **2014**, *15*, 550. [CrossRef]
21. Heinz, S.; Benner, C.; Spann, N.; Bertolino, E.; Lin, Y.C.; Laslo, P.; Cheng, J.X.; Murre, C.; Singh, H.; Glass, C.K. Simple Combinations of Lineage-Determining Transcription Factors Prime Cis-Regulatory Elements Required for Macrophage and B Cell Identities. *Mol. Cell* **2010**, *38*, 576–589. [CrossRef] [PubMed]
22. Chen, E.Y.; Tan, C.M.; Kou, Y.; Duan, Q.; Wang, Z.; Meirelles, G.v.; Clark, N.R.; Ma'ayan, A. Enrichr: Interactive and Collaborative HTML5 Gene List Enrichment Analysis Tool. *BMC Bioinform.* **2013**, *14*, 128. [CrossRef] [PubMed]
23. Chao, R.; Renqi, Y.; Lixue, W.; Xianzhong, X.; Yongming, Y. Minimum Quality Threshold in Pre-Clinical Sepsis Studies (MQTiPSS): Quality Thresholds for Study Design and Humane Modeling Endpoints. *Zhonghua Wei Zhong Bing Ji Jiu Yi Xue* **2019**, *31*, 1061–1071.
24. Langley, R.J.; Tsalik, E.L.; Velkinburgh, J.C.V.; Glickman, S.W.; Rice, B.J.; Wang, C.; Chen, B.; Carin, L.; Suarez, A.; Mohney, R.P.; et al. An Integrated Clinico-Metabolomic Model Improves Prediction of Death in Sepsis. *Sci. Transl. Med.* **2013**, *5*, 195ra95. [CrossRef]
25. Finn, P.F.; Dice, J.F. Proteolytic and Lipolytic Responses to Starvation. *Nutrition* **2006**, *22*, 830–844. [CrossRef] [PubMed]
26. Vandewalle, J.; Timmermans, S.; Paakinaho, V.; Vancraeynest, L.; Dewyse, L.; Vanderhaeghen, T.; Wallaeys, C.; van Wyngene, L.; van Looveren, K.; Nuyttens, L.; et al. Combined Glucocorticoid Resistance and Hyperlactatemia Contributes to Lethal Shock in Sepsis. *Cell Metab.* **2021**, *33*, 1763–1776.e5. [CrossRef]
27. Paumelle, R.; Haas, J.T.; Hennuyer, N.; Baugé, E.; Deleye, Y.; Mesotten, D.; Langouche, L.; Vanhoutte, J.; Cudejko, C.; Wouters, K.; et al. Hepatic PPARα Is Critical in the Metabolic Adaptation to Sepsis. *J. Hepatol.* **2019**, *70*, 963–973. [CrossRef]
28. Wong, H.R.; Cvijanovich, N.; Allen, G.L.; Lin, R.; Anas, N.; Meyer, K.; Freishtat, R.J.; Monaco, M.; Odoms, K.; Sakthivel, B.; et al. Genomic Expression Profiling across the Pediatric Systemic Inflammatory Response Syndrome, Sepsis, and Septic Shock Spectrum. *Crit. Care Med.* **2009**, *37*, 1558. [CrossRef]
29. van der Linden, A.; Blokker, B.M.; Kap, M.; Weustink, A.C.; Riegman, P.H.J.; Oosterhuis, J.W.; Cappello, F. Post-Mortem Tissue Biopsies Obtained at Minimally Invasive Autopsy: An RNA-Quality Analysis. *PLoS ONE* **2014**, *9*, e115675. [CrossRef]
30. van Malenstein, H.; Wauters, J.; Mesotten, D.; Langouche, L.; de Vos, R.; Wilmer, A.; van Pelt, J. Molecular Analysis of Sepsis-Induced Changes in the Liver: Microarray Study in a Porcine Model of Acute Fecal Peritonitis with Fluid Resuscitation. *Shock* **2010**, *34*, 427–436. [CrossRef]

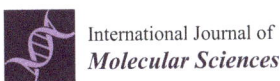

Article

Natural Compound 2,2′,4′-Trihydroxychalcone Suppresses T Helper 17 Cell Differentiation and Disease Progression by Inhibiting Retinoid-Related Orphan Receptor Gamma T

Yana Yang [†], Wenhui Qi [†], Yanyan Zhang, Ruining Wang, Mingyue Bao, Mengyuan Tian, Xing Li and Yuan Zhang *

Key Laboratory of Medicinal Resources and Natural Pharmaceutical Chemistry (Shaanxi Normal University), The Ministry of Education, National Engineering Laboratory for Resource Development of Endangered Crude Drugs in Northwest China, College of Life Sciences, Shaanxi Normal University, Xi'an 710119, China
* Correspondence: yuanzhang@snnu.edu.cn or yuanzhang_bio@126.com; Tel.: +86-29-8531-0266
† These authors contributed equally to this work.

Abstract: Retinoid-related orphan receptor γt (RORγt), a vital transcription factor for the differentiation of the pro-inflammatory Th17 cells, is essential to the inflammatory response and pathological process mediated by Th17 cells. Pharmacological inhibition of the nuclear receptor RORγt provides novel immunomodulators for treating Th17-driven autoimmune diseases and organ transplant rejection. Here, we identified 2,2′,4′-trihydroxychalcone (TDC), a natural chalcone derivant, binds directly to the ligand binding domain (LBD) of RORγt and inhibited its transcriptional activation activity. Using three mice models of Th17-related diseases, it was found that the administration of TDC effectively alleviated the disease development of experimental autoimmune encephalomyelitis (EAE), experimental colitis, and skin allograft rejection. Collectively, these results demonstrated TDC targeting RORγt to suppress Th17 cell polarization, as well as its activity, thus, indicating the potential of this compound in treating of Th17-related autoimmune disorders and organ transplant rejection disorders.

Keywords: chalcone derivant; RORγt; Th17 cell differentiation; experimental autoimmune encephalomyeliti; experimental colitis; skin allograft rejection

1. Introduction

Th17 cells, distinguished by the expression of pro-inflammatory cytokines such as IL-17, IL-22, and IL-21, are an important lineage of CD4$^+$ T effector (Teff) cells [1,2]. There is overwhelming evidence that Th17 cells exert an essential function in autoimmune inflammation, for instance experimental autoimmune encephalomyelitis (EAE), rheumatoid arthritis, inflammatory bowel disease (IBD), and acute allograft rejection [3–5].

The retinoic acid receptor-related orphan receptor gamma t (RORγt; NR1F3), as a ligand-dependent transcriptional factor of Th17 cell differentiation, belongs to the nuclear hormone receptor superfamily. It is reported that RORγt promoted IL-17A production and Th17 polarization. It also taken part in antitumor immunity, autoimmune diseases as well as transplant rejection [6,7]. Based on structural analysis, RORγt regulated target gene expression and physiological function through interacting with both coactivators and corepressors. Therefore, functional inhibitors play a critical role in disease treatment by targeting RORγt, such as digoxin, SR1001, SR1555, ursolic acid and so on [6,8]. However, some drugs discovered did not apply to clinical research due to the severe adverse reactions and low efficacy [9–11]. Hence, our goal is to screen out a safe, effective, and natural drug that targets RORγt to treat Th17-associated inflammatory disease.

In this study, compounds that bind to the active domain of RORγt three-dimensional structure were screened from the ZINC database, and the most promising natural com-

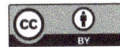

pound 2,2′,4′-trihydroxychalcone (TDC), a natural chalcone derivant, was obtained. Chalcone derivant, as the biogenetic precursors of all known flavonoids, is consist of an uncomplicated chemical framework, which can be broadly identified in vegetables and fruits [12–14]. Recently, more and more findings concerning to TDC application in antioxidant, anti-inflammatory, anti-tumor activity, and improving memory impairment in various animal models [12,15]. Hence, TDC itself might be potentially used as a lead compound by targeting RORγt for further research on autoimmune diseases as well as organ transplant rejection.

Here, we focused on the positive benefits of TDC, which exhibited significant therapeutic effects on EAE, experimental colitis, and skin allograft rejection. In addition, we demonstrated that TDC, as a prospective and novel pharmacological inhibitor of RORγt, provides a candidate for clinical immunomodulator for treating Th17-related autoimmune disorders and organ transplant rejection disorders.

2. Results

2.1. Structure-Based Virtual Screening of Small Molecules Targeting RORγt

In order to screen out novel Retinoid-related orphan receptor γt (RORγt) inhibitors, 60 natural compounds including 2,2′,4′-trihydroxychalcone (TDC) with good binding parameters to RORγt protein were obtained, which have been shown in our previous studies [16] (Figure 1A). The data was showed that TDC formed hydrogen may bond with A496 in RORγt pocket 1. We found that the hydroxybenzene ring of RORγt formed hydrophobic interactions with V494, F506, W317, I492, and L325 in the protein structure. Its o-hydroxybenzene ring can also interact with L501, I328, L505, and the surrounding benzene ring to form hydrophobic interactions (Figure 1B,C).

2.2. TDC Suppressed RORγt Transcription Activity In Vitro

We used lentivirus to co-transfer RORγt and CNS2-PIL-17-TK-luciferase reporter genes into 293T cells to establish a dual-luciferase reporter system for the purpose of evaluating the activity of TDC on RORγt transcriptional level. By measuring the viability of 293T, cells were treated with various concentrations (0–100 μM) of TDC, and we chose TDC up to 25 μM for the luciferase reporting experiment (Figure 1D). It can be clearly seen that, in comparison to the vehicle-treated group, TDC markedly suppressed the luciferase activity. At the same time, when the TDC concentration was 25 μM, the expression of luciferase was reduced to 33.63% of the control group (Figure 1E). In summary, these data demonstrated that TDC notably inhibited the transcriptional level of RORγt.

2.3. TDC Inhibited Th17 Cell Differentiation In Vitro

In order to optimize the treatment dose of TDC on T cells, the CCK8 activity was measured to detect the effect of different concentrations of TDC on the viability of splenocytes. The results showed that 5 μM TDC was not toxic to splenocytes (Figure 1F). Subsequently, we used different concentrations of TDC (1.25, 2.5, and 5 μM) to perform in vitro experiments to measure the production of Th17-related cytokines. The results showed that TDC significantly inhibited Th17 cell polarization and decreased the secretion of IL-17 in a dose-dependent pattern as against the vehicle group (Figure 1G,H,J). qRT-PCR was used to test the effect of TDC on the gene level of cytokines such as IL-17a and IL-17f, in which TDC at 2.5 μM significantly inhibited the gene expression of IL-17a and IL-17f (Figure 1I). Taken together, TDC treatment obviously inhibited Th17 cell differentiation in vitro.

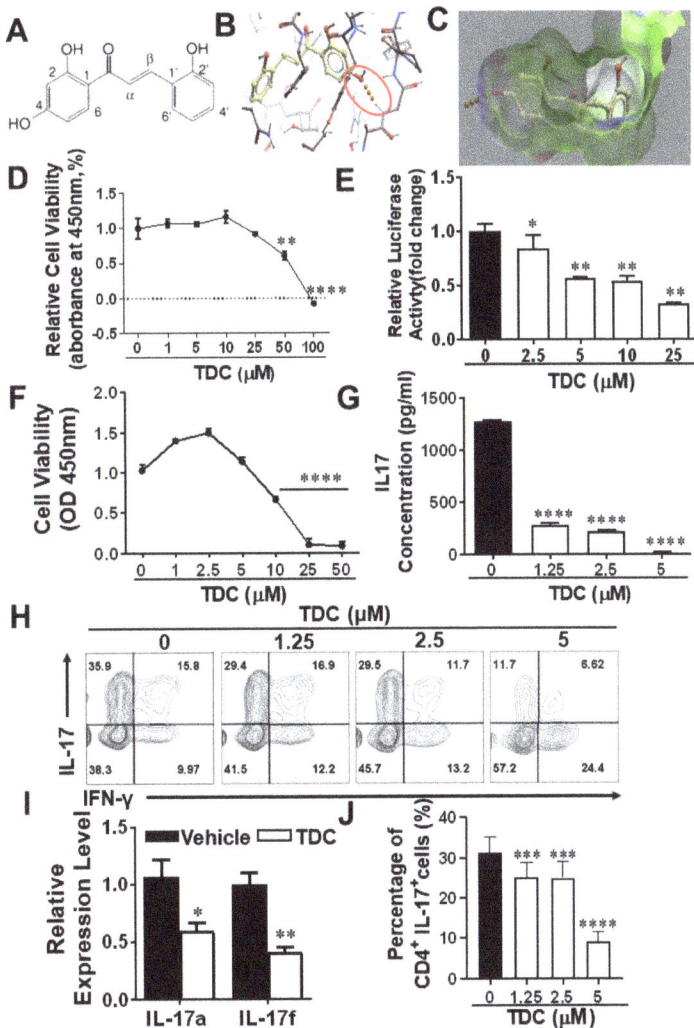

Figure 1. Molecular docking and inhibition of Th17 cell differentiation by TDC targeting RORγt. (**A**) Structural formulas of compound TDC. (**B**) Hydrogen bond connections between TDC and A496 in pocket 1 of RORγt protein (PDB: 5C4T). (**C**) The electron cloud distribution stated TDC binds with V494, F506, W317, I492, and L325 in pocket 1 of 5C4T protein. (**D**) The effect of various concentrations (1–100 μM) of TDC on the viability of HEK293T cells overexpressing mRORγt. (**E**) The impact of TDC on the activity of RORγt luciferase reporter gene. (**F**) The influence of TDC on splenocyte cell viability. (**G**) The level of IL-17 production in Th17 cells after TDC treatment by ELISA. (**I**) qRT-PCR was performed to test *IL-17a* and *IL-17f* genes in TDC and vehicle-treated groups. (**H,J**) Intracellular IL-17 staining was used to evaluate the influence of TDC treatment on Th17 cell differentiation by flow cytometry. Data are shown as mean ± SD (*n* = 3 each group) and representative three experiments. * $p < 0.05$, ** $p < 0.01$, *** $p < 0.001$, **** $p < 0.0001$, compared to control group, and determined by one-way ANOVA with Tukey's multiple comparisons test (**D–H**) or unpaired Student's *t* test (**I**).

2.4. TDC Efficiently Ameliorated the Onset of EAE and Reduced CNS Inflammation

In the prophylactic treatment experiment, TDC or vehicle administration started from day 0 p.i. with a dosage of 10 mg/kg/day in EAE mice by intraperitoneal injection.

Compared with the vehicle group, TDC administration significantly inhibited clinical scores (Figure 2A) and cumulative clinical scores (Figure 2B) of EAE mice. To further assesses the pathological alterations in the TDC-treated group, histological evaluates of lumbar SCs were performed to determine central nervous system (CNS) inflammation and myelin loss on day 18 p.i. As demonstrated in Figure 2C,D, TDC treatment significantly reduced inflammatory infiltration and demyelination.

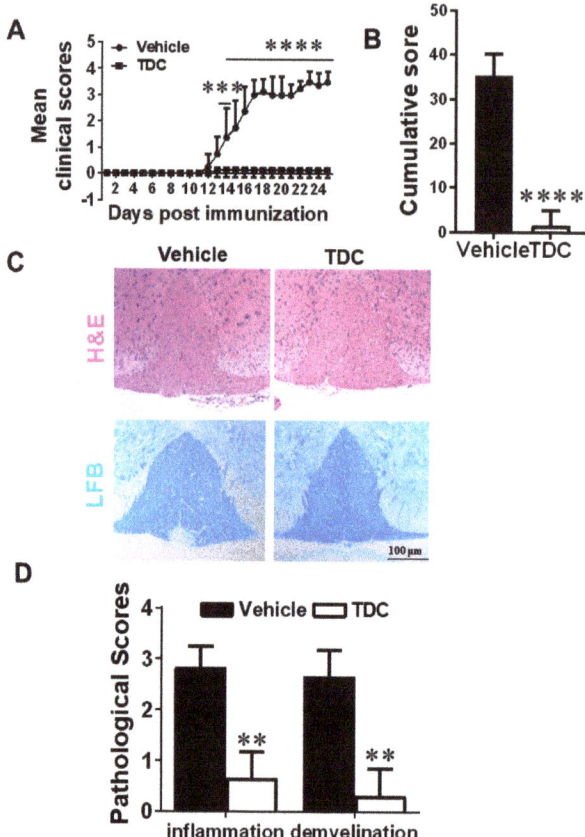

Figure 2. TDC ameliorated the progress of EAE. (**A**) EAE development was evaluated and recorded following a 0–5 scale. (**B**) Cumulative Score of EAE. Clinical scores were cumulated from day 10 p.i. to day 25 p.i. (**C**) Pathological sections at the lumbar level were stained to evaluate the degree of inflammatory infiltration (H&E), (**D**) The pathology scores of inflammation area were evaluated. Data are shown as mean ± SD (n = 3 each group) and representative three experiments. ** $p < 0.01$, *** $p < 0.001$, **** $p < 0.0001$, compared to vehicle-treated group, unpaired t test (**B,D**) or two-way ANOVA with multiple comparisons test (**A**). Scale bar = 100 μm.

2.5. TDC Treatment Blocked the Activation of Debdritic Cells (DCs) and MOG-Reactive T Cells in the CNS

For the purpose of evaluate the impact of TDC on infiltrating pro-inflammatory cells, MNCs in the CNS of EAE mice were harvested on day 20 p.i. and added MOG_{35-55} (10 μg/mL). The number of MNCs, $CD45^+$, $CD4^+$, and $CD8^+$ T cells in the CNS of TDC-treated group was markedly reduced than those of the control group (Figure 3A,B,D). At the same time, the number of pathogenic Th1, Th17, and $CD4^+GM\text{-}CSF^+$ cells was remarkably reduced compared with the vehicle group (Figure 3C,D). In addition, TDC inhibited the transcriptional level of cytokines such as *IL-17a, GM-CSF, IL-23, IFN-γ, IL-1β, IL-6, TNF-α*, and chemokines such as *CXCL1*, *CXCL19*, *CXCL12* and *CXCL10* of the SCs of EAE mice (Figure 3E). During the onset of the disease, inflammatory T cells invading the CNS interact with APCs, which lead to reactivation of T cells and activation of APCs [17]. Dendritic cells (DCs) and microglia (CD11b$^+$CD45hi$^+$), which belong to a class of APCs, played a key role in antigen presentation in innate and adaptive immune mechanism [18,19]. The data demonstrated that the proportion of activated microglia did not change obviously (Supplementary Figure S1A,C). The number of DC cells (CD11c$^+$CD80$^+$ and CD11c$^+$CD86$^+$) (Supplementary Figure S1B,D) in the TDC group was less than in the vehicle group, even if there was no significant difference. The similar outcome could be noted in the peripheral tissues (Supplementary Figure S2).

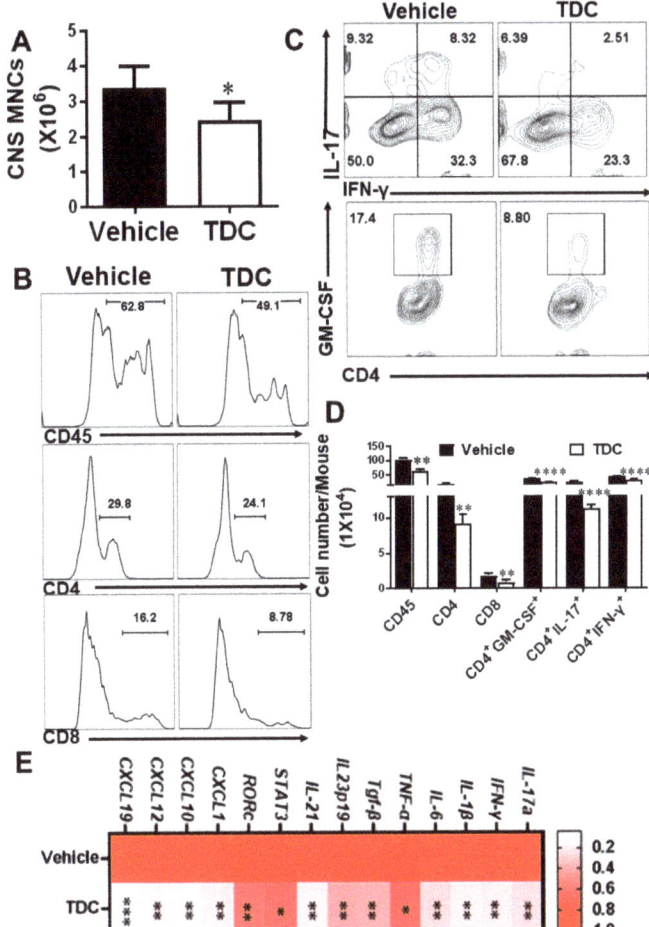

Figure 3. TDC treatment inhibited the inflammatory infiltration of the CNS. (**A**) The number of mononuclear cells in the CNS of EAE mice treated with TDC and vehicle. (**B**) Flow histograms of CD45$^+$ cells, CD4$^+$ T cells, and CD8$^+$ T cells. (**C**) Flow cytometric pseudo-color image of CD4$^+$ GM-CSF$^+$ cells, Th1, and Th17 cells. (**D**) The statistical results of the number of CD45$^+$ cells, CD4$^+$ T cells, CD8$^+$ T cells, CD4$^+$IFN-γ$^+$, CD4$^+$IL-17$^+$, CD4$^+$GM-CSF$^+$ cells. (**E**) The effect of TDC treatment on the expression of inflammation-related genes in the SC of EAE mice. Data are shown as mean ± SD (n = 5 each group) and representative three experiments. * $p < 0.05$, ** $p < 0.01$, *** $p < 0.001$, **** $p < 0.0001$, compared to vehicle-treated group, unpaired t test (**A**,**E**) or two-way ANOVA with multiple comparisons test (**D**).

2.6. TDC Alleviated DSS-Induced Colitis

To study whether TDC has a relief effect on colitis, DSS induced mouse colitis model was employed in this study. As shown in Figure 4, TDC treatment greatly alleviated DSS-induced colitis, as proven by the remarkably relief of weight loss (Figure 4A), and notably ameliorated of colonic shortening (Figure 4C,D). At the same time, DAI score showed a persistent trend with the above data, indicating that DSS-induced colitis was effectively alleviated by TDC (Figure 4B). Subsequently, H&E staining was used to evaluate colonic mucosal lesions. Compared with the naïve group and vehicle group, the TDC group displayed fewer pro-inflammatory cell infiltration, relatively intact colonic architecture, and minor mucosal damage (Figure 4E,F). Taken together, it was obvious that TDC could improve DSS-induced colitis in the animal model.

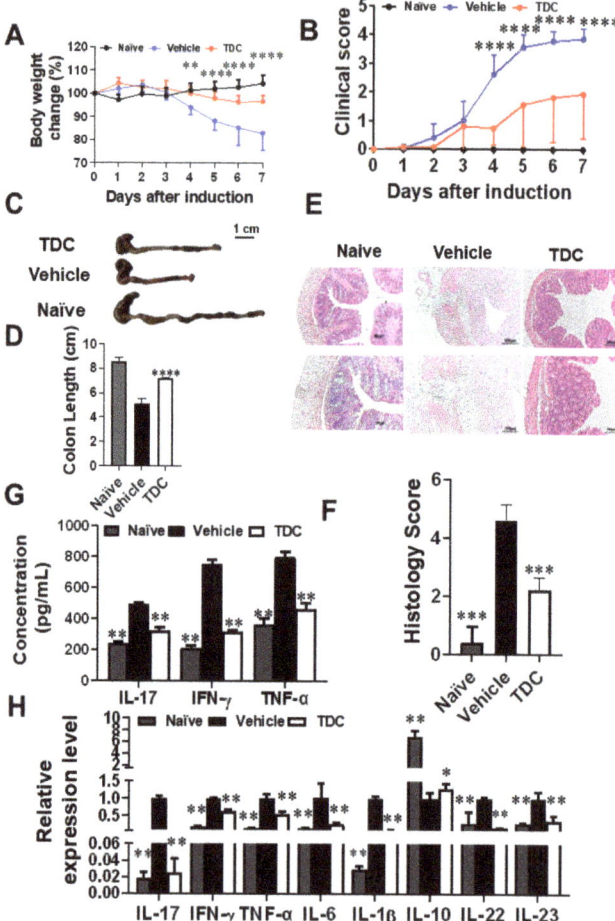

Figure 4. DSS-induced colitis was relieved by TDC. (**A**) The mouse body weight was measured every day during the experiment. (**B**) Clinical score of colitis. (**C,D**) Colon length of mice (n = 6 each group), scale bar = 1 cm. (**E,F**) H&E staining of colonic tissues in the three groups, scale bar = 200 μm (upper row) or 100μm (lower row). (**G**) ELISA assay was used to detect the secretion of IL-17, IL-6, and TNF-α in mouse colon (n = 6 per group) (**H**) qRT-PCR was carried out to test the proinflammatory genes in the colitis colon tissues of TDC and vehicle-treated groups. Data are shown as mean ± SD (n = 3 each group). * $p < 0.05$, ** $p < 0.01$, *** $p < 0.001$, **** $p < 0.0001$, one-way ANOVA with Tukey's multiple comparisons test (**D,F–H**), two-way ANOVA with multiple comparisons test (**A,B**).

2.7. TDC Treatment Decreased the Secretion of Pro-Inflammatory Cytokines and Preserved the Proportion of Th17/Treg Cells

To further investigate the function of TDC on T cells in DSS-induced colitis mice, tissues and cells of colitis mice at 7 days after TDC administration were collected. Flow cytometry data displayed that in comparison to the vehicle group, the proportion of Th17 cells in different types in the TDC group was decreased (Figure 5A,C), and the proportion of Treg cells was increased (Figure 5B,D). We used ELISA to check the production of the pro-inflammatory cytokines in colonic tissues. As shown in Figure 4G, TDC treatment significantly inhibited the release of inflammatory factors such as IL-17, IFN-γ, and TNF-α. Next, qRT-PCR was used to detect the expression of inflammation-related genes in the colon, which TDC inhibited the expression of *IL-17*, *IFN-γ*, *TNF-α*, *IL-1β*, *IL-6*, *IL-22*, and *IL-23* genes in the mouse colon and promoted the expression of *IL-10* gene (Figure 4H). In other words, TDC treatment blocked the production of pro-inflammatory cytokines and maintained the balance of Th17/Treg cells to improve colitis in mice.

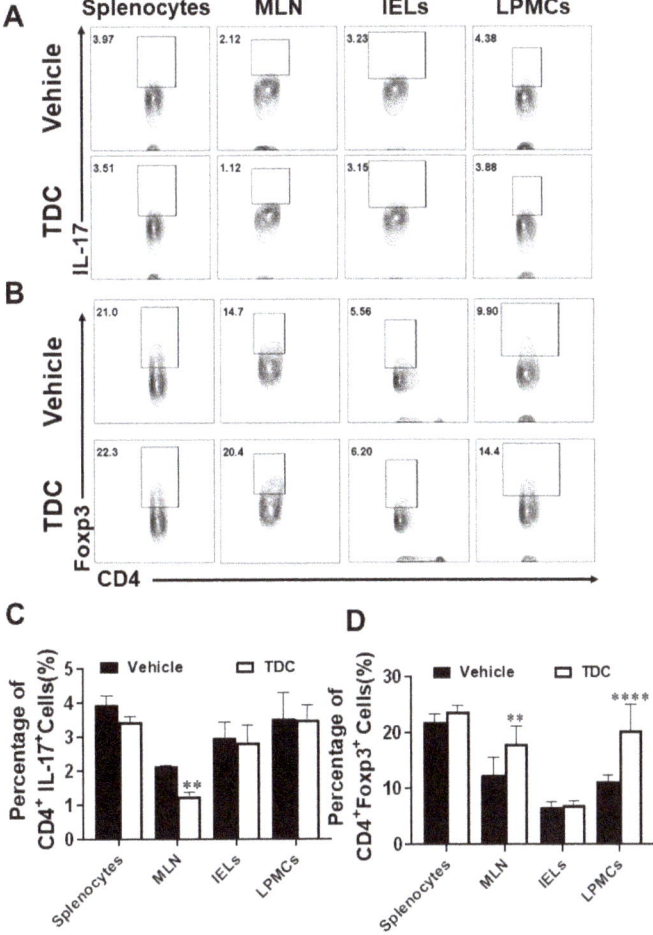

Figure 5. TDC treatment maintained the Th17/Treg balance in DSS-induced colitis mice. (**A**) Flow cytometric pseudo-color images of Th17 cells positive for IL-17 in different organs. (**B**) Flow cytometric pseudo-color images of Treg cells positive for Foxp3 in different organs. (**C,D**) The statistical results of the proportion of CD4$^+$ IL-17$^+$ and CD4$^+$ Foxp3$^+$ cells. Data are shown as mean ± SD (n = 6 each group). ** $p < 0.01$, **** $p < 0.0001$, two-way ANOVA with multiple comparisons test.

2.8. TDC Alleviated the Transplantation Rejection Responses of Skin Graft In Vivo

After 7 days of skin transplantation, the grafts in the vehicle group exhibited scab and necrosis, indicating significant rejection, while the grafts in the CSA group and TDC group survived (Figure 6A). Recipient mice were sacrificed on day 7 of the experiment, and the transplanted skin tissues were stained with H&E. According to the results, inflammatory infiltration in CSA group and TDC group was remarkably reduced compared with the vehicle-treated group (Figure 6B). Corresponding tissues were collected to check the level of related inflammation factors. As shown in Figure 6C, production of IL-17, IFN-γ, and TNF-α were significantly inhibited by TDC. qRT-PCR was employed to measure the expression of inflammation-related genes in the graft. TDC treatment inhibited the expression of *IFN-γ*, *IL-12p35*, *IL-12p40*, *TGF-β*, *TNF-α*, *IL-17C*, and *IL-6* genes in skin transplants, and upregulated the expression level of *Foxp3* and *IL-10* genes (Figure 6D). These results indicated that TDC inhibited allograft rejection and could be a potential immunomodulator.

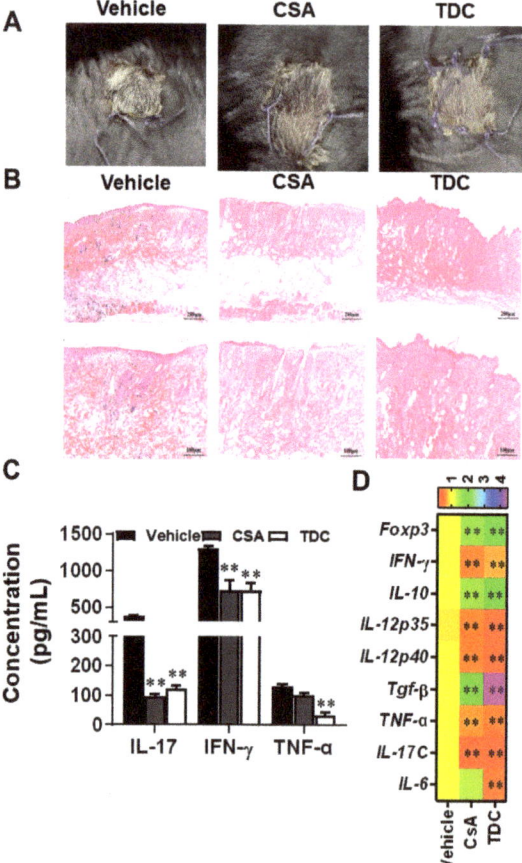

Figure 6. TDC treatment prevented skin allograft rejection. (**A**) The macroscopic aspect of the skin graft 7 days after the skin graft. (**B**) H&E staining of grafted skin slices 7 days after skin transplantation. Scale bar = 200 μm (upper row) or 100 μm (lower row). (**C**) The production of IL-17, IFN-γ and TNF-α in the supernatant of splenocyte culture was detected by ELISA. (**D**) qRT-PCR was performed to test the pro-inflammatory genes in the skin grafts of mice. Data are shown as mean ± SD (n = 3 each group). ** $p < 0.01$, one-way ANOVA with multiple comparisons test (**C**) or unpaired Student's t test (**D**).

2.9. TDC Inhibited Skin Graft Rejection in Allogeneic Mice by Maintaining a Balance between Th17 Cells and Treg Cells

Since Th17 and Treg cells played a critical role in mediating allograft rejection, splenocyte and lymphocyte mononuclear cells of mice were collected for flow cytometry analysis at the 7th day after skin transplantation. In comparison to the vehicle group, the proportion of Th17 cells in the lymphocytes and splenocytes decreased under TDC and CSA treatment (Figure 7A). The proportion of Th1 cells in splenocytes decreased under TDC treatment (Figure 7B). As shown in Figure 7C, the proportion of Treg cells enhanced under CSA and TDC treatment, although there was no significant difference in TDC group. In comparison to the vehicle group, the ratio of CD4$^+$ TNF-α^+ cells decreased, and there was no significant difference in the proportion of IL-4 and IL-10 cells in the CSA and TDC groups (Supplementary Figure S3A,B). These results indicated that TDC played a critical role in suppressing allograft rejection.

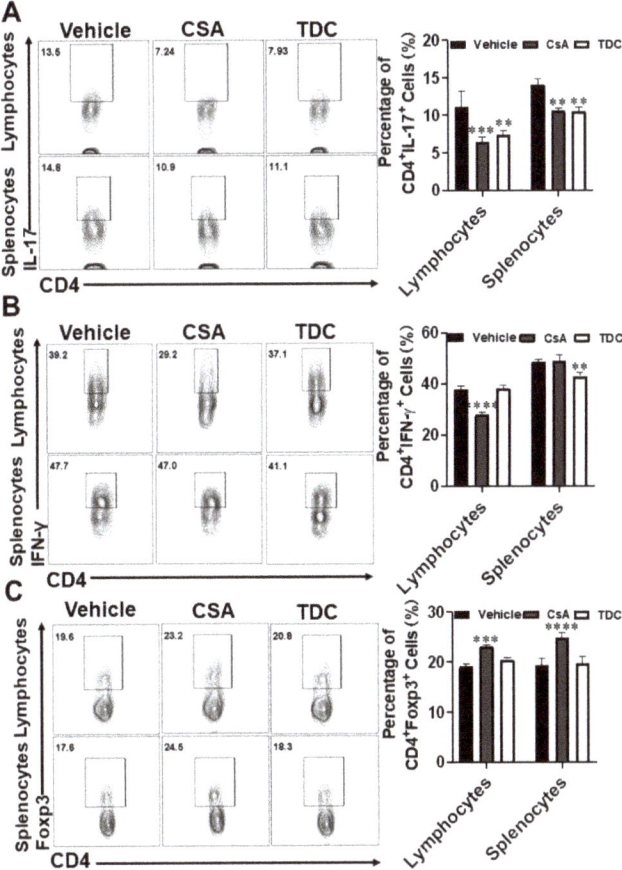

Figure 7. Effects of TDC on Th17, Th1 and Treg cells in splenocytes and lymph nodes of skin transplanted mice. Splenocytes and lymphocytes were prepared in each group at the 8th day after administration. CD4$^+$ IL-17$^+$, CD4$^+$ Foxp3$^+$ and CD4$^+$ IFN-γ^+ were detected by flow cytometry. (**A**) Flow cytometric pseudo-color images and statistical results of Th17 cells in different organs. (**B**) Flow cytometric pseudo-color images and statistical results of Th1 cells. (**C**) Flow cytometric pseudo-color images and statistical results of Treg cells in different organs. The results in the panel are expressed as means ± SD and are representative of three experiments (n = 6 each group), ** $p < 0.01$, *** $p < 0.001$, **** $p < 0.0001$, two-way ANOVA with multiple comparisons test.

3. Discussion

This study identified small molecule compounds for the treatment of Th17-driven autoimmune and transplant rejection disorders by high-throughput virtual screening for high-efficiency RORγt inhibitor. Among the 60 RORγt-targeting compounds found by virtual screening, TDC, as a flavonoid extracted from *Glycyrrhiza glabra*, had attracted our attention due to its extensive sources and high safety. We found that TDC significantly inhibited the clinical symptoms of MOG-induced EAE, and additionally effectively alleviated the symptoms of colitis mice and relieved skin graft rejection. Mechanically, TDC regulated Th17/Treg balance to alleviate the disease.

RORγt played a vital role in driving Th17 cell differentiation and IL-17 production, which indicated in the pathology of multiple autoimmune and inflammatory diseases [7,20,21]. However, currently reported drugs targeting RORγt cannot be applied in clinical practice due to the side effects, poor therapeutic action and off-target effect [22]. Our experimental results demonstrated that RORγt-targeting TDC with anti-inflammatory activity had no obvious toxic and side effects on splenocyte viability within the effective dose range.

CD4$^+$ T helper cells regulated immunity and inflammation by differentiating into effector T cell subsets with different functions, such as Th1, Th2, Th17, and Treg [23]. Th1 and Th17, as pro-inflammatory cells, are involved in the pathogenesis of various inflammatory and autoimmune disorders [24–26]. However, previous research suggested that IL-23, as the main pro-inflammatory factor and associated with the stable differentiation of Th17, seems to be necessary for maintaining chronic inflammation [27]. The inhibitor targeting RORγt may lessen not only the Th17 reaction but also influence the proportion of Tregs [27]. The studies have also shown that there is a balance between the expression level of RORγt and Foxp3, which regulates the balance of Treg and Th17 [28]. In addition, Treg inhibits IL-12 production by producing IL-10 and TGF-β, thereby inhibiting IL-12-induced Th1 cell differentiation. Based on these data, we hypothesized that TDC inhibits Th17 and Th1 differentiation and maintains the balance between T cells and Treg cells by acting as an inhibitor of RORγt.

We found that TDC could alleviate the pathology of EAE disease through reduced Th1 and Th17 in the CNS (Figure 3). Th17 cells not only exhibit a critical function in multiple sclerosis but also in IBD [29]. However, it is reported that some drugs for IBD have too many side effects to be used in the clinic, and there is a failure of anti-IL-17 strategies for the treatment of Crohn's disease [8,30–32]. Previous studies have shown that Foxp3$^+$ RORγt$^+$ Treg cells exist in the intestines of IBD patients and were enhanced by RORγt inhibition [33,34]. We thus chose a colitis animal model which was induced by DSS to assess the function of TDC. In our study, TDC improved DSS-induced colitis, decreased the production of pro-inflammatory cytokines, and maintained the balance of Th17/Treg cells in mice (Figure 4). At last, skin transplantation was used to further confirm the immunomodulatory function of TDC. Similarly, TDC inhibited skin graft rejection in allogeneic mice by maintaining the balance between Th17 cells and Treg cells (Figure 6).

Taking the previous reporters into account, together with our own scientific study, in this work, TDC targeting RORγt was identified through virtual screening and in vitro validation. Furthermore, three animal models of Th17-driven disorders were carried out to evaluate the immunomodulatory potential of TDC in vivo. In terms of mechanism, we found that TDC targeting RORγt can inhibit Th17 cell differentiation and its function. Meanwhile, it could stabilize Foxp3 expression and regulate Th17/Treg balance. The present study suggests that TDC was a prospective immunomodulatory agent for treating autoimmune diseases and transplant rejection which paving the way for a future clinical study.

4. Material and Methods

4.1. Virtual Screening and Molecular Docking

Structure-based virtual screening plays a critical role in drug exploration. Candidate inhibitors targeting RORγt (PDB: 5C4T) were screened out from the zinc natural products database (http://zinc.docking.org) containing 150,000 natural small molecule compounds using Autodock Vina and PyRx software, which acquired on 4 July 2017 [35]. Receptor models and small-molecule libraries were built, followed by scoring and structural docking of small-molecule compounds that fit the receptor-small-molecule structure. Generally speaking, we believe that the higher the score, the more likely the ligand will bind to the active center of the protein.

4.2. Luciferase Reporter Assays

We transfected HEK293T cells with a vector overexpressing of RORγt and expressing an IL-17 promoter-driven luciferase. After cells were treated with TDC (0–25 μM) for 16 h, ONE-Glo™ Luciferase Assay kit (Promega, Madison, WI, USA) was employed to monitor the luciferase activity, which was determined by GloMax [36].

4.3. EAE Induction and Treatment

Female C57BL/6 mice (aged 8 weeks) were purchased from Experimental Animal Center, Air Force Medical University (Xi'an, Shaanxi, China). All experimental protocols on mice were carried out following the standardized guidelines and specifications (No. ECES-2015-0247), which were approved and supported by the Institutional Animal Ethics Committee of Shaanxi Normal University. In order to construct the EAE mouse model, mice were immunized at the two points of spinal cord (SC) cervical expansion and lumbar expansion on the back with 200 μg of myelin oligodendrocyte glycoprotein peptide 35-55 (MOG_{35-55}) (GenScript, Nanjing, China) in 200 μL of hybrid emulsion containing incomplete Freund's adjuvant (Sigma-Aldrich, St. Louis, MO, USA) with 5 mg/mL heat-killed *Mycobacterium tuberculosis* H37Ra (BD, Franklin Lakes, NJ, USA) [37]. All animals were intraperitoneally (i.p.) injected with 200 ng pertussis toxin (Sigma-Aldrich) in PBS on days 0 and 2 post-immunization (p.i.). TDC (10 mg/kg/day), dissolved in a solvent consisting of dimethyl sulfoxide (DMSO, 3%), Kolliphor (10%), and 5% glucose solution (87%), was injected i.p. to EAE mice every day. The clinical scores were recorded daily in a double-blind manner, following a 0–5 scale described previously [36].

4.4. DSS-Induced Colitis

Male C57BL/6 mice (aged 8 weeks) were induced colitis by adding 3% dextran sulfate sodium (DSS) to drinking water for a week [38]. Gavage administered these animals with vehicle or TDC (100 mg/kg/day) during the DSS treatment. During DSS treatment, mice were observed and recorded daily for morbidity and body weight. At the same time, we scored the pathological characteristics of each mouse daily, involving stool consistency, presence of blood in the stool, and weight loss. Disease activity index (DAI) was evaluated by a clinical score of colitis mice in a double-blind manner according to the previous study [39].

4.5. Skin Grafting

BALB/c (aged 8 weeks old, male) and C57BL/6 mice (aged 8 weeks old, male) were used to construct the skin grafting model. Under sterile conditions, back skin of the BALB/c mouse (10 mm × 10 mm) was transplanted to the back of the C57BL/6 mouse. Firstly, we adjust the skin patch and the recipient skin. Next, we suture with 6-0 thread to make them combined tightly, promoting the growth of the skin. Finally, the recipient mice were covered with a sterile gauze and bandaged [40]. We randomly divided the mice into three groups with different treatment [Vehicle, TDC (10 mg/kg/day), or Cyclosporine A (CSA, 20 mg/kg/day)]. The treatment was performed for 7 days from the day of transplantation. The skin grafts on the back of recipient mice were observed daily for inflammation, edema, necrosis, scab, and shedding. We consider more than 80% of the skin necrosis to be complete rejection.

4.6. Histopathological Analysis

Mice in the experimental group were sacrificed at the corresponding time points and perfused with cold phosphate buffered saline (PBS) transcardially. Tissues [brain, spinal cord (SC), distal colon, and grafts] were fixed with 4% paraformaldehyde for 24 h and then sectioned into 5-micron slices. The distal colon and graft skin were stained with hematoxylin-eosin (H&E), and the brain and SC were stained with H&E and Luxol Fast Blue (LFB). Slides were assessed and recorded in a double-blinded fashion to assess inflammatory cell infiltration or demyelination accorded to the previous protocols [38].

4.7. Th17 Cell Polarization

Splenocytes were isolated and co-incubated with Con A (5 µg/mL) and TDC at different concentrations (1, 2.5, 5, 10, 25, and 50 µM) for 18 h. The cell viability was determined by Cell counting kit-8 (ZETA, Arcadia, CA, USA). An optimized dose with no cytotoxicity was used in the subsequent in vitro experiments. Isolation of $CD4^+$ T lymphocytes was carried out following the protocols of the Naïve $CD4^+$ T Cell Separation Kit (Miltenyi Biotec, Bergisch Gladbach, Germany), then incubated with 5 µg/mL of anti-CD3, 2 µg/mL of anti-CD28 (Bioxcell, Lebanon, NH, USA), 2 ng/mL of TGF-β, 20 ng/mL of IL-6, 10 ng/mL of IL-1β (Peprotech, Cranbury, NJ, USA), 10 µg/mL of anti-IL-4, and 10 µg/mL of anti-IFN -γ (Bioxcell, Lebanon, NH, USA) to induce Th17 cell differentiation. Three days later, cells were harvested in order to evaluate the percentage of Th17 cells by flow cytometry. Simultaneously, a cell medium was gathered to determine IL-17 production by ELISA.

4.8. Cytokine Measurement by Flow Cytometry and ELISA

Spleenocytes, mesenteric lymph nodes, intestinal intraepithelial lymphocytes (IELs), lamina propria mononuclear cells (LPMCs), and mononuclear cells (MNCs) were isolated, and the process of cell extraction are described previously [36]. These separated cells were seeded in vitro at different time, and stimulated by PMA (50 ng/mL, Sigma-Aldrich, Steinheim, Germany), ionomycin (500 ng/mL), and GolgiPlug (Thermo Fisher Scientific, Waltham, MA, USA) for 5 h. Subsequently, cells were stained on the surface, fixed, and permeated, and then internally stained with mouse Abs (Bioxcell, Lebanon, NH, USA). Flow cytometry analysis was carried out on the CytoFLEX S Flow Cytometer (Beckman coulter, Brea, CA, USA) and the results were evaluated with FlowJo (Treestar, Ashland, Wilmington, DE, USA). The cell supernatants were gathered and cytokine production (IFN-γ, IL-17, GM-CSF, and TNF-α) were determined by ELISA (R&D Systems, Minneapolis, MN, USA).

4.9. Real-Time Quantitative PCR

RNA Preparation Pure Tissue Kit (Tiangen, Beijing, China) was used to isolate total ribonucleic acid from the spinal cords of EAE experimental mice, the colon of colitis mice, and the skin graft of skin transplanted mice. cDNA was obtained through using Prime Script™ RT Master Mix Kit by using reverse transcription PCR, and then added to ChamQ™ SYBR®qPCR Master Mix (TaKaRa, Shiga, Japan) for real-time quantitative PCR (qRT-PCR). Data were quantitatively analyzed on the LightCycler® 96 system (Roche, Shanghai, China). Mouse glyceraldehyde 3-phosphate dehydrogenase (*GAPDH*) gene, as a housekeeping gene, was used as a standardization control.

4.10. Statistical Analysis

All data are presented as the mean ± SD, and statistical analyses were performed using GraphPad Prism 6 software (GraphPad, La Jolla, CA, USA). When comparing two groups, data were assessed by unpaired Student's *t* test. When comparing multiple groups, experimental results were evaluated by one-way ANOVA with Tukey's multiple comparisons test or two-way ANOVA with multiple comparisons test.

Supplementary Materials: The following supporting information can be downloaded at: https://www.mdpi.com/article/10.3390/ijms232314547/s1.

Author Contributions: Data curation, Y.Y., W.Q. and Y.Z. (Yanyan Zhang); formal analysis, Y.Y., W.Q. and Y.Z. (Yanyan Zhang); methodology, M.T., M.B. and R.W.; resources, Y.Z. (Yuan Zhang); writing—original draft, Y.Y.; writing—review and editing, Y.Z. (Yuan Zhang) and X.L. All authors have read and agreed to the published version of the manuscript.

Funding: This study was supported by the Chinese National Natural Science Foundation (Grant Nos. 82271199, 31970771, 82071396), the Shaanxi Provincial Key R&D Foundation (Grant No. 2021ZDLSF03-09), the Fundamental Research Funds for the Central Universities (Grant Nos. GK202201013, GK202202006, GK202105002).

Institutional Review Board Statement: The study was conducted following the standardized guidelines and specifications (No. ECES-2015-0247), which were approved and supported by the Institutional Animal Ethics Committee of Shaanxi Normal University.

Data Availability Statement: The data presented in this study are available upon request to corresponding author.

Conflicts of Interest: The authors declare no conflict of interest.

Ethics Approval: All experimental procedures on mice were carried out in accordance with the standardized guidelines and specifications (No. ECES-2015-0247), which were approved and supported by the Institutional Animal Ethics Committee of Shaanxi Normal University.

Abbreviations

APCs: Antigen-presenting cells; CSA, Cyclosporine A; CNS, Central nervous system; DCs, Dendritic cells; DAI, Disease activity index; DSS, Dextran sulfate sodium; EAE, Experimental autoimmune encephalomyelitis; H&E, Hematoxylin and eosin; IL-17, Interleukin-17; IBD, Inflammatory bowel disease; IELs, Intraepithelial lymphocytes; i.p., Intraperitoneally; KD, Equilibrium dissociation constant; LFB, Luxol fast blue; LPMCs, Lamina propria mononuclear cells; MST, Microscale thermophoresis; MNCs, Mononuclear cells; MLNs, Mesenteric lymph nodes; MS, Multiple sclerosis; qRT-PCR, Real-time quantitative PCR; RORγt, Retinoic acid receptor-related orphan gamma t; TDC, 2,2′,4′-trihydroxychalcone; Th17, T-helper 17; Th1, T-helper 1; Tregs, Regulatory T cells.

References

1. Park, H.; Li, Z.; Yang, X.O.; Chang, S.H.; Nurieva, R.; Wang, Y.-H.; Wang, Y.; Hood, L.; Zhu, Z.; Tian, Q.; et al. A distinct lineage of CD4 T cells regulates tissue inflammation by producing interleukin 17. *Nat. Immunol.* **2005**, *6*, 1133–1141. [CrossRef] [PubMed]
2. Xiao, S.; Yosef, N.; Yang, J.; Wang, Y.; Zhou, L.; Zhu, C.; Wu, C.; Baloglu, E.; Schmidt, D.; Ramesh, R.; et al. Small-molecule RORγt antagonists inhibit T helper 17 cell transcriptional network by divergent mechanisms. *Immunity* **2014**, *40*, 477–489. [CrossRef] [PubMed]
3. Noack, M.; Miossec, P. Th17 and regulatory T cell balance in autoimmune and inflammatory diseases. *Autoimmun. Rev.* **2014**, *13*, 668–677. [CrossRef] [PubMed]
4. Banerjee, D.; Zhao, L.; Wu, L.; Palanichamy, A.; Ergun, A.; Peng, L.; Quigley, C.; Hamann, S.; Dunstan, R.; Cullen, P.; et al. Small molecule mediated inhibition of RORγ-dependent gene expression and autoimmune disease pathology in vivo. *Immunology* **2016**, *147*, 399–413. [CrossRef] [PubMed]
5. Rostami, A.; Ciric, B. Role of Th17 cells in the pathogenesis of CNS inflammatory demyelination. *J. Neurol. Sci.* **2013**, *333*, 76–87. [CrossRef]
6. Ding, Q.; Zhao, M.; Bai, C.; Yu, B.; Huang, Z. Inhibition of RORγt activity and Th17 differentiation by a set of novel compounds. *BMC Immunol.* **2015**, *16*, 32. [CrossRef]
7. Huang, M.; Bolin, S.; Miller, H.; Ng, H.L. RORγ Structural Plasticity and Druggability. *Int. J. Mol. Sci.* **2020**, *21*, 5329. [CrossRef]
8. Zapadka, T.E.; Lindstrom, S.I.; Taylor, B.E.; Lee, C.A.; Tang, J.; Taylor, Z.R.R.; Howell, S.J.; Taylor, P.R. RORγt Inhibitor-SR1001 Halts Retinal Inflammation, Capillary Degeneration, and the Progression of Diabetic Retinopathy. *Int. J. Mol. Sci.* **2020**, *21*, 3547. [CrossRef]
9. Huh, J.R.; Leung, M.W.L.; Huang, P.; Ryan, D.A.; Krout, M.R.; Malapaka, R.R.V.; Chow, J.; Manel, N.; Ciofani, M.; Kim, S.V.; et al. Digoxin and its derivatives suppress TH17 cell differentiation by antagonizing RORγt activity. *Nature* **2011**, *472*, 486–490. [CrossRef]

10. Xu, T.; Wang, X.; Zhong, B.; Nurieva, R.I.; Ding, S.; Dong, C. Ursolic acid suppresses interleukin-17 (IL-17) production by selectively antagonizing the function of RORgamma t protein. *J. Biol. Chem.* **2011**, *286*, 22707–22710. [CrossRef]
11. Ghoshal, S.; Stevens, J.R.; Billon, C.; Girardet, C.; Sitaula, S.; Leon, A.S.; Rao, D.C.; Skinner, J.S.; Rankinen, T.; Bouchard, C.; et al. Adropin: An endocrine link between the biological clock and cholesterol homeostasis. *Mol. Metab.* **2018**, *8*, 51–64. [CrossRef]
12. Silvestrini, A.; Meucci, E.; Vitali, A.; Giardina, B.; Mordente, A. Chalcone inhibition of anthracycline secondary alcohol metabolite formation in rabbit and human heart cytosol. *Chem. Res. Toxicol.* **2006**, *19*, 1518–1524. [CrossRef] [PubMed]
13. Le Bail, J.C.; Pouget, C.; Fagnere, C.; Basly, J.P.; Chulia, A.J.; Habrioux, G. Chalcones are potent inhibitors of aromatase and 17beta-hydroxysteroid dehydrogenase activities. *Life Sci.* **2001**, *68*, 751–761. [CrossRef]
14. Salehi, B.; Quispe, C.; Chamkhi, I.; El Omari, N.; Balahbib, A.; Sharifi-Rad, J.; Bouyahya, A.; Akram, M.; Iqbal, M.; Docea, A.O.; et al. Pharmacological Properties of Chalcones: A Review of Preclinical Including Molecular Mechanisms and Clinical Evidence. *Front. Pharmacol.* **2020**, *11*, 592654. [CrossRef] [PubMed]
15. Zhu, Z.; Li, C.; Wang, X.; Yang, Z.; Chen, J.; Hu, L.; Jiang, H.; Shen, X. 2,2′,4′-trihydroxychalcone from Glycyrrhiza glabra as a new specific BACE1 inhibitor efficiently ameliorates memory impairment in mice. *J. Neurochem.* **2010**, *114*, 374–385. [CrossRef] [PubMed]
16. Qi, W.-H.; Zhang, Y.-Y.; Xing, K.; Hao, D.-X.; Zhang, F.; Wang, R.-N.; Bao, M.-Y.; Tian, M.-Y.; Yang, Y.-N.; Li, X.; et al. 2′,4′-Dihydroxy-2,3-dimethoxychalcone: A pharmacological inverse agonist of RORγt ameliorating Th17-driven inflammatory diseases by regulating Th17/Treg. *Int. Immunopharmacol.* **2022**, *108*, 108769. [CrossRef]
17. Carson, M.J.; Doose, J.M.; Melchior, B.; Schmid, C.D.; Ploix, C.C. CNS immune privilege: Hiding in plain sight. *Immunol. Rev.* **2006**, *213*, 48–65. [CrossRef]
18. Lee, E.; Eo, J.-C.; Lee, C.; Yu, J.-W. Distinct Features of Brain-Resident Macrophages: Microglia and Non-Parenchymal Brain Macrophages. *Mol. Cells* **2021**, *44*, 281–291. [CrossRef]
19. Nam, J.-H.; Lee, J.-H.; Choi, S.-Y.; Jung, N.-C.; Song, J.-Y.; Seo, H.-G.; Lim, D.-S. Functional Ambivalence of Dendritic Cells: Tolerogenicity and Immunogenicity. *Int. J. Mol. Sci.* **2021**, *22*, 4430. [CrossRef] [PubMed]
20. Wu, J.; Zhou, C.; Chen, W.; Xie, A.; Li, J.; Wang, S.; Ye, P.; Wang, W.; Xia, J. Digoxin attenuates acute cardiac allograft rejection by antagonizing RORγt activity. *Transplantation* **2013**, *95*, 434–441. [CrossRef]
21. Tian, Y.; Han, C.; Wei, Z.; Dong, H.; Shen, X.; Cui, Y.; Fu, X.; Tian, Z.; Wang, S.; Zhou, J.; et al. SOX-5 activates a novel RORγt enhancer to facilitate experimental autoimmune encephalomyelitis by promoting Th17 cell differentiation. *Nat. Commun.* **2021**, *12*, 481. [CrossRef]
22. Cha, H.J.; Park, M.T.; Chung, H.Y.; Kim, N.D.; Sato, H.; Seiki, M.; Kim, K.W. Ursolic acid-induced down-regulation of MMP-9 gene is mediated through the nuclear translocation of glucocorticoid receptor in HT1080 human fibrosarcoma cells. *Oncogene* **1998**, *16*, 771–778. [CrossRef] [PubMed]
23. Manel, N.; Unutmaz, D.; Littman, D.R. The differentiation of human T(H)-17 cells requires transforming growth factor-beta and induction of the nuclear receptor RORgammat. *Nat. Immunol.* **2008**, *9*, 641–649. [CrossRef]
24. Korn, T.; Bettelli, E.; Oukka, M.; Kuchroo, V.K. IL-17 and Th17 Cells. *Annu. Rev. Immunol.* **2009**, *27*, 485–517. [CrossRef] [PubMed]
25. Elson, C.O.; Cong, Y.; Weaver, C.T.; Schoeb, T.R.; McClanahan, T.K.; Fick, R.B.; Kastelein, R.A. Monoclonal anti-interleukin 23 reverses active colitis in a T cell-mediated model in mice. *Gastroenterology* **2007**, *132*, 2359–2370. [CrossRef] [PubMed]
26. Becher, B.; Durell, B.G.; Noelle, R.J. Experimental autoimmune encephalitis and inflammation in the absence of interleukin-12. *J. Clin. Investig.* **2002**, *110*, 493–497. [CrossRef] [PubMed]
27. Cua, D.J.; Sherlock, J.; Chen, Y.; Murphy, C.A.; Joyce, B.; Seymour, B.; Lucian, L.; To, W.; Kwan, S.; Churakova, T.; et al. Interleukin-23 rather than interleukin-12 is the critical cytokine for autoimmune inflammation of the brain. *Nature* **2003**, *421*, 744–748. [CrossRef]
28. Kleinewietfeld, M.; Hafler, D.A. The plasticity of human Treg and Th17 cells and its role in autoimmunity. *Semin. Immunol.* **2013**, *25*, 305–312. [CrossRef]
29. Tan, J.; Liu, H.; Huang, M.; Li, N.; Tang, S.; Meng, J.; Tang, S.; Zhou, H.; Kijlstra, A.; Yang, P.; et al. Small molecules targeting RORγt inhibit autoimmune disease by suppressing Th17 cell differentiation. *Cell Death Dis.* **2020**, *11*, 697. [CrossRef]
30. Moschen, A.R.; Tilg, H.; Raine, T. IL-12, IL-23 and IL-17 in IBD: Immunobiology and therapeutic targeting. *Nat. Rev. Gastroenterol. Hepatol.* **2019**, *16*, 185–196. [CrossRef]
31. Hohenberger, M.; Cardwell, L.A.; Oussedik, E.; Feldman, S.R. Interleukin-17 inhibition: Role in psoriasis and inflammatory bowel disease. *J. Dermatol. Treat.* **2018**, *29*, 13–18. [CrossRef] [PubMed]
32. Lee, J.-Y.; Hall, J.A.; Kroehling, L.; Wu, L.; Najar, T.; Nguyen, H.H.; Lin, W.-Y.; Yeung, S.T.; Silva, H.M.; Li, D.; et al. Serum Amyloid A Proteins Induce Pathogenic Th17 Cells and Promote Inflammatory Disease. *Cell* **2020**, *180*, 79–91. [CrossRef] [PubMed]
33. Mickael, M.E.; Bhaumik, S.; Basu, R. Retinoid-Related Orphan Receptor RORγt in CD4 T-Cell-Mediated Intestinal Homeostasis and Inflammation. *Am. J. Pathol.* **2020**, *190*, 1984–1999. [CrossRef] [PubMed]
34. Martínez-Blanco, M.; Lozano-Ojalvo, D.; Pérez-Rodríguez, L.; Benedé, S.; Molina, E.; López-Fandiño, R. Retinoic Acid Induces Functionally Suppressive Foxp3RORγt T Cells. *Front. Immunol.* **2021**, *12*, 675733. [CrossRef] [PubMed]
35. Wu, X.; Shen, H.; Zhang, Y.; Wang, C.; Li, Q.; Zhang, C.; Zhuang, X.; Li, C.; Shi, Y.; Xing, Y.; et al. Discovery and Characterization of Benzimidazole Derivative XY123 as a Potent, Selective, and Orally Available RORγ Inverse Agonist. *J. Med. Chem.* **2021**, *64*, 8775–8797. [CrossRef] [PubMed]

36. Yang, T.; Li, X.; Yu, J.; Deng, X.; Shen, P.-X.; Jiang, Y.-B.; Zhu, L.; Wang, Z.-Z.; Zhang, Y. Eriodictyol suppresses Th17 differentiation and the pathogenesis of experimental autoimmune encephalomyelitis. *Food Funct.* **2020**, *11*, 6875–6888. [CrossRef]
37. Zhang, Y.; Li, X.; Ciric, B.; Ma, C.-G.; Gran, B.; Rostami, A.; Zhang, G.-X. Therapeutic effect of baicalin on experimental autoimmune encephalomyelitis is mediated by SOCS3 regulatory pathway. *Sci. Rep.* **2015**, *5*, 17407. [CrossRef]
38. Tanaka, K.-I.; Namba, T.; Arai, Y.; Fujimoto, M.; Adachi, H.; Sobue, G.; Takeuchi, K.; Nakai, A.; Mizushima, T. Genetic evidence for a protective role for heat shock factor 1 and heat shock protein 70 against colitis. *J. Biol. Chem.* **2007**, *282*, 23240–23252. [CrossRef]
39. Murano, M.; Maemura, K.; Hirata, I.; Toshina, K.; Nishikawa, T.; Hamamoto, N.; Sasaki, S.; Saitoh, O.; Katsu, K. Therapeutic effect of intracolonically administered nuclear factor kappa B (p65) antisense oligonucleotide on mouse dextran sulphate sodium (DSS)-induced colitis. *Clin. Exp. Immunol.* **2000**, *120*, 51–58. [CrossRef]
40. Qiu, R.; Wang, Y. Retinoic Acid Receptor-Related Orphan Receptor γt (RORγt) Agonists as Potential Small Molecule Therapeutics for Cancer Immunotherapy. *J. Med. Chem.* **2018**, *61*, 5794–5804. [CrossRef]

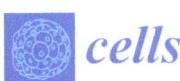

Article

Sanguinarine Enhances the Integrity of the Blood–Milk Barrier and Inhibits Oxidative Stress in Lipopolysaccharide-Stimulated Mastitis

Zhijie Zheng [1], Yonghui Zheng [1], Xiaoben Liang [1], Guanhong Xue [1] and Haichong Wu [1,2,*]

[1] Department of Veterinary Medicine, College of Animal Sciences, Zhejiang University, Hangzhou 310058, China
[2] Key Laboratory of Fujian Universities Preventive Veterinary Medicine and Biotechnology, Longyan University, Longyan 364012, China
* Correspondence: haichongwu@zju.edu.cn

Abstract: Mastitis is a common clinical disease which threatens the welfare and health of dairy cows and causes huge economic losses. Sanguinarine (SG) is a plant-derived alkaloid which has many biological functions, including antibacterial and antioxidant properties. The present study attempted to evaluate the effect of SG on lipopolysaccharide (LPS)-induced oxidative stress reactions and explore its potential mechanisms. The expression profile of SG was analyzed by network pharmacology, and it was found that differentially expressed genes were mainly involved in the Wnt signaling pathway and oxidative stress through GO and KEGG enrichment. In in vitro experiments, the dosage of SG was non-toxic to mouse mammary epithelial cells (mMECs) ($p > 0.05$). SG not only inhibited the increase in ROS induced by LPS, but also enhanced the activity of antioxidant enzymes ($p < 0.05$). Moreover, the results of the in vivo experiments showed that SG alleviated LPS-induced inflammatory damage of mouse mammary glands and enhanced the integrity of the blood–milk barrier ($p < 0.05$). Further studies suggested that SG promoted Nrf2 expression and suppressed the activation of the Wnt signaling pathway ($p < 0.05$). Conclusively, this study clarified the protective effect of SG on mastitis and provided evidence for new potential mechanisms. SG exerted its antioxidant function through activating Nrf2 and inhibiting the Wnt/β-catenin pathway, repairing the blood–milk barrier.

Keywords: sanguinarine; mastitis; blood–milk barrier; oxidative stress; Nrf2; Wnt/β-catenin

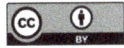

1. Introduction

Mastitis is an epidemic in the global dairy industry, mainly caused by pathogenic microorganism infection, which can lead to the decline of milk production and quality [1,2]. In addition, mastitis can also lead to prolonged estrus and even the death of cows postpartum, which seriously threatens the welfare and health of cows and causes huge economic losses to humans [3,4]. Mammals during the peripartum period, which lasts from 3 weeks before to 3 weeks after parturition, are physiologically unstable and susceptible to a number of metabolic diseases compromising productivity [5,6].

It has been proved that many microorganisms can cause cow mastitis, among which *Escherichia coli* is one of the significant pathogenic microorganisms causing clinical mastitis [7]. Lipopolysaccharides (LSPs) in the cell wall of *E. coli* can cause inflammation and trigger innate immune responses, leading to a series of inflammatory reactions [8]. More and more evidence has shown that the Wnt/β-catenin signaling pathway is related to LPS-induced diseases, which cause the upregulation of inflammatory factors and lead to breast injury [9,10]. In addition, some studies have shown that LPS can also increase the production of reactive oxygen species (ROS) and change mitochondrial membrane potentials [11]. The blood–milk barrier, composed of mammary epithelial cells, is the most important line of defense in the protection of mammary glands [12]. The main structure of the blood–milk barrier is the tight junction (TJ), which forms a tight barrier that only allows the passage of small molecules and prevents the penetration of adjacent cell membranes [13,14]. LPS can destroy tight junction proteins after causing mastitis, leading to the degradation of the barrier, invasion of harmful substances and microorganisms, and aggravation of oxidative stress [15]. Oxidative stress in early-lactation cows exerts an important role in dysfunctional inflammatory response [16]. Therefore, it is particularly important to protect the integrity of the blood–milk barrier and suppress the pathogenic bacteria leading to excessive inflammatory response.

For many years, most dairy farms have mainly used antibiotics to treat mastitis, but over time the pathogens have developed drug resistance, and antibiotic residues in dairy products have become more and more serious, endangering human health [17]. In addition, vaccines for the treatment of bovine mastitis have not produced good results [18]. Therefore, there is an urgent need to find and develop new therapies for bovine mastitis.

Sanguinarine (SG), a plant-derived alkaloid, has many pharmacological functions, such as anti-oxidation, anti-inflammatory, and anti-tumor properties [19,20]. The results of animal experiments have suggested that SG relieved the symptoms of Dextran Sulfate Sodium (DSS)-induced colitis in rats [21]. However, it is not clear whether SG has a protective effect on LPS-induced mastitis. Therefore, we explored the role of SG in an LPS-stimulated mouse mastitis model and explored the possible mechanisms.

2. Materials and Methods

2.1. Reagents

LPS was purchased from Sigma-Aldrich (055:B5, San Diego, CA, USA). The antibodies used in the experiments were purchased from Cell Signaling Technology (CST, Danvers, MA, USA). Sangui-narine (SG, purity ≥98%; Figure 1A) was obtained from Yuanye Biotech Co., Ltd. (Shanghai, China). The purity of the SG was detected by high-performance liquid chromatography (HPLC). The experiment was conducted on the EChrom2000 DAD Data System. Chromatography was performed with a SinoChrom 0DS-BP column (4.6 × 250 mm, 5 μm). An elute with 0.1% phosphoric acid water/acetonitrile at a flow rate of 1.0 mL/min was used, and detection with DAD at 325 nm was performed (Figure 1B). The ELISA kits used (for TNF-α and IL-1β) were purchased from Wuhan Boster Biological Technology, Ltd. (Wuhan, China).

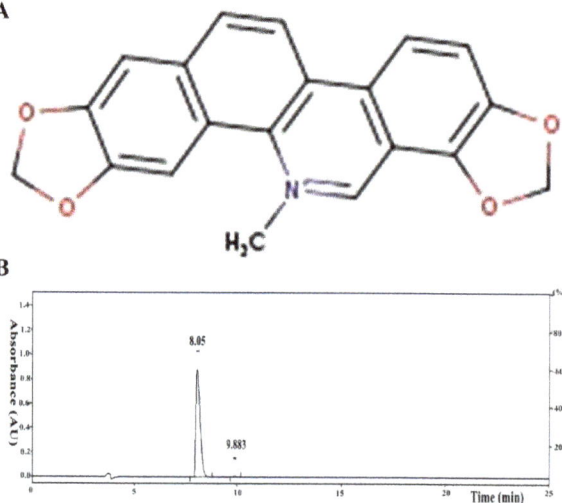

Figure 1. (**A**) The chemical structure of SG. (**B**) HPLC chromatogram of SG.

2.2. Animal Treatment and Experimental Design

Sixty female BALB/c mice (8 weeks old, weighing 20–25 g) were purchased from the Animal Center of Zhejiang University. Before the experiment, all mice were given sufficient water and feed and stored in a 12/12 h dark/light-cycle environment. The whole feeding process was maintained at room temperature and 65% humidity. The animals were cared for humanely; all experiments involving the mice were conducted according to the Guide for the Care and Use of Laboratory Animals of the National Research Council, and all experimental protocols were followed by the Institutional Animal Care and Use Committee of Zhejiang University (approval number: GBT 35892-2018).

The mice were randomly divided into the following six groups: a control group, an LPS group, sanguinarine groups (SG groups: 5, 25, and 50 μM), and a dexamethasone group (5 mg/kg, DEX group). SG was dissolved and diluted in CMC Na (Sigma, San Diego, CA, USA) to give final concentrations of 5, 25, and 50 μM. The mouse mastitis model was prepared as described previously [22]. Briefly, one hour before the onset of LPS-induced mastitis, SG (5, 25, and 50 μM) or dexamethasone (5 mg/kg) was injected intraperitoneally twice every six hours. After pentobarbital anesthesia, LPS was injected into the two abdominal mammary glands for 24 h (the fourth pair of mammary glands, R4 and L4). Finally, the mice were sacrificed by CO_2 inhalation, and the mammary tissues were collected for further study.

2.3. Histopathological Examination

The samples of mammary glands were fixed in 10% formalin. Paraffin sections were prepared by dehydration with graded alcohol. Next, the tissues were sectioned and stained with hematoxylin. Finally, the H&E-stained sections were observed under a light microscope, and images were collected to evaluate pathological changes.

2.4. Myeloperoxidase (MPO) Analysis

The mouse mammary gland tissue samples, weighing 100 mg, were ground in 2 mL PBS solution and centrifuged at 12,000 rpm for 15 min at 4 °C. Then, the supernatants were collected and analyzed using the MPO kit (Nanjing Jiancheng Biotechnology Co., Ltd., Nanjing, China). Finally, according to the calculation formula, the MPO enzyme activity of each sample was calculated.

2.5. Cell Culture and Treatment

As previously described, after collecting mammary gland tissues from the lactating mice, the digested tissues were suspended and passed through a cell filter to remove larger tissue debris. Epithelial cells were obtained by removing fibroblasts, endothelial cells, and other single cells. The isolated mMECs were cultured at 37 °C in a 5% CO_2 humidified incubator containing 10% fetal bovine serum (FBS, Gibco, New York, NY, USA) supplemented with 100 U/mL penicillin and streptomycin and 10 μg/mL insulin. The mMECs were pretreated with different concentrations of SG (5, 25, and 50 μM) for 1 h and then stimulated with LPS (1 μg/mL) for 6 h.

2.6. Cell Biological Detection and Viability Assay

Cells were fixed with paraformaldehyde for 15 min at room temperature and washed three times with PBS. Cells were then blocked with 10% normal goat serum for half an hour at room temperature and incubated with primary antibody overnight at 4 °C. After the completion of primary antibody adsorption, the cells were incubated with fluorescent-labeled secondary antibodies (Bios, Beijing, China) for one hour at room temperature and washed three times in PBS. Nuclei were stained with Hoechst dye and then visualized with a laser scanning confocal microscope (Leica, Wetzlar, Germany).

Cell viability was determined using an MTT kit. Briefly, mMECs (1×10^5 cells/mL) were passed in 96-well plates for 6 h and then treated with different concentrations of SG for 24 h. Finally, MTT (20 μL, 5 mg/mL) was added for 4 h, the supernatant was removed, and 100 µL DMSO was added to each well. The optical density (OD) values were obtained at 570 nm.

2.7. Cytokine and Enzyme Activity Analyses

The cytokine expression levels and enzyme activities (GSH-Px, SOD) were determined using the respective kits, according to the commercial instructions. The samples were handled according to the introductions for each kit, and the OD values were calculated using a full-wavelength microplate reader.

2.8. Western Blot Analysis

Protein lysates were added to tissue homogenates and total protein for each sample was extracted by centrifugation. Total protein concentrations were tested using a Bicinchoninic Acid (BCA) kit, then denatured protein samples were used for subsequent studies. Protein samples were separated on 10% SDS-PAGE, transferred to PVDF membranes (Millipore, Burlington, MA, USA), and blocked with 5% skim milk at room temperature for 2 h. The membranes were then incubated with specific primary antibodies (1:1000 dilution) overnight. Finally, the membranes were incubated with secondary antibodies (1:3000 dilution) and determined using ECL chemiluminescence reagent.

2.9. qRT-PCR Assay

Total RNA in mMECs was extracted using Trizol reagent (Invitrogen, Carlsbad, CA, USA) and then converted into cDNA using a reverse transcription kit (Takara, Otsu, Japan). The primers (Nrf2 and GAPDH) were designed using primer 5.0 software (Premier company, Canada) and are shown in Table 1. GAPDH was used as an internal standard. Relative fold changes in gene expression levels were calculated using the $2^{-\Delta\Delta Ct}$ comparative method.

Table 1. Primers used for qPCR.

Name	Sequence (5′→3′): Forward and Reverse	GenBank Accession No.	Product Size (bp)
Nrf2	GACCTAAAGCACAGCCAACACAT CTTCAATCGGCTTGAATGTTTGTC	NM_010902.5	182
GAPDH	CAATGTGTCCGTCGTGGATCT GTCCTCAGTGTAGCCCAAGATG	NM_001289726.1	124

2.10. Network Pharmacological Analysis

The pharmaceutical property of SG was estimated using network pharmacology technology. The Swisstarget website was used to predict the potential of SG, and metascape software (https://metascape.org/gp/index.html#/main/step1, accessed on 9 September 2022) was used to analyze the target genes via GO and KEGG. Finally, Cytoscape software provided a visual of the SG targeting pathway network.

2.11. Immunofluorescence Analysis

Paraffin slices were immersed in xylene for dewaxing and were dehydrated with ethanol at different concentrations along a gradient. The tissue slices were permeated with PBS appending Triton X-100 (Sigma, San Diego, CA, USA) and 10% BSA, then incubated overnight with special primary antibodies and corresponding secondary antibodies. Nuclei were stained with DAPI reagent. Finally, all sections were observed under a fluorescence microscope.

2.12. ROS Analysis

The production of ROS in mMECs was determined using an ROS Assay Kit (Beyotime, Hangzhou, China). Cells (1×10^5 cells/mL) were passed into 6-well plates and then incubated with control media or LPS in the presence or absence of SG (5, 25, and 50 µM). The cells were incubated with DCFH-DA for 1 h in the dark, and extracellular DCFH-DA solution was removed. Finally, relative levels of fluorescence were quantified using a fluorescence plate reader MTP902 (Olympus, Tokyo, Japan).

2.13. Data Analysis

Statistical analysis was conducted with SPSS software. The results are presented as means ± SDs. All data in the present study were analyzed by one-way ANOVA followed by Dunnett's test, and significant differences were determined at $p < 0.05$.

3. Results

3.1. Network Pharmacological Analysis of SG

The development of bioinformatics technology, especially network pharmacological analysis, allowed for more accurate predictions in this experiment. The results showed 197 common genes in "SG", "inflammation", and "oxidation". GO annotation and KEGG analysis showed that these target genes were related to oxidative stress and inflammatory response (Figure 2).

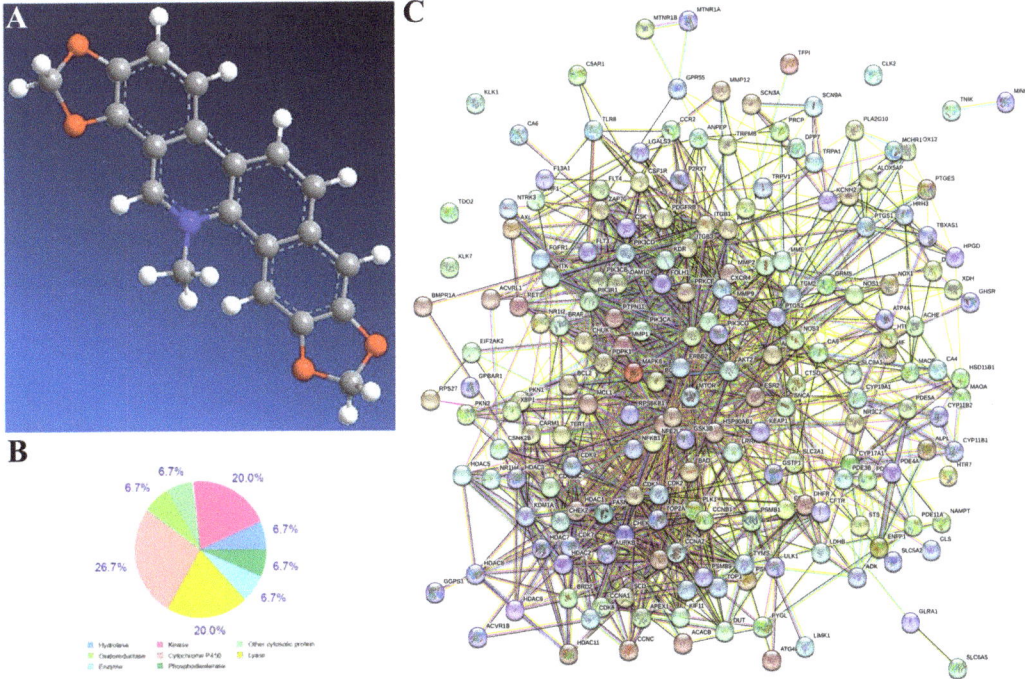

Figure 2. *Cont.*

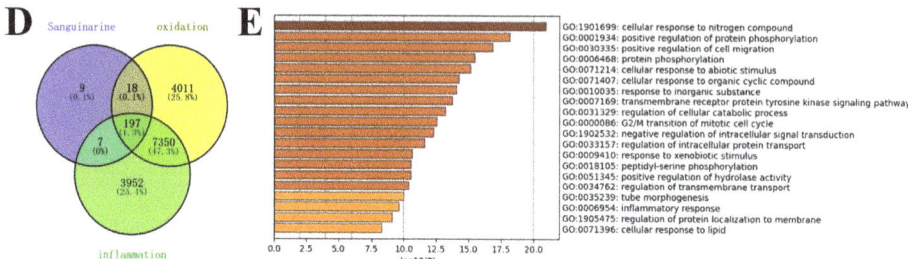

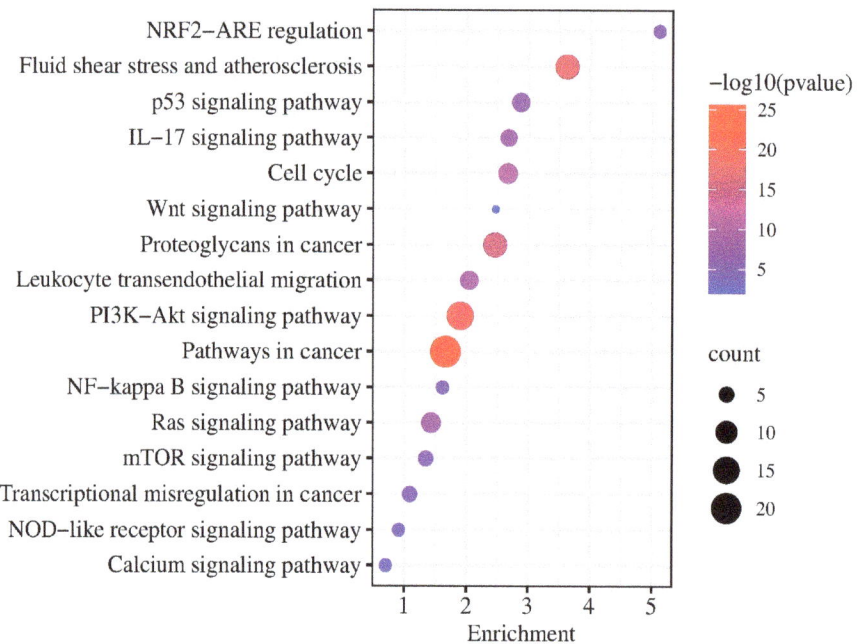

Figure 2. Network pharmacological analysis of SG. (**A**) Three-dimensional structure formula of SG. (**B**) The target classes of SG. (**C**) The potential targets of SG were predicted using the SwissTarget website. (**D**) The common target genes in "SG", "inflammation", and "oxidation". (**E,F**) GO annotation and KEGG were used to analyze these target genes.

3.2. Cell Viability and Biological Assay

Cytokeratin-18 was used to identify the integrity of mMECs (Figure 3A). The cell viability of mMECs was assessed by MTT assay. As shown in Figure 3B, the cell viability of mMECs was not affected by the SG treatment.

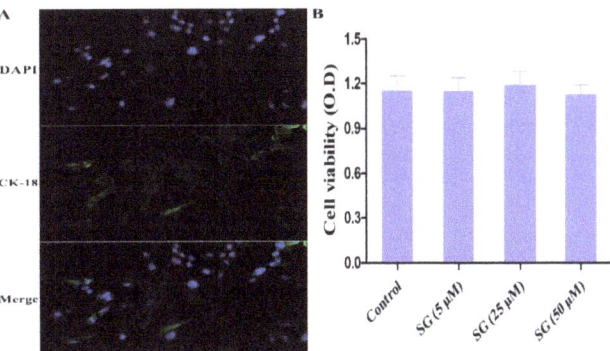

Figure 3. Cell viability and biological detection. (**A**) Cytokeratin-18 was used to identify the integrity of mMECs (scale bar: 20 μm). (**B**) The effect of SG on cell viability was detected by MTT assay. Data are presented as the means ± SEMs of three independent experiments.

3.3. Effect of SG on LPS-Induced Oxidative Stress

The increase in ROS yield caused by LPS was significantly alleviated under SG treatment (Figure 4A). In addition, the enzyme activities of superoxide dismutase (SOD) and glutathione peroxidase (GSH-Px) were also determined using commercial kits (Jiancheng Bioengineering institute, Nanjing, China) in LPS-stimulated mMECs. The results showed that the enzyme activities of SOD and GSH-Px in the LPS challenge group were lower than those in the control group, but SG significantly increased the activities of SOD and GSH-Px (Figure 4B).

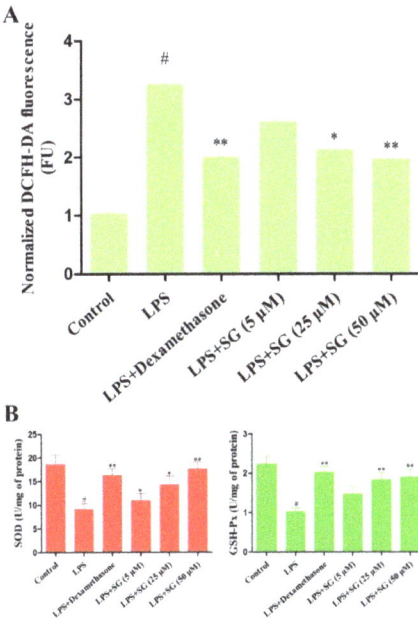

Figure 4. Effect of SG on LPS-stimulated oxidative stress. (**A**) Effect of SG on LPS-triggered ROS production in mMECs. (**B**) The activities of anti-oxidative enzymes were determined using commercial kits. Data are presented as the means ± SEMs of three independent experiments. The symbol # indicates $p < 0.05$ vs. the control group. The symbols * and ** represent significant differences at $p < 0.05$ and $p < 0.01$, respectively.

3.4. SG Alleviated LPS-Induced Mammary Gland Injury in Mice

Histological changes in mouse mastitis stimulated by LPS were evaluated by H&E staining. Morphological changes in mammary glands were observed after the LPS and SG treatments (Figure 5). The results of the histopathological analysis suggested that, compared with the control group, LPS caused obvious pathological changes, including breast tissue congestion, extensive inflammatory cell infiltration, and destruction of acinar structures (Figure 5A,B). However, severe histopathological changes induced by LPS were greatly attenuated by dexamethasone or SG treatment, especially at high concentrations of SG (Figure 5C–F).

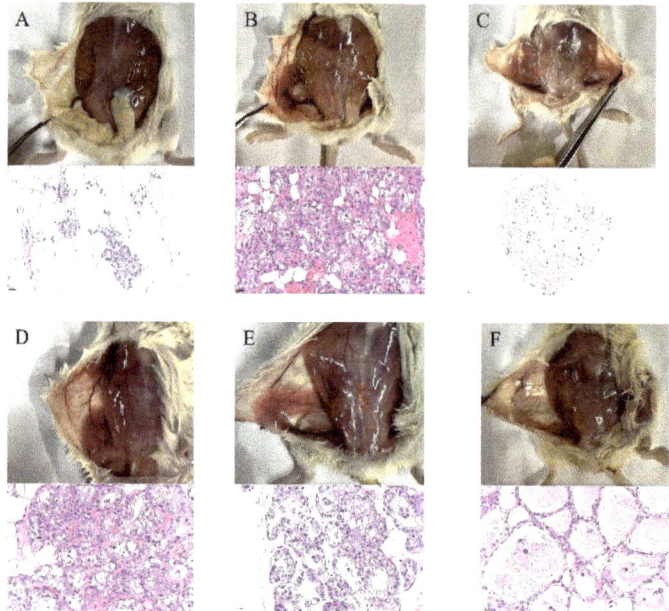

Figure 5. SG alleviated LPS-induced mammary gland injury in mice (HE; scale bar: 50 μm). (**A**) Control group. (**B**) LPS group. (**C**) LPS + dexamethasone group. (**D–F**) LPS + SG groups (5, 25, and 50 μM).

3.5. SG Reduced LPS-Induced Inflammatory Response and Improved the Integrity of the Blood–Milk Marrier

It is well known that TNF-α and IL-1β play vital roles in inflammatory response. In order to analyze the effect of SG on LPS-induced inflammation, the expression levels of TNF-α and IL-1β in tissues were detected by ELISA assays. LPS stimulation could markedly increase the expression of TNF-α and IL-1β. Compared with the LPS group, SG treatment greatly decreased the levels of these pro-inflammatory cytokines (Figure 6A). Moreover, myeloperoxidase (MPO) is a heme protein rich in neutrophils and serves as a marker of neutrophil function and activation [21]. The results showed that SG treatment significantly reduced LPS-induced MPO activity (Figure 6B). The tight junction proteins, such as Claudin-3, play vital roles in the blood–milk barrier [23]. An immunofluorescence technique was used to evaluate the integrity of the blood–milk barrier. The results showed that SG significantly reduced the inhibition by LPS of the expression of the tight junction protein claudin-3 (Figure 6C).

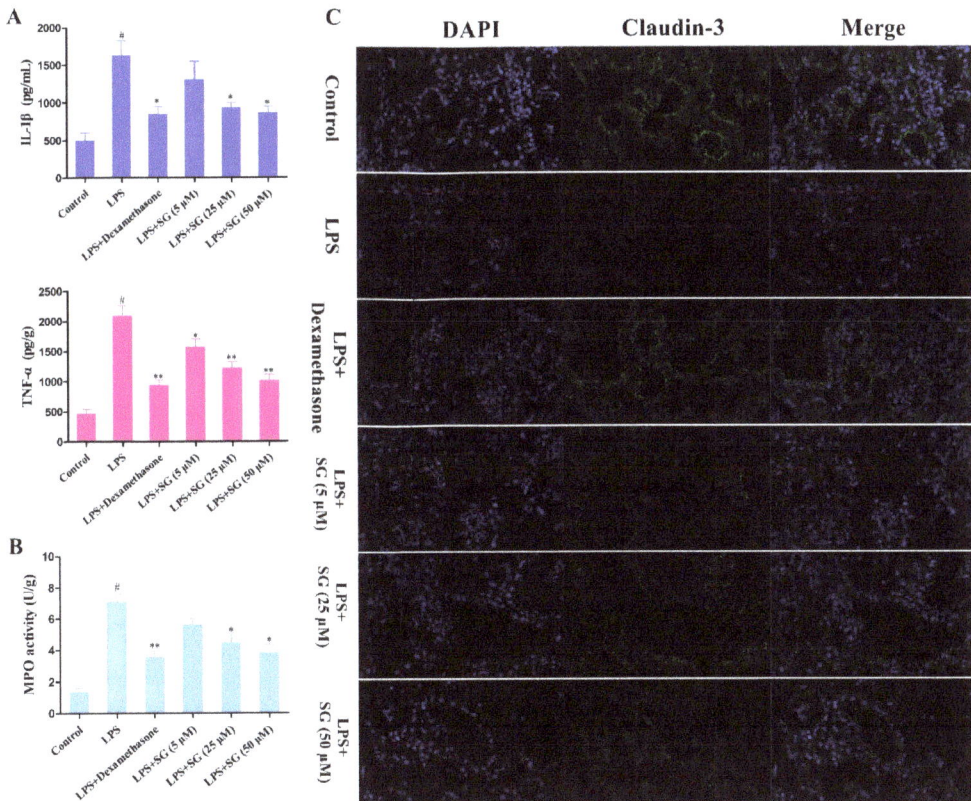

Figure 6. SG reduced LPS-induced inflammatory response and improved the integrity of the blood–milk barrier. (**A**) The expression levels of TNF-α and IL-1β in tissues were detected by ELISA assays. (**B**) MPO activity. (**C**) The tight junction protein Claudin-3 was detected by immunofluorescence assay (Scale bar: 20 μm). Data are presented as the means ± SEMs of three independent experiments. The symbol # indicates $p < 0.05$ vs. the control group. The symbols * and ** represent significant differences at $p < 0.05$ and $p < 0.01$, respectively.

3.6. Effects of SG on the Activation of Nrf2 and the Wnt/β-Catenin Pathway

It has been found that the activation of Nrf2 is related to oxidative stress and inflammatory reaction [24]. An immunofluorescence technique was used to detect the expression levels of Nrf2 protein in the mammary gland tissues. As shown in Figure 7A, SG treatment could significantly increase the activation of Nrf2, but the activation of Nrf2 was reduced by LPS challenge. Additionally, the Wnt/β-catenin signaling pathway plays a crucial role in LPS-induced inflammation [25]. Thus, we also investigated the effect of SG on the Wnt/β-catenin pathway in LPS-induced mouse mastitis. Compared with the control group, LPS challenge significantly increased the expression of wnt3a and β-catenin proteins. In contrast, SG treatment significantly reduced the expression levels of wnt3a and β-catenin (Figure 7B).

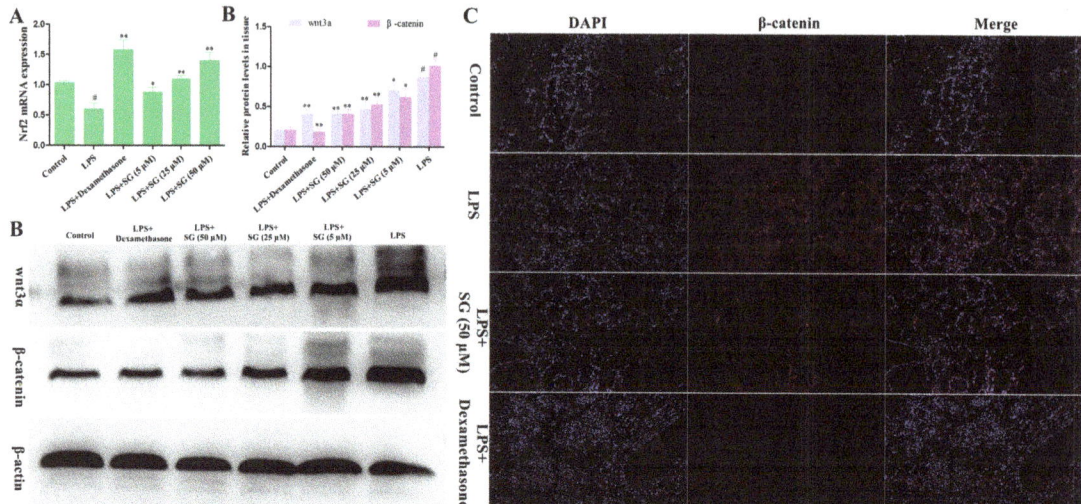

Figure 7. Effects of SG on the activation of Nrf2 and the Wnt/β-catenin pathway. (**A**) The expression of Nrf2 was determined by qRT-PCR assay. (**B**) The levels of proteins in the Wnt/β-catenin pathway were detected by Western blot assay. (**C**) The level of β-catenin protein was determined by an immunofluorescence technique (scale bar: 50 μm). Statistical analysis of the Western blot quantification should be carried out by performing a multiple *t*-test. Data are presented as the means ± SEMs of three independent experiments. The symbol # indicates $p < 0.05$ vs. the control group. The symbols * and ** represent significant differences at $p < 0.05$ and $p < 0.01$, respectively.

4. Discussion

Mastitis is a common clinical disease in dairy cows, which affects the health and welfare of dairy cows and causes huge economic losses to the dairy industry [26,27]. At present, the most commonly used treatment for cow mastitis is antibiotic therapy. However, the nonstandard use of antibiotics leads to drug resistance and drug residues of pathogenic bacteria, which bring greater challenges in the prevention and treatment of mastitis and affect the quality of dairy products [28]. Therefore, it is imperative to reduce the use of antibiotics clinically, and it is urgent to find new drugs to treat mastitis.

SG has been proved to have anti-inflammatory and anti-oxidative-stress effects, with few side effects [29]. We tried to explore the protective role of SG against mastitis in mice and the mechanisms involved. mMECs are the first line of defense for contacting, recognizing, and responding to foreign microorganisms in the mammary glands, and their role is similar to that of sentinel cells [30,31]. The overproduction of ROS will lead to oxidative stress, which damages the immune and anti-inflammatory functions of dairy cows in the transition period [16]. Moreover, the antioxidant enzymes, such as SOD and GSH-Px, play key roles in the antioxidant defense system of dairy cows [32]. In in vitro studies, SG significantly reduced oxidative stress induced by LPS and increased antioxidant enzyme activity.

One of the characteristics of immune response is the release of cytokines, which play an important role in host immune response to infection and disease [33]. It was reported that IL-1β and TNF-α expression levels were critical to the body's immunity, but excessive secretion caused fatal systemic inflammation and damaged breast tissue and cells [34]. SG treatment could down-regulate the LPS-induced production of IL-1β and TNF-α. MPO is a biomarker of neutrophil infiltration, can produce reactive oxidants and diffuse free radicals, and is involved in the immune regulation of inflammation. In the process of inflammation, the activity of MPO increases, which can lead to acute and chronic vascular tissue damage [35]. The present experiments found that the mice in the LPS-treated group exhibited significantly increased MPO activity, but the MPO activity gradually decreased with the increase in SG concentration. The above results indicated that SG could protect against the LPS-induced inflammatory injury process by reducing oxidative stress and improving antioxidant enzyme activity.

Nrf2 is an important antioxidant transcription factor, which can reduce inflammation by promoting the expression of its downstream anti-inflammatory genes [36]. In the present study, it was found that SG promoted the expression of Nrf2. Studies have shown that the Wnt/β-catenin signaling pathway is associated with a variety of diseases, including inflammation [37]. Wnt proteins are a family of secreted adiponectins that play decisive roles in cell proliferation, migration, and differentiation [38]. The Wnt/β-catenin signaling pathway could also promote the expression of cytokines and thus aggravate inflammatory response [39]. The present study showed that SG inhibited the LPS-induced activation of the Wnt/β-catenin signaling pathway.

5. Conclusions

In conclusion, this study clarified the protective effect of SG against mastitis and provided evidence for new potential mechanisms. The dosage of SG used in this experiment was non-toxic to mMECs. SG not only inhibited the increase in ROS induced by LPS, but also enhanced the activities of antioxidant enzymes. Thus, SG exerted its anti-inflammatory and antioxidant functions by activating Nrf2 and inhibiting the Wnt/β-catenin pathway, repairing the blood–milk barrier.

Author Contributions: Conceptualization, Z.Z. and Y.Z.; methodology, G.X. and X.L.; data curation, Z.Z. and Y.Z.; writing, supervision, H.W.; formal analysis, Z.Z., X.L., G.X. and Y.Z.; funding acquisition, H.W. All authors have read and agreed to the published version of the manuscript.

Funding: This research was funded by the National Natural Science Foundation of China (grant no. 32102733), the Zhejiang Provincial Natural Science Foundation of China (grant no. LQ22C180004), and the fund opened by the Key Laboratory of Fujian Universities Preventive Veterinary Medicine and Biotechnology, Longyan University (grant no. 2020KF02).

Institutional Review Board Statement: The animals were cared for humanely, all experiments involving mice were conducted according to the Guide for the Care and Use of Laboratory Animals of the National Research Council, and all experimental protocols were followed by the Institutional Animal Care and Use Committee in Zhejiang University (approval no. GBT 35892-2018).

Informed Consent Statement: Not applicable.

Data Availability Statement: All data are contained in the manuscript.

Conflicts of Interest: The authors declare no conflict of interest.

References

1. Gu, B.; Miao, J.; Fa, Y.; Lu, J.; Zou, S. Retinoic acid attenuates lipopolysaccharide-induced inflammatory responses by suppressing TLR4/NF-kappaB expression in rat mammary tissue. *Int. Immunopharmacol.* **2010**, *10*, 799–805. [CrossRef] [PubMed]
2. Fusco, R.; Cordaro, M.; Siracusa, R.; Peritore, A.F.; D'Amico, R.; Licata, P.; Crupi, R.; Gugliandolo, E. Effects of Hydroxytyrosol against Lipopolysaccharide-Induced Inflammation and Oxidative Stress in Bovine Mammary Epithelial Cells: A Natural Therapeutic Tool for Bovine Mastitis. *Antioxidants* **2020**, *9*, 693. [CrossRef] [PubMed]
3. Petersson-Wolfe, C.S.; Leslie, K.E.; Swartz, T.H. An Update on the Effect of Clinical Mastitis on the Welfare of Dairy Cows and Potential Therapies. *Vet. Clin. N. Am. Food Anim. Pract.* **2018**, *34*, 525–535. [CrossRef] [PubMed]
4. Fiore, E.; Arfuso, F.; Gianesella, M. Metabolic and hormonal adaptation in Bubalus bubalis around calving and early lactation. *PLoS ONE* **2018**, *13*, e0193803. [CrossRef]
5. Bazzano, M.; Giannetto, C.; Fazio, F.; Arfuso, F.; Giudice, E.; Piccione, G. Metabolic profile of broodmares during late pregnancy and early post-partum. *Reprod. Domest. Anim. Zuchthyg.* **2014**, *49*, 947–953. [CrossRef]
6. Mavangira, V.; Kuhn, M.J.; Abuelo, A.; Morisseau, C.; Hammock, B.D.; Sordillo, L.M. Activity of sEH and Oxidant Status during Systemic Bovine Coliform Mastitis. *Antioxidants* **2021**, *10*, 812. [CrossRef]
7. Asaf, S.; Leitner, G.; Furman, O.; Lavon, Y.; Kalo, D.; Wolfenson, D.; Roth, Z. Effects of Escherichia coli- and Staphylococcus aureus-induced mastitis in lactating cows on oocyte developmental competence. *Reproduction* **2014**, *147*, 33–43. [CrossRef]

8. Ibeagha-Awemu, E.M.; Lee, J.W.; Ibeagha, A.E.; Bannerman, D.D.; Paape, M.J.; Zhao, X. Bacterial lipopolysaccharide induces increased expression of toll-like receptor (TLR) 4 and downstream TLR signaling molecules in bovine mammary epithelial cells. *Vet. Res.* **2008**, *39*, 11. [CrossRef]
9. Tang, X.; Liu, C.; Li, T.; Lin, C.; Hao, Z.; Zhang, H.; Zhao, G.; Chen, Y.; Guo, A.; Hu, C. Gambogic acid alleviates inflammation and apoptosis and protects the blood-milk barrier in mastitis induced by LPS. *Int. Immunopharmacol.* **2020**, *86*, 106697. [CrossRef]
10. Yin, H.; Xue, G.; Dai, A.; Wu, H. Protective Effects of Lentinan Against Lipopolysaccharide-Induced Mastitis in Mice. *Front. Pharmacol.* **2021**, *12*, 755768. [CrossRef]
11. Long, E.; Capuco, A.V.; Wood, D.L.; Sonstegard, T.; Tomita, Y.; Paape, M.J.; Zhao, X. Escherichia coli induces apoptosis and proliferation of mammary cells. *Cell Death Differ.* **2001**, *8*, 808–816. [CrossRef] [PubMed]
12. Tsugami, Y.; Matsunaga, K.; Suzuki, T.; Nishimura, T.; Kobayashi, K. Phytoestrogens Weaken the Blood-Milk Barrier in Lactating Mammary Epithelial Cells by Affecting Tight Junctions and Cell Viability. *J. Agric. Food Chem.* **2017**, *65*, 11118–11124. [CrossRef] [PubMed]
13. Stelwagen, K.; Singh, K. The role of tight junctions in mammary gland function. *J. Mammary Gland Biol. Neoplasia* **2014**, *19*, 131–138. [CrossRef] [PubMed]
14. Lam, J.S.; Anderson, E.M.; Hao, Y. LPS quantitation procedures. *Methods Mol. Biol.* **2014**, *1149*, 375–402. [CrossRef]
15. Burvenich, C.; Van Merris, V.; Mehrzad, J.; Diez-Fraile, A.; Duchateau, L. Severity of E. coli mastitis is mainly determined by cow factors. *Vet. Res.* **2003**, *34*, 521–564. [CrossRef]
16. Khan, M.Z.; Ma, Y.; Xiao, J.; Chen, T.; Ma, J.; Liu, S.; Wang, Y.; Khan, A.; Alugongo, G.M.; Cao, Z. Role of Selenium and Vitamins E and B9 in the Alleviation of Bovine Mastitis during the Periparturient Period. *Antioxidants* **2022**, *11*, 657. [CrossRef]
17. Huemer, M.; Mairpady Shambat, S.; Brugger, S.D.; Zinkernagel, A.S. Antibiotic resistance and persistence-Implications for human health and treatment perspectives. *EMBO Rep.* **2020**, *21*, e51034. [CrossRef]
18. Green, M.; Bradley, A. The changing face of mastitis control. *Vet. Rec.* **2013**, *173*, 517–521. [CrossRef]
19. Zhang, F.; Xie, J.; Wang, G.; Zhang, G.; Yang, H. Anti-osteoporosis activity of Sanguinarine in preosteoblast MC3T3-E1 cells and an ovariectomized rat model. *J. Cell. Physiol.* **2018**, *233*, 4626–4633. [CrossRef]
20. Prabhu, K.S.; Bhat, A.A.; Siveen, K.S.; Kuttikrishnan, S.; Raza, S.S.; Raheed, T.; Jochebeth, A.; Khan, A.Q.; Chawdhery, M.Z.; Haris, M.; et al. Sanguinarine mediated apoptosis in Non-Small Cell Lung Cancer via generation of reactive oxygen species and suppression of JAK/STAT pathway. *Biomed. Pharmacother. Biomed. Pharmacother.* **2021**, *144*, 112358. [CrossRef]
21. Li, X.; Wu, X.; Wang, Q.; Xu, W.; Zhao, Q.; Xu, N.; Hu, X.; Ye, Z.; Yu, S.; Liu, J.; et al. Sanguinarine ameliorates DSS induced ulcerative colitis by inhibiting NLRP3 inflammasome activation and modulating intestinal microbiota in C57BL/6 mice. *Phytomed. Int. J. Phytother. Phytopharm.* **2022**, *104*, 154321. [CrossRef]
22. Jiang, K.; Ma, X.; Guo, S.; Zhang, T.; Zhao, G.; Wu, H.; Wang, X.; Deng, G. Anti-inflammatory Effects of Rosmarinic Acid in Lipopolysaccharide-Induced Mastitis in Mice. *Inflammation* **2018**, *41*, 437–448. [CrossRef] [PubMed]
23. Buchan, K.D.; Prajsnar, T.K.; Ogryzko, N.V.; de Jong, N.W.M.; van Gent, M.; Kolata, J.; Foster, S.J.; van Strijp, J.A.G.; Renshaw, S.A. A transgenic zebrafish line for in vivo visualisation of neutrophil myeloperoxidase. *PLoS ONE* **2019**, *14*, e0215592. [CrossRef]
24. Kan, X.; Liu, J.; Cai, X.; Huang, Y.; Xu, P.; Fu, S.; Guo, W.; Hu, G. Tartary buckwheat flavonoids relieve the tendency of mammary fibrosis induced by HFD during pregnancy and lactation. *Aging* **2021**, *13*, 25377–25392. [CrossRef]
25. Ma, N.; Wei, G.; Zhang, H.; Dai, H.; Roy, A.C.; Shi, X.; Chang, G.; Shen, X. Cis-9, Trans-11 CLA Alleviates Lipopolysaccharide-Induced Depression of Fatty Acid Synthesis by Inhibiting Oxidative Stress and Autophagy in Bovine Mammary Epithelial Cells. *Antioxidants* **2021**, *11*, 55. [CrossRef] [PubMed]
26. Chen, C.; Wang, J.; Chen, J.; Zhou, L.; Wang, H.; Chen, J.; Xu, Z.; Zhu, S.; Liu, W.; Yu, R.; et al. Morusin alleviates mycoplasma pneumonia via the inhibition of Wnt/β-catenin and NF-κB signaling. *Biosci. Rep.* **2019**, *39*. [CrossRef]
27. Yang, Z.; Yin, R.; Cong, Y.; Yang, Z.; Zhou, E.; Wei, Z.; Liu, Z.; Cao, Y.; Zhang, N. Oxymatrine lightened the inflammatory response of LPS-induced mastitis in mice through affecting NF-κB and MAPKs signaling pathways. *Inflammation* **2014**, *37*, 2047–2055. [CrossRef]
28. Li, H.; Sun, P. Insight of Melatonin: The Potential of Melatonin to Treat Bacteria-Induced Mastitis. *Antioxidants* **2022**, *11*, 1107. [CrossRef]
29. Krömker, V.; Leimbach, S. Mastitis treatment-Reduction in antibiotic usage in dairy cows. *Reprod. Domest. Anim. Zuchthyg.* **2017**, *52* (Suppl. S3), 21–29. [CrossRef]
30. Mackraj, I.; Govender, T.; Gathiram, P. Sanguinarine. *Cardiovasc. Ther.* **2008**, *26*, 75–83. [CrossRef]
31. Bruckmaier, R.M.; Wellnitz, O. Triennial Lactation Symposium/Bolfa: Pathogen-specific immune response and changes in the blood-milk barrier of the bovine mammary gland. *J. Anim. Sci.* **2017**, *95*, 5720–5728. [CrossRef] [PubMed]
32. O'Brien, J.; Martinson, H.; Durand-Rougely, C.; Schedin, P. Macrophages are crucial for epithelial cell death and adipocyte repopulation during mammary gland involution. *Development* **2012**, *139*, 269–275. [CrossRef] [PubMed]
33. Hall, J.A.; Bobe, G.; Vorachek, W.R.; Kasper, K.; Traber, M.G.; Mosher, W.D.; Pirelli, G.J.; Gamroth, M. Effect of supranutritional organic selenium supplementation on postpartum blood micronutrients, antioxidants, metabolites, and inflammation biomarkers in selenium-replete dairy cows. *Biol. Trace Elem. Res.* **2014**, *161*, 272–287. [CrossRef]
34. Ni, H.; Martínez, Y.; Guan, G.; Rodríguez, R.; Más, D.; Peng, H.; Valdivié Navarro, M.; Liu, G. Analysis of the Impact of Isoquinoline Alkaloids, Derived from Macleaya cordata Extract, on the Development and Innate Immune Response in Swine and Poultry. *BioMed Res. Int.* **2016**, *2016*, 1352146. [CrossRef]

35. Glynn, D.J.; Hutchinson, M.R.; Ingman, W.V. Toll-like receptor 4 regulates lipopolysaccharide-induced inflammation and lactation insufficiency in a mouse model of mastitis. *Biol. Reprod.* **2014**, *90*, 91. [CrossRef] [PubMed]
36. Galijasevic, S. The development of myeloperoxidase inhibitors. *Bioorg. Med. Chem. Lett.* **2019**, *29*, 1–7. [CrossRef] [PubMed]
37. Lv, H.; Liu, Q.; Wen, Z.; Feng, H.; Deng, X.; Ci, X. Xanthohumol ameliorates lipopolysaccharide (LPS)-induced acute lung injury via induction of AMPK/GSK3β-Nrf2 signal axis. *Redox Biol.* **2017**, *12*, 311–324. [CrossRef]
38. Lietman, C.; Wu, B.; Lechner, S.; Shinar, A.; Sehgal, M.; Rossomacha, E.; Datta, P.; Sharma, A.; Gandhi, R.; Kapoor, M.; et al. Inhibition of Wnt/β-catenin signaling ameliorates osteoarthritis in a murine model of experimental osteoarthritis. *JCI Insight* **2018**, *3*, e96308. [CrossRef]
39. Katoh, M. Multi-layered prevention and treatment of chronic inflammation, organ fibrosis and cancer associated with canonical WNT/β-catenin signaling activation (Review). *Int. J. Mol. Med.* **2018**, *42*, 713–725. [CrossRef]

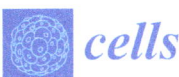

Review

O-GlycNacylation Remission Retards the Progression of Non-Alcoholic Fatty Liver Disease

Yicheng Zhou [1], Zhangwang Li [2], Minxuan Xu [1], Deju Zhang [3], Jitao Ling [1], Peng Yu [1,*] and Yunfeng Shen [1,*,†]

1. Department of Endocrinology and Metabolism, the Second Affiliated Hospital of Nanchang University, Branch of Nationlal Clinical Research Center for Metabolic Diseases, Institute for the Study of Endocrinology and Metabolism in Jiangxi Province, Nanchang 330006, China
2. The Second Clinical Medical College of Nanchang University, Nanchang 330031, China
3. Food and Nutritional Sciences, School of Biological Sciences, The University of Hong Kong, Pokfulam Road, Hong Kong
* Correspondence: ndefy01524@ncu.edu.cn (P.Y.); ndefy97008@ncu.edu.cn (Y.S.)
† Yunfeng Shen is the first corresponding author.

Abstract: Non-alcoholic fatty liver disease (NAFLD) is a metabolic disease spectrum associated with insulin resistance (IR), from non-alcoholic fatty liver (NAFL) to non-alcoholic steatohepatitis (NASH), cirrhosis, and hepatocellular carcinoma (HCC). O-GlcNAcylation is a posttranslational modification, regulated by O-GlcNAc transferase (OGT) and O-GlcNAcase (OGA). Abnormal O-GlcNAcylation plays a key role in IR, fat deposition, inflammatory injury, fibrosis, and tumorigenesis. However, the specific mechanisms and clinical treatments of O-GlcNAcylation and NAFLD are yet to be elucidated. The modification contributes to understanding the pathogenesis and development of NAFLD, thus clarifying the protective effect of O-GlcNAcylation inhibition on liver injury. In this review, the crucial role of O-GlcNAcylation in NAFLD (from NAFL to HCC) is discussed, and the effect of therapeutics on O-GlcNAcylation and its potential mechanisms on NAFLD have been highlighted. These inferences present novel insights into the pathogenesis and treatments of NAFLD.

Keywords: O-GlcNAcylation; insulin resistance; non-alcoholic fatty liver disease; non-alcoholic steatohepatitis; fibrosis; cirrhosis; hepatocellular carcinoma

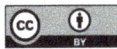

1. Introduction

Non-alcoholic fatty liver disease (NAFLD) is a clinicopathological syndrome with excessive fat deposition in the hepatocytes [1]. It is closely associated with metabolic syndrome, obesity, insulin resistance (IR), and dyslipidemia. Due to the lack of obvious symptoms and starting with simple steatosis in most NAFLD patients, the disease is missed. However, a subset of NAFLD can develop into non-alcoholic steatohepatitis (NASH), and 20% of NASH patients progress to hepatic fibrosis. Once fibrosis occurs, a poor prognosis is developed, such as liver cirrhosis or hepatocellular carcinoma (HCC), the second-most common cause of cancer-related deaths [2]. Nowadays, with the abrupt rising of obesity and diabetes worldwide, the incidence of NAFLD has escalated rapidly [3], with a global prevalence of 25% [4]. Metabolic abnormalities are closely associated with NAFLD, and it was, hence, renamed "metabolic dysfunction-associated fatty liver disease" (MAFLD) in 2020 [5]. (For the convenience of its description, this article has used NAFLD). Moreover, NAFLD is associated with a metabolic imbalance in glucose, lipids, amino acids, bile acids, and iron [6]. Several recent studies have focused on the role of glucose or other metabolisms in NAFLD. Among these, hyperglycemia is a major influencing factor on NAFLD and stimulates insulin secretion and increases the synthesis of triglycerides in the liver. The excessive triglycerides accumulate gradually in the liver and are exported to generate hypertriglyceridemia [7]. In addition, long-term and chronic hyperglycemia-induced hepatocytes injury alters the structure and function of pancreatic β-cells and causes IR, thereby inducing and accelerating the occurrence and progression of NAFLD [8]. Glucose and fructose are the primary mediators of NAFLD, leading to triglyceride production [9]. Therefore, it is of great significance to elucidate the pathogenesis of NAFLD.

One hypothesis of NAFLD pathogenesis has been described by the "2-hit theory" [10], whereby the first hit of hepatic triglyceride accumulation (hepatic steatosis) is induced by IR facilitated by the liver metabolism of fructose. In the second hit, fructose promotes the fructosylation of proteins, the formation of reactive oxygen species (ROS), due to the molecular instability of its five-membered furanose ring [8], endoplasmic reticulum (ER) stress, and inflammation [11], which causes hepatocellular damage and eventually fibrosis [12]. Gradually, the "2-hit theory" has been modified into the "multiple parallel hits" hypothesis for NASH pathogenesis, suggesting that liver damage is caused by multiple parallel pathogenic events [13]. Recently, glycosylation, a posttranslational modification of the proteins in glucose metabolism, has been under intensive focus. The N-glycosylation on the specific peptide sites of serum proteins is a potential marker for the diagnosis of NAFLD-associated hepatocellular carcinoma (NAFLD-HCC) [14]. In addition, the N-glycosylation of the cyclic adenosine monophosphate (AMP)-responsive element-binding protein H (CREBH) improves lipid metabolism and alleviates NAFLD lipotoxicity [15]. Furthermore, some studies have indicated that protein O-GlcNAcylation differentially influences hepatic metabolism and fibrosis [16,17]. Polyphenolic compounds, such as silibinin and curcumin, have reduced NAFLD/NASH by inhibiting O-GlcNAcylation in mouse models [18,19]. Therefore, it can be inferred that O-GlcNAcylation plays a critical role in the pathogenesis of NAFLD.

The modification is also associated with various disorders related to abnormal glucose metabolism, including diabetic cardiomyopathy (DCM). Previous studies focused on the pathogenic mechanism of O-GlcNAcylation in DCM. Protein O-GlcNAcylation is significantly modified in the myocardium in diabetics and is a key regulator of the diabetic cardiac phenotype [20]. Mitigating this posttranslational protein modification improves DCM [21]. Interestingly, aberrant O-GlcNAcylation was detected in obesity, diabetes, cancer, and neurodegenerative diseases [22–24]. Also, the level of O-GlcNAcylation was upregulated in NASH mice [19]. In this review, O-GlcNAcylation in the pathogenesis of NAFLD is discussed and analyzed. Moreover, the application prospect of the intervention of O-GlcNAcylation in the treatment of NAFLD is reviewed for the first time.

2. Role of O-GlcNAc in Normal Liver Tissue

O-GlcNAcylation is a posttranslational modification requiring the attachment of a single O-linked β-N-acetylglucosamine (O-GlcNAc) moiety to the proteins [25–27]. The hexosamine biosynthetic pathway (HBP) regulates the O-GlcNAcylation levels. UDP-GlcNAc, a substrate for the protein O-GlcNAcylation, is produced in this process [28]. The two main enzymes involved in the regulation of protein O-GlcNAcylation modification are as follows: The O-GlcNAc transferase (OGT) catalyzes the transfer of a single N-acetylglucosamine to the proteins from UDP-GlcNAc, leading to their modification with the O-GlcNAc, and the single N-acetylglucosamine is hydrolyzed from the protein by O-GlcNAcase (OGA). O-GlcNAcylation has a reciprocal correlation with O-phosphorylation and modulates many biological processes in eukaryotes; thus, it is considered a critical regulatory modification [29].

O-GlcNAcylation is essential for maintaining the normal physiological homeostasis of the liver; studies have shown that modification acts as a metabolic sensor for liver clock regulation to maintain the circadian control of glucose [30,31]. Some studies have shown that O-GlcNAcylation plays a critical role in gluconeogenesis (Figure 1). The activity of peroxisome proliferator-activated receptor-γ co-activator1α (PGC1α) and FoxO1, key gluconeogenic regulators, is regulated by O-GlcNAcylation [32–34]. PGC1α, an essential coactivator of the transcriptional stimulation of gluconeogenic genes [35–37], further stimulates the expression of gluconeogenic genes. OGT affects PGC1α-mediated gluconeogenesis gene expression by targeting PGC1α via the host cell factor C1 (HCF-1) [34,35].

O-GlcNAcylation also stabilizes PGC1α by recruiting BAP1 for deubiquitination to promote gluconeogenesis [34]. PGC1α promotes OGT to effectuate O-GlcNAcylation and activate FoxO1 and increases the expression of Pepck and G6pc and the transcription of ROS detoxification enzymes, manganese superoxide dismutase (MnSOD) and catalase (CAT), further promoting hepatic glucose production [32]. OGT also increases the expression of Pepck and G6pc, which induces hepatic gluconeogenesis by the O-GlcNAcylation of the cAMP-regulated transcriptional co-activator 2 (CRTC2), a co-activator of the cyclic AMP-responsive element-binding protein (CREB) [38]. It has also been suggested that OGT is involved in glucocorticoid-induced gluconeogenesis [39]. p53 is usually recognized as a tumor suppressor [40]. A recent study reported that insulin sensitivity and liver glucose homeostasis are regulated by integrating the p53 signaling pathways, which depend on p53 O-GlcNAcylation. Subsequently, O-GlcNAcylated p53 binds to the PCK1 promoter to activate the gluconeogenic effect [41].

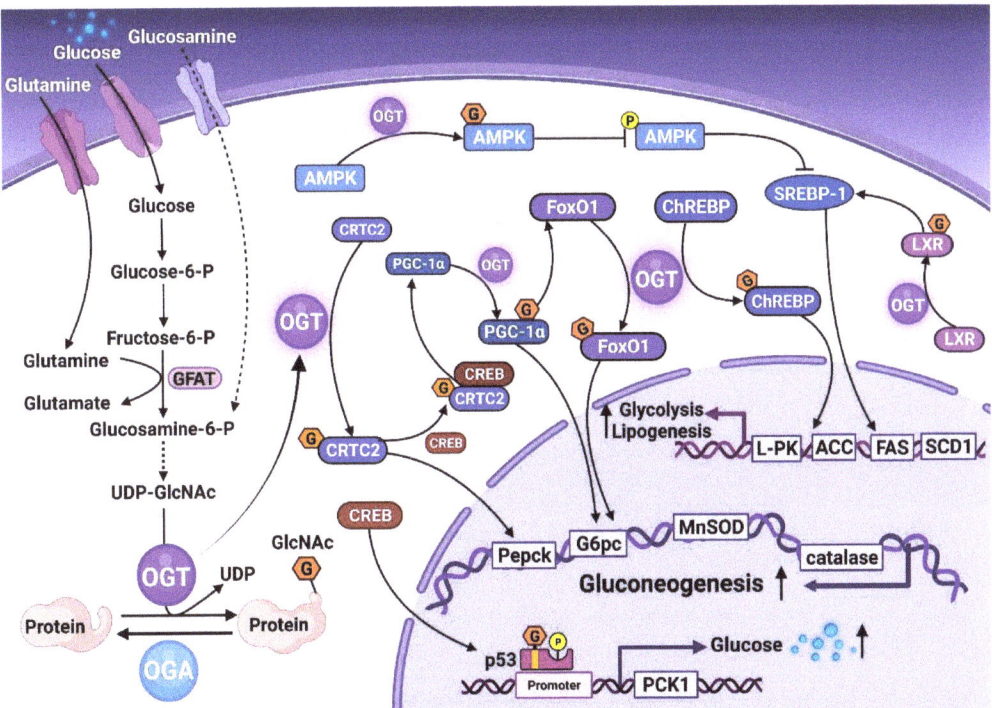

Figure 1. O-GlcNAcylation maintained normal physiological homeostasis in the liver. The HBP regulated the level of O-GlcNAcylation, and OGT catalyzed the transfer of single N-acetyl glucosamine from UDP-GlcNAC to the proteins; hydrolysis of a single N-acetylglucosamine from the proteins by OGA. O-GlcNAcylation of PGC-1α, FoxO1, and CRTC2 increases the expression of gluconeogenic genes and induces hepatic gluconeogenesis. O-GlcNAcylated p53 bound to the PCK1 promoter regulated the PCK1 levels and increased glucose synthesis. LXR, AMPK, ChREBP, and SREBP-1 were directly or indirectly regulated by O-GlcNAcylation, and subsequently, the transcriptional activity of target glycolysis and lipogenic genes was increased. HBP, hexosamine biosynthetic pathway; GFAT, glutamine fructose-6-phosphate amidotransferase; OGT, O-GlcNAc transferase; OGA, O-GlcNAcase; CRTC2, cAMP-regulated transcriptional co-activator 2; CREB, cyclic AMP-responsive element-binding protein; PGC1α, peroxisome proliferator-activated receptor-γ co-activator1α; ChREBP, carbohydrate-responsive element-binding

protein; AMPK, AMP-activated protein kinase; SREBP-1, sterol regulatory element-binding protein 1; LXR, liver X receptors; ACC, acetyl-CoA carboxylase; FAS, fatty acid synthase; SCD1, stearoyl-CoA desaturase1; MnSOD, manganese superoxide dismutase.

Furthermore, whether glucose flux promotes fat production through O-GlcNAcylation needed to be clarified. liver X receptors (LXRs) are lipid metabolism, glucose stability, and inflammation sensors. O-GlcNAcylation of the hepatic LXR was observed in refed mice and streptozotocin-induced diabetic mice [42]. High glucose increases the O-GlcNAcylation of the LXR and the transcriptional activity of the sterol regulatory element-binding protein 1 (SREBP-1) promoter. SREBP-1 is a master transcriptional regulator of hepatic lipogenesis [42], and the O-GlcNAcylation of the LXR upregulates the expression of SREBP-1 in the liver [42]. OGT regulates the phosphorylation and stability of SREBP-1 by increasing AMP-activated protein kinase (AMPK) O-GlcNAcylation in breast cancer [43], followed by the transcriptional activity of acetyl-CoA carboxylase (ACC) and fatty acid synthase (FAS). The carbohydrate-responsive element-binding protein (ChREBP) plays a vital role in glycolysis and lipogenesis. In hepatocytes, the O-GlcNAcylation of the ChREBP stabilizes the protein and increases its transcriptional activity on the target glycolysis [*liver pyruvate kinase (L-PK)*] and lipidogenic genes [*ACC, FAS,* and *stearoyl-CoA desaturase1 (SCD1)*] [44]. Therefore, exploring the mechanistic and kinetic characterization of O-GlcNAcylation on key signaling proteins is promising for an in-depth understanding of normal hepatic metabolism. Finally, some studies have shown that multiple nodes of the insulin signaling pathway were altered by OGT. Under normal physiological conditions, O-GlcNAcylation is responsible for insulin signaling transduction. However, it would be abnormally elevated and induce IR in the state of overnutrition.

Elevated O-GlcNAcylation is not entirely detrimental to the liver. The termination of defective liver regeneration leads to reduced hepatocyte redifferentiation, severe necroinflammation, early fibrotic changes, and the formation of dysplastic nodules leading to the development of hepatocellular carcinoma (HCC) [45]. HNF4a O-GlcNAcylation in hepatocytes plays a key role in the termination of liver regeneration and prevention of hepatic dysplasia [45]. Studies have confirmed that calcium-dependent O-GlcNAc signaling is also critical in driving hepatic autophagy to maintain a nutrient and energy balance in response to starvation [46]. In addition, O-GlcNAc maintains a normal mitochondrial function, and the long-term elevation of o-GlcNAacylation coupled with an increased OGA expression modulates the mitochondrial function and reduces antioxidant responses [47]. For other liver diseases, such as hepatitis B, O-GlcNAcylation promotes the autophagic degradation of hepatitis B virus (HBV) replication virions and proteins through the mTORC1 signaling pathway and autophagosome-lysosome fusion, resulting in reduced HBV replication [48].

3. O-GlcNAcylation Contributes to IR

The liver is an insulin-sensitive organ and essential for maintaining blood glucose. IR also plays a vital role in the occurrence and development of type 2 diabetes mellitus (T2DM) and NAFLD. Strikingly, NAFLD occurs in 70–80% of T2DM and obesity patients, and most NAFLD patients, develop hepatic IR [49]. The pathogenesis of NAFLD is closely related to IR as it is one of the components of the pathogenesis of NAFLD [50]. Additionally, IR is characterized by decreased glucose uptake and utilization in tissues, including liver tissue, adipose tissue, and muscle tissue [51]. IR increases the circulating free fatty acids through dysregulated lipolysis, resulting in an impaired insulin signal, a reduced clearance rate of glucose metabolism, and the dysregulation of lipid aggregation and decomposition [52]. In addition, the body increases lipid synthesis for energy by breaking down fat. Insulin increases lipase activity, thereby elevating the uptake of triglycerides by the adipose tissue and fat storage in the liver [53]. Lipid deposition in the liver further exacerbates IR. Preview studies demonstrated a critical role of O-GlcNAcylation in attenuating insulin signaling [49,50] (Figure 2).

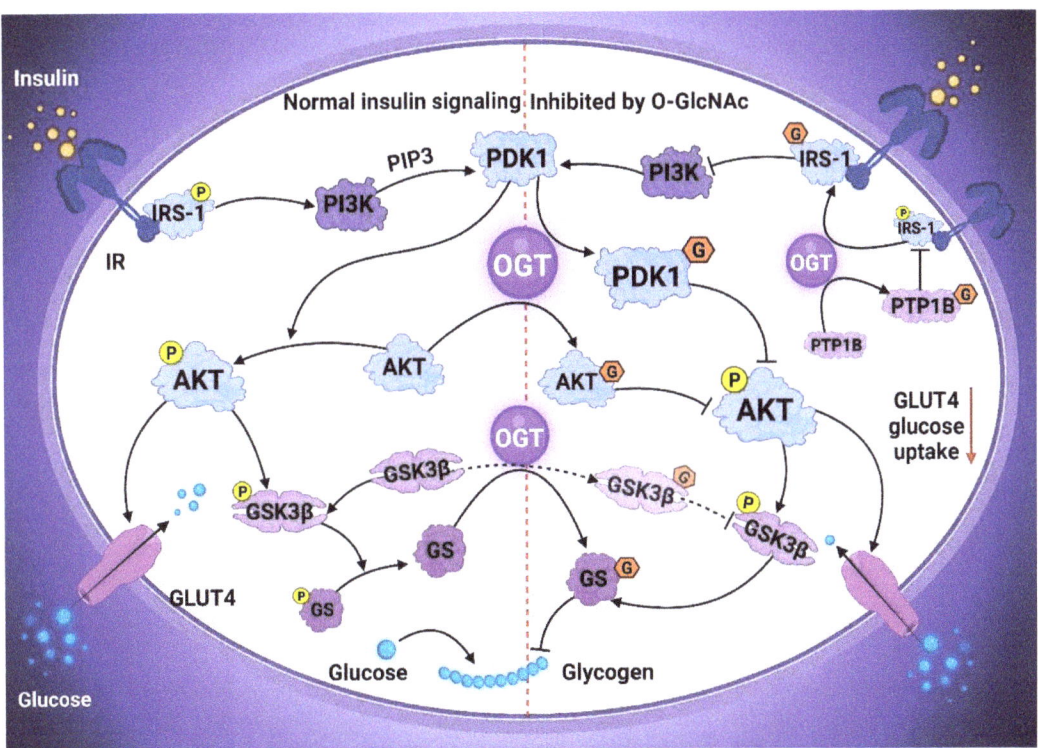

Figure 2. O-GlcNAcylation attenuated insulin signaling. Normal insulin signaling (Left). Insulin binding to the insulin receptor (IR) leads to the recruitment of IRS-1 and activates PI3K, producing PIP3 and activating PDK1 and AKT. The PI3K/AKT pathway induces the expression of GLUT4 and its transport from intracellular vesicles to cell membranes to promote glucose uptake. In addition, the PI3K/AKT pathway activates GSK3β and GS to promote glycogen synthesis. Insulin signaling was inhibited by O-GlcNAcylation (Right). OGT inactivated key insulin signaling proteins, including IRS-1, PI3K, PDK1, AKT, and PTP1B, and attenuated insulin signaling and insulin resistance. PI3K, phosphatidylinositol-3-kinase; PDK1, phosphoinositide-dependent protein kinase 1; AKT, serine/threonine-protein kinase B; GSK3β, glycogen synthase kinase 3 beta; GS, glycogen synthase; PTP1B, protein tyrosine phosphatase 1B; OGT, O-GlcNAc transferase.

A major mechanism for terminating insulin signaling is the inactivation of insulin receptor substrates. OGT inactivates the insulin signaling proteins, including insulin receptor substrate 1 (IRS-1), phosphatidylinositol-3-kinase (PI3K), phosphoinositide-dependent protein kinase 1 (PDK1), serine/threonine-protein kinase B (AKT), and protein tyrosine phosphatase 1B (PTP1B), promoting the attenuation of insulin signaling [50,51]. Interestingly, OGT uses IRS-1 as its direct substrate [54]. In 3T3-L1 adipocytes, the Tyr608 phosphorylation of IRS-1 is inhibited by elevated O-GlcNAcylation, thereby reducing AKT activity [54]. In addition, OGT also uses PDK1 and PI3K as direct substrates in insulin signal attenuation [54,55]. Decreased AKT activity is vital for terminating insulin signaling, and O-GlcNAcylation plays a key role in the regulation of AKT activity. Normal O-GlcNAcylation is valuable for AKT signal transduction, while the O-GlcNAcylation of Thr305/Thr312 disrupts the interaction between AKT and PDK1, resulting in the downregulation of AKT activity [56]. Then, the decreased AKT activity reduces glycogen synthesis via glycogen synthase kinase 3 beta (GSK3β) phosphorylation. GSKβ is modified by O-GlcNAcylation, after the inhibition of GSK3β by lithium, and the overall

O-GlcNAcylation level is significantly increased [57]. However, the function of GSK3β O-GlcNAcylation needs further exploration. In addition, PTP1B controls hepatic insulin signaling by inhibiting PTP1B O-GlcNAcylation, improving insulin sensitivity, and reducing liver lipid deposition [58]. Another study found that the O-GlcNAcylation level of glycogen synthase (GS) is increased, and the activity of GS is decreased after high glucose or glucosamine treatment, thereby leading to IR [59]. Therefore, abnormal glycogenogenesis and gluconeogenesis are closely related to O-GlcNAcylation during the development of hepatic IR.

4. Association of O-GlcNAc with NAFLD Process

O-GlcNAcylation acts as a promoting factor throughout NAFL-NASH-liver fibrosis-HCC. The LXR and the ChREBP are directly modified by O-GlcNAcylation, and SREBP-1 is indirectly regulated by O-GlcNAcylation, resulting in liver fat deposition and NAFL formation [42–44] (Figure 3). During the progression of NAFL to NASH, O-GlcNAcylation modifies I6PK1 and the Nuclear factor-κB (NF-κB) subunit p65 to increase the inflammatory injury, while the NF-κB subunit c-Rel undergoes O-GlcNAcylation to exert an anti-inflammatory effect under hyperglycemic conditions [17,60,61]. Moreover, the O-GlcNAcylation of collagens accelerates fibrosis, while that of the serum response factor (SRF) has an antifibrotic effect [62,63]. It modifies the receptor-interacting protein kinase 3 (RIPK3) to induce NAFLD-HCC [64,65].

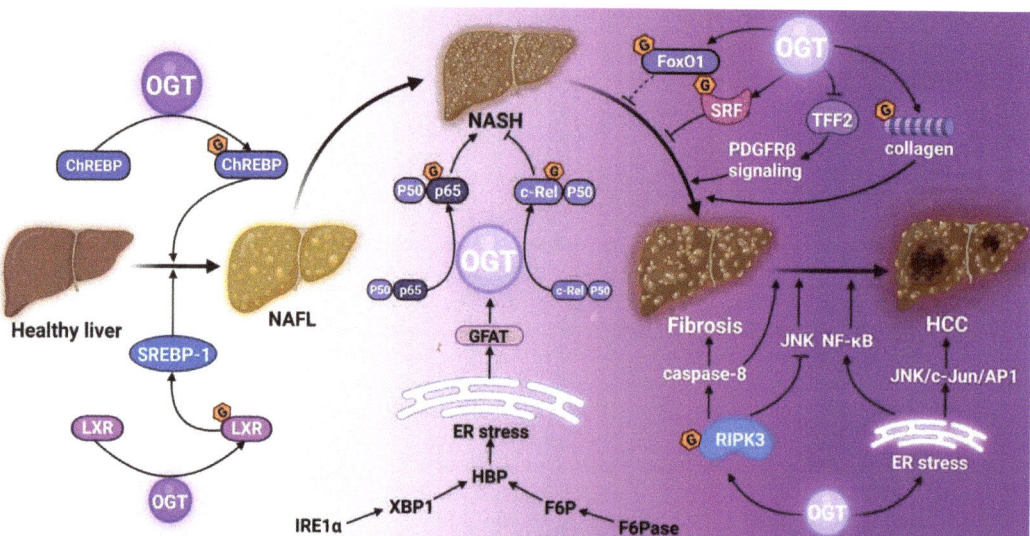

Figure 3. O-GlcNAcylation and NAFL-NASH-liver fibrosis-hepatoma tetralogy. The O-GlcNAcylation of the LXR, the ChREBP, and SREBP-1 promoted NAFL formation. O-GlcNAcylated NF-κB subunit p65 played a role in the progression of NASH by facilitating inflammatory damage, and the O-GlcNAcylated NF-κB subunit c-Rel exerted an anti-inflammatory effect. During liver fibrosis, O-GlcNAcylation of collagens accelerated fibrosis, while O-GlcNAcylation of the SRF represented anti-fibrotic effects. Finally, O-GlcNAcylated RIPK3 contributed to HCC. NAFL, non-alcoholic fatty liver; NASH, non-alcoholic steatohepatitis; LXR, Liver X receptor; carbohydrate-responsive element-binding protein; ChREBP, carbohydrate-responsive element-binding protein; SREBP-1, sterol regulatory element-binding protein 1; NF-κB, Nuclear factor-κB; SRF, serum response factor; HCC, hepatocellular carcinoma; OGT, O-GlcNAc transferase; GFAT, glutamine fructose-6-phosphate amidotransferase; ER stress, endoplasmic reticulum stress; HBP, hexosamine biosynthetic pathway; IRE1α, inositol requiring enzyme 1α; XBP1, X-box-binding protein 1; PDGFRβ, platelet-derived growth factor receptor β; TFF2, trefoil factor 2; JNK, Jun N-terminal kinases.

4.1. O-GlcNAc and NAFL

NAFLD is a generalized term encompassing a range of liver conditions of varying severities resulting in liver fibrosis [52]; a simple steatosis named NAFL resulted from triglyceride accumulation in the cytoplasm of hepatocytes. On the other hand, the ChREBP is a pivotal transcription factor mediating the effects of glucose on glycolysis and lipogenesis genes. A previous study showed that the ChREBP is a regulatory center of adipogenesis in vivo and plays a decisive role in developing hepatic steatosis and IR; the specific inhibition of the ChREBP significantly improves hepatic steatosis in ob/ob mice [66]. A further study demonstrated that O-GlcNAcylation stabilizes the ChREBP and increases the activity on glycolytic lipogenic genes (*L-PK*, *ACC*, *FAS*, and *SCD1*) [44] (Table 1). Importantly, the overexpression of OGT significantly increases the ChREBP in C57BL/6J mice liver, resulting in enhanced lipogenic gene expression and excess hepatic triglyceride deposition [44]. Furthermore, HCF-1 O-GlcNAcylation, in response to glucose or a high-carbohydrate diet (HCD), first recruited OGT to the ChREBP, which led to ChREBP O-GlcNAcylation and activation [67]. Whether the mechanism of O-GlcNAcylation regulates the ChREBP in HCD-induced NAFLD mice needs to be investigated further.

The level of SREBP-1, a transcription factor that activates FAS and ACC1, is elevated [68], accompanied by hepatic steatosis [69]. Mice with the liver-specific overexpression of mature human SREBP-1 develop hepatic lipid accumulation and feature a fatty liver by the age of 6 months [70]. A previous study demonstrated that excessive glucose promotes lipid accumulation by upregulating lipid genes, such as *SREBP-1*, *FAS*, and *ACC1*, in cultured hepatocytes and animal model liver tissues [71]. Previous studies have shown that SREBP-1 protein expression is regulated by O-GlcNAcylation [43]. Also, the overexpression of glutamine fructose-6-phosphate amidotransferase (GFAT) promotes lipid accumulation in hepatic cells as well as inflammatory pathway activation by increasing the ER stress by the HBP [72], which indicates a critical role of the HBP in thyroglobulin (TG) accumulation. However, an updated study did not observe the response of SREBP-1 O-GlcNAcylation to GFAT inhibitors [73]. The correlation between SREBP-1 and the HBP and whether SREBP-1 directly effectuates O-GlcNAcylation is yet to be elucidated.

4.2. O-GlcNAc and NASH

In the preliminary stage, most patients with NAFLD manifest as hepatic steatosis without any symptoms. As the disease progresses, a proportion of the patients show NASH with inflammatory manifestation, hepatocyte injury, and fibrosis [74]. Nevertheless, the molecular mechanisms underlying the development of NAFLD and NASH are poorly understood. Protein O-GlcNAcylation impedes insulin signaling and promotes adipogenesis [16]. A recent study showed that inositol hexakisphosphate kinases 1 (IP6K1) inhibitors improve metabolic disorders, NAFLD/NASH. and fibrosis by altering these pathways [17]. How IP6K1 stimulates the protein O-GlcNAcylation to improve NAFLD by knocking down OGT remains to be explored.

Previous studies have indicated that O-GlcNAcylation is upregulated in NASH mice; however, the causal correlation between the upregulation of O-GlcNAcylation and the pathology of NASH is unclear. NF-κB, a proinflammatory transcription, is related to many pathogenic liver diseases [75], and NF-κB activated by inositol requiring enzyme 1α (IRE1α) causes liver inflammation and promotes NASH [76,77]. In addition, the activity of NF-κB is regulated by O-GlcNAcylation [60], and the upregulated O-GlcNAcylation activates NF-κB and increases inflammatory damage [78].

Table 1. Role of O-GlcNAc on the process of NAFLD.

Experiment Type	Key Factor	Directly Modified or Not	Level of O-GlcNAc	Specific Mechanism	Final Conclusion	Ref.
Animal and Cell	ChREBP	Yes	↑	Transcriptional activity of L-PK, ACC, FAS, and SCD1	Hepatic TG deposition	[44]
Cell and Animal	SREBP-1	No	↑	SREBP-1 phosphorylation and stability via AMPK signaling	TG deposition	[43]
Cell and Animal	IP6K1	No	↑	Unclarified	Promote NASH and fibrosis	[17]
Cell and Animal	NF-κB	Yes	↑	p65 is modified to induce activation of NFκB	Inflammatory damage	[60]
Cell	Collagen	Yes	↑	c-Rel is modified and activated	Anti-inflammatory effect	[61]
Animal & Cell	SRF	Yes	↑	Activate HSCs	Liver fibrosis	[62]
Animal & Cell	RIPK3	Yes	↓	Inhibited SRF activity to induce α-SMA transcription	Prevent liver fibrosis	[63]
			↑	RIPK3 stability, caspase 8 cleavage, and JNK activation	Promote NAFLD-HCC	[64,65]

ChREBP, carbohydrate-responsive element-binding protein; L-PK, liver pyruvate kinase; ACC, acetyl-CoA carboxylase; FAS, fatty acid synthase; SCD1, stearoyl-CoA desaturase1; TG, thyroglobulin; SREBP-1, sterol regulatory element-binding protein 1; AMPK, AMP-activated protein kinase; IP6K1, inositol hexakisphosphate kinases 1; NASH, non-alcoholic steatohepatitis; NF-κB, Nuclear factor-κB; HSCs, hepatic stellate cells; SRF, serum response factor; α-SMA, α-smooth muscle actin; RIPK3, receptor-interacting protein kinase 3; JNK, c-Jun N-terminal kinases; NAFLD-HCC, NAFLD-associated hepatocellular carcinoma. Up arrow represents up-regulation, Down arrow represents down-regulation.

ROS accumulation and related ER stresses are caused by fat toxicity [79,80]. The transcription of GTAT is upregulated under ER stress, increasing protein O-GlcNAcylation [81]. Another study showed that O-GlcNAcylation, OGT, and GFAT levels are increased in mice with a methionine-choline deficient (MCD) diet, and the upregulated OGT and GFAT originate from the upstream target IRE1α induced via ER stress [19]. Currently, transcription factor X-box-binding protein 1 (XBP1) is the only known transcription factor downstream of IRE1α [82], and a key transcription factor is involved in hepatic adipogenesis and inflammation through ER stress [83]. These studies suggested that the upstream activator of the HBP is regulated by the transcription of XBP1 and is a positive regulatory loop for the onset of NASH. In another study, the expression of fructose-1,6-bisphosphatase (FBPase) was upregulated in NASH mice, leading to elevated F6P levels, HBP flux, and upregulated O-GlcNAcylation [18]. The increased level of protein O-GlcNAcylation by elevating the HBP flux in the liver plays a critical role in establishing a correlation between the increase in liver FBPase and NASH [84].

4.3. O-GlcNAc and Hepatic Fibrosis

Hepatic fibrosis is the most critical predictor of mortality in NAFLD, and the risk of liver-associated mortality increases exponentially with the increase in the fibrosis stage [85]. NASH patients with liver fibrosis are prone to develop cirrhosis [86]. Currently, only a few studies are related to O-GlcNAcylation and liver fibrosis. Hepatic stellate cells (HSCs) are the major source of the extracellular matrix in the liver [87]. Activated HSCs contribute to fibrogenesis. Interestingly, O-GlcNAcylation is involved in activating HSCs and collagen expression [62]. HSC activation originates from FoxO1 inactivation, leading to NAFLD fibrosis [88]. Paradoxically, the expression and activity of FoxO1 are increased in NASH patients [89]. Since FoxO1 plays a critical role in fibrosis and could be O-GlcNAcylated, it is essential to elucidate the role of FoxO1 O-GlcNAacylation on liver fibrosis through gene knockdown.

It was found that OGT-deficient hepatocytes are prone to hepatocyte ballooning, inflammation, and liver fibrosis [65]. OGT, a negative regulator of HSC activation, exerts a protective effect against hepatic fibrosis by boosting SRF O-GlcNAcylation. Therefore, the OGT expression and O-GlcNAcylation were decreased in HSCs isolated from MCD-fed mice livers [63]. In contrast, a recent study reported that OGT-deficient necroptotic hepatocytes secrete trefoil factor 2 (TFF2), which induces HSC activation, proliferation, and migration via platelet-derived growth factor receptorβ (PDGFRβ) signaling [90]. Thus, it is essential to clarify whether O-GlcNAc could be used as a biomarker for liver disease.

4.4. O-GlcNAc and NAFLD-HCC

NAFLD is becoming the leading cause of HCCs. NAFLD/NASH-HCC incidence and mortality rates are rising worldwide [91]. Furthermore, a retrospective cohort study from 2002 to 2012 indicated that NASH-related HCC increased significantly, and the number of patients undergoing liver transplantation for HCCs secondary to NASH increased by nearly four-fold, while the number of patients with HCCs secondary to chronic hepatitis C virus (HCV) increases only by two-fold [92]. NAFLD-HCC patients exhibit upregulated levels of OGT, which plays an oncogenic role by activating the oncogenic c-jun N-terminal kinases (JNK)/c-Jun/AP-1 and nuclear factor-kappa B (NF-κB) cascades [93]. Another study demonstrated that OGT is a key inhibitor of hepatocyte necroptosis in alcoholic fatty liver disease, and the lack of O-GlcNAcylation induces necroptosis in hepatocytes [65]. However, the specific pathogenesis mechanisms of NAFLD-HCC have not yet been totally revealed.

The mutual inhibition of caspase 8 and RIPK3 is essential for the development of NASH and hepatocarcinogenesis [64,94], and RIPK3 prevents cell proliferation from limiting the development of HCCs by inhibiting caspase 8 cleavage and JNK activation [64]. A study discovered that O-GlcNAcylation inhibits RIPK3 protein expression and stability [65]. Further investigation would analyze the molecular mechanism underlying OGT-regulated-*RIPK3* gene transcription by O-GlcNAcylation. Nonetheless, only a few studies have elaborated on the role of OGA in the liver. Targeting O-GlcNAcylation is a potential therapy for NAFLD-HCC.

Furthermore, OGT overexpression in the liver increased intracellular palmitic acid levels and promoted HCC by activating ER stress-associated oncogenic signaling cascades, including the JNK/c-Jun/AP1 and NF-κB signaling pathways [93]. Typically, 2/3 of NAFLD-HCC tumors show OGT overexpression, while 1/3 of no change in OGT expression is seen, suggesting that OGT expression is associated with gene polymorphism related to the occurrence and progression of NAFLD and NASH, such as *PNOLA3* p.I148M, *TM6SF2* p.E167K, and *MBOAT7* rs641738 [95,96]. Further studies should investigate whether OGT has a prognostic value for NAFLD-HCC.

5. Drugs Ameliorates NAFLD through Inhibition of O-GlcNAcylation

Metformin (MET) inhibits the proliferation of cervical cancer cells by reducing the O-GlcNAcylation of AMPK and increasing the level of phospho-AMPK [97] (Table 2). Another study indicated that MET inhibits the O-GlcNAc modification of NF-κB p65 and the ChREBP in the diabetic retina [98]. In addition, MET has been shown to have a protective effect on NAFLD, but the specific mechanism is yet unclear [99]. Furthermore, O-GlcNAcylation is activated, and AMPK/ACC pathway phosphorylation is inhibited in high-fat diet (HFD)-fed mice [100]. It has also been suggested that MET reduces hepatic TG accumulation and improves obesity-related NAFLD by inhibiting hepatic apolipoprotein A5 (ApoA5) synthesis through the AMPK/LXRα signaling pathway [101]. Therefore, it was speculated that MET promotes AMPK phosphorylation in the NAFLD liver by regulating AMPK O-GlcNAcylation and inhibiting the O-GlcNAc modification of the ChREBP, further increasing fat mobilization and reducing fat deposition in the liver. Also, inflammatory damage is alleviated by inhibiting the O-GlcNAc modification of NF-κB p65 in NAFLD patients.

The glucagon-like peptide-1 (GLP-1) receptor agonist, liraglutide, improves NASH by lowering liver enzyme levels and reducing liver fat [103]. Also, liraglutide and semaglutide improved NASH in clinical trials [114,115]. Yu et al. [116] proposed that GLP-1 inhibits the activation of the NLR family, pyrin domain-containing 3 (NLRP3) inflammasome, and reduced the production of ROS by enhancing mitophagy in hepatocytes, eventually improving NAFLD and delaying the progression of NASH. In addition, the activity of GLP-1 was enhanced by the inhibition of proteolysis due to O-GlcNAcylation [102]. However, the mechanisms underlying the elevated protein O-GlcNAcylation induced by GLP-1 that alleviated NAFLD/NASH are yet to be elaborated.

Goldberg et al., and Park et al. [117,118] speculated that increased O-GlcNAcylation enhances the pro-fibrotic signaling in mesangial cells exposed to high glucose. Sodium-glucose cotransporter 2 inhibitor (SGLT-2i) exerts antifibrotic effects in the diabetic kidney by reducing protein O-GlcNacylation [104]. In a clinical study, NAFLD patients treated with SGLT-2i experienced a remission of hepatic steatosis and improvement in liver fibrosis [105]. Some animal studies have also shown improvements in hepatic steatosis and steatohepatitis with various SGLT-2is, including remogliflozin, luseogliflozin, empagliflozin (EMPA), ipragliflozin, and NGI001 [119–124]. EMPA attenuated NAFLD in HFD-fed mice by activating autophagy and reducing ER stress and apoptosis [125]. Another study suggested that EMPA significantly improves NAFLD-related liver injury by enhancing the autophagy of hepatic macrophages through the AMPK/mammalian target of the rapamycin (mTOR) signaling pathway and further inhibiting the interleukin (IL)-17/IL-23 axis-mediated inflammatory response [126]. Presumably, SGLT-2i exerts an antifibrotic effect in NAFLD patients by reducing the protein O-GlcNacylation. It also ameliorates NAFLD/NASH by reducing ER stress and activates hepatocyte autophagy by inhibiting O-GlcNacylation.

Table 2. Drug interactions with O-GlcNAcylation and NAFLD.

Drug.	Correlation with O-GlcNAcylation	Effects on NAFLD	Ref.
MET	↑ O-GlcNAcylation of AMP, NF-κB, and ChREBP	↓ Liver TG accumulation and improved NAFLD	[97–99,101]
GLP-1	O-GlcNAcylation enhance GLP-1 activity	↓ Liver enzyme levels and liver fat	[102,103]
SGLT-2I	Reduced O-GlcNAcylation exerts an anti-fibrotic effect	↓ Liver steatosis and liver fibrosis	[104,105]
ACEI	Enhancement of Ang1-7 axis to reduce O-GlcNAcylation	↓ Incidence of liver cancer and cirrhosis	[106,107]
GSH	Positive correlation between c-Jun O-GlcNAcylation and GSH synthesis	supported liver metabolism and improved NAFLD	[108,109]
ALA	↑ O-GlcNAcylation of ERK, p38, CuZnSOD, CAT, HSP70, and HSP90	↓ Liver TG accumulation and improved NAFLD	[110–113]
Curcumin	Inhibition O-GlcNAcylation and blocked NF-κB signaling pathway	Exert anti-inflammatory effect, alleviated NAFLD/NASH	[19]
Silibinin	Inhibition of O-GlcNAcylation and blocked NF-κB signaling pathway	Anti-inflammatory effect, alleviated NASH	[18]

NAFLD, non-alcoholic fatty liver disease; MET, metformin; AMP, cyclic adenosine monophosphate; NF-κB, Nuclear factor-κB; ChREBP, carbohydrate-responsive element-binding protein; GLP-1, glucagon-like peptide-1; SGLT-2I, sodium-glucose cotransporter 2 inhibitor; Ang, angiotensin; ACEI, Ang converting enzyme inhibitors; GSH, glutathione; ALA, alpha-lipoic acid; CuZnSOD, Cu/Zn-superoxide dismutase; CAT, catalase; HSP, heat shock proteins. Up arrow represents up-regulation, Down arrow represents down-regulation.

The positive cardiovascular and metabolic effects of angiotensin (Ang)-converting enzyme inhibitors (ACEIs) are mainly dependent on the reduction of AngII formation and the increase in the negatively regulated Ang 1-7 axis of the renin-angiotensin system (RAS) [127,128]. Some studies have shown that ACE/AngII/AT1 contributes to the occurrence and progression of NAFLD [129]. The activation of the ACE2/Ang-(1-7)/Mas axis ameliorates hepatic IR through the Akt/PI3K/IRS-1/JNK insulin signaling pathway [130]. Moreover, Ang1-7 contributes to the correction of diabetic retinopathy by reducing the O-GlcNAcylation of the retinal protein in HFD-fed mice through the Mas/EPAC/Rap1/OGT signaling axis [106]. Also, ACEI therapy has been shown to reduce the incidence of liver cancer and cirrhosis in NAFLD patients [107].

Acetaminophen (APAP) overdose is a common cause of acute liver failure (ALF) in North American and European countries [131,132]. The increase in the hepatic O-GlcNacylated protein leads to the dysregulation of the hepatic glutathione (GSH) supplement response and increases the APAP-induced hepatic injury, while reduced O-GlcNacylation causes rapid GSH replenishment and the subsequent inhibition of APAP-induced liver injury [133]. Increased hepatic O-GlcNacylation as a response to excessive APAP increases and delays JNK activation, which is correlated to pronounced liver damage [133]. Moreover, Chen et al. [108] displayed a positive correlation between O-GlcNacylated c-Jun and GSH synthesis in clinical liver cancer samples. The overexpression of O-GlcNAcylated c-Jun inhibits ferroptosis by inducing GSH synthesis and blocking c-Jun O-GlcNacylation, which is beneficial for the treatment of iron apoptosis-related HCC [108]. Also, oral GSH exhibits a therapeutic effect on NAFLD patients; however, the mechanisms are remained unknown [109].

Alpha-lipoic acid (ALA) protects the kidney from oxidative damage in diabetic rats by reducing the O-GlcNAcylation of ERK and p38 [110]. In another study, ALA slowed the development of diabetic complications and ensured the function and health of red blood cells by reducing the O-GlcNAcylation modification levels of antioxidant enzymes: CuZn-superoxide dismutase (SOD), CAT, heat shock protein (HSP) 70, and HSP 90 [111]. Furthermore, it confirmed that the O-GlcNAcylation of the thioredoxin interacting protein (TXNIP) activates the NLRP3 inflammasome by interacting with the NLRP3 [134]. In a clinical trial, ALA was demonstrated to improve IL-6 and serum adiponectin levels in NAFLD patients [135]. Recently, two studies showed that ALA attenuates hepatic triglyceride accumulation and NAFLD by inhibiting the NLRP3 inflammasome [112,113]. Whether ALA plays a crucial role in NAFLD by changing the total level of O-GlcNAcylation or directly reducing the O-GlcNAcylation of NLRP3 and the role of O-GlcNAcylation in NAFLD, although drugs such as ALA, GSH, and ACEI exert a protective effect through anti-inflammatory and antioxidant effects, are yet to be clarified.

Hitherto, the pharmacological treatment of NAFLD by directly inhibiting O-GlcNAc has rarely been studied. Lee et al., showed that curcumin regulates the expression of SIRT1 and SOD1 through O-GlcNAcylation signaling [19]. It also reduces hepatitis by blocking the HBP flux signaling pathway; the anti-inflammatory effect of curcumin was achieved by inhibiting O-GlcNAcylation and blocking the NF-κB signaling pathway [19]. Silibinin blocks the NF-κB signaling pathway by inhibiting O-GlcNAcylation and alleviates inflammation in NASH mice [18]. Therefore, additional drug studies are required to further explore the treatment of NAFLD/NASH by targeting O-GlcNAcylation.

6. Conclusions

In this study, elevated O-GlcNAcylation promoted the development and exacerbation of IR and was eventually involved in the progression of NAFL-NASH-cirrhosis-hepatoma tetralogy. In addition, the potential drugs targeted at O-GlcNAcylation in the NAFLD intervention were reviewed. Thus, elucidating the molecular mechanisms of O-GlcNAcylation provided additional strategies and ideas for preventing and treating NAFLD.

Author Contributions: Y.S. and P.Y.: study concept, design, methodology, and funding acquisition. Y.Z.: drafting of the manuscript, critical revision of the manuscript for important intellectual content, and validation. Z.L.: visualization, editing, and supervision. M.X., D.Z. and J.L.: acquisition of data, analysis, and interpretation of data. All authors have read and agreed to the published version of the manuscript.

Funding: This work was supported by the National Natural Science Foundation of China [grant number No.82160170 and No.81860151]; the National Key R&D Program of China, Synthetic Biology Research [No.2019YFA0904500]; the Key R&D Program of Jiangxi Province [No. 20192BBG70027]; the National Clinical Research Center for Geriatrics—JiangXi branch center [No. 2021ZDG02001]; [No. 20212BAB216047 and No. 202004BCJL23049], and the National Natural Science Foundation of China [grant number No. 82100869].

Acknowledgments: The graphical abstracts were created with BioRender software (BioRender.com).

Conflicts of Interest: The authors declare no conflict of interest.

Abbreviations

Ang	angiotensin
APAP	acetaminophen
ALF	acute liver failure
ALA	alpha-lipoic acid
ApoA5	apolipoprotein A5
ACC	acetyl-CoA carboxylase
AMP	adenosine monophosphate
AMPK	AMP-activated protein kinase
AKT	serine/threonine-protein kinase B
ACEI	Angiotensin-converting enzyme inhibitors
CAT	catalase
CRTC2	cAMP-regulated transcriptional co-activator 2
CREB	cyclic AMP-responsive element-binding protein
CREBH	cyclic AMP-responsive element-binding protein H
ChREBP	carbohydrate-responsive element-binding protein
DCM	diabetic cardiomyopathy
EMPA	empagliflozin
ER	endoplasmic reticulum
FAS	fatty acid synthase
FBPase	fructose-1,6-bisphosphatase
GSH	glutathione
GS	glycogen synthase
GLP-1	glucagon-like peptide-1
GSK3β	glycogen synthase kinase 3 beta
GFAT	glutamine fructose-6-phosphate amidotransferase
HCV	hepatitis C virus
HSP	heat shock protein
HCF-1	host cell factor C1
HSCs	hepatic stellate cells
HCD	high-carbohydrate diet
HCC	hepatocellular carcinoma
HBP	hexosamine biosynthetic pathway
IL	interleukin
IR	insulin resistance
IRS-1	insulin receptor substrate 1
IRE1α	inositol requiring enzyme 1α
IP6K1	inositol hexakisphosphate kinases 1
JNK	Jun N-terminal kinases

LXRs	liver X receptors
L-PK	liver pyruvate kinase
MET	metformin
MCD	methionine-choline deficient
mTOR	mammalian target of rapamycin
MnSOD	manganese superoxide dismutase
MAFLD	metabolic dysfunction-associated fatty liver disease
NASH	non-alcoholic steatohepatitis
NAFLD	non-alcoholic fatty liver disease
NLRP3	NLR family, pyrin domain containing 3
OGA	GlcNAcase
OGT	O-GlcNAc transferase
O-GlcNAc	O-linked β-N-acetylglucosamine
PI3K	phosphatidylinositol-3-kinase
PTP1B	protein tyrosine phosphatase 1B
PDGFRβ	platelet-derived growth factor receptor β
PDK1	phosphoinositide-dependent protein kinase 1
PGC1α	peroxisome proliferator-activated receptor-γ co-activator1α
ROS	reactive oxygen species
RAS	renin-angiotensin system
RIPK3	receptor-interacting protein kinase 3
SRF	serum response factor
SOD	superoxide dismutase
SCD1	stearoyl-CoA desaturase1
SGLT-2i	sodium-glucose cotransporter 2 inhibitor
SREBP-1	sterol regulatory element-binding protein 1
TG	thyroglobulin
TFF2	trefoil factor 2
T2DM	type 2 diabetes mellitus
TXNIP	thioredoxin interacting protein
XBP1	X-box-binding protein 1

References

1. Angulo, P. Nonalcoholic fatty liver disease. *N. Engl. J. Med.* **2002**, *346*, 1221–1231. [CrossRef] [PubMed]
2. Khamphaya, T.; Chukijrungroat, N.; Saengsirisuwan, V.; Mitchell-Richards, K.A.; Robert, M.E.; Mennone, A.; Ananthanarayanan, M.; Nathanson, M.H.; Weerachayaphorn, J. Nonalcoholic fatty liver disease impairs expression of the type II inositol 1,4,5-trisphosphate receptor. *Hepatology* **2018**, *67*, 560–574. [CrossRef] [PubMed]
3. Allen, A.M.; Therneau, T.M.; Larson, J.J.; Coward, A.; Somers, V.K.; Kamath, P.S. Nonalcoholic fatty liver disease incidence and impact on metabolic burden and death: A 20 year-community study. *Hepatology* **2018**, *67*, 1726–1736. [CrossRef] [PubMed]
4. Cotter, T.G.; Rinella, M. Nonalcoholic Fatty Liver Disease 2020: The State of the Disease. *Gastroenterology* **2020**, *158*, 1851–1864. [CrossRef] [PubMed]
5. Eslam, M.; Newsome, P.N.; Sarin, S.K.; Anstee, Q.M.; Targher, G.; Romero-Gomez, M.; Zelber-Sagi, S.; Wai-Sun Wong, V.; Dufour, J.F.; Schattenberg, J.M.; et al. A new definition for metabolic dysfunction-associated fatty liver disease: An international expert consensus statement. *J. Hepatol.* **2020**, *73*, 202–209. [CrossRef]
6. Gawrieh, S.; Marion, M.C.; Komorowski, R.; Wallace, J.; Charlton, M.; Kissebah, A.; Langefeld, C.D.; Olivier, M. Genetic variation in the peroxisome proliferator activated receptor-gamma gene is associated with histologically advanced NAFLD. *Dig. Dis. Sci.* **2012**, *57*, 952–957. [CrossRef]
7. Shao, M.; Ye, Z.; Qin, Y.; Wu, T. Abnormal metabolic processes involved in the pathogenesis of non-alcoholic fatty liver disease (Review). *Exp. Ther. Med.* **2020**, *20*, 26. [CrossRef]
8. Lim, J.S.; Mietus-Snyder, M.; Valente, A.; Schwarz, J.M.; Lustig, R.H. The role of fructose in the pathogenesis of NAFLD and the metabolic syndrome. *Nat. Rev. Gastroenterol. Hepatol.* **2010**, *7*, 251–264. [CrossRef]
9. Jensen, T.; Abdelmalek, M.F.; Sullivan, S.; Nadeau, K.J.; Green, M.; Roncal, C.; Nakagawa, T.; Kuwabara, M.; Sato, Y.; Kang, D.H.; et al. Fructose and sugar: A major mediator of non-alcoholic fatty liver disease. *J. Hepatol.* **2018**, *68*, 1063–1075. [CrossRef]
10. Browning, J.D.; Horton, J.D. Molecular mediators of hepatic steatosis and liver injury. *J. Clin. Investig.* **2004**, *114*, 147–152. [CrossRef]
11. Park, J.S.; Lee, D.H.; Lee, Y.S.; Oh, E.; Bae, K.H.; Oh, K.J.; Kim, H.; Bae, S.H. Dual roles of ULK1 (unc-51 like autophagy activating kinase 1) in cytoprotection against lipotoxicity. *Autophagy* **2020**, *16*, 86–105. [CrossRef]

12. Navarro, L.A.; Wree, A.; Povero, D.; Berk, M.P.; Eguchi, A.; Ghosh, S.; Papouchado, B.G.; Erzurum, S.C.; Feldstein, A.E. Arginase 2 deficiency results in spontaneous steatohepatitis: A novel link between innate immune activation and hepatic de novo lipogenesis. *J. Hepatol.* **2015**, *62*, 412–420. [CrossRef]
13. Kim, S.H.; Kim, G.; Han, D.H.; Lee, M.; Kim, I.; Kim, B.; Kim, K.H.; Song, Y.M.; Yoo, J.E.; Wang, H.J.; et al. Ezetimibe ameliorates steatohepatitis via AMP activated protein kinase-TFEB-mediated activation of autophagy and NLRP3 inflammasome inhibition. *Autophagy* **2017**, *13*, 1767–1781. [CrossRef]
14. Lin, Y.; Zhu, J.; Pan, L.; Zhang, J.; Tan, Z.; Olivares, J.; Singal, A.G.; Parikh, N.D.; Lubman, D.M. A Panel of Glycopeptides as Candidate Biomarkers for Early Diagnosis of NASH Hepatocellular Carcinoma Using a Stepped HCD Method and PRM Evaluation. *J. Proteome Res.* **2021**, *20*, 3278–3289. [CrossRef]
15. Zhang, N.; Wang, Y.; Zhang, J.; Liu, B.; Deng, X.; Xin, S.; Xu, K. N-glycosylation of CREBH improves lipid metabolism and attenuates lipotoxicity in NAFLD by modulating PPARalpha and SCD-1. *FASEB J.* **2020**, *34*, 15338–15363. [CrossRef]
16. Zhang, K.; Yin, R.; Yang, X. O-GlcNAc: A Bittersweet Switch in Liver. *Front. Endocrinol.* **2014**, *5*, 221. [CrossRef]
17. Mukherjee, S.; Chakraborty, M.; Ulmasov, B.; McCommis, K.; Zhang, J.; Carpenter, D.; Msengi, E.N.; Haubner, J.; Guo, C.; Pike, D.P.; et al. Pleiotropic actions of IP6K1 mediate hepatic metabolic dysfunction to promote nonalcoholic fatty liver disease and steatohepatitis. *Mol. Metab.* **2021**, *54*, 101364. [CrossRef]
18. Lee, S.J.; Nam, M.J.; Lee, D.E.; Park, J.W.; Kang, B.S.; Lee, D.S.; Lee, H.S.; Kwon, O.S. Silibinin Ameliorates O-GlcNAcylation and Inflammation in a Mouse Model of Nonalcoholic Steatohepatitis. *Int. J. Mol. Sci.* **2018**, *19*, 2165. [CrossRef]
19. Lee, D.E.; Lee, S.J.; Kim, S.J.; Lee, H.S.; Kwon, O.S. Curcumin Ameliorates Nonalcoholic Fatty Liver Disease through Inhibition of O-GlcNAcylation. *Nutrients* **2019**, *11*, 2702. [CrossRef]
20. Prakoso, D.; Lim, S.Y.; Erickson, J.R.; Wallace, R.S.; Lees, J.G.; Tate, M.; Kiriazis, H.; Donner, D.G.; Henstridge, D.C.; Davey, J.R.; et al. Fine-tuning the cardiac O-GlcNAcylation regulatory enzymes governs the functional and structural phenotype of the diabetic heart. *Cardiovasc. Res.* **2022**, *118*, 212–225. [CrossRef]
21. Qin, L.; Wang, J.; Zhao, R.; Zhang, X.; Mei, Y. Ginsenoside-Rb1 Improved Diabetic Cardiomyopathy through Regulating Calcium Signaling by Alleviating Protein O-GlcNAcylation. *J. Agric. Food Chem.* **2019**, *67*, 14074–14085. [CrossRef] [PubMed]
22. Olivier-Van Stichelen, S.; Hanover, J.A. You are what you eat: O-linked N-acetylglucosamine in disease, development and epigenetics. *Curr. Opin. Clin. Nutr. Metab. Care* **2015**, *18*, 339–345. [CrossRef] [PubMed]
23. Peterson, S.B.; Hart, G.W. New insights: A role for O-GlcNAcylation in diabetic complications. *Crit. Rev. Biochem. Mol. Biol.* **2016**, *51*, 150–161. [CrossRef] [PubMed]
24. Wright, J.N.; Collins, H.E.; Wende, A.R.; Chatham, J.C. O-GlcNAcylation and cardiovascular disease. *Biochem. Soc. Trans.* **2017**, *45*, 545–553. [CrossRef]
25. Bond, M.R.; Hanover, J.A. A little sugar goes a long way: The cell biology of O-GlcNAc. *J. Cell Biol.* **2015**, *208*, 869–880. [CrossRef]
26. Hardiville, S.; Hart, G.W. Nutrient regulation of gene expression by O-GlcNAcylation of chromatin. *Curr. Opin. Chem. Biol.* **2016**, *33*, 88–94. [CrossRef]
27. Yang, X.; Qian, K. Protein O-GlcNAcylation: Emerging mechanisms and functions. *Nat. Rev. Mol. Cell Biol.* **2017**, *18*, 452–465. [CrossRef]
28. Pekkurnaz, G.; Trinidad, J.C.; Wang, X.; Kong, D.; Schwarz, T.L. Glucose regulates mitochondrial motility via Milton modification by O-GlcNAc transferase. *Cell* **2014**, *158*, 54–68. [CrossRef]
29. Hart, G.W. Dynamic O-linked glycosylation of nuclear and cytoskeletal proteins. *Annu. Rev. Biochem.* **1997**, *66*, 315–335. [CrossRef]
30. Kaasik, K.; Kivimae, S.; Allen, J.J.; Chalkley, R.J.; Huang, Y.; Baer, K.; Kissel, H.; Burlingame, A.L.; Shokat, K.M.; Ptacek, L.J.; et al. Glucose sensor O-GlcNAcylation coordinates with phosphorylation to regulate circadian clock. *Cell Metab.* **2013**, *17*, 291–302. [CrossRef]
31. Li, M.D.; Ruan, H.B.; Hughes, M.E.; Lee, J.S.; Singh, J.P.; Jones, S.P.; Nitabach, M.N.; Yang, X. O-GlcNAc signaling entrains the circadian clock by inhibiting BMAL1/CLOCK ubiquitination. *Cell Metab.* **2013**, *17*, 303–310. [CrossRef] [PubMed]
32. Housley, M.P.; Udeshi, N.D.; Rodgers, J.T.; Shabanowitz, J.; Puigserver, P.; Hunt, D.F.; Hart, G.W. A PGC-1alpha-O-GlcNAc transferase complex regulates FoxO transcription factor activity in response to glucose. *J. Biol. Chem.* **2009**, *284*, 5148–5157. [CrossRef] [PubMed]
33. Housley, M.P.; Rodgers, J.T.; Udeshi, N.D.; Kelly, T.J.; Shabanowitz, J.; Hunt, D.F.; Puigserver, P.; Hart, G.W. O-GlcNAc regulates FoxO activation in response to glucose. *J. Biol. Chem.* **2008**, *283*, 16283–16292. [CrossRef] [PubMed]
34. Ruan, H.B.; Han, X.; Li, M.D.; Singh, J.P.; Qian, K.; Azarhoush, S.; Zhao, L.; Bennett, A.M.; Samuel, V.T.; Wu, J.; et al. O-GlcNAc transferase/host cell factor C1 complex regulates gluconeogenesis by modulating PGC-1alpha stability. *Cell Metab.* **2012**, *16*, 226–237. [CrossRef] [PubMed]
35. Herzig, S.; Long, F.; Jhala, U.S.; Hedrick, S.; Quinn, R.; Bauer, A.; Rudolph, D.; Schutz, G.; Yoon, C.; Puigserver, P.; et al. CREB regulates hepatic gluconeogenesis through the coactivator PGC-1. *Nature* **2001**, *413*, 179–183. [CrossRef] [PubMed]
36. Dominy, J.E., Jr.; Lee, Y.; Jedrychowski, M.P.; Chim, H.; Jurczak, M.J.; Camporez, J.P.; Ruan, H.B.; Feldman, J.; Pierce, K.; Mostoslavsky, R.; et al. The deacetylase Sirt6 activates the acetyltransferase GCN5 and suppresses hepatic gluconeogenesis. *Mol. Cell* **2012**, *48*, 900–913. [CrossRef]
37. Wu, Z.; Jiao, P.; Huang, X.; Feng, B.; Feng, Y.; Yang, S.; Hwang, P.; Du, J.; Nie, Y.; Xiao, G.; et al. MAPK phosphatase-3 promotes hepatic gluconeogenesis through dephosphorylation of forkhead box O1 in mice. *J. Clin. Investig.* **2010**, *120*, 3901–3911. [CrossRef]

38. Dentin, R.; Hedrick, S.; Xie, J.; Yates, J., 3rd; Montminy, M. Hepatic glucose sensing via the CREB coactivator CRTC2. *Science* **2008**, *319*, 1402–1405. [CrossRef]
39. Li, M.D.; Ruan, H.B.; Singh, J.P.; Zhao, L.; Zhao, T.; Azarhoush, S.; Wu, J.; Evans, R.M.; Yang, X. O-GlcNAc transferase is involved in glucocorticoid receptor-mediated transrepression. *J. Biol. Chem.* **2012**, *287*, 12904–12912. [CrossRef]
40. Efeyan, A.; Serrano, M. p53: Guardian of the genome and policeman of the oncogenes. *Cell Cycle* **2007**, *6*, 1006–1010. [CrossRef]
41. Gonzalez-Rellan, M.J.; Fondevila, M.F.; Fernandez, U.; Rodriguez, A.; Varela-Rey, M.; Veyrat-Durebex, C.; Seoane, S.; Bernardo, G.; Lopitz-Otsoa, F.; Fernandez-Ramos, D.; et al. O-GlcNAcylated p53 in the liver modulates hepatic glucose production. *Nat. Commun.* **2021**, *12*, 5068. [CrossRef]
42. Anthonisen, E.H.; Berven, L.; Holm, S.; Nygard, M.; Nebb, H.I.; Gronning-Wang, L.M. Nuclear receptor liver X receptor is O-GlcNAc-modified in response to glucose. *J. Biol. Chem.* **2010**, *285*, 1607–1615. [CrossRef]
43. Sodi, V.L.; Bacigalupa, Z.A.; Ferrer, C.M.; Lee, J.V.; Gocal, W.A.; Mukhopadhyay, D.; Wellen, K.E.; Ivan, M.; Reginato, M.J. Nutrient sensor O-GlcNAc transferase controls cancer lipid metabolism via SREBP-1 regulation. *Oncogene* **2018**, *37*, 924–934. [CrossRef]
44. Guinez, C.; Filhoulaud, G.; Rayah-Benhamed, F.; Marmier, S.; Dubuquoy, C.; Dentin, R.; Moldes, M.; Burnol, A.F.; Yang, X.; Lefebvre, T.; et al. O-GlcNAcylation increases ChREBP protein content and transcriptional activity in the liver. *Diabetes* **2011**, *60*, 1399–1413. [CrossRef]
45. Robarts, D.R.; McGreal, S.R.; Umbaugh, D.S.; Parkes, W.S.; Kotulkar, M.; Abernathy, S.; Lee, N.; Jaeschke, H.; Gunewardena, S.; Whelan, S.A.; et al. Regulation of Liver Regeneration by Hepatocyte O-GlcNAcylation in Mice. *Cell. Mol. Gastroenterol. Hepatol.* **2022**, *13*, 1510–1529. [CrossRef]
46. Ruan, H.B.; Ma, Y.; Torres, S.; Zhang, B.; Feriod, C.; Heck, R.M.; Qian, K.; Fu, M.; Li, X.; Nathanson, M.H.; et al. Calcium-dependent O-GlcNAc signaling drives liver autophagy in adaptation to starvation. *Genes Dev.* **2017**, *31*, 1655–1665. [CrossRef]
47. Tan, E.P.; McGreal, S.R.; Graw, S.; Tessman, R.; Koppel, S.J.; Dhakal, P.; Zhang, Z.; Machacek, M.; Zachara, N.E.; Koestler, D.C.; et al. Sustained O-GlcNAcylation reprograms mitochondrial function to regulate energy metabolism. *J. Biol. Chem.* **2017**, *292*, 14940–14962. [CrossRef]
48. Wang, X.; Lin, Y.; Liu, S.; Zhu, Y.; Lu, K.; Broering, R.; Lu, M. O-GlcNAcylation modulates HBV replication through regulating cellular autophagy at multiple levels. *FASEB J.* **2020**, *34*, 14473–14489. [CrossRef]
49. Tolman, K.G.; Fonseca, V.; Dalpiaz, A.; Tan, M.H. Spectrum of liver disease in type 2 diabetes and management of patients with diabetes and liver disease. *Diabetes Care* **2007**, *30*, 734–743. [CrossRef]
50. Choudhury, J.; Sanyal, A.J. Insulin resistance and the pathogenesis of nonalcoholic fatty liver disease. *Clin. Liver Dis.* **2004**, *8*, 575–594. [CrossRef]
51. Bugianesi, E.; McCullough, A.J.; Marchesini, G. Insulin resistance: A metabolic pathway to chronic liver disease. *Hepatology* **2005**, *42*, 987–1000. [CrossRef] [PubMed]
52. Friedman, S.L.; Neuschwander-Tetri, B.A.; Rinella, M.; Sanyal, A.J. Mechanisms of NAFLD development and therapeutic strategies. *Nat. Med.* **2018**, *24*, 908–922. [CrossRef] [PubMed]
53. Schuster, S.; Cabrera, D.; Arrese, M.; Feldstein, A.E. Triggering and resolution of inflammation in NASH. *Nat. Rev. Gastroenterol. Hepatol.* **2018**, *15*, 349–364. [CrossRef] [PubMed]
54. Whelan, S.A.; Dias, W.B.; Thiruneelakantapillai, L.; Lane, M.D.; Hart, G.W. Regulation of insulin receptor substrate 1 (IRS-1)/AKT kinase-mediated insulin signaling by O-Linked beta-N-acetylglucosamine in 3T3-L1 adipocytes. *J. Biol. Chem.* **2010**, *285*, 5204–5211. [CrossRef] [PubMed]
55. Whelan, S.A.; Lane, M.D.; Hart, G.W. Regulation of the O-linked beta-N-acetylglucosamine transferase by insulin signaling. *J. Biol. Chem.* **2008**, *283*, 21411–21417. [CrossRef]
56. Wang, S.; Huang, X.; Sun, D.; Xin, X.; Pan, Q.; Peng, S.; Liang, Z.; Luo, C.; Yang, Y.; Jiang, H.; et al. Extensive crosstalk between O-GlcNAcylation and phosphorylation regulates Akt signaling. *PLoS ONE* **2012**, *7*, e37427. [CrossRef]
57. Wang, Z.; Pandey, A.; Hart, G.W. Dynamic interplay between O-linked N-acetylglucosaminylation and glycogen synthase kinase-3-dependent phosphorylation. *Mol. Cell. Proteom.* **2007**, *6*, 1365–1379. [CrossRef]
58. Zhao, Y.; Tang, Z.; Shen, A.; Tao, T.; Wan, C.; Zhu, X.; Huang, J.; Zhang, W.; Xia, N.; Wang, S.; et al. The Role of PTP1B O-GlcNAcylation in Hepatic Insulin Resistance. *Int. J. Mol. Sci.* **2015**, *16*, 22856–22869. [CrossRef]
59. Parker, G.J.; Lund, K.C.; Taylor, R.P.; McClain, D.A. Insulin resistance of glycogen synthase mediated by o-linked N-acetylglucosamine. *J. Biol. Chem.* **2003**, *278*, 10022–10027. [CrossRef]
60. Yang, W.H.; Park, S.Y.; Nam, H.W.; Kim, D.H.; Kang, J.G.; Kang, E.S.; Kim, Y.S.; Lee, H.C.; Kim, K.S.; Cho, J.W. NFkappaB activation is associated with its O-GlcNAcylation state under hyperglycemic conditions. *Proc. Natl. Acad. Sci. USA* **2008**, *105*, 17345–17350. [CrossRef]
61. Ramakrishnan, P.; Clark, P.M.; Mason, D.E.; Peters, E.C.; Hsieh-Wilson, L.C.; Baltimore, D. Activation of the transcriptional function of the NF-kappaB protein c-Rel by O-GlcNAc glycosylation. *Sci. Signal.* **2013**, *6*, ra75. [CrossRef]
62. Fan, X.; Chuan, S.; Hongshan, W. Protein O glycosylation regulates activation of hepatic stellate cells. *Inflammation* **2013**, *36*, 1248–1252. [CrossRef]
63. Li, R.; Ong, Q.; Wong, C.C.; Chu, E.S.H.; Sung, J.J.Y.; Yang, X.; Yu, J. O-GlcNAcylation inhibits hepatic stellate cell activation. *J. Gastroenterol. Hepatol.* **2021**, *36*, 3477–3486. [CrossRef]

64. Vucur, M.; Reisinger, F.; Gautheron, J.; Janssen, J.; Roderburg, C.; Cardenas, D.V.; Kreggenwinkel, K.; Koppe, C.; Hammerich, L.; Hakem, R.; et al. RIP3 inhibits inflammatory hepatocarcinogenesis but promotes cholestasis by controlling caspase-8- and JNK-dependent compensatory cell proliferation. *Cell Rep.* **2013**, *4*, 776–790. [CrossRef]
65. Zhang, B.; Li, M.D.; Yin, R.; Liu, Y.; Yang, Y.; Mitchell-Richards, K.A.; Nam, J.H.; Li, R.; Wang, L.; Iwakiri, Y.; et al. O-GlcNAc transferase suppresses necroptosis and liver fibrosis. *JCI Insight* **2019**, *4*, e127709. [CrossRef]
66. Dentin, R.; Benhamed, F.; Hainault, I.; Fauveau, V.; Foufelle, F.; Dyck, J.R.; Girard, J.; Postic, C. Liver-specific inhibition of ChREBP improves hepatic steatosis and insulin resistance in ob/ob mice. *Diabetes* **2006**, *55*, 2159–2170. [CrossRef]
67. Lane, E.A.; Choi, D.W.; Garcia-Haro, L.; Levine, Z.G.; Tedoldi, M.; Walker, S.; Danial, N.N. HCF-1 Regulates De Novo Lipogenesis through a Nutrient-Sensitive Complex with ChREBP. *Mol. Cell* **2019**, *75*, 357–371.e7. [CrossRef]
68. Horton, J.D.; Goldstein, J.L.; Brown, M.S. SREBPs: Activators of the complete program of cholesterol and fatty acid synthesis in the liver. *J. Clin. Investig.* **2002**, *109*, 1125–1131. [CrossRef]
69. Kawano, Y.; Cohen, D.E. Mechanisms of hepatic triglyceride accumulation in non-alcoholic fatty liver disease. *J. Gastroenterol.* **2013**, *48*, 434–441. [CrossRef]
70. Knebel, B.; Haas, J.; Hartwig, S.; Jacob, S.; Kollmer, C.; Nitzgen, U.; Muller-Wieland, D.; Kotzka, J. Liver-specific expression of transcriptionally active SREBP-1c is associated with fatty liver and increased visceral fat mass. *PLoS ONE* **2012**, *7*, e31812. [CrossRef]
71. Gorgani-Firuzjaee, S.; Meshkani, R. SH2 domain-containing inositol 5-phosphatase (SHIP2) inhibition ameliorates high glucose-induced de-novo lipogenesis and VLDL production through regulating AMPK/mTOR/SREBP1 pathway and ROS production in HepG2 cells. *Free Radic. Biol. Med.* **2015**, *89*, 679–689. [CrossRef] [PubMed]
72. Sage, A.T.; Walter, L.A.; Shi, Y.; Khan, M.I.; Kaneto, H.; Capretta, A.; Werstuck, G.H. Hexosamine biosynthesis pathway flux promotes endoplasmic reticulum stress, lipid accumulation, and inflammatory gene expression in hepatic cells. *Am. J. Physiol. Endocrinol. Metab.* **2010**, *298*, E499–E511. [CrossRef] [PubMed]
73. Park, J.; Lee, Y.; Jung, E.H.; Kim, S.M.; Cho, H.; Han, I.O. Glucosamine regulates hepatic lipid accumulation by sensing glucose levels or feeding states of normal and excess. *Biochim. Biophys. Acta Mol. Cell Biol. Lipids* **2020**, *1865*, 158764. [CrossRef] [PubMed]
74. Kleiner, D.E.; Brunt, E.M.; Van Natta, M.; Behling, C.; Contos, M.J.; Cummings, O.W.; Ferrell, L.D.; Liu, Y.C.; Torbenson, M.S.; Unalp-Arida, A.; et al. Design and validation of a histological scoring system for nonalcoholic fatty liver disease. *Hepatology* **2005**, *41*, 1313–1321. [CrossRef] [PubMed]
75. Elsharkawy, A.M.; Mann, D.A. Nuclear factor-kappaB and the hepatic inflammation-fibrosis-cancer axis. *Hepatology* **2007**, *46*, 590–597. [CrossRef]
76. Malhi, H.; Kaufman, R.J. Endoplasmic reticulum stress in liver disease. *J. Hepatol.* **2011**, *54*, 795–809. [CrossRef]
77. Lake, A.D.; Novak, P.; Hardwick, R.N.; Flores-Keown, B.; Zhao, F.; Klimecki, W.T.; Cherrington, N.J. The adaptive endoplasmic reticulum stress response to lipotoxicity in progressive human nonalcoholic fatty liver disease. *Toxicol. Sci.* **2014**, *137*, 26–35. [CrossRef]
78. Baudoin, L.; Issad, T. O-GlcNAcylation and Inflammation: A Vast Territory to Explore. *Front. Endocrinol.* **2014**, *5*, 235. [CrossRef]
79. Ron, D.; Walter, P. Signal integration in the endoplasmic reticulum unfolded protein response. *Nat. Rev. Mol. Cell Biol.* **2007**, *8*, 519–529. [CrossRef]
80. Ni, M.; Zhang, Y.; Lee, A.S. Beyond the endoplasmic reticulum: Atypical GRP78 in cell viability, signalling and therapeutic targeting. *Biochem. J.* **2011**, *434*, 181–188. [CrossRef]
81. Ngoh, G.A.; Hamid, T.; Prabhu, S.D.; Jones, S.P. O-GlcNAc signaling attenuates ER stress-induced cardiomyocyte death. *Am. J. Physiol. Heart Circ. Physiol.* **2009**, *297*, H1711–H1719. [CrossRef]
82. So, J.S.; Hur, K.Y.; Tarrio, M.; Ruda, V.; Frank-Kamenetsky, M.; Fitzgerald, K.; Koteliansky, V.; Lichtman, A.H.; Iwawaki, T.; Glimcher, L.H.; et al. Silencing of lipid metabolism genes through IRE1alpha-mediated mRNA decay lowers plasma lipids in mice. *Cell Metab.* **2012**, *16*, 487–499. [CrossRef]
83. Kim, I.; Xu, W.; Reed, J.C. Cell death and endoplasmic reticulum stress: Disease relevance and therapeutic opportunities. *Nat. Rev. Drug Discov.* **2008**, *7*, 1013–1030. [CrossRef]
84. Visinoni, S.; Khalid, N.F.; Joannides, C.N.; Shulkes, A.; Yim, M.; Whitehead, J.; Tiganis, T.; Lamont, B.J.; Favaloro, J.M.; Proietto, J.; et al. The role of liver fructose-1,6-bisphosphatase in regulating appetite and adiposity. *Diabetes* **2012**, *61*, 1122–1132. [CrossRef]
85. Dulai, P.S.; Singh, S.; Patel, J.; Soni, M.; Prokop, L.J.; Younossi, Z.; Sebastiani, G.; Ekstedt, M.; Hagstrom, H.; Nasr, P.; et al. Increased risk of mortality by fibrosis stage in nonalcoholic fatty liver disease: Systematic review and meta-analysis. *Hepatology* **2017**, *65*, 1557–1565. [CrossRef]
86. Hui, J.M.; Kench, J.G.; Chitturi, S.; Sud, A.; Farrell, G.C.; Byth, K.; Hall, P.; Khan, M.; George, J. Long-term outcomes of cirrhosis in nonalcoholic steatohepatitis compared with hepatitis C. *Hepatology* **2003**, *38*, 420–427. [CrossRef]
87. Pinzani, M.; Rombouts, K. Liver fibrosis: From the bench to clinical targets. *Dig. Liver Dis.* **2004**, *36*, 231–242. [CrossRef]
88. Adachi, M.; Osawa, Y.; Uchinami, H.; Kitamura, T.; Accili, D.; Brenner, D.A. The forkhead transcription factor FoxO1 regulates proliferation and transdifferentiation of hepatic stellate cells. *Gastroenterology* **2007**, *132*, 1434–1446. [CrossRef]
89. Valenti, L.; Rametta, R.; Dongiovanni, P.; Maggioni, M.; Fracanzani, A.L.; Zappa, M.; Lattuada, E.; Roviaro, G.; Fargion, S. Increased expression and activity of the transcription factor FOXO1 in nonalcoholic steatohepatitis. *Diabetes* **2008**, *57*, 1355–1362. [CrossRef]

90. Zhang, B.; Lapenta, K.; Wang, Q.; Nam, J.H.; Chung, D.; Robert, M.E.; Nathanson, M.H.; Yang, X. Trefoil factor 2 secreted from damaged hepatocytes activates hepatic stellate cells to induce fibrogenesis. *J. Biol. Chem.* **2021**, *297*, 100887. [CrossRef]
91. Paik, J.M.; Golabi, P.; Younossi, Y.; Mishra, A.; Younossi, Z.M. Changes in the Global Burden of Chronic Liver Diseases from 2012 to 2017: The Growing Impact of NAFLD. *Hepatology* **2020**, *72*, 1605–1616. [CrossRef] [PubMed]
92. Wong, R.J.; Cheung, R.; Ahmed, A. Nonalcoholic steatohepatitis is the most rapidly growing indication for liver transplantation in patients with hepatocellular carcinoma in the U.S. *Hepatology* **2014**, *59*, 2188–2195. [CrossRef] [PubMed]
93. Xu, W.; Zhang, X.; Wu, J.L.; Fu, L.; Liu, K.; Liu, D.; Chen, G.G.; Lai, P.B.; Wong, N.; Yu, J. O-GlcNAc transferase promotes fatty liver-associated liver cancer through inducing palmitic acid and activating endoplasmic reticulum stress. *J. Hepatol.* **2017**, *67*, 310–320. [CrossRef] [PubMed]
94. Gautheron, J.; Vucur, M.; Reisinger, F.; Cardenas, D.V.; Roderburg, C.; Koppe, C.; Kreggenwinkel, K.; Schneider, A.T.; Bartneck, M.; Neumann, U.P.; et al. A positive feedback loop between RIP3 and JNK controls non-alcoholic steatohepatitis. *EMBO Mol. Med.* **2014**, *6*, 1062–1074. [CrossRef] [PubMed]
95. Krawczyk, M.; Jimenez-Aguero, R.; Alustiza, J.M.; Emparanza, J.I.; Perugorria, M.J.; Bujanda, L.; Lammert, F.; Banales, J.M. PNPLA3 p.I148M variant is associated with greater reduction of liver fat content after bariatric surgery. *Surg. Obes. Relat. Dis.* **2016**, *12*, 1838–1846. [CrossRef]
96. Miyaaki, H.; Nakao, K. Significance of genetic polymorphisms in patients with nonalcoholic fatty liver disease. *Clin. J. Gastroenterol.* **2017**, *10*, 201–207. [CrossRef]
97. Kim, M.Y.; Kim, Y.S.; Kim, M.; Choi, M.Y.; Roh, G.S.; Lee, D.H.; Kim, H.J.; Kang, S.S.; Cho, G.J.; Shin, J.K.; et al. Metformin inhibits cervical cancer cell proliferation via decreased AMPK O-GlcNAcylation. *Anim. Cells Syst.* **2019**, *23*, 302–309. [CrossRef]
98. Kim, Y.S.; Kim, M.; Choi, M.Y.; Lee, D.H.; Roh, G.S.; Kim, H.J.; Kang, S.S.; Cho, G.J.; Kim, S.J.; Yoo, J.M.; et al. Metformin protects against retinal cell death in diabetic mice. *Biochem. Biophys. Res. Commun.* **2017**, *492*, 397–403. [CrossRef]
99. Barbero-Becerra, V.J.; Santiago-Hernandez, J.J.; Villegas-Lopez, F.A.; Mendez-Sanchez, N.; Uribe, M.; Chavez-Tapia, N.C. Mechanisms involved in the protective effects of metformin against nonalcoholic fatty liver disease. *Curr. Med. Chem.* **2012**, *19*, 2918–2923. [CrossRef]
100. Pang, Y.; Xu, X.; Xiang, X.; Li, Y.; Zhao, Z.; Li, J.; Gao, S.; Liu, Q.; Mai, K.; Ai, Q. High Fat Activates O-GlcNAcylation and Affects AMPK/ACC Pathway to Regulate Lipid Metabolism. *Nutrients* **2021**, *13*, 1740. [CrossRef]
101. Lin, M.J.; Dai, W.; Scott, M.J.; Li, R.; Zhang, Y.Q.; Yang, Y.; Chen, L.Z.; Huang, X.S. Metformin improves nonalcoholic fatty liver disease in obese mice via down-regulation of apolipoprotein A5 as part of the AMPK/LXRalpha signaling pathway. *Oncotarget* **2017**, *8*, 108802–108809. [CrossRef]
102. Levine, P.M.; Balana, A.T.; Sturchler, E.; Koole, C.; Noda, H.; Zarzycka, B.; Daley, E.J.; Truong, T.T.; Katritch, V.; Gardella, T.J.; et al. O-GlcNAc Engineering of GPCR Peptide-Agonists Improves Their Stability and in Vivo Activity. *J. Am. Chem. Soc.* **2019**, *141*, 14210–14219. [CrossRef]
103. Cusi, K. Incretin-Based Therapies for the Management of Nonalcoholic Fatty Liver Disease in Patients with Type 2 Diabetes. *Hepatology* **2019**, *69*, 2318–2322. [CrossRef]
104. Hodrea, J.; Balogh, D.B.; Hosszu, A.; Lenart, L.; Besztercei, B.; Koszegi, S.; Sparding, N.; Genovese, F.; Wagner, L.J.; Szabo, A.J.; et al. Reduced O-GlcNAcylation and tubular hypoxia contribute to the antifibrotic effect of SGLT2 inhibitor dapagliflozin in the diabetic kidney. *Am. J. Physiol. Ren. Physiol.* **2020**, *318*, F1017–F1029. [CrossRef]
105. Akuta, N.; Watanabe, C.; Kawamura, Y.; Arase, Y.; Saitoh, S.; Fujiyama, S.; Sezaki, H.; Hosaka, T.; Kobayashi, M.; Kobayashi, M.; et al. Effects of a sodium-glucose cotransporter 2 inhibitor in nonalcoholic fatty liver disease complicated by diabetes mellitus: Preliminary prospective study based on serial liver biopsies. *Hepatol. Commun.* **2017**, *1*, 46–52. [CrossRef]
106. Dierschke, S.K.; Toro, A.L.; Barber, A.J.; Arnold, A.C.; Dennis, M.D. Angiotensin-(1-7) Attenuates Protein O-GlcNAcylation in the Retina by EPAC/Rap1-Dependent Inhibition of O-GlcNAc Transferase. *Investig. Ophthalmol. Vis. Sci.* **2020**, *61*, 24. [CrossRef]
107. Zhang, X.; Wong, G.L.; Yip, T.C.; Tse, Y.K.; Liang, L.Y.; Hui, V.W.; Lin, H.; Li, G.L.; Lai, J.C.; Chan, H.L.; et al. Angiotensin-converting enzyme inhibitors prevent liver-related events in nonalcoholic fatty liver disease. *Hepatology* **2022**, *76*, 469–482. [CrossRef]
108. Chen, Y.; Zhu, G.; Liu, Y.; Wu, Q.; Zhang, X.; Bian, Z.; Zhang, Y.; Pan, Q.; Sun, F. O-GlcNAcylated c-Jun antagonizes ferroptosis via inhibiting GSH synthesis in liver cancer. *Cell Signal.* **2019**, *63*, 109384. [CrossRef]
109. Honda, Y.; Kessoku, T.; Sumida, Y.; Kobayashi, T.; Kato, T.; Ogawa, Y.; Tomeno, W.; Imajo, K.; Fujita, K.; Yoneda, M.; et al. Efficacy of glutathione for the treatment of nonalcoholic fatty liver disease: An open-label, single-arm, multicenter, pilot study. *BMC Gastroenterol.* **2017**, *17*, 96. [CrossRef]
110. Arambasic, J.; Mihailovic, M.; Uskokovic, A.; Dinic, S.; Grdovic, N.; Markovic, J.; Poznanovic, G.; Bajec, D.; Vidakovic, M. Alpha-lipoic acid upregulates antioxidant enzyme gene expression and enzymatic activity in diabetic rat kidneys through an O-GlcNAc-dependent mechanism. *Eur. J. Nutr.* **2013**, *52*, 1461–1473. [CrossRef]
111. Mirjana, M.; Jelena, A.; Aleksandra, U.; Svetlana, D.; Nevena, G.; Jelena, M.; Goran, P.; Melita, V. Alpha-lipoic acid preserves the structural and functional integrity of red blood cells by adjusting the redox disturbance and decreasing O-GlcNAc modifications of antioxidant enzymes and heat shock proteins in diabetic rats. *Eur. J. Nutr.* **2012**, *51*, 975–986. [CrossRef] [PubMed]
112. Ko, C.Y.; Lo, Y.M.; Xu, J.H.; Chang, W.C.; Huang, D.W.; Wu, J.S.; Yang, C.H.; Huang, W.C.; Shen, S.C. Alpha-lipoic acid alleviates NAFLD and triglyceride accumulation in liver via modulating hepatic NLRP3 inflammasome activation pathway in type 2 diabetic rats. *Food Sci. Nutr.* **2021**, *9*, 2733–2742. [CrossRef] [PubMed]

113. Rahmanabadi, A.; Mahboob, S.; Amirkhizi, F.; Hosseinpour-Arjmand, S.; Ebrahimi-Mameghani, M. Oral alpha-lipoic acid supplementation in patients with non-alcoholic fatty liver disease: Effects on adipokines and liver histology features. *Food Funct.* **2019**, *10*, 4941–4952. [CrossRef] [PubMed]
114. Armstrong, M.J.; Gaunt, P.; Aithal, G.P.; Barton, D.; Hull, D.; Parker, R.; Hazlehurst, J.M.; Guo, K.; LEAN Trial Team; Abouda, G.; et al. Liraglutide safety and efficacy in patients with non-alcoholic steatohepatitis (LEAN): A multicentre, double-blind, randomised, placebo-controlled phase 2 study. *Lancet* **2016**, *387*, 679–690. [CrossRef]
115. Newsome, P.N.; Buchholtz, K.; Cusi, K.; Linder, M.; Okanoue, T.; Ratziu, V.; Sanyal, A.J.; Sejling, A.S.; Harrison, S.A.; Investigators, N.N. A Placebo-Controlled Trial of Subcutaneous Semaglutide in Nonalcoholic Steatohepatitis. *N. Engl. J. Med.* **2021**, *384*, 1113–1124. [CrossRef]
116. Yu, X.; Hao, M.; Liu, Y.; Ma, X.; Lin, W.; Xu, Q.; Zhou, H.; Shao, N.; Kuang, H. Liraglutide ameliorates non-alcoholic steatohepatitis by inhibiting NLRP3 inflammasome and pyroptosis activation via mitophagy. *Eur. J. Pharmacol.* **2019**, *864*, 172715. [CrossRef]
117. Goldberg, H.; Whiteside, C.; Fantus, I.G. O-linked beta-N-acetylglucosamine supports p38 MAPK activation by high glucose in glomerular mesangial cells. *Am. J. Physiol. Endocrinol. Metab.* **2011**, *301*, E713–E726. [CrossRef]
118. Park, M.J.; Kim, D.I.; Lim, S.K.; Choi, J.H.; Han, H.J.; Yoon, K.C.; Park, S.H. High glucose-induced O-GlcNAcylated carbohydrate response element-binding protein (ChREBP) mediates mesangial cell lipogenesis and fibrosis: The possible role in the development of diabetic nephropathy. *J. Biol. Chem.* **2014**, *289*, 13519–13530. [CrossRef]
119. Nakano, S.; Katsuno, K.; Isaji, M.; Nagasawa, T.; Buehrer, B.; Walker, S.; Wilkison, W.O.; Cheatham, B. Remogliflozin Etabonate Improves Fatty Liver Disease in Diet-Induced Obese Male Mice. *J. Clin. Exp. Hepatol.* **2015**, *5*, 190–198. [CrossRef]
120. Qiang, S.; Nakatsu, Y.; Seno, Y.; Fujishiro, M.; Sakoda, H.; Kushiyama, A.; Mori, K.; Matsunaga, Y.; Yamamotoya, T.; Kamata, H.; et al. Treatment with the SGLT2 inhibitor luseogliflozin improves nonalcoholic steatohepatitis in a rodent model with diabetes mellitus. *Diabetol. Metab. Syndr.* **2015**, *7*, 104. [CrossRef]
121. Jojima, T.; Tomotsune, T.; Iijima, T.; Akimoto, K.; Suzuki, K.; Aso, Y. Empagliflozin (an SGLT2 inhibitor), alone or in combination with linagliptin (a DPP-4 inhibitor), prevents steatohepatitis in a novel mouse model of non-alcoholic steatohepatitis and diabetes. *Diabetol. Metab. Syndr.* **2016**, *8*, 45. [CrossRef]
122. Petito-da-Silva, T.I.; Souza-Mello, V.; Barbosa-da-Silva, S. Empagliflozin mitigates NAFLD in high-fat-fed mice by alleviating insulin resistance, lipogenesis and ER stress. *Mol. Cell. Endocrinol.* **2019**, *498*, 110539. [CrossRef]
123. Tahara, A.; Takasu, T. SGLT2 inhibitor ipragliflozin alone and combined with pioglitazone prevents progression of nonalcoholic steatohepatitis in a type 2 diabetes rodent model. *Physiol. Rep.* **2019**, *7*, e14286. [CrossRef]
124. Chiang, H.; Lee, J.C.; Huang, H.C.; Huang, H.; Liu, H.K.; Huang, C. Delayed intervention with a novel SGLT2 inhibitor NGI001 suppresses diet-induced metabolic dysfunction and non-alcoholic fatty liver disease in mice. *Br. J. Pharmacol.* **2020**, *177*, 239–253. [CrossRef]
125. Nasiri-Ansari, N.; Nikolopoulou, C.; Papoutsi, K.; Kyrou, I.; Mantzoros, C.S.; Kyriakopoulos, G.; Chatzigeorgiou, A.; Kalotychou, V.; Randeva, M.S.; Chatha, K.; et al. Empagliflozin Attenuates Non-Alcoholic Fatty Liver Disease (NAFLD) in High Fat Diet Fed ApoE$^{(-/-)}$ Mice by Activating Autophagy and Reducing ER Stress and Apoptosis. *Int. J. Mol. Sci.* **2021**, *22*, 818. [CrossRef]
126. Meng, Z.; Liu, X.; Li, T.; Fang, T.; Cheng, Y.; Han, L.; Sun, B.; Chen, L. The SGLT2 inhibitor empagliflozin negatively regulates IL-17/IL-23 axis-mediated inflammatory responses in T2DM with NAFLD via the AMPK/mTOR/autophagy pathway. *Int. Immunopharmacol.* **2021**, *94*, 107492. [CrossRef]
127. Kucharewicz, I.; Pawlak, R.; Matys, T.; Pawlak, D.; Buczko, W. Antithrombotic effect of captopril and losartan is mediated by angiotensin-(1-7). *Hypertension* **2002**, *40*, 774–779. [CrossRef]
128. Ishiyama, Y.; Gallagher, P.E.; Averill, D.B.; Tallant, E.A.; Brosnihan, K.B.; Ferrario, C.M. Upregulation of angiotensin-converting enzyme 2 after myocardial infarction by blockade of angiotensin II receptors. *Hypertension* **2004**, *43*, 970–976. [CrossRef]
129. Xu, Y.Z.; Zhang, X.; Wang, L.; Zhang, F.; Qiu, Q.; Liu, M.L.; Zhang, G.R.; Wu, X.L. An increased circulating angiotensin II concentration is associated with hypoadiponectinemia and postprandial hyperglycemia in men with nonalcoholic fatty liver disease. *Intern. Med.* **2013**, *52*, 855–861. [CrossRef]
130. Cao, X.; Yang, F.Y.; Xin, Z.; Xie, R.R.; Yang, J.K. The ACE2/Ang-(1-7)/Mas axis can inhibit hepatic insulin resistance. *Mol. Cell. Endocrinol.* **2014**, *393*, 30–38. [CrossRef]
131. Nourjah, P.; Ahmad, S.R.; Karwoski, C.; Willy, M. Estimates of acetaminophen (Paracetomal)-associated overdoses in the United States. *Pharmacoepidemiol. Drug Saf.* **2006**, *15*, 398–405. [CrossRef] [PubMed]
132. Lee, W.M. Etiologies of acute liver failure. *Semin. Liver Dis.* **2008**, *28*, 142–152. [CrossRef] [PubMed]
133. McGreal, S.R.; Bhushan, B.; Walesky, C.; McGill, M.R.; Lebofsky, M.; Kandel, S.E.; Winefield, R.D.; Jaeschke, H.; Zachara, N.E.; Zhang, Z.; et al. Modulation of O-GlcNAc Levels in the Liver Impacts Acetaminophen-Induced Liver Injury by Affecting Protein Adduct Formation and Glutathione Synthesis. *Toxicol. Sci.* **2018**, *162*, 599–610. [CrossRef] [PubMed]
134. Filhoulaud, G.; Benhamed, F.; Pagesy, P.; Bonner, C.; Fardini, Y.; Ilias, A.; Movassat, J.; Burnol, A.F.; Guilmeau, S.; Kerr-Conte, J.; et al. O-GlcNacylation Links TxNIP to Inflammasome Activation in Pancreatic beta Cells. *Front. Endocrinol.* **2019**, *10*, 291. [CrossRef]
135. Hosseinpour-Arjmand, S.; Amirkhizi, F.; Ebrahimi-Mameghani, M. The effect of alpha-lipoic acid on inflammatory markers and body composition in obese patients with non-alcoholic fatty liver disease: A randomized, double-blind, placebo-controlled trial. *J. Clin. Pharm. Ther.* **2019**, *44*, 258–267. [CrossRef]

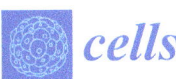

Article

Decreased CSTB, RAGE, and Axl Receptor Are Associated with Zika Infection in the Human Placenta

Gabriel Borges-Vélez [1], Juan A. Arroyo [2], Yadira M. Cantres-Rosario [3], Ana Rodriguez de Jesus [4], Abiel Roche-Lima [4], Julio Rosado-Philippi [1], Lester J. Rosario-Rodríguez [1], María S. Correa-Rivas [5], Maribel Campos-Rivera [6] and Loyda M. Meléndez [1,4,*]

[1] Department of Microbiology and Medical Zoology, School of Medicine, University of Puerto Rico Medical Sciences Campus, San Juan, PR 00936, USA
[2] Department of Cell Biology and Physiology, College of Life Sciences, Brigham Young University, Provo, UT 84602, USA
[3] Comprehensive Cancer Center, University of Puerto Rico, San Juan, PR 00936, USA
[4] Center for Collaborative Research in Health Disparities, University of Puerto Rico Medical Sciences Campus, San Juan, PR 00936, USA
[5] Department of Pathology and Laboratory Medicine, School of Medicine, University of Puerto Rico Medical Sciences Campus, San Juan, PR 00936, USA
[6] School of Dental Medicine, University of Puerto Rico Medical Sciences Campus, San Juan, PR 00936, USA
* Correspondence: loyda.melendez@upr.edu; Tel.: +1-787-777-0079; Fax: +1-787-777-0078

Abstract: Zika virus (ZIKV) compromises placental integrity, infecting the fetus. However, the mechanisms associated with ZIKV penetration into the placenta leading to fetal infection are unknown. Cystatin B (CSTB), the receptor for advanced glycation end products (RAGE), and tyrosine-protein kinase receptor UFO (AXL) have been implicated in ZIKV infection and inflammation. This work investigates CSTB, RAGE, and AXL receptor expression and activation pathways in ZIKV-infected placental tissues at term. The hypothesis is that there is overexpression of CSTB and increased inflammation affecting RAGE and AXL receptor expression in ZIKV-infected placentas. Pathological analyses of 22 placentas were performed to determine changes caused by ZIKV infection. Quantitative proteomics, immunofluorescence, and western blot were performed to analyze proteins and pathways affected by ZIKV infection in frozen placentas. The pathological analysis confirmed decreased size of capillaries, hyperplasia of Hofbauer cells, disruption in the trophoblast layer, cell agglutination, and ZIKV localization to the trophoblast layer. In addition, there was a significant decrease in CSTB, RAGE, and AXL expression and upregulation of caspase 1, tubulin beta, and heat shock protein 27. Modulation of these proteins and activation of inflammasome and pyroptosis pathways suggest targets for modulation of ZIKV infection in the placenta.

Keywords: placenta; trophoblast; Hofbauer cells (HC); Zika virus (ZIKV); tandem mass tagging (TMT)

1. Introduction

The Zika virus (ZIKV) is a mosquito-borne flavivirus with high global relevance [1]. This virus is known to cause fever, rash, joint pain, and conjunctivitis [2]. Viral infection can occur in several ways, including mosquito bites, sexual contact, and blood transfusion. Importantly, ZIKV can be transmitted vertically from a pregnant mother to the developing fetus, causing fetal abnormalities known as congenital Zika virus syndrome (CZS) [3]. CZS includes microcephaly, hearing loss, intracranial calcifications, ocular dysfunction, and seizures in newborns [4–6]. ZIKV can be attracted to the placenta via direct and contiguous infection of the cell layers, virion transit through a breach, or cell-associated transport [5–7]. This virus evades innate human defenses and compromises the placental integrity of the maternal–fetal barriers [6,7]. However, the molecular mechanisms associated with ZIKV penetration into the placenta leading to fetal infection are unknown.

The main structure of the placenta is the chorionic villi which act as a continuous selective barrier that provides gas exchange, nutrient uptake, waste elimination, thermoregulation, hormones, and immunity. This barrier is composed of different trophoblast cell layers. The trophoblast cells mature into syncytiotrophoblasts, which fuse to form the syncytium, the outer layer of the chorionic villi. The cytotrophoblasts are precursors to the syncytiotrophoblasts and the extravillous trophoblasts that anchor the placenta to the endometrium [8]. The syncytiotrophoblast external layer is less permissive to ZIKV infection than the cytotrophoblast layer. This layer is more profound in a healthy placenta and should not be exposed to infection [9]. Placental Hofbauer cells (HCs) are fetal–placental macrophages situated in the intervillous space close to fetal capillaries and provide a conduit for the vertical transmission of some viruses, including ZIKV. Multiple ZIKV strains, including the Puerto Rico strain, successfully infect primary cultures of HCs obtained from term human placentas [4,5]. Due to the proximity of chorionic villi to the fetal blood supply, simple viral multiplication inside HCs may act as a source of virus transmission through fetal blood. However, the mechanism by which ZIKV is resistant to destruction in the placenta is unknown. In recent studies, the lysosomal protease inhibitor cystatin B (CSTB) was found down-regulated in the proteomes of in-vitro-HIV-infected HCs compared to blood-derived macrophages [10]. This suggested an association with HIV-1 restriction in HCs compared to bloodborne monocyte-derived macrophages (MDM) [10]. Further studies confirmed differences in STAT-1 signaling between HC and MDM [11]. In addition, high levels of CSTB interfered with STAT-1 and IFN antiviral responses in MDM, promoting viral replication [12]. However, the role of CSTB in ZIKV placental infection has not been elucidated.

A known hallmark of ZIKV infection is the development of placental inflammation [13,14]. Placental inflammation is associated with fetal and neonatal health and disease [15]. The receptor for advanced glycation end-products (RAGE) is a member of the immunoglobulin superfamily of cell surface receptors expressed in the placenta [16–18]. RAGE activation is implicated in inflammation and cell migration processes and is low under physiological settings but can be upregulated in response to inflammation [19]. In this process, activation of RAGE by advanced glycation end products or by damage-associated molecular patterns leads to increased expression and secretion of a variety of inflammatory-response-related molecules, such as TNF α (tumor necrosis factor α), INF γ (interferon γ), and IL-6 (interleukin-6) [19]. In addition, RAGE activation in the placenta is associated with inflammatory diseases such as preeclampsia and intrauterine growth restriction [18]. Interestingly, RAGE receptor activation has been correlated with the activation of the AXL tyrosine kinase receptor [20]. AXL receptors are broadly expressed, and increased activity of this receptor has been implicated in various cellular signaling pathways, including those that influence survival, growth, migration, invasion, and inflammatory responses [21,22]. In the placenta, increased AXL has been implicated in ZIKV infection and inflammatory-associated obstetrics complications, suggesting its essential role in disease development [23–27]. Activation of the RAGE and AXL receptors in the ZIKV-infected placenta as well as the inflammatory pathways affected by the infection still must be elucidated to better understand virus transmission during pregnancy.

If novel preventative and therapeutic strategies are to be created, the mechanism by which ZIKV affects the placental host immune system must be discovered. This work aims to investigate CSTB, RAGE receptor, and AXL receptor expression in ZIKV-infected placental tissues. This will enable the identification of possible mechanisms activated by ZIKV infection of the placenta. We also performed quantitative proteomics and pathway analyses to elucidate the mechanisms and pathways of ZIKV transplacental transmission.

2. Materials and Methods

Placental samples: This study was approved by the University of Puerto Rico Medical Sciences Institutional Review Board (IRB). Placentas were collected with approval from subjects of legal age, 21 years or more. Zika virus infection during pregnancy was determined via RT-PCR performed at the Puerto Rico Department of Health. One set of placenta samples (n = 12) was collected from already-processed/examined placentas stored at the Laboratory of Anatomic Pathology, ASEM, Puerto Rico Medical Center, and paraffin blocks were prepared and labeled with a unique number without patient identifiers. Samples were divided into two groups: positive and negative for ZIKV infection. We randomly chose placental tissue from six ZIKV-infected and six negative control women for this study. Placental pathology sections containing chorionic villi were processed overnight (at 4°) and cut into 4 µm thick sections. The second group of fresh frozen placental tissue samples (n = 10) were obtained from the repository of a pilot project, Dental and Craniofacial Effects of Intrauterine Zika Infection (1R21DE027235-01). Proteins from 5 positive and 5 negative ZIKV-infected placentas were extracted for proteomics and for western blot experiments.

Immunofluorescence: Immunofluorescence (IF) was performed on paraffin-embedded placental sections (n = 12) as previously published by our laboratory [28]. Briefly, slides were deparaffinized, followed by treatment with eBioscience™ IHC Antigen Retrieval Solution—Low pH (1X) (Invitrogen, Waltham, MA, USA). Next, slides were incubated overnight (at 4°) with antibodies for NS1 (ZIKV protein; Arigo Biolaboratories Corp., Hsinchu City, Taiwan), cytokeratin (for trophoblast identification; Fitzgerald, Acton, MA, USA), IBA-1 (for macrophages identification; FUJIFILM Wako Pure Chemical Corporation, Osaka, Japan), CSTB (for cystatin B; Abcam plc., Cambridge, UK), AXL (Abcam plc., Cambridge, UK), or RAGE (Abcam plc., Cambridge, UK). Secondary antibodies used were goat anti-mouse Alexa Fluor™ 488, goat anti-rabbit Alexa Fluor™ 546, and goat anti-guinea pig Alexa Fluor™ 647 (Thermo Fisher Scientific, Whatman, MA, USA). Slides were mounted with VECTASHIELD antifade mounting medium with DAPI (Vector Laboratories Inc., Newark, CA, USA) (for nuclear staining). IF was examined using the Eclipse E400 microscope (Nikon Inc., Melville, NY, USA). Pictures were taken with a DS-Qi2 Monochrome Camera (Nikon Inc., Melville, NY, USA) using the NIS-Elements Imaging Software (Nikon Inc., Melville, NY, USA).

Trophoblast cells and ZIKV infection: The trophoblast cell line JEG-3 (HTB-36™) was purchased from ATCC® and cultured in ATCC-formulated Eagle's Minimum Essential Medium in 10% fetal bovine serum at 37 °C with 5% CO_2 in T25 and T75 (Corning, Corning, NY, USA) vented tissue culture treated flasks. Cells were exposed for two hours to ZIKV PRVAB59 virus (MOI 0.1) at 50% cell confluency. After two hours, the media containing the virus was removed, replaced with fresh medium, and incubated for 24 h. At the conclusion of the exposure, total cell lysates were obtained.

Western Blot: Western blot was performed as previously published by our laboratory [29]. Briefly, whole tissue homogenates were obtained from frozen placenta using Tissue PE LB™ (G-Biosciences, St. Louis, MO, USA). Cultured cells were lysed, and proteins were extracted with RIPA Lysis and Extraction Buffer (Thermo Scientific, Whatman, MA, USA). Tissues and cell protein lysates (40 µg; n = 5 per group) were centrifuged and dried overnight using a Speed Vac (at 4°). Pellets were rehydrated in sample buffer and water, followed by heat at 95 °C for 5 min. Samples were run in a 4–20% TGX gels (Bio-Rad) and transferred to PVDF membranes. Membranes were blocked with EveryBlot Blocking Buffer (Bio-Rad, Hercules, CA, USA) and incubated overnight (at 4°) with antibodies against CTSB (Abcam plc., Cambridge, UK), AXL (Abcam plc., Cambridge, UK), RAGE (Abcam plc., Cambridge, UK), HSP27 (Abcam plc., Cambridge, UK), Tubulin (TUBB; Abcam plc., Cambridge, UK), CASP1 (Abcam plc., Cambridge, UK), and Vinculin (Abcam plc., Cambridge, UK). Membranes were developed using ChemiDoc XRS+ (Bio-Rad) equipment. Band densities were normalized to Vinculin, and comparison between groups were performed.

Statistical analysis of Western blot data: Data are shown as means ± SE. Differences in CTSB, AXL, RAGE, HSP27, TUBB, and CASP1 protein expression were determined between control and ZIKV-positive placentas. Data were analyzed for outliers using ROUT at Q = 1%. Normality was determined using a Shapiro–Wilk test with alpha = 0.05. Statistical differences were determined using an unpaired t-test with $p < 0.05$.

Proteomics Sample Processing: Proteins were isolated from frozen placentas, and concentration was determined as described in the western blot section. Quantitative proteomics protocols were based on Borges et al. 2021 [28]. A total of 10 placentas were processed, and protein extracts (100 µg) were obtained and separated using SDS-PAGE in a Coomassie stained gel for proteomics processing and quantitation. Proteome bands were cut out, and gel pieces were distained by incubation with 50 mM ammonium bicarbonate/50% acetonitrile solution at 37 °C for 2 to 3 h. Proteins were reduced with dithiothreitol (25 mM DTT in 50 mM ammonium bicarbonate) at 55 °C, alkylated with iodoacetamide (10 mM IAA in 50 mM ammonium bicarbonate) at room temperature in the dark, and digested with trypsin (Promega, Madison, WI, USA) overnight at 37 °C at a trypsin/protein ratio of 1:50. The next day, digested peptides were extracted out of the gel pieces using a mixture of 50% acetonitrile/2.5% formic acid in water. Extracted peptides were dried and stored at –80 °C until TMT labeling.

TMT Labeling: TMT reagents are reconstituted in acetonitrile (41 µL for 0.8 mg) on the day of use. As specified by the manufacturer's protocol (Thermo Scientific, Wathman, MA, USA), dried digests were reconstituted in 100 mM TEAB (triethyl ammonium bicarbonate), TMT labels were added according to the experimental design followed by one-hour incubation with occasional vortexing and a quenching step of 15 min. Finally, equal amounts of each labeled sample were mixed to generate a final pool later submitted to fractionation.

Fractionation: This method was performed using the Pierce High pH Reversed-Phase Peptide Fractionation Kit (REF 89875) and following the manufacturer's instructions. Briefly, the column was conditioned twice using 300 µL of acetonitrile and centrifuged at $5000 \times g$ for 2 min, and the steps were repeated using 0.1% trifluoroacetic acid (TFA). Next, each TMT-labeled pool was reconstituted in 300 µL of 0.1% TFA, loaded onto the column, washed, and then eluted 16 times using a series of elution solutions with different acetonitrile/0.1% triethylamine percentages and centrifugation of $3000 \times g$ for 2 min, generating 16 fractions for analysis. The flow-through step was stored as suggested in the protocol. In case of peptide loss, these can be analyzed if requested.

LC-MS/MS Analysis: Fractions were reconstituted in 0.1% formic acid in water (Buffer A), and a small portion was transferred to autosampler vials for MS/MS analysis using the Easy-nLC1200 (Thermo Fisher Scientific, Wathman, MA, USA). A PicoChip H354 REPROSIL-Pur C18-AQ 3 µm 120 A (75 µm × 105 mm) chromatographic column (New Objective) was used for peptide separation. The separation was obtained using a gradient of 7–25% of 0.1% of formic acid in acetonitrile (Buffer B) for 102 min, 25–60% of Buffer B for 20 min, and 60–95% Buffer B for 6 min. This resulted in a total gradient time of 128 min at a flow rate of 300 nL/min, with an injection volume of 2 µL per sample. Q-Exactive Plus (Thermo Fisher Scientific, Whatman, MA, USA) operates in positive polarity mode and data-dependent mode. The full scan (MS1) was measured over the range of 375 to 1400 at resolution of 70,000. The MS2 (MS/MS) analysis was configured to select the ten (10) most intense ions (Top10) for HCD fragmentation with a resolution of 35,000. A dynamic exclusion parameter was set for 30 s.

Database Search and Results: Mass spectrometric raw data were analyzed using Proteome Discoverer (PD) software, version 2.5. Files were searched against a human database downloaded using the PD Protein Center tool (tax ID = 9606). The modifications included a dynamic modification for oxidation +15.995 Da (M), a static modification of +57.021 Da (C), and static modifications from the TMT reagents +229.163 Da (Any N Term, K). Channel 126 was marked as the control channel, enabling data normalization against the internal pool. The TMT certificate of analysis (Lot: WD312186) was used to correct for isotopic impurities of reporter ions. A series of filters was applied to the PD result file to use those with the highest confidence level, eliminate keratins, and only consider proteins with two or more protein-unique peptides. These filtering parameters reduced protein hits from 4778 proteins to 2881 proteins. These results were exported to Excel for statistics, bioinformatics, and ingenuity pathway analyses.

Statistics, Bioinformatics, and Ingenuity Pathway Analyses: The bioinformatic analysis was performed for the proteomic datasets associated with Zika Virus (5 Zika (+) vs. 5 Zika (−)). The analysis was performed with the Bioconductor software Limma [30,31]. A total of 2797 proteins were processed prior to the statistical analysis. The statistical analysis performed was a single-channel analysis between cases and controls. The results from the statistical analysis were considered to be proteins differentially abundant between groups based on FC ≥ |1.5| and p-value ≤ 0.05. For ingenuity pathway analyses (IPA), we selected pathways based on the most significant fold changes and p-values together with protein function related to inflammation, tissue remodeling, and protein–protein interactions with CSTB, RAGE, and AXL. IPA tools were canonical pathways, pathway predictions (using the Molecule Activity Predictor tools (MAP)), and protein–protein interaction networks. Ingenuity pathway analysis (IPA) was generated using their software (IPA®) (networks, functional analyses, etc.) (QIAGEN Inc., Hilden, DE, USA, https://www.qiagenbioinformatics.com/products/ingenuity-pathway-analysis (accessed on 17 October 2022)) and used for enrichment pathway proteome analysis.

3. Results

Zika Virus Placenta infection: We first confirmed placental infection by staining for ZIKV non-structural protein 1 (NS1). NS1 is a protein necessary for viral replication and infection [32]. Immunofluorescence confirmed the presence of NS1 in the placenta of ZIKV-infected mothers (Figure 1A). Interestingly, this protein was localized mainly in the villi trophoblast of infected placentas. This localization was more prominent in the syncytiotrophoblast layer of the placenta (Figure 1A).

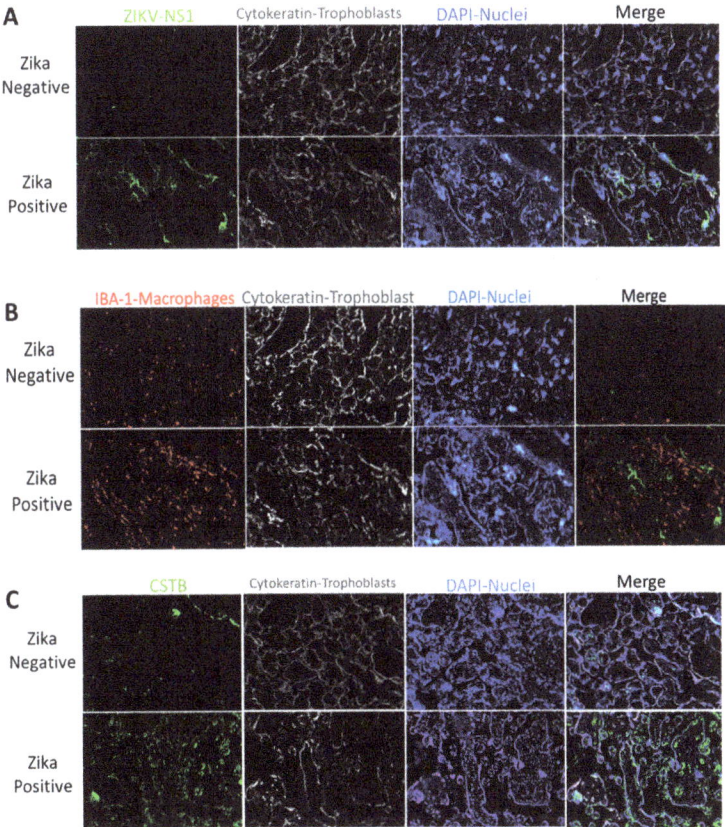

Figure 1. *Cont.*

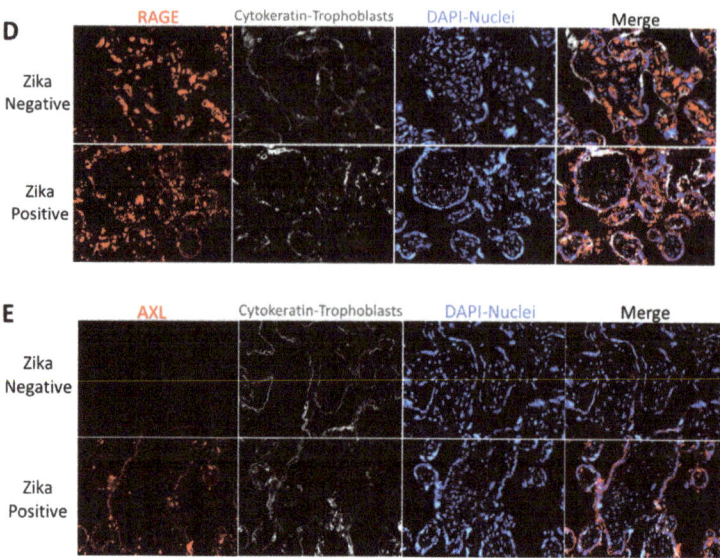

Figure 1. Expression of ZIKV protein and inflammatory proteins in ZIKV-positive and negative placental villi. (**A**) Viral non-structural protein 1 (NS1) labeling of trophoblasts in ZIKV-negative and positive placentas. Representative fluorescence immunohistochemistry of ZIKV-negative placental tissue (upper panel) and ZIKV-infected tissue (lower panel). From left to right, tissue is labeled for anti-NS1 (green), anti-cytokeratin 8 + 18 (white), DAPI for nuclei (blue), and merged figure. Pictures were captured at a magnification of 20×. (**B**) Macrophage labeling of ZIKV-negative and positive placentas. Representative fluorescence immunohistochemistry of ZIKV-negative (upper panel) and positive placentas (lower panel). The tissue is labeled with anti-Iba1 for placental macrophages or Hofbauer cells (red), with anti-cytokeratin 8 + 18 (white) for trophoblast cells, DAPI for nuclei (blue) and anti-NS1 (green). Pictures were captured at a magnification of 20×. (**C**) Cystatin B labeling of ZIKV-negative and positive placentas. Protein labeling of ZIKV-positive (upper panel) and negative placentas (lower panel). Placenta tissue was labeled with anti-cystatin B or CSTB (green), anti-cytokeratin 8 + 18 (white) for trophoblast cells, DAPI for nuclei (blue). Pictures were captured at a magnification of 20×. (**D**) RAGE expression in ZIKV-negative and positive placentas. Representative fluorescence immunohistochemistry of ZIKV-negative (upper panel) and positive placentas (lower panel). Protein is labeled with anti-RAGE (red), anti-cytokeratin 8 + 18 (white) for trophoblast cells, and DAPI for nuclei (blue). Pictures were captured at a magnification of 40×. (**E**) AXL expression in ZIKV-negative and positive placentas. Representative fluorescence immunohistochemistry of ZIKV-negative (upper panel) and positive placenta (lower panel). Protein labeled with anti-AXL (red), anti-cytokeratin 8 + 18 (white) for trophoblast cells, and DAPI for nuclei (Blue). Pictures were captured at a magnification of 40×.

Zika Virus infection associated molecules: Macrophages participate in innate immunity and are present in most tissues, such as the liver, skin, gut, lung, and placenta [33]. In the placenta, macrophage hyperplasia was observed during placental infections [34]. We observed increased macrophage infiltration in the ZIKV-infected placentas compared to controls (Figure 1B and Figure S1). This infiltration was observed in the stroma of the placental villi (Figure 1B and Figure S1). Interestingly, when we compared macrophage infiltration with Iba-1 antibody and the expression of ZIKV NS1 protein in the placenta, we observed no colocalization (Figure 1B and Figure S2). The macrophage hyperplasia was observed in the stroma of the placental villi, while ZIKV infection was observed mainly in the outer syncytiotrophoblast layer of the villi (Figures 1A,B, S1 and S2).

Cystatin B (CSTB) is a cysteine protease inhibitor that facilitates HIV infection of placental macrophages [10–12,35]. In the ZIKV-infected placenta, we detected increased CSTB expression compared to controls (Figure 1C). This increase seems to be distributed in the syncytiotrophoblast layer and in a few in the villi macrophages (Figures 1C and S3).

We decided to investigate the expression of two receptors participating in innate immune responses. RAGE receptor is associated with increased inflammation in several organs [18]. Placental staining showed increased RAGE expression in the ZIKV-infected placenta compared to controls (Figure 1D). This receptor was localized to the stroma in ZIKV-negative placentas, while in ZIKV-positive samples was localized to the placenta's trophoblast layer, demonstrating increased expression in the syncytiotrophoblast layer (Figure 1D). Interestingly, there was a very low AXL presence in the stroma of ZIKV-negative placentas and no expression in the syncytiotrophoblast layer. However, in ZIKV-positive placentas, an increased AXL expression was observed mainly in the syncytiotrophoblast layer (Figure 1E). To quantify the expression of CSTB, AXL, and RAGE in the placenta, tissue lysates were used to perform western blots. We determined that in ZIKV-infected placentas, there was a significant decrease in CSTB (2.9-fold; $p < 0.0003$), AXL (2.2-fold; $p < 0.0002$) and RAGE (9.7-fold; $p < 0.0002$) expression as compared to controls (Figure 2A). When we examined trophoblast cells infected in vitro with ZIKV, there was a significant decrease in CSTB (1.4-fold; $p < 0.008$) and an increase in AXL (1.4-fold; $p < 0.008$) and RAGE (1.7-fold; $p < 0.008$) expression compared to controls.

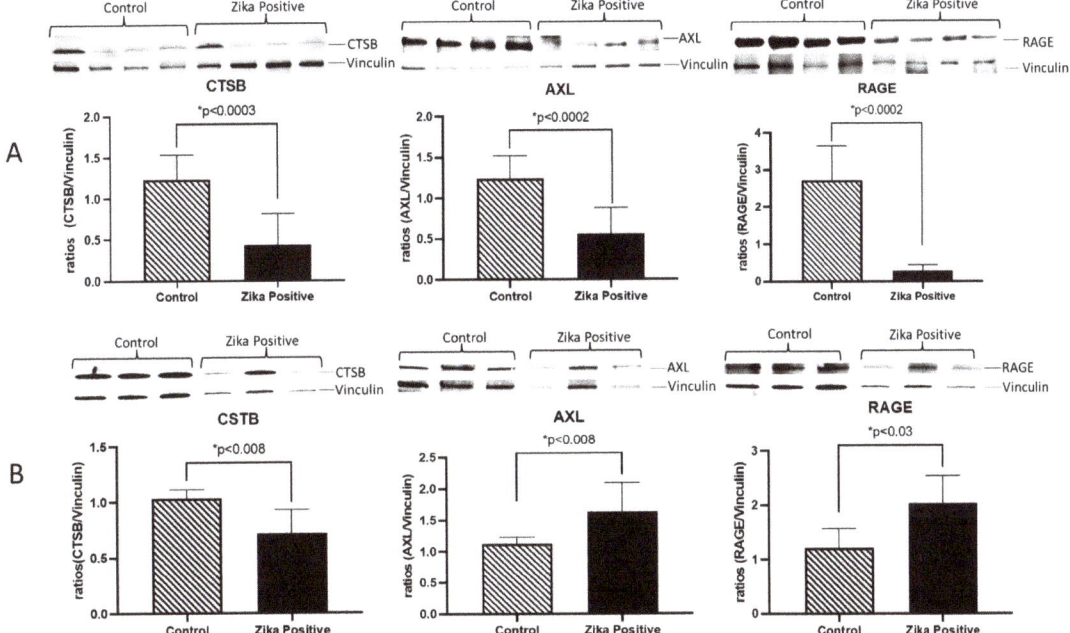

Figure 2. Expression of CSTB, AXL, and RAGE in ZIKV-positive and negative placentas and infected trophoblasts cells. Western blot results from placenta tissue samples showed decreased CSTB, AXL, and RAGE protein levels in the infected placental tissues compared to controls (**A**). Western blot showed decreased CSTB, while AXL and RAGE proteins were increased in infected trophoblast cells compared to controls (**B**). Statistical analysis was performed using Graph Pad 8 from Prism. Statistical differences were determined using an unpaired t-test with $p < 0.05$.

To further investigate the inflammatory pathways activated by ZIKV in the placenta, we conducted a quantitative proteomics analysis of frozen placentas from five ZIKV-positive and negative controls using limma Bioconductor software and IPA analyses. As a result, we found 44 differentially more abundant proteins in ZIKV-positive compared to ZIKV-negative placentas, as illustrated in the volcano plot (Figure S4). The list of proteins is described in Table S1.

Pathway analyses revealed upregulation of proteins associated with the inflammasome (Figure 3), pyroptosis signaling (Figure 4), and the remodeling of the epithelial adherent junction pathway (see Figure S5). The upregulation of these proteins predicts an activation of the pathways mentioned, which could lead to an impaired inflammatory immune response. The upregulated proteins observed in our pathway analysis are caspase-1 (CASP1), serine/threonine-protein kinase Nek7 (NEK7), ubiquitin-associated protein 2-like (Ub), tubulin alpha-1C chain (TUBA1C), and tubulin beta chain (TUBB).

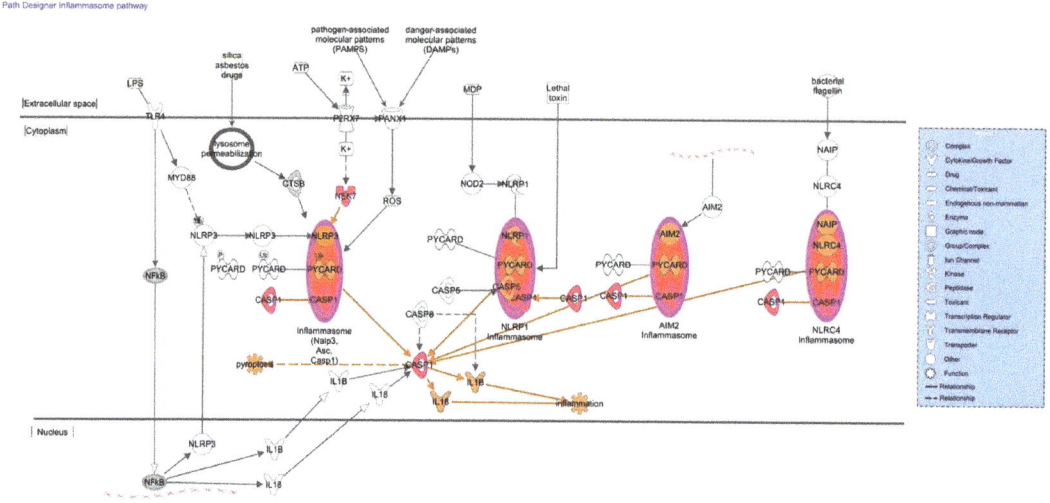

Figure 3. Inflammasome pathways of differentially expressed proteins from ZIKV-positive and negative placentas. Prediction legend: the intensity of red corresponds to higher upregulation of the protein. These proteins are caspase-1 (CASP1), serine/threonine-protein kinase Nek7 (NEK7) and ubiquitin-associated protein 2-like (Ub). The color grey means that the protein was identified but there was no significant increase in expression. Proteins in orange in the diagrams were not detected by our proteomics experiments. The orange means predicted activation of the protein or interaction leading to activation. The protein gene name is used in the diagrams. To identify proteins, refer to Supplementary Table S1's gene name column. Data were analyzed using IPA (QIAGEN Inc., Hilden, Germany, https://www.qiagenbioinformatics.com/products/ingenuitypathway-analysis; accessed 15 September 2022).

Protein interaction analysis revealed that phosphofurin acidic cluster sorting protein 1 (PACS1) and CASP1 indirectly interact with CSTB and were upregulated (Figure 5). PACS1 indirectly affects the expression of CSTB, and CSTB indirectly activates CASP1. Poly(rC)-binding protein 1 (PCBP1) and small heat shock protein beta 1 (HSPB1/HSP27), which were upregulated in ZIKV-positive placenta, interact directly with AXL (Figure 5). PCBP1 can bind directly with AXL in protein–protein interactions and, AXL activates HSP27 via phosphorylation cascades. These results suggest that infection of ZIKV in the placenta is causing impaired immune responses.

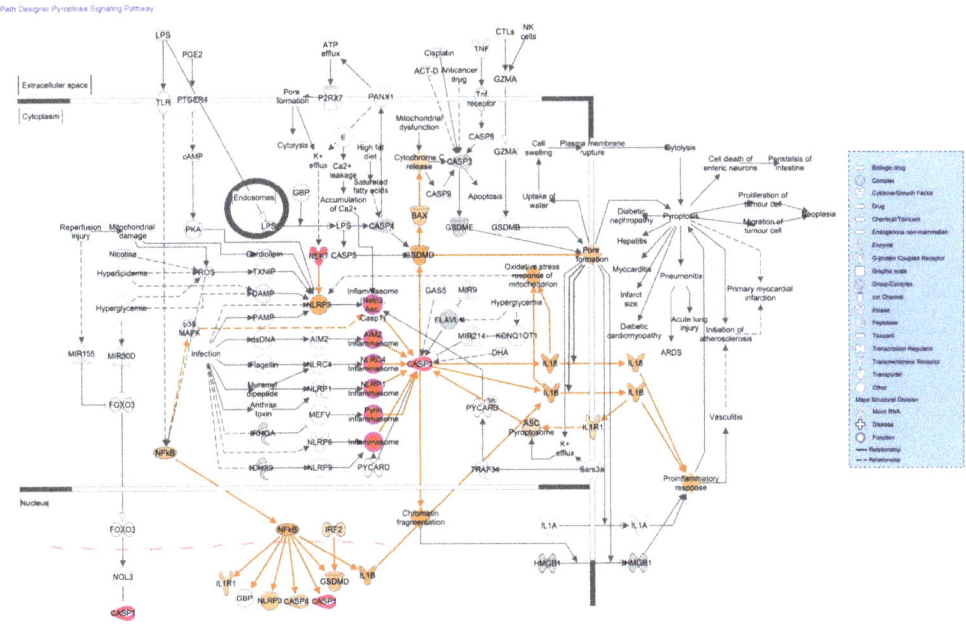

Figure 4. Pyroptosis signaling pathways of differentially expressed proteins from ZIKV-positive and negative placentas. Prediction legend: the intensity of red corresponds to higher upregulation of the protein. These proteins are the caspase-1 (CASP1) inflammasome component and the serine/threonine-protein kinase Nek7 (NEK7). Grey means that the protein was identified but there was no significant increase in expression. Our proteomics experiments did not detect proteins in orange in the diagrams. Orange means predicted activation of the protein or interaction leading to activation. The protein gene name is used in the diagrams. Data were analyzed using of IPA (QIAGEN Inc., https://www.qiagenbioinformatics.com/products/ingenuitypathway-analysis; accessed 15 September 2022).

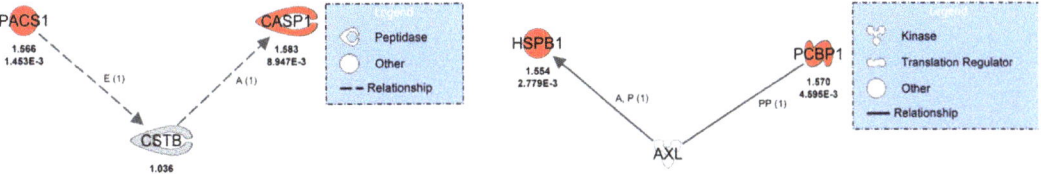

Figure 5. CSTB and AXL protein interactions from differentially expressed proteins from ZIKV-positive and negative placentas are upregulated protein interactions. Prediction legend: the intensity of red corresponds to higher upregulation of the protein. Upregulated proteins are phosphofurin acidic cluster sorting protein 1 (PACS1), caspase 1 (CASP1), poly(rC)-binding protein 1 (PCBP1), and small heat shock protein beta 1 (HSPB1/HSP27). The grey color means that the protein was identified but there was no significant increase in expression. A constant line means direct interaction, and a dashed line is indirect interaction. The letter E means expression; A means activation; P means phosphorylation/dephosphorylation and PP protein–protein binding. Arrowhead means acts on, and a line without an arrow refers to binding only. Data were analyzed using IPA (QIAGEN Inc., https://www.qiagenbioinformatics.com/products/ingenuitypathway-analysis; accessed 15 September 2022).

HSP27, TUBB, and CASP1 were selected for further validation using western blot analyses of ZIKV-positive and negative placental tissues. These proteins were selected based on involvement in the pathway analysis literature involving ZIKV interaction and inflammation (Table 1). We found that HSP27 was increased (3.2-fold; $p < 0.002$) in ZIKV-infected placental tissue compared to the negative control (Figure 6). Interestingly, in contrast to quantitative proteomics results, TUBB and CASP1 protein levels were significantly decreased (2.1-fold; $p < 0.002$ and 3.1-fold; $p < 0.0002$) in the western blots (Figure 6).

Table 1. Differentially expressed proteins from ZIKV-positive and negative placenta were selected for validation. Proteins selected for validation of quantitative proteomics. Quantitative proteomics results are included for the selected proteins and brief descriptions.

Protein	Gene Name	Fold-Change	p-Value	Function
Caspase-1	CASP1	1.583	0.0089	Thiol protease is involved in various inflammatory processes by proteolytically cleaving other proteins [36].
Small heat shock protein beta 1 (HSP27)	HSPB1	1.554	0.0028	Molecular chaperone probably maintaining denatured proteins in a folding-competent state [37].
Tubulin beta chain	TUBB	1.542	0.0096	A principal constituent of microtubules [38].

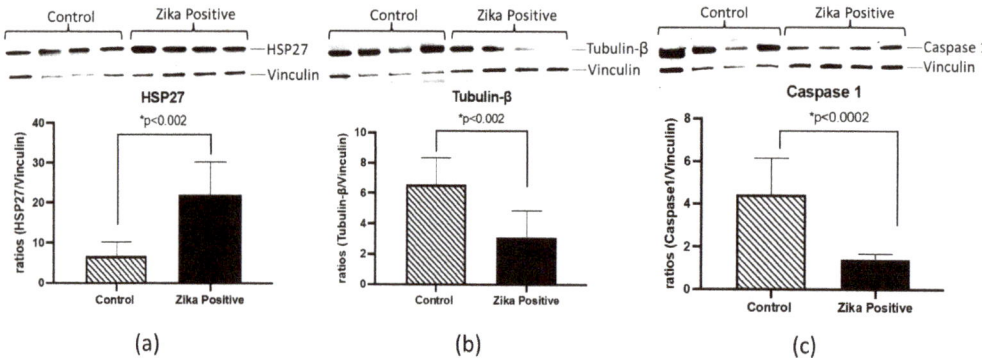

Figure 6. Validation of proteomics data of differentially expressed proteins from ZIKV-positive and negative frozen placentas by western blot. From left to right, we have the densitometry analysis of HSP27, TUBB, and CASP1. Results from relative intensity analysis of protein of interest and representative western blot bands (top of each figure) for this experiment are shown in (**a**–**c**). Relative intensity values for each band were determined using Image Lab Software from Bio-Rad, and ratios were determined using vinculin as a loading control. Statistical analysis was performed using Graph Pad 8 from Prism. Statistical differences were determined using an unpaired t-test with $p < 0.05$.

4. Discussion

The Zika virus (ZIKV) is a flavivirus known to infect the placenta and induce fetal abnormalities [39,40]. Although much progress has been made in researching this virus, the mechanism of placental infection remains to be elucidated. Many placental-oriented ZIKV studies have been performed in cell culture models, but actual ZIKV-infected placental tissues are scarce. Therefore, in our laboratory, we became interested in determining signaling molecules associated with this viral infection in the placenta. Concerning the information about the pregnancies, we recognize that it would be ideal to have the data on medical details and the corresponding children. However, these tissues were obtained from the Puerto Rico Department of Health, and no other information was provided to the investigators. The only information obtained was if they were affected by Zika virus or not.

The first step of our study included pathological analysis of our placental tissue. Previous pathology analysis in our laboratory revealed decreased size of capillaries, hyperplasia of Hofbauer cells, disruption in the trophoblast layer, and tissue and cell agglutination [41]. Subsequently, we performed proteomics analyses of nine placentas stored in formalin collected during the Puerto Rico 2016 ZIKV epidemic. Quantitative proteomics and ingenuity pathway analysis revealed that 45 of the deregulated proteins in ZIKV-positive compared to ZIKV-negative placentas were cellular components of the extracellular matrix, and 16 played a role in its structure and organization [28]. Of these, fibrinogen was further validated by immunohistochemistry in 12 additional placenta samples and found a significant increase in ZIKV-infected placentas, indicating that infection promotes the coagulation of placental tissue and restructuration of ECM potentially affecting the integrity of the tissue and facilitating the dissemination of the virus from mother to the fetus.

In the current studies, we used frozen placenta tissue from another local repository of ZIKV-infected placentas. We first confirmed ZIKV infection in tissue using immunofluorescence with an antibody against a ZIKV protein, NS1. NS1 protein was mainly localized to the trophoblast layers of the placental tissue compared to the stromal macrophages or HC. These results demonstrated that ZIKV NS1 protein persists in placental tissue until term and is localized in the trophoblast barrier. This result suggests that NS1 protein could contribute to the pathology observed in placental tissue since it has been confirmed that it activates innate immunity, causing cytokine storms, and is involved in immune evasion by binding to the complement system proteins [42]. As expected from previous proteomics analyses [28], the placenta cytokeratin labeling of the trophoblast cell layers confirmed damage in the villi layer of the trophoblasts. This is important as this layer provides a barrier to the developing fetus and is damaged by ZIKV, allowing the exchange of virus-infected cells between the mother and developing fetus [43]. To better understand the role of inflammatory proteins in placental infection by ZIKV, we decided to perform protein expression studies in placental macrophages and trophoblasts from infected and control samples using immunofluorescence. Placental macrophages (Hofbauer cells) are generally present in the placental chorionic villi from as early as 18 days of gestation up to delivery [44]. Macrophage hyperplasia has been reported in ZIKV-infected placentas [41,45]. We confirmed ZIKV-induced macrophage hyperplasia in the stroma of disease patients' placental tissue compared to negative controls (IBA-1 staining). Unexpectedly, when we compared ZIKV viral protein to macrophage hyperplasia, infection was observed mainly in the trophoblast layer and not in the macrophages. These results and the disruption of extracellular matrix proteins observed previously [28] suggested that macrophage hyperplasia is not caused by direct infection of ZIKV but by the invasion of cells from the blood. To define the players that could be involved in ZIKV infection in the placenta, we explored the expression of proteins previously associated with other viral infections and innate immunity, namely CSTB, RAGE, and AXL. We first wanted to determine the localization and expression of these molecules within the placenta. While CSTB is known to modulate macrophage HIV infection by affecting IFN responses [12], RAGE and AXL are receptors involved in tissue immune responses through nuclear factor kappa B, tumor necrosis factor, and IFN alpha and beta [16,46,47]. We determined that CSTB, RAGE, and AXL localization were primarily expressed in the trophoblast layer that protects the placenta. Interestingly, expression of these molecules was increased in the villi of infected placentas compared to controls. We performed immunoblotting to confirm protein levels in the placental tissues during infection. Interestingly, we determined that expression of these three proteins was significantly decreased in ZIKV-infected placentas compared to controls. This was unexpected as previous bioinformatic analyses have seen an increase in transcriptomic signatures in ZIKV infection of neural cells [48]. However, protein expression can change in different tissues. Previous reports of CSTB protein have shown that this protein is decreased in the proteome of Hofbauer cells compared to blood-derived macrophages [10]. The expression of this protein increases with viral infection and is related to increased STAT-1 signaling and decreased IFN responses [12]. In our studies, we also observed decreased CSTB and

ZIKV infection in Hofbauer cells, suggesting a possible mechanism of ZIKV restriction in the placenta. However, ZIKV infection and CSTB expression were concentrated in the trophoblast villi. RAGE receptor has been found in ZIKV infection of monocytes to mediate transmigration in vitro [49]. We expected RAGE to increase due to Hofbauer hyperplasia, but it decreased significantly. Perhaps this could be a mechanism induced by the virus to evade viral immune response in the ZIKV-infected placenta. AXL receptor has been designated as one of the receptors of entry for ZIKV into the placenta, but recent studies showed that it is not required for entry in mouse models of ZIKV infection [26,27,50–52]. In our study, AXL shows a significant decrease in expression in ZIKV-positive placentas compared to controls. Although the decrease in AXL receptor was unexpected, it can also suggest a possible mechanism of viral internalization and immune response evasion since AXL is involved in the activation of inflammation and cell survival.

Proteomics analyses revealed important information about a possible activation of the inflammasome and the pyroptosis signaling pathway. Both these pathways are essential in promoting a robust immune response to clear viral infections. Three essential proteins are upregulated in these pathways and contribute to the possible activation of these pathways. These proteins are caspase-1 (CASP1), serine/threonine-protein kinase Nek7 (NEK7), and ubiquitin-associated protein 2-like (Ub). CASP1 plays a central role in the execution phase of cell apoptosis. ZIKV recruits host deubiquitinase to cleave CASP1 [53]. This could explain why we see increased peptides of CASP1 in quantitative proteomics and a decrease of CASP1 in western blot. CASP1 attenuates ZIKV replication [54], and degradation of this protein would be beneficial to the viral propagation. In contrast, activation of an inflammatory response by NEK7 in placental tissue is ideal for ZIKV propagation since cell death caused by the inflammasome and pyroptosis will activate tissue remodeling pathways that were found upregulated in our previous study [28]. Quantitative proteomics detects peptides of the proteins digested while western blot detects antigens linked to a PVDF membrane following antibody treatment. It is possible that the antibody selected did not bind the peptides found in proteomics. Our results also could suggest that overexpression and degradation of CASP1 and TUBB are occurring in ZIKV-infected placental tissue to escape from immune response.

In our previous study [28], we saw how the acute response and coagulation pathways of extracellular proteins are upregulated in a ZIKV infection of the placenta. In our current results, we observed TUBA1C and TUBB, two proteins associated with the remodeling of the epithelial adherent junctions pathway, upregulated. The placental structure's integrity depends on tight and adherent junctions to protect the developing fetus [55]. Therefore, upregulations of the tubulin proteins could compensate for the loss of integrity caused by ZIKV infection by activating and impairing the immune response.

Our quantitative proteomics results further validate the involvement of the proteins CSTB and AXL in ZIKV infection of the placenta. PACS1 and CASP1 are indirectly associated with CSTB; expression PACS1 affects CSTB and CSTB indirectly activates CASP1 by inflammatory pathways. The expression of PACS1 is beneficial for ZIKV since it directs the localization of furin, a protease that cleaves ZIKV polyprotein, permitting the formation of viral particles [56].

PACS could also play a role in downregulating MHC-1 in the placenta, thus impairing the immune response. Our results show a discrepancy between immunohistochemistry and western blot of CSTB. Immunohistochemistry shows increased CSTB in the trophoblast layers. In contrast, our western blot of whole placental tissue shows a decrease in CSTB in ZIKV-positive cases. It is important to emphasize that immunohistochemistry is better for determining localization since areas with lower expression of proteins of interest can be masked due to saturation in other areas. With our labeling, we cannot distinguish the different types of trophoblast cells and their maturation states. CSTB accumulation can only be observed in the outer layer of the placenta, the syncytiotrophoblasts layers, but the placenta is composed of different types of cells that are in different maturation stages. The western blot was performed on a mixture of proteins that come from all the different types of cells that compose the placenta. CSTB observed in whole placental tissue was decreased. To address the limitation of having a mixture of different cell types in ex vivo tissue, we decided to use the trophoblast cell line JEG-3 in vitro infected with ZIKV. Western blot results show a decreased expression of CSTB in this trophoblast cell line. This contrasts with our immunohistochemistry results, which show expression in the syncytiotrophoblast. It appears that CSTB expression increases only in mature syncytiotrophoblasts and not in cytotrophoblasts. It is important to emphasize that the JEG-3 in vitro model has the limitation of being a single type of cytotrophoblast cell in contrast to the placental tissue having different stages of maturation and different types of cells working as a system. It is also difficult to contrast results of a full-term placenta that has been exposed to ZIKV infection for more time against a cell line that was exposed to ZIKV for a few hours. Taken together, these results demonstrated that ZIKV infection induced a shift in the expression of these inflammatory molecules in trophoblasts and Hofbauer cells, with a significant decrease in their expression in whole placental tissue, while increasing the expression of AXL and RAGE in the trophoblast cell layers. Future experiments should address CSTB expression in the placental tissue by isolating the different cell types of the placenta in an ex vivo model. The decrease in CSTB in whole placental tissue and trophoblasts could be an alternative tissue defense mechanism for suppressing the expression of CASP1 and the formation of the inflammasome [57]. We emphasize that the placenta is an organ that avoids inflammation because it is detrimental to the developing fetus. In contrast, ZIKV uses the host inflammatory system while avoiding it and promoting persistence of infection.

Furthermore, we found two upregulated proteins directly associated with AXL, poly(rC)-binding protein 1 (PCBP1) and HSPB1/HSP27. PCBP1 in other flaviviruses has been seen to benefit in the accumulation of viral RNA [58], leading to more viral particles. HSP27 upregulation was detected previously in our study [28] and in ZIKV-infected cells [59]. HSP27 is a chaperone that responds to environmental stress and causes actin remodeling, cytoskeleton, and membrane organization. AXL could activate the HSP27 and cause an upregulation due to response to impaired inflammation and the tissue damage caused by ZIKV infection. Knockout of HSP70 has provided a protection strategy against ZIKV infection [60]. Upregulation confirmation of HSP27 suggests that placental tissue is goes through stress that could be induced by ZIKV infection in the placenta. Our results suggest that HSP27 could play an important role directly or indirectly in ZIKV infection of the placenta, as seen in our previous quantitative proteomics results and confirmed in our current quantitative proteomics analyses and validation using western blot. Future experiments should be directed at the knockout or downregulation of HSP27 and how ZIKV infection and its pathology are affected in placental cell lines and models.

Taken together, these results suggest that a decrease in CSTB, RAGE, and AXL facilitates viral evasion of immune response to ensure its persistence in the trophoblast layer of the placenta. Our study provides insight into possible key molecules exploited by ZIKV infection to ensure its persistence in the host. Pathology findings may be a secondary effect of ZIKV deregulation of host proteins used in immune evasion, survival, and proliferation.

Supplementary Materials: The following supporting information can be downloaded at: https://www.mdpi.com/article/10.3390/cells11223627/s1, Figure S1: Macrophage labeling of placental tissue in Zika negative and Zika positive placentas. Representative fluorescence immunohistochemistry of ZIKV uninfected placental tissue and ZIKV infected tissue.; Figure S2: Localization of Zika Non-Structural Protein 1 of placental tissue in Zika negative and Zika positive placentas.; Figure S3: Localization of Cystatin B in placental tissue of Zika negative and Zika positive placentas.; Figure S4: Volcano plot for comparison between Zika(+) vs. Zika(−).; Figure S5: Overexpression of Tubulin in Remodeling of Epithelial Adherent Junctions pathway. Table S1: Differentially abundant proteins were identified per group comparison with a Fold Change $\geq |1.5|$ and p-value ≤ 0.05.

Author Contributions: The conceptualization of this research was completed through the work of G.B.-V., J.A.A., Y.M.C.-R., A.R.d.J. and L.M.M.; methodology, G.B.-V., J.A.A., J.R.-P., Y.M.C.-R., A.R.d.J. and L.J.R.-R.; formal analysis, G.B.-V., J.A.A., L.J.R.-R. and A.R.-L.; investigation, G.B.-V. and J.A.A.; resources, L.M.M., M.S.C.-R. and M.C.-R.; data curation, G.B.-V., L.J.R.-R. and A.R.-L.; writing—original draft preparation, G.B.-V., J.A.A. and J.R.-P.; writing—review and editing, G.B.-V., J.A.A., J.R.-P., L.J.R.-R., A.R.-L. and L.M.M.; visualization, G.B.-V. and J.A.A.; supervision, J.A.A. and L.M.M.; project administration, L.M.M.; funding acquisition, G.B.-V., J.A.A. and L.M.M. All authors have read and agreed to the published version of the manuscript.

Funding: This research was supported in part by grants from the National Institutes of Health-National Institute of General Medical Sciences (NIGMS) SC1GM11369 (L.M.M.), NIGMS-RISE R25 GM061838 RISE Program (G.B.V.), 1R15HD108743 and PR-INBRE-Institutional Developmental Award (IDEA) P20GM103475 (L.M.M.). Translational Proteomics Center (L.M.M.), and Bioinformatics and Health Informatics (A.R.L., K.C.C.) Research Infrastructure Core components supported by the National Institute on Minority Health and Health Disparities (NIMHD) U54-MD007600 from the Center for Collaborative Research Health Disparities. In addition, the fluorescent microscope used in this research was supported by the Hispanic Alliance for Clinical and Translational Research of the National Institutes of Health under award number U54GM133807-01.

Institutional Review Board Statement: This study was approved by the Institutional Review Board (IRB) of the University of Puerto Rico Medical Sciences Campus (UPR-MSC), Protocol Number 0720119, entitled Role of placenta cystatin B in mother to child transmission of Zika virus. The principal investigator of the protocol is Loyda M. Meléndez. This protocol did not involve direct interaction with human subjects. We did not perform recruitment because the 21 placenta samples were provided by Maria Correa from the UPR-MSC Department of Pathology and given to us with no patient identifiers. Placentas were collected with approval from subjects of legal age, 21 years or more. Information provided to us included gestational age, mode of delivery, and if Zika virus infection occurred during gestation. With this information, we divided our samples into two groups: positive and negative for Zika virus infection. No other information about the placental samples was available to us, and no knowledge of congenital Zika syndrome (CZS) was an outcome. No staff member or student has any financial interest, such as royalty or other payments in sponsor or other entities having a financial interest in intellectual property, product, or services. The research was performed complying with all the University of Puerto Rico Medical Sciences Campus policies and procedures as well as with all applicable Federal and State laws regarding the protection of human participants in research, protecting the rights and welfare of human participants, the conduct of the study, and the ethical performance of the project.

Informed Consent Statement: Patient consent was waived since no information was collected from patients, only from stored placentas that are usually discarded.

Data Availability Statement: The mass spectrometry proteomics data have been deposited to the ProteomeXchange Consortium via the PRIDE partner repository with the dataset identifier PXD037388 and 10.6019/PXD037388. Data are available via ProteomeXchange with identifier PXD037388.

Acknowledgments: This research was supported in part by grants of the National Institutes of Health National Institute of General Medical Sciences (NIGMS) SC1GM11369 (LMM), NIGMS-RISE R25 GM061838 RISE Program (GBV), and PR-INBRE-Institutional Developmental Award (IDEA) P20GM103475 (LMM). Translational Proteomics Center (LMM) and Bioinformatics and Health Informatics (ARL, KCC) Research Infrastructure Core components supported by the National Institute on Minority Health and Health Disparities (NIMHD) U54-MD007600 from the Center for Collaborative Research Health Disparities. The fluorescent microscope used in this research was supported by the Hispanic Alliance for Clinical and Translational Research of the National Institutes of Health under award number U54GM133807-01. We thank the Comprehensive Cancer Center for its research facilities and technical support (YCR). We also acknowledge Yisel M. Cantres-Rosario for her feedback on this manuscript's research design and writing. We acknowledge Bismark Madera-Soro (MS, MT, MLS (ASCP)CM) from the Neuroimaging and Electrophysiology Facility UPR-Molecular Sciences Research Center supported by NIH-NIGMS grant P20GM103642, for helping us with Nis-Elements A software Imaging Software and imaging analysis feedback. We thank the ASEM director, María J. Marcos-Martinez, for providing the placenta samples used in this study to the Pathology Department. We also thank Maribel Campos's staff, who shared collected fresh frozen placentas from the pilot project Dental and Craniofacial Effects of Intrauterine Zika Infection (1R21DE027235-01).

Conflicts of Interest: The authors have no conflicts of interest to declare relevant to this article's content.

References

1. Nobrega, G.M.; Samogim, A.P.; Parise, P.L.; Venceslau, E.M.; Guida, J.P.S.; Japecanga, R.R.; Amorim, M.R.; Toledo-Teixeira, D.A.; Forato, J.; Consonni, S.R.; et al. TAM and TIM Receptors MRNA Expression in Zika Virus Infected Placentas. *Placenta* **2020**, *101*, 204–207. [CrossRef] [PubMed]
2. Rawal, G.; Yadav, S.; Kumar, R. Zika Virus: An Overview. *J. Fam. Med. Prim. Care* **2016**, *5*, 523. [CrossRef] [PubMed]
3. Freitas, D.A.; Souza-Santos, R.; Carvalho, L.M.A.; Barros, W.B.; Neves, L.M.; Brasil, P.; Wakimoto, M.D. Congenital Zika Syndrome: A Systematic Review. *PLoS ONE* **2020**, *15*, e0242367. [CrossRef] [PubMed]
4. De Noronha, L.; Zanluca, C.; Burger, M.; Suzukawa, A.A.; Azevedo, M.; Rebutini, P.Z.; Novadzki, I.M.; Tanabe, L.S.; Presibella, M.M.; Dos Santos, C.N.D. Zika Virus Infection at Different Pregnancy Stages: Anatomopathological Findings, Target Cells and Viral Persistence in Placental Tissues. *Front. Microbiol.* **2018**, *9*, 2266. [CrossRef] [PubMed]
5. Simoni, M.K.; Jurado, K.A.; Abrahams, V.M.; Fikrig, E.; Guller, S. Zika Virus Infection of Hofbauer Cells. *Am. J. Reprod. Immunol.* **2017**, *77*, e12613. [CrossRef] [PubMed]
6. Quicke, K.M.; Bowen, J.R.; Johnson, E.L.; McDonald, C.E.; Ma, H.; O'Neal, J.T.; Rajakumar, A.; Wrammert, J.; Rimawi, B.H.; Pulendran, B.; et al. Zika Virus Infects Human Placental Macrophages. *Cell Host Microbe* **2016**, *20*, 83–90. [CrossRef]
7. Miner, J.J.; Diamond, M.S. Review Zika Virus Pathogenesis and Tissue Tropism. *Cell Host Microbe* **2017**, *21*, 134–142. [CrossRef]
8. Knöfler, M.; Pollheimer, J. Human Placental Trophoblast Invasion and Differentiation: A Particular Focus on Wnt Signaling. *Front. Genet.* **2013**, *4*, 190. [CrossRef]
9. Guzeloglu-Kayisli, O.; Kayisli, U.A.; Schatz, F.; Lockwood, C.J. Vertical Zika Virus Transmission at the Maternal-Fetal Interface. *Front. Virol.* **2022**, *2*, 801778. [CrossRef]
10. Luciano-Montalvo, C.; Ciborowski, P.; Duan, F.; Gendelman, H.E.; Meléndez, L.M. Proteomic Analyses Associate Cystatin B with Restricted HIV-1 Replication in Placental Macrophages. *Placenta* **2008**, *29*, 1016–1023. [CrossRef]
11. Luciano-Montalvo, C.; Meléndez, L.M. Cystatin B Associates with Signal Transducer and Activator of Transcription 1 in Monocyte-Derived and Placental Macrophages. *Placenta* **2009**, *30*, 464–467. [CrossRef] [PubMed]
12. Rivera, L.E.; Kraiselburd, E.; Meléndez, L.M. Cystatin B and HIV Regulate the STAT-1 Signaling Circuit in HIV-Infected and INF-β-Treated Human Macrophages. *J. Neurovirol.* **2016**, *22*, 666–673. [CrossRef] [PubMed]
13. Chen, Q.; Gouilly, J.; Ferrat, Y.J.; Espino, A.; Glaziou, Q.; Cartron, G.; El Costa, H.; Al-Daccak, R.; Jabrane-Ferrat, N. Metabolic Reprogramming by Zika Virus Provokes Inflammation in Human Placenta. *Nat. Commun.* **2020**, *11*, 2967. [CrossRef]
14. Ribeiro, M.R.; Moreli, J.B.; Marques, R.E.; Papa, M.P.; Meuren, L.M.; Rahal, P.; de Arruda, L.B.; Oliani, A.H.; Oliani, D.C.M.V.; Oliani, S.M.; et al. Zika-Virus-Infected Human Full-Term Placental Explants Display pro-Inflammatory Responses and Undergo Apoptosis. *Arch. Virol.* **2018**, *163*, 2687–2699. [CrossRef]
15. Goldstein, J.A.; Gallagher, K.; Beck, C.; Kumar, R.; Gernand, A.D. Maternal-Fetal Inflammation in the Placenta and the Developmental Origins of Health and Disease. *Front. Immunol.* **2020**, *11*, 531543. [CrossRef] [PubMed]
16. Buckley, S.T.; Ehrhardt, C. The Receptor for Advanced Glycation End Products (RAGE) and the Lung. *J. Biomed. Biotechnol.* **2010**, *2010*, 917108. [CrossRef] [PubMed]
17. Warburton, D.; Bellusci, S.; De Langhe, S.; Del Moral, P.-M.; Fleury, V.; Mailleux, A.; Tefft, D.; Unbekandt, M.; Wang, K.; Shi, W. Molecular Mechanisms of Early Lung Specification and Branching Morphogenesis. *Pediatr. Res.* **2005**, *57*, 26–37. [CrossRef]
18. Alexander, K.L.; Mejia, C.A.; Jordan, C.; Nelson, M.B.; Howell, B.M.; Jones, C.M.; Reynolds, P.R.; Arroyo, J.A. Differential Receptor for Advanced Glycation End Products Expression in Preeclamptic, Intrauterine Growth Restricted, and Gestational Diabetic Placentas. *Am. J. Reprod. Immunol.* **2016**, *75*, 172–180. [CrossRef]
19. Xie, J.; Méndez, J.D.; Méndez-Valenzuela, V.; Aguilar-Hernández, M.M. Cellular Signalling of the Receptor for Advanced Glycation End Products (RAGE). *Cell Signal.* **2013**, *25*, 2185–2197. [CrossRef]
20. Tsai, K.Y.F.; Hirschi Budge, K.M.; Llavina, S.; Davis, T.; Long, M.; Bennett, A.; Sitton, B.; Arroyo, J.A.; Reynolds, P.R. RAGE and AXL Expression Following Secondhand Smoke (SHS) Exposure in Mice. *Exp. Lung Res.* **2019**, *45*, 297–309. [CrossRef]
21. Laurance, S.; Lemarié, C.A.; Blostein, M.D. Growth Arrest-Specific Gene 6 (Gas6) and Vascular Hemostasis. *Adv. Nutr.* **2012**, *3*, 196–203. [CrossRef] [PubMed]
22. Korshunov, V.A. Axl-Dependent Signalling: A Clinical Update. *Clin. Sci.* **2012**, *122*, 361–368. [CrossRef] [PubMed]
23. Gui, S.; Zhou, S.; Liu, M.; Zhang, Y.; Gao, L.; Wang, T.; Zhou, R. Elevated Levels of Soluble Axl (SAxl) Regulates Key Angiogenic Molecules to Induce Placental Endothelial Dysfunction and a Preeclampsia-Like Phenotype. *Front. Physiol.* **2021**, *12*, 619137. [CrossRef] [PubMed]
24. Hirschi, K.M.; Tsai, K.Y.F.; Davis, T.; Clark, J.C.; Knowlton, M.N.; Bikman, B.T.; Reynolds, P.R.; Arroyo, J.A. Growth Arrest-Specific Protein-6/AXL Signaling Induces Preeclampsia in Rats. *Biol. Reprod.* **2020**, *102*, 199–210. [CrossRef]
25. Peng, S.; Sun, M.; Sun, X.; Wang, X.; Jin, T.; Wang, H.; Han, C.; Meng, T.; Li, C. Plasma Levels of TAM Receptors and Ligands in Severe Preeclampsia. *Pregnancy Hypertens.* **2018**, *13*, 116–120. [CrossRef]
26. Xie, S.; Zhang, H.; Liang, Z.; Yang, X.; Cao, R. AXL, an Important Host Factor for DENV and ZIKV Replication. *Front. Cell. Infect. Microbiol.* **2021**, *11*, 575346. [CrossRef]
27. Strange, D.P.; Jiyarom, B.; Pourhabibi Zarandi, N.; Xie, X.; Baker, C.; Sadri-Ardekani, H.; Shi, P.-Y.; Verma, S. Axl Promotes Zika Virus Entry and Modulates the Antiviral State of Human Sertoli Cells. *MBio* **2019**, *10*, 4. [CrossRef]

28. Borges-Vélez, G.; Rosado-Philippi, J.; Cantres-Rosario, Y.M.; Carrasquillo-Carrion, K.; Roche-Lima, A.; Pérez-Vargas, J.; González-Martínez, A.; Correa-Rivas, M.S.; Meléndez, L.M. Zika Virus Infection of the Placenta Alters Extracellular Matrix Proteome. *J. Mol. Histol.* **2021**, *53*, 199–214. [CrossRef]
29. Cantres-Rosario, Y.M.; Ortiz-Rodríguez, S.C.; Santos-Figueroa, A.G.; Plaud, M.; Negron, K.; Cotto, B.; Langford, D.; Melendez, L.M. HIV Infection Induces Extracellular Cathepsin B Uptake and Damage to Neurons. *Sci. Rep.* **2019**, *9*, 8006. [CrossRef]
30. Ritchie, M.E.; Phipson, B.; Wu, D.; Hu, Y.; Law, C.W.; Shi, W.; Smyth, G.K. Limma Powers Differential Expression Analyses for RNA-Sequencing and Microarray Studies. *Nucleic Acids Res.* **2015**, *43*, e47. [CrossRef]
31. Kammers, K.; Cole, R.N.; Tiengwe, C.; Ruczinski, I. Detecting Significant Changes in Protein Abundance. *EuPA Open Proteom.* **2015**, *7*, 11–19. [CrossRef]
32. Magalhães, I.C.L.; Marques, L.E.C.; Souza, P.F.N.; Girão, N.M.; Herazo, M.M.A.; Costa, H.P.S.; van Tilburg, M.F.; Florean, E.O.P.T.; Dutra, R.F.; Guedes, M.I.F. Non-Structural Protein 1 from Zika Virus: Heterologous Expression, Purification, and Potential for Diagnosis of Zika Infections. *Int. J. Biol. Macromol.* **2021**, *186*, 984–993. [CrossRef] [PubMed]
33. Melendez, L.M. SARS-CoV-2: Biology, Detection, Macrophage Mediated Pathogenesis and Potential Treatments. *Virol. Immunol. J.* **2020**, *4*, 1–13. [CrossRef]
34. Fakonti, G.; Pantazi, P.; Bokun, V.; Holder, B. Placental Macrophage (Hofbauer Cell) Responses to Infection During Pregnancy: A Systematic Scoping Review. *Front. Immunol.* **2022**, *12*, 756035. [CrossRef]
35. Rivera, L.E.; Colon, K.; Cantres-Rosario, Y.M.; Zenon, F.M.; Melendez, L.M. Macrophage Derived Cystatin B/Cathepsin B in HIV Replication and Neuropathogenesis. *Curr. HIV Res.* **2014**, *12*, 111–120. [CrossRef] [PubMed]
36. Chakraborty, K.; Bhattacharyya, A. Role of Proteases in Inflammatory Lung Diseases. In *Proteases in Health and Disease*; Springer: New York, NY, USA, 2013; pp. 361–385.
37. Rogalla, T.; Ehrnsperger, M.; Preville, X.; Kotlyarov, A.; Lutsch, G.; Ducasse, C.; Paul, C.; Wieske, M.; Arrigo, A.-P.; Buchner, J.; et al. Regulation of Hsp27 Oligomerization, Chaperone Function, and Protective Activity against Oxidative Stress/Tumor Necrosis Factor α by Phosphorylation. *J. Biol. Chem.* **1999**, *274*, 18947–18956. [CrossRef]
38. Li, D.; Shen, K.M.; Zackai, E.H.; Bhoj, E.J. Clinical Variability of TUBB-Associated Disorders: Diagnosis through Reanalysis. *Am. J. Med. Genet. A* **2020**, *182*, 3035–3039. [CrossRef]
39. Auriti, C.; De Rose, D.U.; Santisi, A.; Martini, L.; Piersigilli, F.; Bersani, I.; Ronchetti, M.P.; Caforio, L. Pregnancy and Viral Infections: Mechanisms of Fetal Damage, Diagnosis and Prevention of Neonatal Adverse Outcomes from Cytomegalovirus to SARS-CoV-2 and Zika Virus. *Biochim. Biophys. Acta-Mol. Basis Dis.* **2021**, *1867*, 166198. [CrossRef]
40. Guzeloglu-Kayisli, O.; Guo, X.; Tang, Z.; Semerci, N.; Ozmen, A.; Larsen, K.; Mutluay, D.; Guller, S.; Schatz, F.; Kayisli, U.A.; et al. Zika Virus–Infected Decidual Cells Elicit a Gestational Age–Dependent Innate Immune Response and Exaggerate Trophoblast Zika Permissiveness: Implication for Vertical Transmission. *J. Immunol.* **2020**, *205*, 3083–3094. [CrossRef]
41. Rosenberg, A.Z.; Weiying, Y.; Hill, D.A.; Reyes, C.A.; Schwartz, D.A. Placental Pathology of Zika Virus: Viral Infection of the Placenta Induces Villous Stromal Macrophage (Hofbauer Cell) Proliferation and Hyperplasia. *Arch. Pathol. Lab. Med.* **2017**, *141*, 43–48. [CrossRef]
42. Hilgenfeld, R. Zika Virus NS 1, a Pathogenicity Factor with Many Faces. *EMBO J.* **2016**, *35*, 2631–2633. [CrossRef] [PubMed]
43. Bhatnagar, J.; Rabeneck, D.B.; Martines, R.B.; Reagan-Steiner, S.; Ermias, Y.; Estetter, L.B.C.; Suzuki, T.; Ritter, J.; Keating, M.K.; Hale, G.; et al. Zika Virus RNA Replication and Persistence in Brain and Placental Tissue. *Emerg. Infect. Dis.* **2017**, *23*, 405–414. [CrossRef] [PubMed]
44. Schwartz, D.A.; Baldewijns, M.; Benachi, A.; Bugatti, M.; Bulfamante, G.; Cheng, K.; Collins, R.R.J.; Debelenko, L.; de Luca, D.; Facchetti, F.; et al. Hofbauer Cells and COVID-19 in Pregnancy: Molecular Pathology Analysis of Villous Macrophages, Endothelial Cells, and Placental Findings from 22 Placentas Infected by SARS-CoV-2 with and without Fetal Transmission. *Arch. Pathol. Lab. Med.* **2021**, *145*, 1328–1340. [CrossRef]
45. Schwartz, D.A. Viral Infection, Proliferation, and Hyperplasia of Hofbauer Cells and Absence of Inflammation Characterize the Placental Pathology of Fetuses with Congenital Zika Virus Infection. *Arch. Gynecol. Obstet.* **2017**, *295*, 1361–1368. [CrossRef] [PubMed]
46. Huang, M.T.; Liu, W.L.; Lu, C.W.; Huang, J.J.; Chuang, H.L.; Huang, Y.T.; Horng, J.H.; Liu, P.; Han, D.S.; Chiang, B.L.; et al. Feedback Regulation of IFN-α/β Signaling by Axl Receptor Tyrosine Kinase Modulates HBV Immunity. *Eur. J. Immunol.* **2015**, *45*, 1696–1705. [CrossRef]
47. Son, H.Y.; Jeong, H.K. Immune Evasion Mechanism and AXL. *Front. Oncol.* **2021**, *11*, 756225. [CrossRef]
48. Rolfe, A.J.; Bosco, D.B.; Wang, J.; Nowakowski, R.S.; Fan, J.; Ren, Y. Bioinformatic Analysis Reveals the Expression of Unique Transcriptomic Signatures in Zika Virus Infected Human Neural Stem Cells. *Cell Biosci.* **2016**, *6*, 42. [CrossRef]
49. de Carvalho, G.C.; Borget, M.Y.; Bernier, S.; Garneau, D.; da Silva Duarte, A.J.; Dumais, N. RAGE and CCR7 Mediate the Transmigration of Zika-Infected Monocytes through the Blood-Brain Barrier. *Immunobiology* **2019**, *224*, 792–803. [CrossRef]
50. Rausch, K.; Hackett, B.A.; Weinbren, N.L.; Reeder, S.M.; Sadovsky, Y.; Hunter, C.A.; Schultz, D.C.; Coyne, C.B.; Cherry, S. Screening Bioactives Reveals Nanchangmycin as a Broad Spectrum Antiviral Active against Zika Virus. *Cell Rep.* **2017**, *18*, 804–815. [CrossRef]
51. Tabata, T.; Petitt, M.; Puerta-Guardo, H.; Michlmayr, D.; Wang, C.; Fang-Hoover, J.; Harris, E.; Pereira, L. Zika Virus Targets Different Primary Human Placental Cells, Suggesting Two Routes for Vertical Transmission. *Cell Host Microbe* **2016**, *20*, 155–166. [CrossRef]

52. Hastings, A.K.; Yockey, L.J.; Jagger, B.W.; Hwang, J.; Uraki, R.; Gaitsch, H.F.; Parnell, L.A.; Cao, B.; Mysorekar, I.U.; Rothlin, C.V.; et al. TAM Receptors Are Not Required for Zika Virus Infection in Mice. *Cell Rep.* **2017**, *19*, 558–568. [CrossRef] [PubMed]
53. Zheng, Y.; Liu, Q.; Wu, Y.; Ma, L.; Zhang, Z.; Liu, T.; Jin, S.; She, Y.; Li, Y.; Cui, J. Zika Virus Elicits Inflammation to Evade Antiviral Response by Cleaving cGAS via NS_1-caspase-$_1$ Axis. *EMBO J.* **2018**, *37*, e99347. [CrossRef] [PubMed]
54. Wang, W.; Li, G.; Wu, D.; Luo, Z.; Pan, P.; Tian, M.; Wang, Y.; Xiao, F.; Li, A.; Wu, K.; et al. Zika Virus Infection Induces Host Inflammatory Responses by Facilitating NLRP3 Inflammasome Assembly and Interleukin-1β Secretion. *Nat. Commun.* **2018**, *9*, 106. [CrossRef] [PubMed]
55. Leach, L. The Phenotype of the Human Materno-Fetal Endothelial Barrier: Molecular Occupancy of Paracellular Junctions Dictate Permeability and Angiogenic Plasticity*. *J. Anat.* **2002**, *200*, 599–606. [CrossRef] [PubMed]
56. Owczarek, K.; Chykunova, Y.; Jassoy, C.; Maksym, B.; Rajfur, Z.; Pyrc, K. Zika Virus: Mapping and Reprogramming the Entry. *Cell Commun. Signal.* **2019**, *17*, 41. [CrossRef] [PubMed]
57. Tang, Y.; Cao, G.; Min, X.; Wang, T.; Sun, S.; Du, X.; Zhang, W. Cathepsin B Inhibition Ameliorates the Non-Alcoholic Steatohepatitis through Suppressing Caspase-1 Activation. *J. Physiol. Biochem.* **2018**, *74*, 503–510. [CrossRef]
58. Cousineau, S.E.; Rheault, M.; Sagan, S.M. Poly(RC)-Binding Protein 1 Limits Hepatitis C Virus Virion Assembly and Secretion. *Viruses* **2022**, *14*, 291. [CrossRef]
59. Glover, K.K.M.; Gao, A.; Zahedi-Amiri, A.; Coombs, K.M. Vero Cell Proteomic Changes Induced by Zika Virus Infection. *Proteomics* **2019**, *19*, 1800309. [CrossRef]
60. Taguwa, S.; Yeh, M.-T.; Rainbolt, T.K.; Nayak, A.; Shao, H.; Gestwicki, J.E.; Andino, R.; Frydman, J. Zika Virus Dependence on Host Hsp70 Provides a Protective Strategy against Infection and Disease. *Cell Rep.* **2019**, *26*, 906–920.e3. [CrossRef]

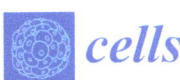

Article

S100A8-Mediated NLRP3 Inflammasome-Dependent Pyroptosis in Macrophages Facilitates Liver Fibrosis Progression

Yan Liu [1,†], Xuehua Kong [1,†], Yan You [2], Linwei Xiang [1], Yan Zhang [1], Rui Wu [3], Lan Zhou [1,*] and Liang Duan [4,*]

1. Key Laboratory of Laboratory Medical Diagnostics, Ministry of Education, Department of Laboratory Medicine, Chongqing Medical University, Chongqing 400016, China
2. Department of Pathology, The Second Affiliated Hospital of Chongqing Medical University, Chongqing 400010, China
3. Department of Laboratory Medicine, The First Affiliated Hospital of Chongqing Medical University, Chongqing 400016, China
4. Department of Laboratory Medicine, The Second Affiliated Hospital of Chongqing Medical University, Chongqing 400010, China
* Correspondence: zhoulan@cqmu.edu.cn (L.Z.); duanliang@cqmu.edu.cn (L.D.); Tel.: +23-68485388 (L.Z.); +23-63693193 (L.D.)
† These authors contributed equally to this work.

Citation: Liu, Y.; Kong, X.; You, Y.; Xiang, L.; Zhang, Y.; Wu, R.; Zhou, L.; Duan, L. S100A8-Mediated NLRP3 Inflammasome-Dependent Pyroptosis in Macrophages Facilitates Liver Fibrosis Progression. *Cells* **2022**, *11*, 3579. https://doi.org/10.3390/cells11223579

Academic Editors: Vasso Apostolopoulos, Jack Feehan and Vivek P. Chavda

Received: 19 October 2022
Accepted: 10 November 2022
Published: 12 November 2022

Publisher's Note: MDPI stays neutral with regard to jurisdictional claims in published maps and institutional affiliations.

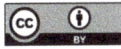

Copyright: © 2022 by the authors. Licensee MDPI, Basel, Switzerland. This article is an open access article distributed under the terms and conditions of the Creative Commons Attribution (CC BY) license (https://creativecommons.org/licenses/by/4.0/).

Abstract: NLRP3 inflammasome-dependent pyroptosis has been implicated in liver fibrosis progression. However, the definite intrahepatic cell types that undergo pyroptosis and the underlying mechanism as well as the clinical importance remain unclear. Here, augmented levels of pyroptosis-related indicators GSDMD, IL-1β, and IL-18 were verified in both liver fibrosis patients and CCl4-induced fibrotic mouse model. Confocal imaging of NLRP3 with albumin, F4/80 or α-SMA revealed that enhanced NLRP3 was mainly localized to kupffer cells (KCs), indicating that KCs are major cell types that undergo pyroptosis. Targeting pyroptosis by inhibitor MCC950 attenuated the severity and ameliorated liver function in fibrosis models. In addition, elevated S100A8 in liver fibrosis patients was correlated with pyroptosis-related indicators. S100A8 stimulated pyroptotic death of macrophages, which resulted in activation of human hepatic stellate cell line LX-2 cells and increased collagen deposition. Mechanistically, S100A8 activated TLR4/NF-κB signaling and upregulated its target genes NLRP3, pro-IL-1β, and pro-IL-18 expression, and induced reactive oxygen (ROS) abundance to activate NLRP3 inflammasome, finally leading to pyroptotic cell death in macrophages. More importantly, circulating GSDMD had the optimal predicting value for liver fibrosis progression. In conclusion, S100A8-mediated NLRP3 inflammasome-dependent pyroptosis by TLR4/NF-κB activation and ROS production in macrophages facilitates liver fibrosis progression. The identified GSDMD has the potential to be a biomarker for liver fibrosis evaluation.

Keywords: NLRP3; S100A8; GSDMD; liver fibrosis

1. Introduction

Hepatic fibrosis is a wound-healing response characterized by the accumulation of extracellular matrix (ECM) following excessive cell death and chronic liver inflammation due to a variety of etiological factors, including virus infection, alcohol abuse, non-alcoholic steatohepatitis, parasitemia, metabolic disorders, and drugs [1,2]. Early stage liver fibrosis can be stopped or reversed by removing the insults that triggered liver damage and inflammation [3,4]. However, in many cases, liver fibrosis progresses to cirrhosis over time and increases the risk of liver failure and hepatocellular carcinoma [1]. At present, serology examination represents one of the frequently used methods for the diagnosis and evaluation of liver fibrosis, but several limitations still exist, including low sensitivity and specificity, inaccurate disease assessment, and even misdiagnosis. In addition, despite decades of efforts by clinical research, there is no effective therapy for liver fibrosis. Therefore, further elucidating the pathogenesis of liver fibrosis and identifying novel biomarkers that closely reflect disease progression are urgently needed.

NLRP3 (NACHT, LRR, and PYD domains-containing protein 3, cryoporin) inflammasome-dependent pyroptosis, a newly identified inflammatory cell death, participates in multiple diseases, including infection, metabolic disorders, and cancer [5,6]. It starts with the recognition of pathogen-associated molecular patterns (PAMPs) or damage-associated molecular patterns (DAMPs) by extracellular pattern recognition receptors (PRRs) leading to enhanced transcription of NLRP3, pro-IL (interleukin)-1β, and pro-IL-18, continues with the activation of NLRP3 and caspase-1 by multiple intracellular stimulus, and ends with gasdermin D (GSDMD)-mediated formation of membrane pores and the maturation and release of proinflammatory cytokines IL-1β and IL-18 [7]. Due to the proinflammatory property of pyroptosis, the role of uncontrolled pyroptosis caused by aberrant inflammasome activation in inflammation-associated diseases has received considerable attention. Pyroptosis has recently been reported to be associated with pulmonary, renal, and cardiovascular fibrosis [8–10]. More importantly, growing evidence suggests a close correlation between NLRP3 inflammasome activation as well as its downstream effectors and liver fibrosis progression. One study reported that hyperactivation of the NLRP3 inflammasome in mice results in hepatocyte pyroptotic death, severe liver inflammation, and fibrosis [11]. Moreover, in a mouse model of non-alcoholic fatty liver disease and non-alcoholic steatohepatitis, NLRP3 inflammasome activation is required for liver inflammation and fibrosis [12,13]. In addition, an in vitro mechanistic study showed that the pyroptosis products IL-1β and IL-18 regulate the activation of hepatic stellate cells (HSCs) and facilitate the development of liver fibrosis [14]. Notably, patients with liver cirrhosis also exhibited elevated levels of circulating GSDMD, IL-1β, and IL-18 in our previous clinical research [15]. Therefore, NLRP3 inflammasome-dependent pyroptosis may serve as a crucial mechanism for the development of liver injury and fibrosis. Nevertheless, the primary occurrence of NLRP3 inflammasome-dependent pyroptosis in which type of cells (hepatocytes, KCs or HSCs), the detailed molecular mechanism regarding how pyroptosis occurs, and its clinical importance during liver fibrosis progression, are still unclear.

S100A8 and S100A9, belonging to the S100 protein family (S100s), are secreted mainly by inflammatory, tumor, and stromal cells exhibiting proinflammatory functions. As two DAMPs, S100A8 and S100A9 have been implicated as inflammation triggers participating in the progression of multiple inflammatory diseases, including rheumatoid arthritis [16], inflammatory bowel [17], and lung disease [18]. Recently, S100A8 and S100A9 were reported to activate NLRP3 inflammasome signaling to promote the pathogenesis of myelodysplastic syndromes [19] and airway obstructive diseases [20]. It is worth noting that our previous study demonstrated an elevated S100A9 in liver fibrosis [21]. Given this, we hypothesized that S100A8 and/or S100A9 may regulate NLRP3 inflammasome-dependent pyroptosis to establish a proinflammatory microenvironment, thereby potentiating the progression of liver fibrosis.

In the present study, the definite cell types that undergo pyroptosis and the underlying mechanism as well as the clinical importance were investigated, aiming to further reveal the pathogenesis of liver fibrosis and identify novel markers and intervention targets. Here, we observed that the macrophage was the major cell type that underwent NLRP3 inflammasome-dependent pyroptosis in liver fibrosis, which could be mediated by S100A8-induced Toll-like receptor 4 (TLR4)/NF-κB activation and ROS generation. Furthermore, inhibiting NLRP3 inflammasome-dependent pyroptosis effectively attenuated liver injury and fibrosis severity in a carbon tetrachloride (CCl4)-induced liver fibrosis mouse model. More importantly, the pyroptosis-related indicator GSDMD had a high predictive value for the onset and progression of liver fibrosis.

2. Materials and Methods

2.1. Human Samples

A total of eighty-nine patients with liver fibrosis were enrolled in the current study between March 2020 and December 2021 at the Second Affiliated Hospital of Chongqing Medical University. Diagnosis was primarily established by histology as well as other methods, such as serological, imaging examination, and medical history. Etiologies, such as viral infection, alcohol consumption, and autoimmunity were determined according to serological and histological findings. The sections for liver histology were examined independently by two experienced pathologists who were unaware of the clinical status. Liver fibrosis grading was assessed according to Batts-Ludwing scores (Fibrosis F0 to F4) [22]. Additionally, sixty age- and gender-matched healthy volunteers who did not have evidence of liver diseases or other chronic disorders were enrolled as healthy controls (HCs). Moreover, five normal liver samples were obtained from healthy controls who underwent liver biopsy to exclude malignancy. The peripheral blood was centrifuged for 10 min to obtain serum. Then, the serum was stored at −80 °C for further examination. This study protocol was in accordance with the ethical guidelines of the Declaration of Helsinki Principles. Informed written consent was obtained from all patients and the study was approved by the Institutional Ethics Committee at the Second Hospital affiliated with Chongqing Medical University (No. 2020-65). Patient characteristics are summarized in Table 1.

Table 1. The characteristics of enrolled individuals.

Parameters	Liver fibrosis	HCs	
	Serum/tissue Specimen ($n = 89$)	Serum specimen ($n = 60$)	Tissue Specimen ($n = 5$)
Gender			
Male n (%)	47 (52.81)	34 (56.66)	3 (60)
Fale n (%)	42 (47.19)	26 (43.33)	2 (40)
Age (years) (IQR)	57 (12.75)	57 (14.5)	59 (17.5)
Aetiology			
Viral hepatitis n (%)	42 (47.19)	NA	NA
Cholestatic /Autoimmune n (%)	25 (28.08)	NA	NA
Alcohol n (%)	16 (17.97)	NA	NA
Others n (%)	6 (6.74)	NA	NA
Stage of fibrosis (F)			
F0 n (%)	9 (10.11)	NA	NA
F1 n (%)	10 (11.23)	NA	NA
F2 n (%)	20 (22.47)	NA	NA
F3 n (%)	29 (32.58)	NA	NA
F4 n (%)	21 (23.59)	NA	NA

Abbreviations: IQR, interquartile range; HCs, healthy controls; NA, not applicable.

2.2. CCl4-Induced Liver Fibrosis Mouse Models

Herein, 6 to 8-week-old male C57BL/6 mice were randomly grouped. For toxic liver fibrosis, they were given intraperitoneal (i.p.) injections of CCl4 (2.5 mL/kg body weight, dissolved in olive oil at a ratio of 1:5) or vehicle (olive oil) (O108686, Aladdin, Fengxian, Shanghai, China) two times per week for 4, 6 or 8 weeks ($n = 5$/group). The mice were sacrificed at 72 h after the final CCl4 injection.

To assess the role of NLRP3 signaling in the mouse model of liver fibrosis, 6 to 8-week-old male mice were randomly divided into three groups. The CCl4 group were given intraperitoneal (i.p.) injections of CCl4 (2.5 mL/kg body weight, dissolved in olive oil at a ratio of 1:5). The (CCl4+MCC950) group were injected (i.p.) with MCC950 (10 mg/kg body weight in 0.9% NaCl) (CP-456773, Selleck, Houston, TX, USA) every second day at the same time as the CCl4 injection up to 8 weeks, while the control group (CCl4+saline) was administrated a comparable volume of 0.9% NaCl (n = 5/group). The mice were sacrificed at 72 h after the final CCl4 injection. All animal experiments were approved and conducted in accordance with the guidelines established by the Hospital Animal Care and Use Committee for Laboratory Animal Research in the Second Affiliated Hospital of Chongqing Medical University (No. 2020-65).

2.3. Mouse Serum and Liver Samples Preparation

At the end of the treatment, all mice were anesthetized and the blood samples were taken via cardiac puncture. The mouse blood was centrifuged at 3500× g rpm at 4 °C for 15 min and then for 10 min to remove any remaining cellular debris. Finally, the serum was stored at −80 °C for further examination. Then, the liver was harvested. A representative section was fixed in 4% paraformaldehyde for 24 h and embedded in paraffin, and the rest of the liver tissue was stored in liquid nitrogen.

2.4. Analysis of Liver Function, Liver Pathology, and Fibrosis

The serum alanine aminotransferase (ALT), aspartate aminotransferase (AST), and total proteins (TP) were assayed by the Autoanalyzer Hitachi 7600-110. H&E staining was used to assess the pathological morphology of the liver. Sirius Red staining was used to demonstrate collagen deposition. The stained sections were observed and photographed under a light microscope (Nikon E400, Chiyoda, Tokyo, Japan).

2.5. Immunohistochemical Staining

The formalin-fixed, paraffin-embedded human and mouse liver tissue sections were subjected to IHC staining. Briefly, the sections were deparaffinized, hydrated, and subjected to antigen retrieval by incubating the slides in a pressure cooker for 15 min in 0.01 M citrate buffer and then incubated with 0.3% hydrogen peroxide (H_2O_2) in methanol for 10 min to block endogenous peroxidase activity. Then, the sections were incubated with primary antibodies against α-smooth muscle actin (α-SMA) (14395-1-AP, Proteintech, Wuhan, Hubei, China), NLRP3 (19771-1-AP, Proteintech, Wuhan, Hubei, China), GSDMD (20770-1-AP, Proteintech, Wuhan, Hubei, China), IL-1β (16806-1-AP, Proteintech, Wuhan, Hubei, China), S100A8 (ab92331, Abcam, Cambridge, England, UK) or S100A9 (ab63818, Abcam, Cambridge, England, UK) overnight at 4 °C. The cells were washed with PBS and stained with anti-rabbit IHC Secondary Antibody Kit (SP-9001, Zhongshan Golden Bridge, Haidian, Beijing, China). Finally, the sections were visualized with 0.05% 3,3-diamino-benzidine tetrachloride (DAB) until the desired brown reaction product was obtained. The stained sections were observed and photographed under a light microscope (Nikon E400, Chiyoda, Tokyo, Japan).

2.6. Immunofluorescence Staining

The formalin-fixed, paraffin-embedded human and mouse liver tissue sections were processed for immunofluorescence staining. In brief, the liver sections were deparaffinized, hydrated, subjected to antigen retrieval, permeabilization, and serum blocking, and then incubated with primary antibody overnight at 4 °C for double immunofluorescence staining. The primary antibodies used were as follows: Rabbit anti-NLRP3 (19771-1-AP, Proteintech, Wuhan, Hubei, China) with rat anti-albumin (MAB1455-SP, R&D, Minneapolis, MN, USA) or with mouse anti-F4/80 (14-4801-85, Invitrogen, Carlsbad, CA, USA), rat anti-NLRP3 (MAB7578-SP, R&D, Minneapolis, Minnesota, USA) with rabbit anti-α-SMA (14395-1-AP, Proteintech, Wuhan, Hubei, China). Then, the sections were washed three times with PBS. Alexa Fluor 647-conjugated goat anti-rabbit secondary antibody (bs-0295G-AF647, Bioss, Tongzhou, Beijing, China) and Alexa Fluor 488-conjugated goat anti-mouse secondary antibody (bs-0296G-AF488, Bioss, Tongzhou, Beijing, China) or goat anti-rat secondary antibody (bs-0293G-AF488, Bioss, Tongzhou, Beijing, China), Alexa Fluor 647-conjugated goat anti-rat secondary antibody (bs-0293G-AF647, Bioss, Tongzhou, Beijing, China) and

Alexa Fluor 488-conjugated goat anti-rabbit secondary antibody (bs-0295G-AF488, Bioss, Tongzhou, Beijing, China) were used for 1 h at room temperature in the dark. Then, the sections were washed with PBS three times, and nuclei were stained with DAPI for 5 min. The sections were washed with PBS three times and mounted with antifade mounting medium (Beyotime, Songjiang, Shanghai, China). Finally, the sections were observed under a confocal microscope (Lecia, Weztlar, Germany).

2.7. Enzyme-Linked Immunosorbent Assay (ELISA)

Protein of interest in serum or cell supernatant was detected by ELISA according to the manufacturer's instructions. Detailed ELISA kits were as follows: Mouse S100A8 (E-EL-M3048, elabscience, Wuhan, Hubei, China), mouse IL-1β (VAL601, Novus, Littleton, CO, USA), mouse IL-18 (E-EL-M0730c, elabscience, Wuhan, Hubei, China), mouse GSDMD (JL46371-96T, JiangLai, Baoshan, Shanghai, China), human S100A8 (E-EL-H1289c, elabscience, Wuhan, Hubei, China), human IL-1β (Mengbio, Shapingba, Chongqing, China), human IL-18 (Mengbio, Shapingba, Chongqing, China), and human GSDMD (Mengbio, Shapingba, Chongqing, China).

2.8. Preparation of Recombinant Proteins

The pGST-moluc and pGST-moluc-S100A8 have been described previously [23]. Briefly, the two plasmids were cloned into E. coil (BL21) by calcium chloride transformation. Then, 0.1 mM isopropylthio-β-D-galactoside was used to induce the expression of GST and GST-hS100A8 protein for 8 h at 14 °C. After incubation, the bacteria were centrifuged at $5000 \times g$ for 10 min and the pellet was resuspended in PBS supplemented with protease inhibitor and 0.1% Triton X-100 and lysed by sonication. Then, the supernatant was collected and incubated with glutathione-sepharose 4B beads (Amersham Biosciences) for 3 h at 4 °C. Recombinant GST-hS100A8 (rhS100A8) or GST bound to the beads was eluted by an elution buffer with reduced glutathione on ice. Finally, the recombinant rhS100A8 or control GST protein was filtered with a 0.22 μm membrane and stored at −80 °C.

2.9. Cell Culture and In Vitro Treatment

Human monocyte THP-1 cells were cultured in 5% CO_2 at 37 °C in 1640-RPMI medium supplemented with 10% fetal bovine serum (FBS, HyClone, Logan, UT, USA), 100 U/mL penicillin, and 100 μg/mL streptomycin (HyClone). THP-1 cells were stimulated with PMA (50 μg/mL) (Sigma, Saint Louis, MO, USA) for 4 h to differentiate them into macrophages, then washed two times with PBS and maintained in fresh medium for further experiments.

To induce pyroptosis in THP-1 differentiated macrophages, high dose of lipopolysaccharide (LPS) (1 μg/mL, L2630, Sigma-Aldrich, Saint Louis, MO, USA) was added to the culture media. In certain experiments, THP-1 differentiated macrophages were stimulated with 2, 5 or 10 μg/mL rhS100A8 for 24 h to extract RNA or for 48 h to extract protein. To explore the role of NF-κB signaling and ROS production in S100A8-induced pyroptosis, THP-1 differentiated macrophages were treated with the NF-κB inhibitor BAY 11-7082 (10 μM, Beyotime, Songjiang, Shanghai, China) or NADPH oxidase (NOX) inhibitor diphenylene iodonium (DPI, 10 μM, S8639, Selleck, Houston, Texas, USA) for 1 h prior to rhS100A8 stimulation (5 μg/mL). To investigate the endogenous PRR of S100A8, THP-1 differentiated macrophages were pretreated with the TLR4 inhibitor TAK-242 (10 μM, S7455, Selleck, Houston, Texas, USA) or the receptor for advanced end products (RAGE) inhibitor FPS-ZM1 (10 μM, S8185, Selleck, Houston, Texas, USA) for 1 h and then stimulated with rhS100A8 (5 μg/mL).

The human hepatic stellate cell line LX-2 was maintained in 5% CO_2 at 37 °C in Dulbecco's modified Eagle medium (DMEM, Gibco, Grand Island, NY, USA) with 10% fetal bovine serum (FBS, HyClone, Logan, UT, USA), 100 U/mL penicillin, and 100 μg/mL streptomycin (HyClone, Logan, UT, USA). LX-2 cells were exposed to conditioned media (CM) from rhS100A8-treated THP-1 macrophages and an equal volume of new DMEM medium for 24 h to extract RNA or for 48 h to extract protein. To confirm that macrophage pyroptosis triggers the activation of HSCs, LX-2 cells were treated with the conditioned medium from THP-1 macrophages exposed to 5 μ/mL of rhS100A8 with or without 1 h of MCC950 pretreatment (1 μM).

2.10. RNA Extraction and Quantitative Real-Time PCR

Total cellular RNA was isolated using Trizol (Invitrogen, Carlsbad, CA, USA) according to the manufacturer's instructions. Briefly, 1 μg of total RNA was reverse-transcribed to cDNA via an Evo M-MLV RT mix kit with gDNA clean (AG11728, Accurate Biotechnology, Changsha, Hunan, China) according to the manufacturer's protocol. The mRNA levels of NLRP3, pro-IL-1β, pro-IL-18, collagen I (COL1A1), α-SMA, and transforming growth factor-β (TGF-β) were analyzed with the CFX96 real-time PCR detection system (Bio-Rad, Richmond, CA, USA) using SYBR Green dye (Biomake, Houston, TX, USA). Primer sequences are summarized in Table 2. GAPDH was used as a reference control. The fold changes in gene expression were calculated by the 2-ΔΔCT method.

Table 2. Sequence of primers used for quantitative RT-PCR.

Genes	Forward (5'-3')	Reverse (5'-3')
NLRP3	CTTCTCTGATGAGGCCCAAG	GCAGCAAACTGGAAAGGAAG
pro-IL-1β	TCCAGGGACAGGATATGGAG	TCTTTCAACACGCAGGACAG
pro-IL-18	AAGATGGCTGCTGAACCAGT	GAGGCCGATTTCCTTGGTCA
Col1a1	AAGAGTGGAGAGTACTGGATT	GTTCTTGCTGATGTACCAGT
α-SMA	CGTGGGTGACGAAGCACAG	GGTGGGATGCTCTTCAGGG
TGF-β	GGCCAGATCCTGTCCAAGC	GTGGGTTTCCACCATTAGCAC
GAPDH	CCACTCCTCCACCTTTGAC	ACCCTGTTGCTGTAGCCA

Abbreviations: NLRP3, nod-like receptor protein-3; COL1A1, collagen I; α-SMA, α-smooth muscle actin; TGF-β, transforming growth factor beta; GAPDH, glyceraldehyde-3-phosphate dehydrogenase.

2.11. Western Blot

Treated cells were collected and lysed in RIPA lysis buffer containing phosphatase and protease inhibitors. The BCA protein assay (abs9232, Absin, Pudong New District, Shanghai, China) was used to assess the protein concentrations. Samples containing equal amounts (30 μg) of proteins were separated by 10% SDS-PAGE and then transferred to polyvinylidene fluoride membranes. Then, the membranes were blocked with 5% bovine serum albumin and incubated overnight at 4 °C with primary antibody against NLRP3 (19771-1-AP, Proteintech, Wuhan, Hubei, China), GSDMD (20770-1-AP, Proteintech, Wuhan, Hubei, China), IL-1β (16806-1-AP, Proteintech, Wuhan, Hubei, China), cleaved caspase-1 (4199T, Cell Signaling Technology, Boston, MA, USA), α-SMA (14395-1-AP, Proteintech, Wuhan, Hubei, China), COL1A1 (66761-1-lg, Proteintech, Wuhan, Hubei, China), TGF-β (MAB1835-SP, R&D, Minneapolis, Minnesota, USA), total NF-κB p65 (10745-1-AP, Proteintech, Wuhan, Hubei, China), phospho-NF-κB p65 (p-p65) (3033, Cell Signaling Technology, Boston, Massachusetts, USA), total IKKα (db2315, diagbio, Hangzhou, Zhejiang, China), phospho-IKKα (p-IKKα) (2697, Cell Signaling Technology, Boston, MA, USA), and β-actin (Zoonbio Biotechnology, Nanjing, Jiangsu, China). The next day, after incubation with goat-anti-rabbit or goat-anti-mouse secondary antibodies, the samples were conjugated with horseradish peroxidase for 1 h at 37 °C, and the immune complexes were detected by enhanced chemiluminescence (ECL, Millipore, Boston, MA, USA).

2.12. Flow Cytometry

The production of ROS in THP-1 macrophages was measured using the dichlorodihydrofluorescein diacetate (H2DCFDA) probe (S9687, Selleck, USA) according to the manufacturer's recommendation. In brief, THP-1 macrophages were stimulated with rhS100A8 (5 μg/mL) or the control protein GST (5 μg/mL) for 6 h. THP-1 macrophages were collected and washed three times with serum-free medium, and subsequently incubated in serum-free medium containing 10 μM H2DCFDA probe at 37 °C for 30 min in the dark.

Then, the media containing H2DCFDA was removed and washed two times with PBS, and the fluorescence intensity of the cells was analyzed by flow cytometry (CytoFLEX). Cells that had been incubated without H2DCFDA were used as negative controls. To detect pyroptotic death in THP-1 macrophages that had been treated with rhS100A8 or control protein GST for 24 h, FLICA 660-YVAD-FMK (FLICA 660 in vitro Active Caspase-1 Detection Kit; ImmunoChemistry Technologies, Davis, CA, USA) was used according to the manufacturer's instructions and propidium iodide (PI) was used to mark cells with membrane pores (Life Technologies, Carlsbad, CA, USA). Flow cytometry measurements were performed three times for each treatment. The mean fluorescence intensity was quantified usingFlowJo v10.8.1 (FlowJo LLC, Ashland, OR, USA).

2.13. Statistical Analysis

All data were analyzed using SPSS 17.0 (IBM Corp., Armonk, NY, USA). Human data were not normally distributed continuous variables and were expressed as the median and interquartile range (IQR). Animal data were expressed as the mean ± standard deviation (SD). Statistical analysis of serum levels of GSDMD, IL-1β, and IL-18 in liver fibrosis patients was determined by the Kruskal-Wallis or Mann-Whitney test. Correlation coefficients (r) were calculated using Spearman correlation. ROC curves were generated to classify patients into different groups, as well as to evaluate the predictive power of serum GSDMD, IL-1β, and IL-18 levels via the calculation of AUC. Differences between multiple groups in the in vitro cell experiments were evaluated using a t-test or one-way analysis of variance. A p-value < 0.05 was considered statistically significant.

3. Results

3.1. NLRP3 Inflammasome-Dependent Pyroptosis Occurs in Liver Fibrosis

Herein, we examined the pyroptosis-related indicators NLRP3, GSDMD, IL-18, and IL-1β. Immunohistochemical (IHC) analysis revealed that the expression of hepatic GSDMD, IL-1β, and IL-18 was significantly upregulated in patients with liver fibrosis compared to HCs (Figures 1A and S1A). Moreover, serological data of GSDMD, IL-1β, and IL-18 supported this IHC result (Figure 1B–D). To further investigate in which types of cells (hepatocytes, KCs, or HSCs) NLRP3 inflammasome-dependent pyroptosis mainly occurs during the process of liver fibrosis, we examined the co-location of NLRP3 with the hepatocyte marker albumin, the KC marker F4/80 or the HSC marker α-smooth muscle actin (α-SMA) in human fibrotic liver tissues. We observed the enhanced expression of NLRP3 in patients with liver fibrosis compared to HCs and NLRP3 was mainly localized to hepatocytes and KCs but not HSCs, especially KCs, indicating that KCs are major cell types that undergo pyroptosis (Figure 1E). Then, we further validated the above results with a CCl4-induced liver fibrosis mouse model (Figure 1F). H&E, Sirius Red, and α-SMA staining proved that we successfully established a mouse model of liver fibrosis (Figures 1G and S1B). Moreover, consistent with the human data, GSDMD and IL-1β expression were significantly increased in the liver from the liver fibrosis mouse model compared with the control (Figures 1G and S1B). Furthermore, serum levels of GSDMD, IL-18, and IL-1β were markedly enhanced in mouse models of liver fibrosis (Figure 1H–J). As expected, double immunolabelling in mouse liver sections also indicated that the activation of NLRP3 occurred mainly in KCs (Figure 1K). To investigate the effects of macrophage pyroptosis on the activation of HSCs and liver fibrosis in vitro, we induced pyroptotic death in THP-1 macrophages using the pyroptosis inducer lipopolysaccharide (LPS) and collected the CM to treat LX-2 cells. The protein levels of IL-1β in the cells and supernatants were confirmed (Figure 1M). The protein levels of HSC activation and the collagen deposition markers COLIA1, α-SMA, and TGF-β were significantly higher in LPS-CM-cultured LX-2 cells than in the control group (Figure 1N).

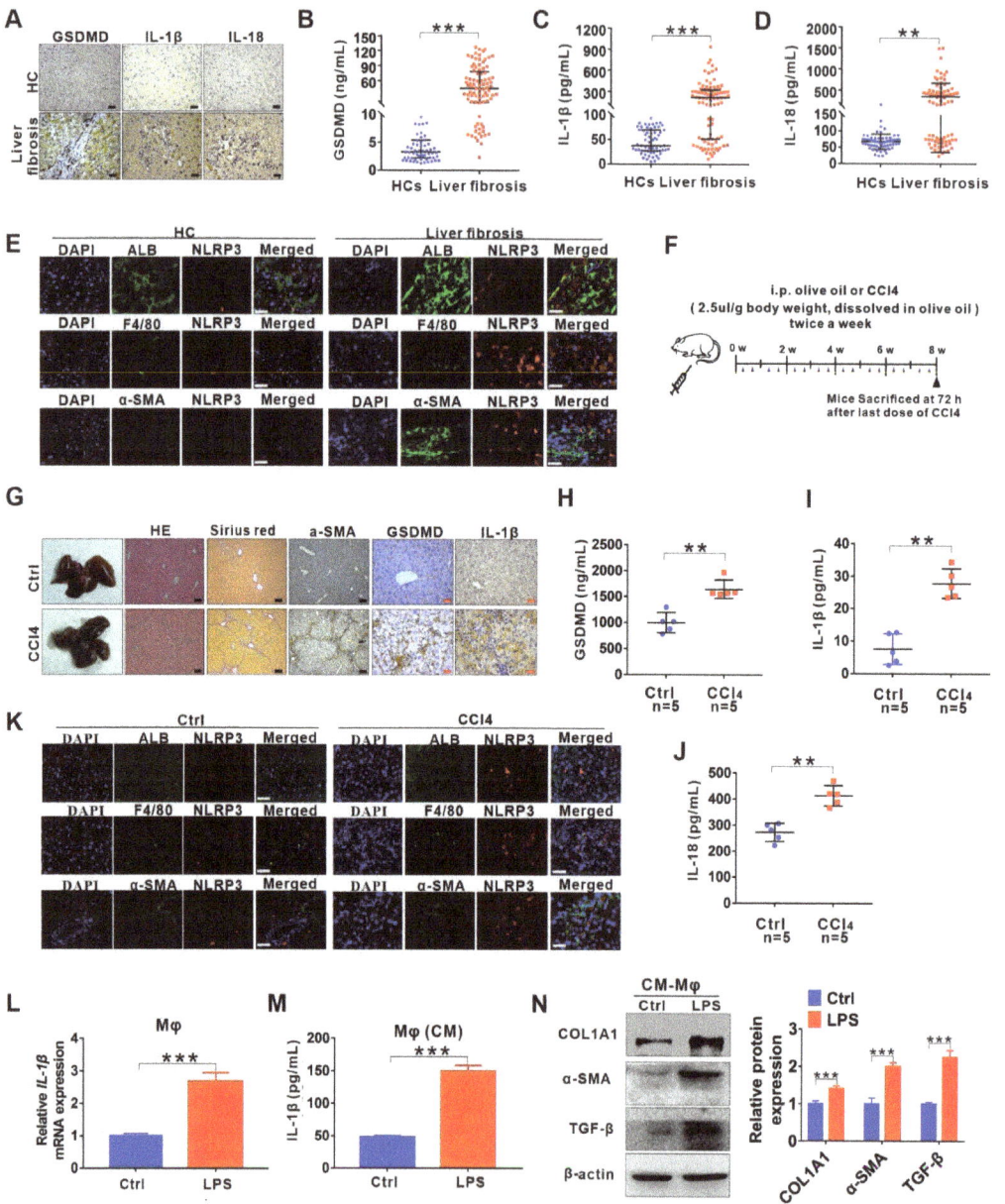

Figure 1. NLRP3 inflammasome-dependent pyroptosis occurs in liver fibrosis. (**A**) IHC staining for GSDMD, IL-1β, and IL-18 in liver sections from liver fibrosis patients and HCs. Scale bar: 40 μm. (**B–D**) ELISA analyses of serum levels of GSDMD (**B**), IL-1β (**C**), and IL-18 (**D**) in liver fibrosis patients (n = 89) and HCs (n = 60). (**E**) Representative immunofluorescence images of NLRP3 (red) and albumin (hepatocyte marker) (top), F4/80 (KC marker) (middle) or α-SMA (HSC marker) (bottom) (green) from the human fibrotic liver tissues. Scale bar: 40 μm. (**F**) Schematic diagram of the study. Liver fibrosis was induced by CCl4 injection for 8 weeks. (**G**) Representative mouse liver histology of H&E, Sirius Red staining, and IHC staining for α-SMA, GSDMD, and IL-1β. Black scale

bar: 100 µm; Red scale bar: 50 µm. (**H–J**) ELISA analyses for serum levels of GSDMD (H), IL-1β (I), and IL-18 (J) in CCl4 group mouse (n = 5) and vehicle group mouse (n = 5). (**K**) Representative immunofluorescence images of NLRP3 (red) and albumin (hepatocyte marker) (top), F4/80 (KC marker) (middle) or α-SMA (HSC marker) (bottom) (green) from the 8-week CCl4-treated mouse liver. The vehicle group mouse liver was used as a control. Scale bar: 40 µm. (**L**) The qRT-PCR analysis for mRNA levels of IL-1β in THP-1 macrophages treated with LPS to induce pyroptosis. (**M**) ELISA analysis for IL-1β expression in supernatants from THP-1. (**N**) Western blot analysis of COL1A1, α-SMA, and TGF-β expression in LX-2 cells which were exposed to CM from LPS-treated THP-1 macrophages. The protein expression was quantified by densitometry and normalized to β-actin and are shown as fold changes relative to the control group (right panel). ** $p < 0.01$, *** $p < 0.001$.

3.2. Inhibition of NLRP3 Inflammasome-Dependent Pyroptosis Alleviates Liver Fibrosis Progression

Given that NLRP3 inflammasome-dependent pyroptosis was involved in the liver fibrosis, we used a specific molecular inhibitor of NLRP3 (MCC950) to treat the liver fibrosis mouse model (Figure 2A), aiming to explore whether targeting the NLRP3 inflammasome-dependent pyroptosis can attenuate liver fibrosis progression. IHC analysis demonstrated that the MCC950 treatment significantly decreased the expression of pyroptosis-related indicators NLRP3, GSDMD, and IL-1β in the fibrotic livers (Figures 2B and S1C). Importantly, the MCC950 treatment reduced liver injury and fibrosis severity, as analyzed by histology, collagen, and α-SMA via HE, Sirius Red, and IHC staining, respectively (Figures 2B and S1C). Serum ALT and AST levels in the serum were notably lower in the MCC950-treated group than in the saline-treated group, while the serum levels of total proteins (TP) were significantly increased in the MCC950-treated group compared to the saline-treated group, indicating an improvement in liver function after MCC950 treatment (Figure 2C–E).

3.3. DAMP S100A8 along with NLRP3 Inflammasome-Dependent Pyroptosis Is Positively Related to the Progression of Liver Fibrosis

Hepatic inflammation is the main initiator of liver injury and fibrosis. As two members of DAMPs, S100A8 and S100A9, can serve as triggering factors and amplifiers of inflammation [24], and we have previously found that S100A9 increases in liver fibrosis [21]. Therefore, we further addressed their relationship with hepatic inflammation and fibrosis. IHC and enzyme-linked immunosorbent assay (ELISA) results showed that S100A8 and S100A9 were both significantly elevated in liver fibrosis patients compared to HCs (Figure 3A–C and Figure S1D). Notably, S100A8 increased more dramatically than S100A9 during the progression of liver fibrosis from fibrosis F0 to F4 (Figure 3D). Additionally, the levels of the pyroptosis-related indicators GSDMD, IL-18, and IL-1β were consistent with those of S100A8, exhibiting a gradual elevation from F0 to F4 (3E–G). Moreover, S100A8 levels were found to be positively correlated with the pyroptosis-related indicators GSDMD, IL-18, and IL-1β levels in LF patients (Figure 3H–J). Then, we conducted CCl4-induced mouse liver fibrosis models (4/6/8 weeks) to further verify the results mentioned above. The progression of liver fibrosis was proven by H&E, Sirius Red, and α-SMA staining from 4 to 8 weeks (Figure 3K). Staining signals of the pyroptosis mediator NLRP3 alone with S100A8 were gradually increased with the aggravation of liver fibrosis in mouse models from 4 to 8 weeks (Figure 3K and Figure S1E,F). Similar to the human data, the increase in S100A9 was not dramatic during the progression (Figure 3K and Figure S1G). Furthermore, serum S100A8 and pyroptosis-related indicators GSDMD, IL-1β, and IL-18 levels were all gradually augmented during the progression of the liver fibrosis model (Figure 3L–O).

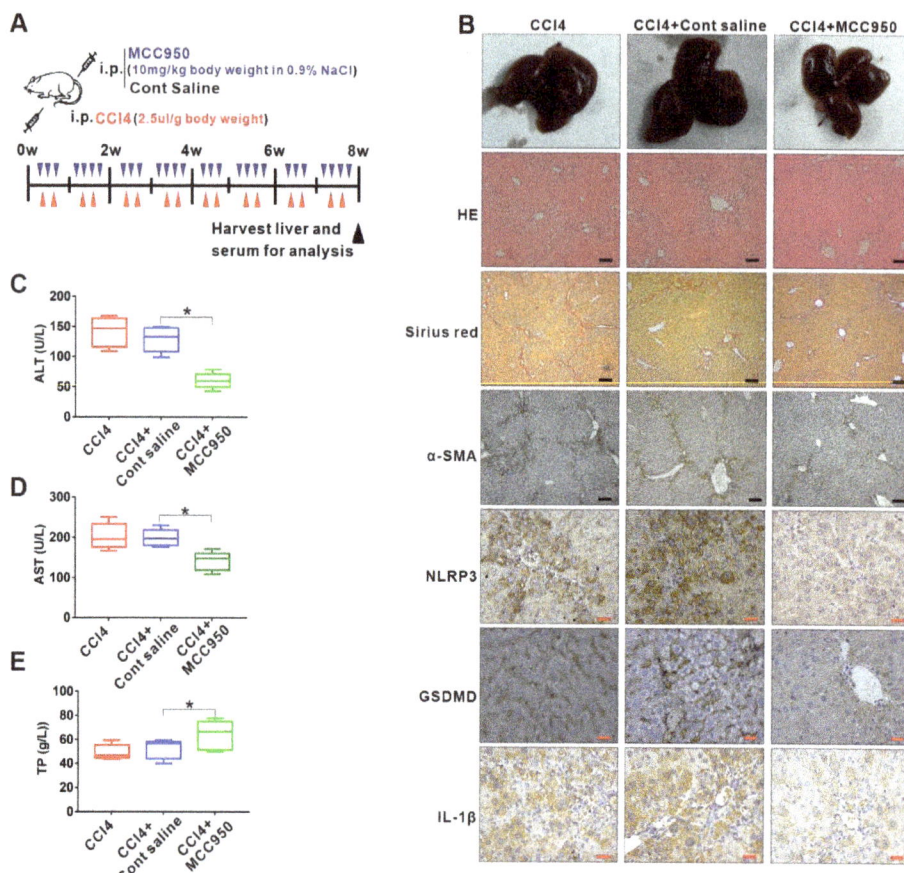

Figure 2. Inhibition of NLRP3 inflammasome-dependent pyroptosis alleviates liver fibrosis progression. (**A**) Experimental protocol of NLRP3 inhibitor MCC950 or saline application based on CCl4 injection in mice. (**B**) Representative liver histology of H&E and Sirius Red staining. The expression of α-SMA, NLRP3, GSDMD, and IL-1β was determined by immunohistochemistry. Black scale bar: 100 μm; Red scale bar: 50 μm. (**C–E**) Serum levels of ALT, AST, and TP were measured. * $p < 0.05$.

3.4. S100A8-Mediated NLRP3 Inflammasome-Dependent Pyroptotic Macrophage Death Amplifies the Activation of Human Hepatic Stellate Cells

DAMPs can activate the NLRP3 inflammasome and trigger persistent inflammation, contributing to fibrogenesis of the kidney [25] and lung [26]. Here, we further explored whether S100A8 can promote liver fibrosis by inducing NLRP3 inflammasome-dependent pyroptotic death in macrophages. The mRNA levels of NLRP3, pro-IL-1β, and pro-IL-18 for priming the NLRP3 inflammasome were upregulated by various concentrations of recombinant human GST-hS100A8 (rhS100A8) protein (2, 5, 10 μg/mL) treatment (Figure 4A–C). In addition, rhS100A8 (5 μg/mL) markedly increased the expression of proteins downstream of NLRP3 inflammasome activation, including cleaved GSDMD (GSDMD p30), cleaved caspase-1, and bioactive IL-1β in THP-1 macrophages (Figure 4D), as well as elevated IL-1β levels in supernatants (Figure S2). Moreover, the rhS100A8 treatment resulted in a significant increase in the number of proptotic THP-1 macrophages detected by caspase-1/PI double staining using FCM (Figure 4E). These data suggested that S100A8 could induce the activation of NLRP3 inflammasome signaling and finally lead to pyroptotic cell death in THP-1 macrophages. Furthermore, to determine whether pyroptoic cell death in macrophages induced by S100A8 was involved in HSC hyperactivation, LX-2 cells were treated with CM from rhS100A8-stimulated THP-1 macrophages, and the fibrotic markers TGF-β, COLIA1, and α-SMA were analyzed. The mRNA and protein levels of the COL1A1, α-SMA, and TGF-β in LX-2 cells were elevated by CM from various concentrations of rhS100A8-treated THP-1 macrophages (Figure 4F–I), which could be blocked by the NLRP3 inhibitor MCC950 (Figure 4J).

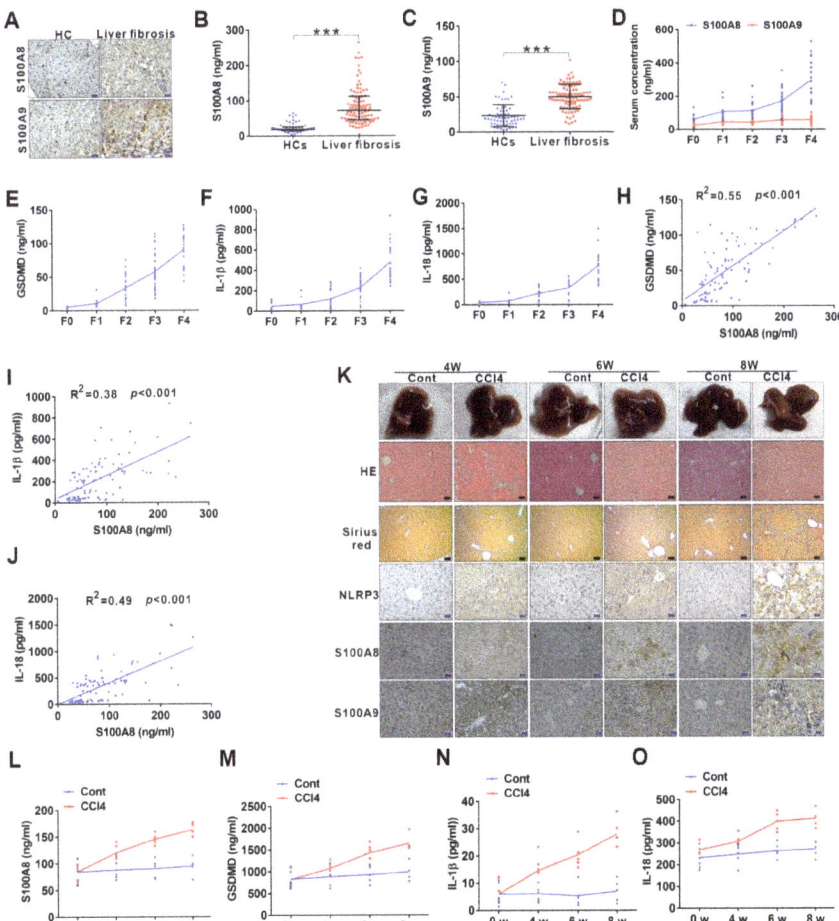

Figure 3. DAMP S100A8 along with NLRP3 inflammasome-dependent pyroptosis is positively related to the progression of liver fibrosis. (A) Representative IHC images for S100A8 and S100A9 in liver sections from liver fibrosis patients and HCs. (B,C) ELISA analyses for serum levels of S100A8 and S100A9 in liver fibrosis patients and HCs. (D) Comparison of serum S100A8 and S100A9 levels in liver fibrosis patients with different phases. (E–G) Distribution of serum GSDMD (E), IL-1β (F), and IL-18 (G) levels in liver fibrosis patients with different phases (F0–4). (H–J) Correlation between serum S100A8 levels and GSDMD (H), IL-1β (I) or IL-18 (J) levels in liver fibrosis patients. (K) Representative mouse liver morphology and staining with H&E and Sirius Red. (L–O) IHC staining of mouse liver sections for NLRP3, S100A8, and S100A9. Black scale bar: 100 μm; Red scale bar: 50 μm. ELISA analyses for serum levels of S100A8 (L), GSDMD (M), IL-1β (n), and IL-18 (O) in 4-, 6-, and 8 week-mouse models of liver fibrosis. *** $p < 0.001$.

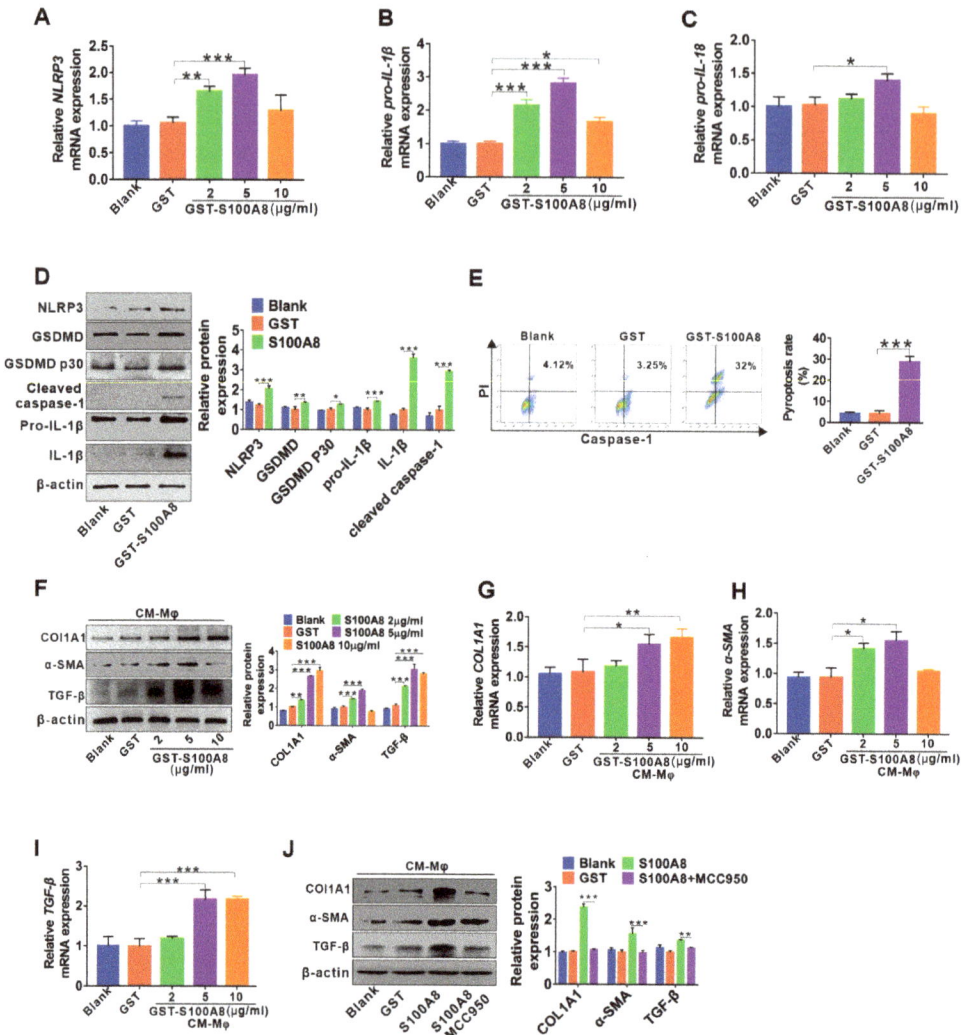

Figure 4. S100A8-mediated NLRP3 inflammasome-dependent pyroptotic macrophage death amplify the activation of human hepatic stellate cells. (**A–C**) The qRT–PCR analysis for the mRNA levels of NLRP3, pro-IL-1β, and pro-IL-18 in THP-1 macrophages treated with 0, 2, 5 or 10 μg/mL rhS100A8 or 5 μg/mL GST for 24 h. (**D**) The protein levels of NLRP3, GSDMD, GSDMD P30, pro-IL-1β, mature IL-1β, and cleaved caspase-1 were detected by Western blot in THP-1 macrophages treated with 5 μg/mL GST or rhS100A8. The protein expression was quantified by densitometry and normalized to β-actin and are shown as fold changes relative to the GST group (right panel). (**E**) PI and active caspase-1 double staining of pyroptotic cell death by flow cytometry in THP-1 macrophages treated with 5 μg/mL GST or rhS100A8. (**F–I**) Western blot analysis (**F**) and qRT-PCR analysis (**G–I**) of COL1A1, α-SMA, and TGF-β in LX-2 cells exposed to CM from THP-1 macrophages that were treated with 0, 2, 5 or 10 μg/mL of rhS100A8 or 5 μg/mL GST. (**J**) Western blot analysis of COL1A1, α-SMA, and TGF-β in LX-2 cells exposed to CM from THP-1 macrophages that were treated with 5 μg/mL of rhS100A8 with or without 1 h of MCC950 pretreatment. The protein expression was quantified by densitometry and normalized to β-actin and are shown as fold changes relative to the GST group (right panel). * $p < 0.05$, ** $p < 0.01$, *** $p < 0.001$.

3.5. TLR4/NF-κB Signaling Cascade and ROS Abundance Are Responsible for S100A8-Induced NLRP3 Inflammasome-Dependent Pyroptotic Death in Macrophages

Since we have observed that S100A8 could induce pyroptotic death in macrophages, we then investigated the potential molecular mechanism. First, we focused on NF-κB activation, a crucial mediator of the priming step for NLRP3 inflammasome-mediated pyroptosis. The protein levels of p-IKKα and p-p65 were enhanced in response to GST-rhS100A8 but not the control GST treatment within 60 min (Figure 5A). In addition, treatment with the NF-κB inhibitor BAY 11-7082 notably reversed S100A8-induced upregulation of the mRNA levels of NLRP3, pro-IL-1β, and pro-IL-18 (Figure 5B–D). Moreover, a similar tendency was confirmed by analysis for protein levels of pyroptosis-related indicators, including NLRP3, GSDMD, GSDMD P30, pro-IL-1β, IL-1β, and cleaved caspase-1 (Figure 5E), suggesting that activation of NF-κB participates in S100A8-induced pyroptosis. It is known that S100A8 is an endogenous ligand of PRRs, including TLR4 [24] and RAGE [27]. Then, we searched whether TLR4 or RAGE transduces S100A8-induced activation of NF-κB signaling as well as the NLRP3 inflammasome. Increased levels of p-p65 and p-IKKα stimulated by S100A8 were partially inhibited by the TLR4 inhibitor TAK-242, while the RAGE inhibitor FPS-ZM1 had fewer effects (Figure 5F). Similarly, inhibition of TLR4 by TAK-242 markedly reduced the mRNA expression of NLRP3, pro-IL-1β, and pro-IL-18, while inhibition of RAGE had minor effects (Figure 5B–D).

As a direct trigger and amplifier of NLRP3 inflammasome activation, ROS is reported to be closely associated with liver fibrosis progression [28]. In peripheral blood of mononuclear cells and HaCaT keratinocytes, ROS production can be induced by S100A8 via increasing NADPH oxidase (NOX) activity [29,30]. Then, we investigated whether S100A8 can directly induce ROS production and mediate NLRP3 inflammasome-dependent pyroptosis. Here, the augmentation of overall ROS levels in THP-1 macrophages was detected after stimulation with S100A8 by DCFH-DA fluorescent probe analysis (Figure 5G). In contrast, suppressing ROS production with the inhibitor DPI clearly attenuated the S100A8-mediated expression of pyroptosis-related indicators NLRP3, GSDMD, pro-IL-1β, mature IL-1β, and GSDMD p30 (Figure 5H), suggesting the important role of ROS in S100A8-mediated NLRP3 inflammasome-dependent pyroptosis.

3.6. The Potential Predictive Powers of S100A8, GSDMD, IL-1β, and IL-18 for the Occurrence and Severity of Liver Fibrosis

Based on the role of S100A8-elicited NLRP3 pyroptosis in liver fibrosis, we chose a well-defined cohort of liver fibrosis patients to assess the clinical importance of circulating S100A8, GSDMD, IL-1β, and IL-18 for predicting the occurrence and progression of disease. The ROC analysis indicated that the circulating GSDMD had the strongest diagnostic value for the occurrence of liver fibrosis with an area under the ROC curve (AUC) of 0.95 (95% CI, 0.9279–0.9842) compared to S100A8, IL-1β or IL-18 with AUCs of 0.93 (95% CI, 0.9011–0.9766), 0.81 (95% CI, 07523–0.8849), and 0.81 (95% CI, 0.7425–0.8803), respectively (Figure 6A). Moreover, we explored the predictive ability of these indicators for liver fibrosis severity. Furthermore, circulating GSDMD had the highest diagnostic value for identifying severe liver fibrosis, which yielded an AUC of 0.91 (95% CI, 0.8614–0.9725) compared to IL-1β, S100A8, and IL-18 with AUCs of 0.90 (95% CI, 0.8523–0.9677), 0.89 (95% CI, 0.8209–0.9606), and 0.89 (95% CI, 0.8348–0.9591), respectively (Figure 6B). These data implied that the identified GSDMD may be used as a potential biomarker during the occurrence and progression of liver fibrosis.

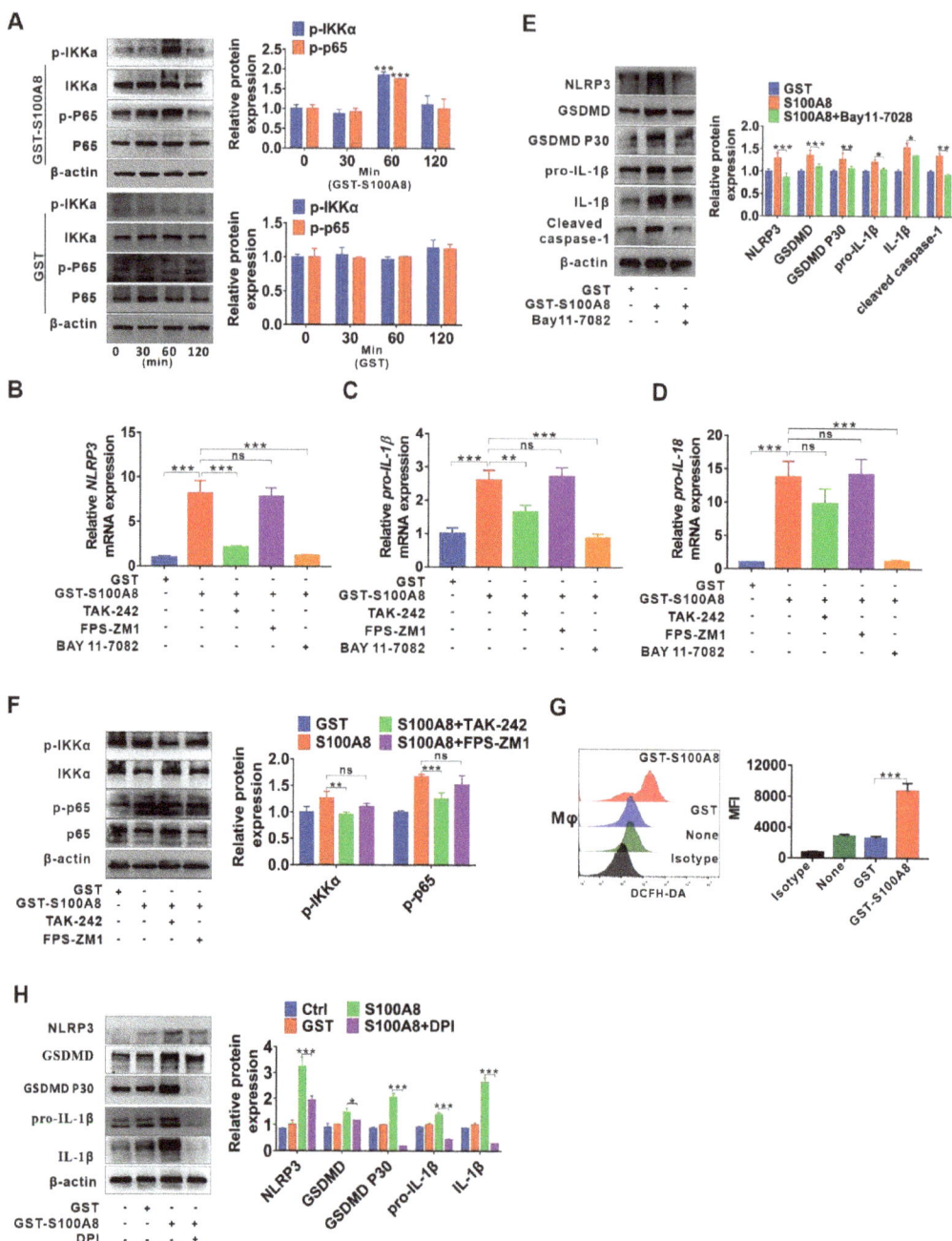

Figure 5. TLR4/NF-κB signaling cascade and ROS abundance are responsible for S100A8-induced NLRP3 inflammasome-dependent pyroptotic death in macrophages. (**A**) Western blot analysis of p65, p-p65, IKKα, and p-IKKα expression in THP-1 macrophages treated with GST-rhS100A8 or GST for 0, 30, 60 or 120 min. The protein expression was quantified by densitometry and normalized to β-actin and are shown as fold changes relative to the 0 min group (right panel). (**B–E**) THP-1 macrophages

were exposed to 5 μg/mL rhS100A8 with or without 1 h of BAY 11-7082, TAK-242 or FPS-ZM1 pretreatment. The qRT-PCR analysis was performed to detect the mRNA levels of NLRP3 (**B**), pro-IL-1β (**C**), and pro-IL-18 (**D**). Western blot analysis was used to determine the protein expression of NLRP3, GSDMD, GSDMD P30, pro-IL-1β, mature IL-1β, and cleaved caspase-1 (**E**). The protein expression was quantified by densitometry and normalized to β-actin and are shown as fold changes relative to the GST group (right panel). (**F**) THP-1 macrophages were pretreated with TAK-242 or FPS-ZM1 for 1 h and then exposed to 5 μg/mL of rhS100A8. Western blot analysis was used to determine the expression of p-p65 and p-IKKα. The protein expression was quantified by densitometry and normalized to β-actin and are shown as fold changes relative to the GST group (right panel). (**G**) Flow cytometry analysis of ROS levels in THP-1 macrophages treated with rhS100A8 for 6 h. (**H**) THP-1 macrophages were exposed to 5 μg/mL of rhS100A8 with or without 1 h of DPI pretreatment. Protein expression levels of NLRP3, GSDMD, GSDMD P30, pro-IL-1β, and mature IL-1β were determined by Western blot. The protein expression was quantified by densitometry and normalized to β-actin and are shown as fold changes relative to the GST group (right panel); ns, not significant; * $p < 0.05$, ** $p < 0.01$, *** $p < 0.001$.

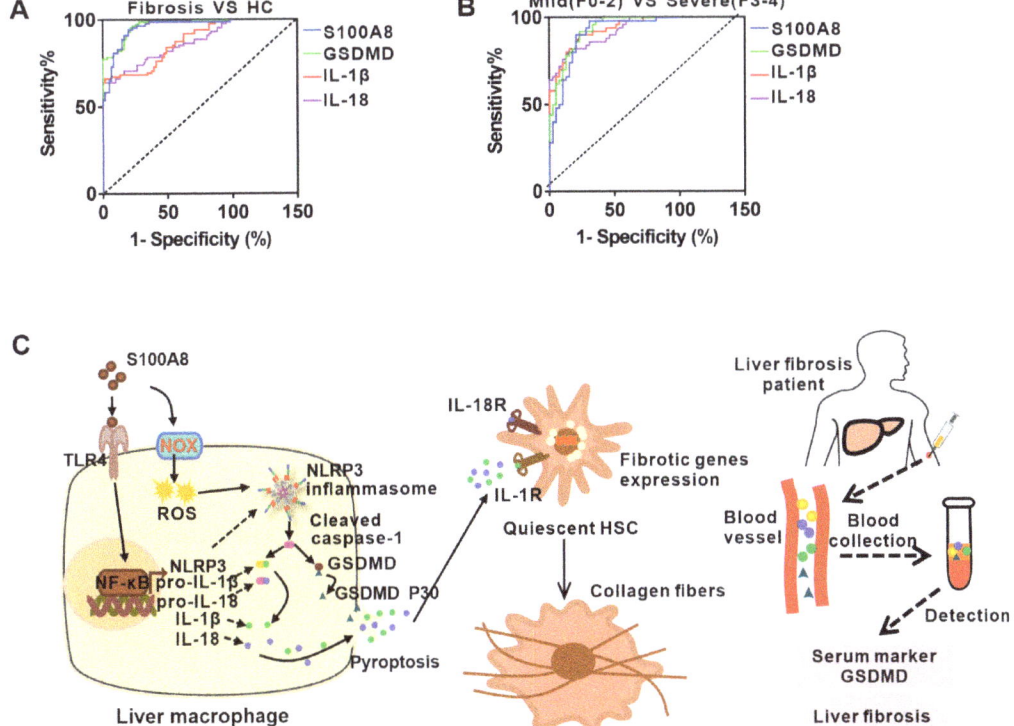

Figure 6. The potential predictive powers of S100A8, GSDMD, IL-1β, and IL-18 for the occurrence and severity of liver fibrosis. (**A**) ROC curves of serum S100A8, GSDMD, IL-1β, and IL-18 for distinguishing liver fibrosis patients from HCs. (**B**) ROC curve, of serum S100A8, GSDMD, IL-1β, and IL-18 for detecting moderate-to-severe liver fibrosis from no or mild liver fibrosis in liver fibrosis patients. (**C**) A working model illustrating that S100A8-mediated NLRP3 inflammasome-dependent pyroptosis in macrophages facilitates liver fibrosis progression, and that the identified GSDMD may be used as a potential biomarker during liver fibrosis onset and progression.

4. Discussion

NLRP3 inflammasome-dependent pyroptosis, an identified inflammatory form of cell death, is activated by two signals; namely, priming and activating signals, leading to persistent inflammation via activation and release of IL-1β, IL-18, and other intracellular contents [7]. Recently, pyroptosis has attracted interest due to its crucial role in inflammation-related diseases [31]. Intrahepatic cell death and persistent inflammation triggered by various etiological factors are two central elements in the occurrence and progression of liver fibrosis. Evidence supports that NLRP3 inflammasome-dependent pyroptosis is involved in the development of liver fibrosis [32]. Nevertheless, the definite cell types that undergo pyroptosis and the underlying mechanism as well as their clinical importance are still unclear. In the present study, we demonstrated that S100A8 as a crucial DAMP could stimulate NLRP3 inflammasome-dependent pyroptotic macrophage death by activating TLR4-dependent NF-κB and inducing ROS abundance, finally facilitating liver fibrosis progression. In addition, we identified that the pyroptosis-related indicator GSDMD may be a potential biomarker for the occurrence and progression of liver fibrosis (Figure 6C).

The role of pyroptosis has been extensively confirmed in a wide range of fibrotic responses ranging from the lung, kidney, heart, and skin. In these fibrotic diseases, the interaction between the NF-κB/NLRP3/caspase-1/IL-1β axis and TGF-β signaling appears to be the main mechanism relevant to fibrosis [8–10,33,34]. Here, elevated levels of the pyroptosis-related indicators GSDMD, IL-1β, and IL-18 were confirmed in both clinical specimens from liver fibrosis patients and CCl4-induced liver fibrosis mouse models. Additionally, their serum levels strongly correlated with the severity of liver fibrosis, suggesting the essential role of pyroptosis during the progression of liver fibrosis. Furthermore, double immunofluorescence staining of NLRP3 with albumin, F4/80 or with α-SMA in human and mouse fibrotic liver tissues demonstrated that enhanced NLRP3 was mainly localized to KCs and hepatocytes, especially KCs, indicating that KCs are major cell types that undergo pyroptosis, which is consistent with other studies regarding these cell types [35]. Targeting the NLRP3 inflammasome and its downstream effectors may be a potent therapeutic strategy for inflammatory diseases [36]. Here, we investigated whether NLRP3 inflammasome-dependent pyroptosis could be an intervention target for liver fibrosis. We used a specific inhibitor of NLRP3, MCC950, to treat CCl4-induced liver fibrosis mouse models. As expected, injection of MCC950 significantly attenuated liver injury, especially liver fibrosis and improved liver function, indicating that NLRP3, as the executor of pyroptosis, is an advancing prevention target for liver fibrosis. Additionally, the effectiveness of the NLRP3 inhibitor was confirmed by the CM (pyroptotic macrophages)-LX-2 culture model. In previous studies, inhibitors of IL-1 signaling and caspase-1 were also effective in treating NLRP3-driven diseases [36]. Therefore, further studies are still needed to compare the effects of these inhibitors with MCC950 to screen out the optimal inhibitors for liver fibrosis.

DAMPs refer to many endogenous molecules with immunomodulatory activity released from stressed, malfunctioning or dead cells and damaged tissues [37]. It has been reported that DAMPs released from dying tubule cells, including HGMB1, contribute to the macrophage infiltration and IL-1β release, which markedly facilitates renal fibrogenesis [25]. Another study also suggested the involvement of citrullinated vimentin derived from lung macrophages as a DAMP during the progression of lung fibrosis [26]. As two members of DAMP, S100A8 and S100A9, were reported to correlate with the onset and progression of bone marrow fibrosis [38] and renal fibrosis [39]. Similarly, elevated levels of S100A8 and S100A9 were verified in clinical samples and CCl4-induced mouse model studies, and their levels were strongly related to the severity of liver fibrosis. Specifically, S100A8 increased more dramatically than S100A9 during the progression of liver fibrosis, implying an important role of S100A8 in the pathogenesis of liver fibrosis. The present data, together with the above-mentioned results from other studies, further emphasize the significance of DAMPs in fibrotic disease. S100A8 and S100A9 are mainly derived from activated immunocytes (neutrophils, macrophages, etc.) and cells in local lesions in many inflammatory processes [40]. Studies have shown that numerous pro-inflammatory cytokines, including tumor necrosis factor-a (TNF-a) and interleukin-1 (IL-1), strongly induce the expression of S100A8/A9 [41]. Moreover, LPS activates caspase-4/5 inflammasome and promotes the secretion of S100A8 from macrophages. The proximal promoter regions of S100A8 and S100A9 have common binding sites for different transcription factors (e.g., AP-1, NF-κB, and C/EBP) [41]. However, the detailed molecular mechanism controlling the transcription of S100A8/A9 genes during liver fibrosis process is necessary for further extended analysis in future studies.

Recently, S100A8 and S100A9 were reported to activate NLRP3 inflammasome signaling to promote the pathogenesis of several diseases [29,42]. Given that the NLRP3 inflammasome can respond to DAMPs as a classical PRR, we focused on whether S100A8 could activate the NLRP3 inflammasome and subsequently lead to pyroptosis. In the present study, we observed a close correlation between S100A8 and pyroptosis, and found a direct effect of S100A8 on macrophage pyroptosis. Additionally, pyroptotic products were able to induce the activation of HSCs. The augmenting inflammatory factor IL-1β was detected in CM, which is a critical profibrotic cytokine that acts on HSCs in previous reports [43]. In addition to IL-1β, other profibrotic cytokines released from damaged cells, such as HGMB1, ATP, and DNA, can trigger HSC activation and collagen production [44], which needs further study for confirmation. Activation of NLRP3 inflammasome-dependent pyroptosis requires two signals, the priming signal and the activating signal. With regard to the priming signal, our data showed that S100A8 interacted with TLR4 and then activated downstream NF-κB with transcriptional upregulation of NLRP3, pro-IL-1β, and pro-IL-18. ROS have been proposed as the second signal for NLRP3 activation [45], and they also appear to play a crucial role in fibrotic progression [46]. In addition, S100A8 was reported to regulate ROS production by increasing NADPH oxidase activity [29,30]. Therefore, we focused on the ROS-mediated second activation signal. In this study, S100A8 significantly enhanced ROS levels in THP-1 macrophages. Furthermore, suppressing ROS generation with the NOX specific inhibitor DPI markedly attenuated S100A8-induced NLRP3 activation. Interestingly, the use of DPI also decreased the levels of the priming signaling molecules pro-IL-1β and total GSDMD mediated by S100A8, suggesting that S100A8-induced ROS production may exhibit a crosstalk with the priming signal NF-κB activation, which was supported by other studies [29,47]. A previous study also suggested that ROS can be generated from mitochondria in a TLR4-dependent manner [48]. Here, it is still unclear whether S100A8-induced ROS production is dependent on TLR4, which requires confirmation in further studies. Collectively, we demonstrated that S100A8 not only induced transcriptional upregulation of NLRP3, pro-IL-1β, and pro-IL-18 via TLR4/NF-κB signaling, but also facilitated oligomerization of NLRP3 proteins and cleavage of caspase-1 through NOX/ROS signaling, finally leading to pyroptotic cell death in macrophages. Recently, we discovered that CD36, which is expressed on the surface of a variety of cells, including macrophages, hepatocytes, enterocytes, myocytes, and adipocytes, also acts as a receptor of S100 family proteins (S100A8, S100A9, and S100A12) [49]. CD36 is involved in many pathophysiological processes, such as cardiovascular, thrombotic, and metabolic phenotypes [50]. However, there are few reports on its role in liver fibrosis. It has been shown that in the presence of DAMPs, CD36 assembles and interacts with other membrane receptors, leading to ROS production and transcription factor activation [51]. Therefore, we wondered whether CD36 mediates S100A8-induced ROS production and NF-κB pathway activation in liver fibrosis progression, which requires further studies to investigate.

Currently, the diagnosis of liver fibrosis mainly depends on liver biopsy supplemented with serology tests and imaging examinations [52]. However, liver biopsy is an invasive method with potential associated complications and mortality [53], and conventional ultrasonography, CT and MRI have little diagnostic significance for early-stage liver fibrosis [54]. Due to their high applicability, good interlaboratory reproducibility, and potential widespread use, serum biomarkers are still the optimal option for liver fibrosis examination. Although there are some identified serum biomarkers, none are liver-specific [54]. Therefore, it is still necessary to identify several new promising serum biomarkers for the diagnosis and staging of liver fibrosis in combination with known good indicators to improve diagnostic power. In this study, since S100A8-induced NLRP3 inflammasome-dependent pyroptosis is correlated with liver fibrosis, its diagnostic value for the onset and progression of liver fibrosis was analyzed. The identified circulating GSDMD had the highest diagnostic value for the diagnosis and staging of liver fibrosis, suggesting that GSDMD may have the potential to be an alternative biomarker for liver fibrosis evaluation. Nevertheless, there are still limitations in our study. Due to the small sample size and lack of specific investigation of liver fibrosis with different etiologies, further research is required in more liver fibrosis patients with different etiologies to confirm these data.

In conclusion, the current study suggests that S100A8 stimulates NLRP3 inflammasome-dependent pyroptosis in macrophages via activating TLR4/NF-κB signaling and inducing ROS abundance, which finally facilitates the progression of liver fibrosis. In addition, the NLRP3 inhibitor MCC950 treatment reduced the development of liver fibrosis in CCl4-induced liver fibrosis mouse models, indicating that blocking NLRP3 inflammasome-dependent pyroptosis may be a promising therapeutic strategy. More importantly, the identified pyroptosis-related indicator GSDMD has the potential to be an alternative biomarker for liver fibrosis evaluation.

Supplementary Materials: The following supporting information can be downloaded at: https://www.mdpi.com/article/10.3390/cells11223579/s1, Figure S1: The mean of IOD analysis for all IHC staining utilizing the Image Pro Plus 6.0 (MediaCybernetics, Silver Spring, MD, USA). Figure S2: ELISA analysis for IL-1β levels in supernatants from THP-1 treated with 5 μg/mL GST or rhS100A8.

Author Contributions: L.D. and L.Z. conceived the study and supervised and coordinated all aspects of the work. R.W. and Y.Y. coordinated the investigation of the subjects' sample analysis. Y.L., X.K., and L.X. performed the experiments and interpreted the data. L.D. and Y.Z. performed the statistical analysis. L.D. drafted the manuscript. L.D. and R.W. contributed to the funding acquisition. All authors have read and agreed to the published version of the manuscript.

Funding: This work was supported by grants from the National Natural Science Foundation of China (82002152 and 82072364), Natural Science Foundation of Chongqing (cstc2019jcyj-msxmX0859), Chongqing Medical Scientific Research Project (Joint Project of Chongqing Health Commission and Science and Technology Bureau) (2020FYYX038), and Senior Medical Talents Program of Chongqing for Young and Middle-Aged.

Institutional Review Board Statement: All animal procedures were approved by the Institutional Ethics Committee at the Second Hospital affiliated with Chongqing Medical University. The protocol of human sample was approved by the Institutional Ethics Committee at the Second Hospital affiliated with Chongqing Medical University (No. 2020-65).

Informed Consent Statement: In compliance with the Declaration of Helsinki, informed written consent for this study was obtained for the participated individuals.

Data Availability Statement: The datasets used and/or analyzed during the current study are available from the corresponding author on reasonable request.

Conflicts of Interest: The authors declare no conflict of interest.

References

1. Hernandez-Gea, V.; Friedman, S.L. Pathogenesis of liver fibrosis. *Annu. Rev. Pathol.* **2011**, *6*, 425–456. [CrossRef] [PubMed]
2. Iredale, J.P. Models of liver fibrosis: Exploring the dynamic nature of inflammation and repair in a solid organ. *J. Clin. Investig.* **2007**, *117*, 539–548. [CrossRef] [PubMed]
3. Lo, R.C.; Kim, H. Histopathological evaluation of liver fibrosis and cirrhosis regression. *Clin. Mol. Hepatol.* **2017**, *23*, 302–307. [CrossRef]
4. Schuppan, D.; Kim, Y.O. Evolving therapies for liver fibrosis. *J. Clin. Investig.* **2013**, *123*, 1887–1901. [CrossRef] [PubMed]
5. Strowig, T.; Henao-Mejia, J.; Elinav, E.; Flavell, R. Inflammasomes in health and disease. *Nature* **2012**, *481*, 278–286. [CrossRef]
6. Sharma, B.R.; Kanneganti, T.-D. NLRP3 inflammasome in cancer and metabolic diseases. *Nat. Immunol.* **2021**, *22*, 550–559. [CrossRef]

7. He, Y.; Hara, H.; Núñez, G. Mechanism and Regulation of NLRP3 Inflammasome Activation. *Trends Biochem. Sci.* **2016**, *41*, 1012–1021. [CrossRef]
8. Tian, R.; Zhu, Y.; Yao, J.; Meng, X.; Wang, J.; Xie, H.; Wang, R. NLRP3 participates in the regulation of EMT in bleomycin-induced pulmonary fibrosis. *Exp. Cell Res.* **2017**, *357*, 328–334. [CrossRef]
9. Wu, M.; Han, W.; Song, S.; Du, Y.; Liu, C.; Chen, N.; Wu, H.; Shi, Y.; Duan, H. NLRP3 deficiency ameliorates renal inflammation and fibrosis in diabetic mice. *Mol. Cell. Endocrinol.* **2018**, *478*, 115–125. [CrossRef]
10. Pinar, A.A.; Scott, T.E.; Huuskes, B.M.; Cáceres, F.E.T.; Kemp-Harper, B.K.; Samuel, C.S. Targeting the NLRP3 inflammasome to treat cardiovascular fibrosis. *Pharmacol. Ther.* **2020**, *209*, 107511. [CrossRef]
11. Wree, A.; Eguchi, A.; McGeough, M.D.; Pena, C.A.; Johnson, C.D.; Canbay, A.; Hoffman, H.M.; Feldstein, A.E. NLRP3 inflammasome activation results in hepatocyte pyroptosis, liver inflammation, and fibrosis in mice. *Hepatology* **2013**, *59*, 898–910. [CrossRef] [PubMed]
12. Wree, A.; McGeough, M.D.; Peña, C.A.; Schlattjan, M.; Li, H.; Inzaugarat, M.E.; Messer, K.; Canbay, A.; Hoffman, H.M.; Feldstein, A.E. NLRP3 inflammasome activation is required for fibrosis development in NAFLD. *Klin. Wochenschr.* **2014**, *92*, 1069–1082. [CrossRef] [PubMed]
13. Mridha, A.R.; Wree, A.; Robertson, A.A.; Yeh, M.M.; Johnson, C.D.; Van Rooyen, D.M.; Haczeyni, F.; Teoh, N.C.-H.; Savard, C.; Ioannou, G.N.; et al. NLRP3 inflammasome blockade reduces liver inflammation and fibrosis in experimental NASH in mice. *J. Hepatol.* **2017**, *66*, 1037–1046. [CrossRef]
14. Reiter, F.P.; Wimmer, R.; Wottke, L.; Artmann, R.; Nagel, J.M.; Carranza, M.O.; Mayr, D.; Rust, C.; Fickert, P.; Trauner, M.; et al. Role of interleukin-1 and its antagonism of hepatic stellate cell proliferation and liver fibrosis in the Abcb4(-/-) mouse model. *World J. Hepatol.* **2016**, *8*, 401–410. [CrossRef] [PubMed]
15. Wang, D.; Zhan, X.; Wu, R.; You, Y.; Chen, W.; Duan, L. Assessment of Pyroptosis-Related Indicators as Potential Biomarkers and Their Association with Severity in Patients with Liver Cirrhosis. *J. Inflamm. Res.* **2021**, *ume 14*, 3185–3196. [CrossRef]
16. Youssef, P.; Roth, J.; Frosch, M.; Costello, P.; Fitzgerald, O.; Sorg, C. Expression of myeloid related proteins (MRP) 8 and 14 and the MRP8/14 heterodimer in rheumatoid arthritis synovial membrane. *J. Rheumatol.* **1999**, *26*, 2523–2528.
17. Sands, B.E. Biomarkers of Inflammation in Inflammatory Bowel Disease. *Gastroenterology* **2015**, *149*, 1275–1285.e2. [CrossRef]
18. Achouiti, A.; Vogl, T.; Endeman, H.; Mortensen, B.L.; Laterre, P.F.; Wittebole, X.; van Zoelen, M.A.; Zhang, Y.; Hoogerwerf, J.J.; Florquin, S.; et al. Myeloid-related protein-8/14 facilitates bacterial growth during pneumococcal pneumonia. *Thorax* **2014**, *69*, 1034–1042. [CrossRef]
19. Sallman, D.A.; Cluzeau, T.; Basiorka, A.A.; List, A. Unraveling the Pathogenesis of MDS: The NLRP3 inflammasome and Py-roptosis Drive the MDS Phenotype. *Front. Oncol.* **2016**, *6*, 151. [CrossRef]
20. Kim, K.; Kim, H.J.; Binas, B.; Kang, J.H.; Chung, I.Y. Inflammatory mediators ATP and S100A12 activate the NLRP3 inflammasome to induce MUC5AC production in airway epithelial cells. *Biochem. Biophys. Res. Commun.* **2018**, *503*, 657–664. [CrossRef]
21. Wu, R.; Zhang, Y.; Xiang, Y.; Tang, Y.; Cui, F.; Cao, J.; Zhou, L.; You, Y.; Duan, L. Association between serum S100A9 levels and liver necroin-flammation in chronic hepatitis B. *J. Transl. Med.* **2018**, *16*, 83. [CrossRef] [PubMed]
22. Batts, K.P.; Ludwig, J. Chronic hepatitis. An update on terminology and reporting. *Am. J. Surg. Pathol.* **1995**, *19*, 1409–1417. [CrossRef] [PubMed]
23. Duan, L.; Wu, R.; Ye, L.; Wang, H.; Yang, X.; Zhang, Y.; Chen, X.; Zuo, G.; Zhang, Y.; Weng, Y.; et al. S100A8 and S100A9 are associated with colorectal carcinoma pro-gression and contribute to colorectal carcinoma cell survival and migration via Wnt/beta-catenin pathway. *PLoS ONE* **2013**, *8*, e62092. [CrossRef] [PubMed]
24. Vogl, T.; Tenbrock, K.; Ludwig, S.; Leukert, N.; Ehrhardt, C.; van Zoelen, M.A.; Nacken, W.; Foell, D.; van der Pol, l.T.; Sorg, C.; et al. Mrp8 and Mrp14 are endogenous activators of Toll- like receptor 4, promoting lethal, endotoxin-induced shock. *Nat. Med.* **2007**, *13*, 1042–1049. [CrossRef] [PubMed]
25. Li, Y.; Yuan, Y.; Huang, Z.-X.; Chen, H.; Lan, R.; Wang, Z.; Lai, K.; Chen, H.; Chen, Z.; Zou, Z.; et al. GSDME-mediated pyroptosis promotes inflammation and fibrosis in obstructive nephropathy. *Cell Death Differ.* **2021**, *28*, 2333–2350. [CrossRef]
26. Li, F.J.; Surolia, R.; Li, H.; Wang, Z.; Liu, G.; Kulkarni, T.; Massicano, A.V.F.; Mobley, J.A.; Mondal, S.; de Andrade, J.A.; et al. Citrullinated vimentin mediates development and progression of lung fibrosis. *Sci. Transl. Med.* **2021**, *13*. [CrossRef]
27. Hofmann, M.A.; Drury, S.; Fu, C.; Qu, W.; Taguchi, A.; Lu, Y.; Avila, C.; Kambham, N.; Bierhaus, A.; Nawroth, P.; et al. RAGE mediates a novel proinflammatory axis: A central cell surface receptor for S100/calgranulin polypeptides. *Cell* **1999**, *97*, 889–901. [CrossRef]
28. Jiang, J.X.; Chen, X.; Serizawa, N.; Szyndralewiez, C.; Page, P.; Schröder, K.; Brandes, R.P.; Devaraj, S.; Török, N.J. Liver fibrosis and hepatocyte apoptosis are attenuated by GKT137831, a novel NOX4/NOX1 inhibitor in vivo. *Free Radic. Biol. Med.* **2012**, *53*, 289–296. [CrossRef]
29. Simard, J.C.; Cesaro, A.; Chapeton-Montes, J.; Tardif, M.; Antoine, F.; Girard, D.; Tessier, P.A. S100A8 and S100A9 Induce Cytokine Ex-pression and Regulate the NLRP3 Inflammasome via ROS-Dependent Activation of NF-kappa B. *PLoS ONE* **2013**, *8*, e72138. [CrossRef]
30. Benedyk, M.; Sopalla, C.; Nacken, W.; Bode, G.; Melkonyan, H.; Banfi, B.; Kerkhoff, C. HaCaT keratinocytes overexpressing the S100 proteins S100A8 and S100A9 show increased NADPH oxidase and NF-kappa B activities. *J. Investig. Dermatol.* **2007**, *127*, 2001–2011. [CrossRef]

31. Liang, F.Q.; Zhang, F.; Zhang, L.L.; Wei, W. The advances in pyroptosis initiated by inflammasome in inflammatory and im-mune diseases. *Inflamm. Res.* **2020**, *69*, 159–166. [CrossRef] [PubMed]
32. Alegre, F.; Pelegrin, P.; Feldstein, A.E. Inflammasomes in Liver Fibrosis. *Semin. Liver Dis.* **2017**, *37*, 119–127. [CrossRef] [PubMed]
33. Song, C.; He, L.; Zhang, J.; Ma, H.; Yuan, X.; Hu, G.; Tao, L.; Zhang, J.; Meng, J. Fluorofenidone attenuates pulmonary inflammation and fibrosis via inhibiting the activation of NALP3 inflammasome and IL-1/IL-1R1/MyD88/NF-B pathway. *J. Cell. Mol. Med.* **2016**, *20*, 2064–2077. [CrossRef] [PubMed]
34. Artlett, C.M.; Sassi-Gaha, S.; Rieger, J.L.; Boesteanu, A.C.; Feghali-Bostwick, C.A.; Katsikis, P. The inflammasome activating caspase 1 mediates fibrosis and myofibroblast differentiation in systemic sclerosis. *Arthritis Care Res.* **2011**, *63*, 3563–3574. [CrossRef] [PubMed]
35. Pan, J.; Ou, Z.; Cai, C.; Li, P.; Gong, J.; Ruan, X.Z.; He, K. Fatty acid activates NLRP3 inflammasomes in mouse Kupffer cells through mitochondrial DNA release. *Cell. Immunol.* **2018**, *332*, 111–120. [CrossRef] [PubMed]
36. Mangan, M.S.J.; Olhava, E.J.; Roush, W.R.; Seidel, H.M.; Glick, G.D.; Latz, E. Targeting the NLRP3 inflammasome in in-flammatory diseases. *Nat. Rev. Drug Discov.* **2018**, *17*, 688. [CrossRef]
37. Medzhitov, R. Origin and physiological roles of inflammation. *Nature* **2008**, *454*, 428–435. [CrossRef]
38. Leimkühler, N.B.; Gleitz, H.F.; Ronghui, L.; Snoeren, I.A.; Fuchs, S.N.; Nagai, J.S.; Banjanin, B.; Lam, K.H.; Vogl, T.; Kuppe, C.; et al. Heterogeneous bone-marrow stromal pro-genitors drive myelofibrosis via a druggable alarmin axis. *Cell Stem Cell* **2021**, *28*, 637–652.e8. [CrossRef]
39. Tammaro, A.; Florquin, S.; Brok, M.; Claessen, N.; Butter, L.M.; Teske, G.J.D.; de Boer, O.J.; Vogl, T.; Leemans, J.C.; Dessing, M.C. S100A8/A9 promotes parenchymal damage and renal fibrosis in obstructive nephropathy. *Clin. Exp. Immunol.* **2018**, *193*, 361–375. [CrossRef]
40. Wang, S.; Song, R.; Wang, Z.; Jing, Z.; Wang, S.; Ma, J. S100A8/A9 in Inflammation. *Front. Immunol.* **2018**, *9*, 1298. [CrossRef]
41. Gebhardt, C.; Németh, J.; Angel, P.; Hess, J. S100A8 and S100A9 in inflammation and cancer. *Biochem. Pharmacol.* **2006**, *72*, 1622–1631. [CrossRef] [PubMed]
42. Tan, X.X.; Zheng, X.H.; Huang, Z.N.; Lin, J.Q.; Xie, C.L.; Lin, Y. Involvement of S100A8/A9-TLR4-NLRP3 Inflammasome Pathway in Contrast-Induced Acute Kidney Injury. *Cell Physiol. Biochem.* **2017**, *43*, 209–222. [CrossRef] [PubMed]
43. Zhang, Y.P.; Di Luqin, W.Y.; Tang, N.; Ai, X.M.; Yao, X.X. Mechanism of interleukin-1b-induced proliferation in rat hepatic stellate cells from different levels of signal transduction. *Apmis* **2014**, *122*, 392–398.
44. Mihm, S. Danger-Associated Molecular Patterns (DAMPs): Molecular Triggers for Sterile Inflammation in the Liver. *Int. J. Mol. Sci.* **2018**, *19*, 3104. [CrossRef]
45. Xue, Y.; Tuipulotu, D.E.; Tan, W.H.; Kay, C.; Man, S.M. Emerging Activators and Regulators of Inflammasomes and Pyroptosis. *Trends Immunol.* **2019**, *40*, 1035–1052. [CrossRef] [PubMed]
46. Artlett, C.M.; Thacker, J.D. Molecular Activation of the NLRP3 Inflammasome in Fibrosis: Common Threads Linking Divergent Fibrogenic Diseases. *Antioxidants Redox Signal.* **2015**, *22*, 1162–1175. [CrossRef]
47. Morgan, M.J.; Liu, Z.G. Crosstalk of reactive oxygen species and NF-kappa B signaling. *Cell Res.* **2011**, *21*, 103–115. [CrossRef] [PubMed]
48. West, A.P.; Brodsky, I.E.; Rahner, C.; Woo, D.K.; Erdjument-Bromage, H.; Tempst, P.; Walsh, M.C.; Choi, Y.; Shadel, G.S.; Ghosh, S. TLR signalling augments macrophage bactericidal activity through mitochondrial ROS. *Nature* **2011**, *472*, 476–480. [CrossRef]
49. Yang, X.; Okamura, D.M.; Lu, X.; Chen, Y.; Moorhead, J.; Varghese, Z.; Ruan, X.Z. CD36 in chronic kidney disease: Novel insights and therapeutic opportunities. *Nat. Rev. Nephrol.* **2017**, *13*, 769–781. [CrossRef]
50. Shu, H.; Peng, Y.; Hang, W.; Nie, J.; Zhou, N.; Wang, D.W. The role of CD36 in cardiovascular disease. *Cardiovasc. Res.* **2020**, *118*, 115–129. [CrossRef]
51. Chen, Y.; Zhang, J.; Cui, W.; Silverstein, R.L. CD36, a signaling receptor and fatty acid transporter that regulates immune cell metabolism and fate. *J. Exp. Med.* **2022**, *219*, e20211314. [CrossRef] [PubMed]
52. Patel, K.; Bedossa, P.; Castera, L. Diagnosis of Liver Fibrosis: Present and Future. *Semin. Liver Dis.* **2015**, *35*, 166–183. [CrossRef] [PubMed]
53. Saadeh, S.; Cammell, G.; M.D., W.D.C.; Younossi, Z.; Barnes, D.; Easley, K. The role of liver biopsy in chronic hepatitis C. *Hepatology* **2001**, *33*, 196–200. [CrossRef] [PubMed]
54. Vilar-Gomez, E.; Chalasani, N. Non-invasive assessment of non-alcoholic fatty liver disease: Clinical prediction rules and blood-based biomarkers. *J. Hepatol.* **2018**, *68*, 305–315. [CrossRef] [PubMed]

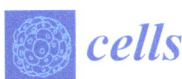

Review

Advanced Glycation End Products and Inflammation in Type 1 Diabetes Development

Chenping Du [1,2], Rani O. Whiddett [1], Irina Buckle [1,3], Chen Chen [2], Josephine M. Forbes [1,3,4,*] and Amelia K. Fotheringham [1,3]

1. Glycation and Diabetes Complications Group, Mater Research Institute-The University of Queensland, Translational Research Institute, Woolloongabba 4102, Australia
2. School of Biomedical Sciences, Faculty of Medicine, The University of Queensland, St Lucia 4072, Australia
3. Faculty of Medicine, The University of Queensland, St Lucia 4072, Australia
4. Department of Medicine, The University of Melbourne, Austin Health, Heidelberg 3084, Australia
* Correspondence: josephine.forbes@mater.uq.edu.au

Abstract: Type 1 diabetes (T1D) is an autoimmune disease in which the β-cells of the pancreas are attacked by the host's immune system, ultimately resulting in hyperglycemia. It is a complex multifactorial disease postulated to result from a combination of genetic and environmental factors. In parallel with increasing prevalence of T1D in genetically stable populations, highlighting an environmental component, consumption of advanced glycation end products (AGEs) commonly found in in Western diets has increased significantly over the past decades. AGEs can bind to cell surface receptors including the receptor for advanced glycation end products (RAGE). RAGE has proinflammatory roles including in host–pathogen defense, thereby influencing immune cell behavior and can activate and cause proliferation of immune cells such as islet infiltrating $CD8^+$ and $CD4^+$ T cells and suppress the activity of T regulatory cells, contributing to β-cell injury and hyperglycemia. Insights from studies of individuals at risk of T1D have demonstrated that progression to symptomatic onset and diagnosis can vary, ranging from months to years, providing a window of opportunity for prevention strategies. Interaction between AGEs and RAGE is believed to be a major environmental risk factor for T1D and targeting the AGE-RAGE axis may act as a potential therapeutic strategy for T1D prevention.

Keywords: type 1 diabetes; dietary AGEs; RAGE; autoimmunity

1. Introduction

Type 1 diabetes (T1D) is an autoimmune disease that comprises 5–10% of all cases of diabetes globally [1]. It is most commonly diagnosed in younger individuals, although the prevalence of adults diagnosed with T1D has increased significantly over the past decades [2]. Although T1D is the most common form of diabetes in children, the incidence continues to increase by about 2–3% per year globally across all age groups, with the most significant increase in prevalence observed in adults [3,4]. Many therapies targeting inflammatory and immune pathways such as anti-CD3 monoclonal antibodies [5] and IL-1 receptor antagonists [6] have been tested over the past decade but have only been shown to slow disease progression in early stages prior to clinical onset [5,7,8]. Currently, there is no cure for T1D. The only approved first-line therapy for T1D is exogenous insulin, the only way to manage disease symptoms and enable most individuals to lead a relatively healthy and long life. However, variations in blood sugar concentrations can be life-threatening and are associated with increased risk for complications. Approximately 40% of individuals with type 1 experience microvascular and macrovascular complications leading to premature mortality and commonly have ongoing mental health impacts due to complex disease management [9].

Due to the lifelong nature of T1D, there is significant interest in preventing, or delaying, the onset and progression of this disease. Disease pathogenesis occurs over many years prior to diagnosis, suggesting that there could be a therapeutic window of opportunity for prevention before specific clinical diagnosis of "overt" disease. A pathway suggested as important for the onset and progression of T1D is the advanced glycation end products (AGEs) and their receptor, the receptor for advanced glycation end products (RAGE) (AGE-RAGE) axis. This review will discuss the pathogenesis of TID, the contribution of genetic susceptibility and environment, how AGEs and RAGE might be involved and how reducing AGE and RAGE signaling through dietary restriction of AGEs may be crucial for T1D prevention.

2. Main Text
2.1. Pathophysiology of Type 1 Diabetes

T1D is a chronic autoimmune disease where β-cells in the islets of Langerhans of the pancreas are progressively damaged, leading to a critical loss of insulin production resulting in life-threatening high glucose concentrations in the blood (hyperglycemia; Figure 1)[2]. Individuals with T1D often present with common symptoms such as frequent urination (polyuria), fatigue, and weight loss [10]. In addition, individuals with T1D also present with islet-specific antibodies against self-antigens signifying pancreatic autoimmunity. Although antibodies are not postulated to have pathological roles, they indicate disease progression and the presence of 2 or more islet antibodies confers a significantly increased risk of developing T1D [11]. The most common autoantibodies in both children and adults are against insulin (IAA), glutamic acid decarboxylase (GADA), insulinoma antigen-2 (IA-2A), and zinc transporter 8 (ZnT8A) [12]. However, IAA usually presents early in life while GADA often appears much later in childhood [12]. In addition, autoantibodies are not detectable at any stage in some individuals, which complicates diagnosis of diabetes type [13], particularly in adults.

2.2. Genetic Susceptibility

T1D is a very heterogeneous disease with over 90 loci encoded on different regions of the genome implicated in autoimmunity [14]. In particular, genes encoding for human leukocyte antigen (HLA) class II haplotypes, including alleles DR3/4 and DQ8 are most commonly associated with T1D [15]. HLA class I and II molecules are involved in control of self-antigens and recognition of pathogens [15]. The different HLA variants influence the presentation of antigens to T cells and signal transduction post-antigen binding, which alters immune tolerance and likely changes the threshold for reactions to self-antigens leading to autoimmunity [16]. Although genetic factors are important, the increasing prevalence of T1D in genetically stable populations suggests that environmental factors are also necessary for precipitation of disease. The individual contributions of and interaction between genetic and environmental factors in T1D are commonly studied in population-based twin cohorts and diabetic animal models. Studies examining monozygotic and dizygotic twins showed that the majority of twins, approximately 70% were discordant for T1D, further supporting that environmental triggers are essential for T1D development [17,18]. The Non-obese diabetic (NOD) mouse model of autoimmune diabetes has contributed significantly to the understanding of T1D, as the progression of diabetes shows similarity to that in humans [19]. Autoantibodies against "self" islet antigens appear in early life and precede progressive defects in insulin secretion and islet invasion and destruction by cells of the immune system [20]. NOD mice also have genetic susceptibility linked to MHC class II alleles as is seen in humans and the presence of antigen-specific immune cells, especially the CD4$^+$ and CD8$^+$ T cells in lymphoid organs and the pancreatic islets [21]. Due to the barriers in obtaining human pancreata to study all possible pathogenic mechanisms of T1D, NOD mice present a useful starting point for rationalization of potential therapeutic targets.

2.3. Autoimmunity and Role of the Immune System

Tolerance is an essential process in the development of the adaptive immune system where regulated unresponsiveness of the immune system to self-antigens is achieved [22]. In healthy individuals, it is common for some autoreactive T cells to escape central tolerance. Normally, when this occurs, antigen-specific cells recognizing "self"-antigens are usually deleted, neutralized or suppressed by processes such as secondary selection in the peripheral tissues, including at sites such as the local lymph nodes and spleen [23]. However, in individuals with T1D, there is a loss of tolerance to self-antigens due to defects in central and peripheral tolerance, which is elegantly reviewed here [21,24]. The reasons for this are not well understood. Some theories suggest that various environmental factors such as viral infections and dietary factors in combination with genetic risk, can result in inflammation of the pancreas and/or pancreatic islets leading to cell death and presentation of self-islet antigens by MHC molecules to the immune system [10,21,25–27]. Hence, the postulate is that in T1D, abnormalities in central and peripheral tolerance then allow antigen specific self-reactive T cells to escape these processes and go on to interact with self-antigens in the pancreas and other sites, leading to autoimmunity and autoantibody production [28].

Development of T1D commonly occurs over several years and is divided into stages (Figure 1) involving both the innate and adaptive immune systems. Stages one and two occur before the clinical diagnosis and hence are termed as "prediabetes" and are detected by the appearance of two or more autoantibodies, followed by dysglycaemia (where blood glucose concentrations are above the normal range following tolerance testing but do not meet the criteria for diagnosis) [29]. The third stage, where the diagnosis is made, is characterized by high blood glucose concentrations (hyperglycemia) and symptomatic onset [30]. It is generally believed that β-cell damage occurs prior to symptomatic onset and autoantibody levels should reduce over time. However, this has been challenged in some studies [31] where there was a positive relationship between T cell autoimmunity to islet antigens and disease duration, suggesting that T1D is very heterogenous and progression of the disease can be dependent on many factors such as age at diagnosis, family history immunogenetic profile and disease duration. Factors such as obesity, BMI and energy intake also appear to influence the progression of type 1 diabetes, with higher BMI and obesity associated with earlier onset of T1D [32–34] and progression of islet autoimmunity [35]. This has been attributed to factors such as insulin resistance and chronic inflammation acting as accelerating factors in type 1 diabetes pathogenesis [33,36]. Although clinical management of individuals with T1D continue to improve, individuals diagnosed with T1D are still limited to exogenous insulin therapy, with only a few individuals (18% of children and 13% of adults) achieving the recommended glycemic target of <7% for glycated hemoglobin (HbA1c) [37,38]. Once individuals are diagnosed, there are currently no therapies to reverse β-cell loss nor improve β-cell function. Therefore, prevention strategies for T1D in the early stages are a major goal of current research.

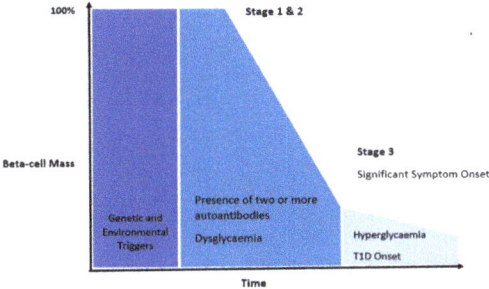

Figure 1. Stages of T1D according to classical theories. Genetic susceptibility and environmental

factors can influence the onset of T1D. T1D has two preclinical stages which are present before clinical diagnosis. Stage 1 is characterized by the presence of two or more autoantibodies specific to β-cell antigens. People in this stage are generally asymptomatic and have normal glycemic control. Stage 2 involves changes in glycemic control (dysglycemia) measured as a loss in insulin secretion (by C-peptide) during a mixed meal tolerance test in combination with the presence of 2 or more autoantibodies. Stage 3 involves significant clinical symptomatic onset and commonly, people at this stage have severe β-cell loss/damage. Individuals in Stage 3 can present with symptoms such as polyuria, weight loss and fatigue and require exogenous insulin therapies. The progression from Stage 1 to 3 can vary between several months to years since many individual have a so called "honeymoon" period where their pancreas is still able to produce a significant amount of its own insulin reducing exogenous insulin requirements [39].

Early in T1D development in NOD mice, islet inflammation termed insulitis occurs, where infiltration of immune cells such as T and B lymphocytes, macrophages, and dendritic cells (DCs) around and into the Islets of Langerhans is seen [40]. Following the study of human pancreata using resources such as the Juvenile Diabetes Research Foundation (JDRF) Network for Pancreatic Organ Donors with Diabetes (nPOD) [41–43], it has been discovered that the number of immune cells infiltrating the islets is often more variable than in mice. Indeed, it is more commonly present in individuals with a younger age of onset and with short disease duration [44]. As suggested above, the loss of β-cell specific tolerance can lead to β-cell damage and destruction by immune cells, facilitating the release of self-antigens by the pancreas. These are endocytosed by antigen-presenting cells (APCs) such as resident DCs and macrophages. Several studies have supported the role of both these cell types in the precipitation of T1D. When macrophages phagocytose antigens or cell fragments, activation of the innate immune system likely triggers inflammatory pathways, further exacerbating damage to β-cells and potentially recruiting the adaptive immune system [45–48]. Whether this process is an early event, occurring prediabetes in response to an environmental trigger such as a viral infection or involved in perpetuation of immune cell damage to β-cells in the longer term remains to be determined. In addition to their role in antigen presentation, dendritic cells (DCs) also play important roles in maintaining tolerance through the suppression of auto-reactive T cells and induction of Tregs [49,50]. This is not discussed further in this review but has been elegantly summarized previously [51,52]. In T1D pathogenesis, the perpetuation of self-antigen presentation and inflammation due to aberrant macrophage and DC function have been identified both in murine models [51,53,54] and in individuals who later develop diabetes [55–57]. Resident DCs in the pancreas also recognize danger signals from the damaged β-cells, leading to the release of chemokines which attract other immune cells. DCs then migrate to the pancreatic lymph node, presenting β-cell antigens to T cells, thereby activating effector CD4$^+$ and CD8$^+$ T cells (Figure 2) [58]. It is also postulated that DCs can do this in situ in the pancreas [59].

Many studies have shown that T cells (Figure 2) play an essential role in both the progression and development of T1D [41,48,60]. CD4$^+$ T cells can secrete proinflammatory cytokines, attracting additional T and B cells and other immune cells to surround or enter the pancreatic islets [61]. CD4$^+$ T cells also provide help to support effector CD8$^+$ T cell activation which are postulated as the β-cell assassins in T1D. CD8$^+$ T cells, generally mediate β-cell death directly via perforins, granzymes and FAS-FAS ligand death pathways [61,62]. Studies in NOD mice have shown that T1D can only be developed in the presence of both CD4$^+$ and CD8$^+$ T cells, but not by either population alone [60]. An early study found that anti-CD3 monoclonal antibodies act as immunosuppressants by reducing T cell activation and can prevent T1D onset in NOD mice [63]. This has led to the development of a promising therapy using the anti-CD3 monoclonal antibody, teplizumab in humans, the first drug that has been shown to delay T1D diagnosis in individuals at high risk (defined as having more than two autoantibodies and relatives of individuals with T1D) [5]. In humans, studies of pancreatic sections show significant infiltration by CD4$^+$ and CD8$^+$ T cells [41,64]. In an early study, increases in both CD8$^+$ T cells and MHC class I expression were seen in individuals newly diagnosed with T1D [65]. Studies have also observed the recurrence of T1D in recipients who received pancreas transplantation from an HLA identical donor, with immune infiltration consisting predominantly of CD8+ T cells, a few CD4+ T cells and near-total destruction of β-cells [66]. Taken together, these studies further highlight the importance of T cells in T1D development and onset, and provide evidence that CD8+ T cells may be the primary effector immune cells responsible for the destruction of β-cells in T1D.

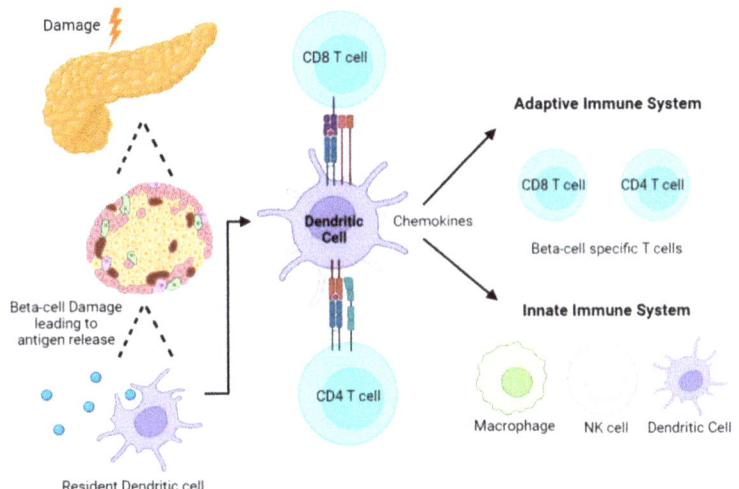

Figure 2. **Major Immune Cells Implicated in T1D Pathogenesis.** Damage to the β-cells of the pancreas can lead to the release of antigens. Antigens can be recognized by resident DCs which leads to the uptake and presentation of islet specific antigens to T cell. DCs will present antigens to T cells in the pancreatic lymph node leading to the release of chemokines which attract additional β-cell specific T cells and innate immune cells. If these β-cell autoantigen specific T cells are not removed by peripheral tolerance, they can further enhance inflammation and contribute to β-cell death.

Studies of immune infiltration in T1D have mostly focused on infiltration into the islets or the endocrine compartment of the pancreas, and often the areas surrounding the islets, but the exocrine structures are often overlooked in T1D development. However, it has become increasingly clear that individuals with T1D also have exocrine insufficiency. The major function of the exocrine pancreas is the production of digestive enzymes. Studies have shown that in individuals with T1D, the exocrine pancreas is reduced by approximately 30% [67]. Studies in the human pancreas have also observed more DCs and T cell infiltration into the exocrine pancreas in organ donors with T1D [68]. These findings suggest that there may be pathological connections between the endocrine and exocrine pancreas. Further understanding of immune cell behavior and accumulation in the exocrine pancreas may provide new insights into the reasons for islet damage and infiltration, and assist in the generation of effective and long-lasting therapies to prevent T1D onset.

Another key component of peripheral immune regulation involves regulatory T cells (Tregs). Forkhead box P3 protein (FOXP3) positive Tregs are regulatory T cells responsible for maintaining homeostasis by suppressing the activity of effector T cells, including CD4+ and CD8+ T cells. Increased inflammatory cytokine production by effector T cells may alter the phenotype of Tregs, reducing their suppressive abilities [69]. In humans, a rare disorder known as the immunodysregulation polyendocrinopathy enteropathy X-linked syndrome (IPEX), due to the loss of function of the *FOXP3* gene, can lead to the onset of many autoimmune diseases, especially T1D, in which is diagnosed in >80% of affected individuals before two years of age [70]. This highlights the importance of Tregs in maintaining tolerance, and the importance of functional Tregs in preventing T1D development. Imbalances between regulatory and effector T cells is thought to contribute to autoimmunity and T1D development [69], and individuals are often reported with a deficiency in interleukin 2 (IL-2) production [71]. IL-2 is arguably the most important growth factor for T regulatory cell function and increases the expression of FOXP3 and Treg suppression molecules with the ability to inhibit the activation of perforin or granzymes released from killer CD8$^+$ T cells, limiting autoimmunity [72]. Studies found that a low-dose IL-2 injection can stimulate pancreatic Treg function and proliferation and reduce production of the proinflammatory cytokines such as interferon-gamma (IFN-γ) [71]. Increasing Treg cells in the pancreas by administration of IL-2 has been found to reverse disease in NOD mice. Several clinical studies have found that although frequent low-dose IL-2 therapy increased Tregs population, they were transient and returned to pretreatment levels after treatment [73]. Another study examined a slightly higher IL-2 dose and observed an increased expansion of non-Tregs such as Natural Killer (NK) cell populations, potentially shifting from immune tolerance to activation [74]. The off-target effects limit the therapeutic potential of IL-2 in individuals at high risk and established T1D [71]. Although T cells are pivotal for T1D development, it is postulated that other immune cells such as B cells and NK cells [75] also have important roles in the pathogenesis of T1D. These cells' involvement in T1D is not discussed further here but elegantly reviewed in Lehuen et al. (2010) [48].

2.4. Environmental Triggers, Dietary AGEs, Inflammation and T1D Risk

Several environmental factors have been postulated to trigger inflammation and potentially β-cell autoimmunity in T1D. Enteroviral infection is one of the most well studied environmental factors and is associated with insulitis and β-cell loss, in particular those of the Coxsackievirus B family. Enteroviruses elicit strong immune responses by targeting β-cells surface receptors, inducing inflammation and promoting autoimmunity [60]. Several human prospective studies [76,77] have observed positive associations between enteroviral infections and progression to autoimmunity and clinical diagnosis of T1D, however, there are also studies that have found no association [78]. With the recent COVID-19 pandemic, the incidence of T1D appeared to be higher than in previous years with increases in both incidence and severity at diagnosis, measured as diabetic ketoacidosis [79,80]. Although clearly implicated in disease pathogenesis, more research is required to elucidate the mechanisms by which viral infections induce β-cells specific autoimmunity and damage. Other environmental factors suspected to contribute to alter risk for T1D development include vaccinations, lower vitamin D levels, and exposure to toxins. These are not further discussed here but are elegantly reviewed in Rewers & Ludvigsson (2016) [25].

Another major environmental factor which may influence the risk for T1D is increased consumption of highly processed foods. Food processing imparts commercially desirable properties such as increased shelf-life, flavor and digestibility, using methods such as dry heat baking [81]. This, in combination with the higher sugar, fat, refined carbohydrate and lower wholegrain content of highly processed foods, amplifies the production of chemical compounds known as advanced glycation end products (AGEs). The most common and well-studied AGE ligands in vivo are carboxymethyl lysine (CML) and methyl-glyoxal derived hydroimidazolones (MG-H1), which are both known to bind to AGE receptors such as RAGE [82]. Scheijen et al. (2016) found that food items with short heating times that are low in protein and carbohydrates and high in water, such as fruits and vegetables, have the lowest AGE content [83]. AGEs are formed via non-enzymatic reactions, where reducing sugars such as glucose react with amine residues on proteins [84] (reviewed in detail here, [85]). This process involves the Maillard reaction which can be subdivided into three steps (Figure 3), with the first step producing Schiff bases before rearranging into more stable Amadori products which are reversible, followed by the formation of AGEs which are irreversible [86]. Exogenous AGEs in foods can be absorbed across the gastrointestinal tract, contributing to the body's AGE pool [87]. Based on human and animal studies, approximately 10% of total AGEs eaten are thought to be absorbed into the blood, with two-thirds remaining in the body for more than three days [88]. Studies in mice have confirmed that consumption of dietary AGEs can elevate serum and tissue AGE levels [81].

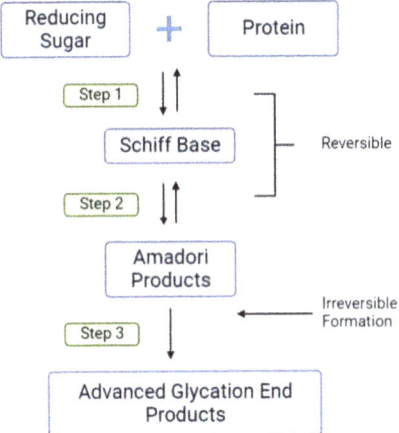

Figure 3. The basic chemistry of AGE Formation. Reducing sugars such as D-glucose, fructose, ribose and reactive dicarbonyls, including methylglyoxal, interact with amine groups such as lysine, tyrosine and arginine on proteins and peptides. Following various reversible chemical transition stages, the irreversible formation of advanced glycation end products such as Nε carboxymethyllysine modifications, HbA_{1C}, fructosamine albumin and methylglyoxal hydroimidazolones occurs.

In addition to ingestion from the diet, AGEs are also formed endogenously in the body, an example of which is HbA1c and fructosamine albumin, used clinically to track long term blood sugar control. Endogenous AGEs are produced as a natural consequence of cellular metabolism, particularly in environments with high oxidative stress [89]. In diabetes, the abundance of glucose in the bloodstream accelerates and exacerbates the formation of AGEs [90]. Clearance of AGEs from the body occurs via the gastrointestinal tract (GIT) and liver into the feces, and via the kidneys into the urine. As such, the AGE content in the body at any time is influenced by the amount of AGEs formed endogenously, AGEs ingested, their biodistribution, metabolism and the rate of excretion into the urine and feces [91]. Dietary AGE digestion and absorption in the GIT may interact with and change the composition of gut microbiome, as the gut microbiome is largely influenced by diet. The gut microbiome has increasingly been recognized as one of the key factors contributing to T1D onset by altering gut permeability and immune homeostasis [92]. Many studies in vitro and in vivo have observed that high dietary AGEs can alter the microbial composition, though the specific microbial changes require further validation [93–95]. Microbial dysbiosis can mediate immunological responses resulting in β-cell damage and T1D onset. The impact of AGEs on gut homeostasis is not further discussed, but is reviewed in Zhou et al. (2020) [96] and Snelson & Coughlan (2019) [97].

AGE research over the past decades has focused mainly on their role in the development and progression of various chronic complications of diabetes [98]. Due to the long half-life and abundance of plasma proteins and components of the extracellular matrix (ECM) including albumin, fibrinogen, and collagen, they are the predominant targets for glycation [84]. Increased glycation and accumulation of AGE modified proteins has been implicated in both microvascular and macrovascular complications of diabetes including kidney disease, retinopathy, cardiovascular disease and wound healing [98]. AGE accumulation on long lived proteins such as collagen in the skin have also emerged as biomarkers for the development of diabetic complications. AGE skin autofluorescence is a non-invasive, fast, and reliable method of measuring AGEs which has excellent associations to actual measured skin and body AGE accumulation, and is reviewed elegantly here [99]. In general, studies show that accumulation and/or higher AGE concentrations are associated with the development or presence of one or more diabetes complications.

Recent studies have highlighted the importance of dietary consumption of AGEs as risk factors for T1D onset. Firstly, high circulating concentrations of the AGE are an important environmental risk factor for T1D when added to the known risk factor, the presence of autoantibodies, to help identify individuals who are most likely to develop the disease [100]. Murine studies have suggested that AGEs initiate β-cell dysfunction via ligation to their receptor RAGE resulting in oxidative stress and insulin deficiency [101]. Studies in isolated islets have found that chronic administration of AGEs reduced insulin content within the islet and insulin secretion in response to glucose stimulation and increased infiltration of immune cells into the pancreatic islets which are via effects on mitochondrial superoxide production and ATP production [101,102]. High AGEs were also found to inhibit ATP synthesis, inhibiting the ATP-dependent K+ channel from opening, leading to impaired glucose-stimulated insulin secretion [102]. Here, AGEs impaired insulin secretion by elevating nitric oxide synthase (NOS) and thus nitric oxide concentrations in the pancreatic islets and INS cells. This subsequently resulted in inhibition of electron transport chain component cytochrome c oxidase, resulting in reduced ATP synthesis and reduced insulin secretion [102]. When healthy rats were exposed chronically to a high AGE diet, insulin secretory defects and islet infiltration in the absence of diabetes were observed [101]. Similarly, increased islet hormone content including insulin, proinsulin, and glucagon, and reduced immune infiltration were observed in mice fed with a low AGE diet compared to a high AGE diet [103,104]. A study in humans found that a higher serum AGE concentration was seen in at risk children who progressed to T1D compared to non-progressors [101]. This suggests that increased AGE consumption can impair β-cell function contributing to T1D development.

In addition, other studies have shown that the effects of dietary AGEs are not limited to postnatally, but also affect β-cell function during the perinatal and gestational period. Maternal-blood and food-derived AGE burden in early life are reported to prematurely raise babies' circulating AGE concentrations, influencing their risk for inflammatory conditions such as T1D [105]. Studies using dietary AGE restriction in NOD mouse models have found that lowering consumption of dietary AGEs in mothers from conception to weaning significantly decreased fasting blood glucose concentrations and improved insulin responses to glucose in offspring [103,104]. Further, pancreatic islets from offspring mice where the mothers consumed a high AGE diet during and post gestation showed increased immune cell infiltration compared to those infants whose mothers consumed a low AGE diet [103]. Importantly, intergenerational dietary AGE study observed a significant reduction of T1D incidence in mice fed with the low AGE diet compared to the high AGEs diet [104]. Further, inflammatory changes induced by high dietary AGE consumption can be ameliorated by AGEs lowering therapy alagebrium chloride [101,106].

Finally, in healthy individuals, there is a positive relationship between the circulating concentrations of AGEs and insulin secretion [107]. However, the rate of AGEs clearance is often greatly altered in individuals with diabetes who also have impairments in either kidney or liver function influencing insulin secretion and sensitivity [108]. Increased prevalence of obesity in individuals with T1D could also increase the likelihood of developing liver diseases such as Non-alcoholic steatohepatitis (NASH) and Non-alcoholic fatty liver disease (NAFLD) [109,110], impacting AGEs clearance. Obesity has been increasingly recognized to be associated with earlier onset of T1D and development of a "T1D like" phenotype characterized by immune infiltration and islet autoimmunity [36]. Perhaps not surprising is that lower dietary AGE intake improves insulin sensitivity in overweight individuals [111,112] as well as decreasing chronic low-grade inflammation. Low AGE diets also impact renal function in overweight and obese individuals [113] and hepatic function in rodent models of obesity and liver fibrosis [114,115]. Obesity has long been recognized as a risk factor for type 2 diabetes (T2D) but the increasing prevalence of obesity in individuals at risk for and diagnosed with T1D draws highlights the need for therapies that not only lower blood glucose but also provide greater weight management. Taken together, these findings suggest that increasing AGEs concentrations in the body can lead to β-cell damage and impaired β-cell function, possibly by influencing immunoregulation, contributing to T1D. Although the loss of β-cells through autoimmunity is unique in T1D, the mechanisms by which dietary AGEs induce β-cells dysfunction could also apply to T2D, but this is not further discussed in this review.

2.5. AGE Binding to RAGE

RAGE is a member of the immunoglobulin superfamily encoded by the *AGER* gene [116]. It is a proinflammatory receptor expressed in many cell types including immune cells and is important for host–pathogen defense [117]. AGEs bind to the cell surface AGE receptor RAGE [118] and upregulate its expression, a process exacerbated in diabetes via a positive-feedback loop [119]. However, RAGE is a multiligand receptor which can be stimulated by various ligands other than AGEs, including amyloid-B, amphoterin, and S100-calgranulins (Figure 3) [84]. Compared to other ligands of RAGE, AGEs have a relatively low affinity, and at low serum concentrations are unlikely to induce strong RAGE signaling [120]. However, in diabetes, AGEs concentration increases significantly due to the abundance of glucose in the bloodstream, therefore significantly upregulating RAGE signaling [116].

Another group of receptors known as the scavenger receptors also exhibit binding affinity for AGEs. Scavenger receptors are also multiligand receptors expressed on different cell types including the endothelial cells and immune cells such as macrophages. Research into scavenger receptor proteins has mainly been focused on the link to macrovascular and microvascular complications of diabetes, in particular atherosclerosis [121]. For example, class B scavenger receptor SR-B1 plays an important atheroprotective role, binding cholesteryl esters from high density lipoprotein (HDL-CE) and eliminating excessive cholesterol from peripheral tissues through cholesterol efflux [122]. However, in vitro AGEs inhibit SR-B1 selective cholesterol efflux to HDL [123] and HDL-CE uptake, suggesting pathological roles of AGEs binding to scavenger receptors. Similarly, the SR-B family receptor CD36 also binds AGEs [121,124] and has garnered substantial interest in the context of diabetes and its complications [125]. Like RAGE, CD36 is expressed on a wide variety of cells, including pancreatic β-cells, monocytes, macrophages and subsets of T and B cells [126] and binds a wide variety of ligands. CD36 and associated downstream signaling has been implicated in the development of insulin resistance, β-cell dysfunction and loss of β-cell mass in metabolic syndrome and type 2 diabetes (reviewed here [125]). Further CD36 has been implicated in a reduction in Treg and CD8+ T cell functionality in the tumor microenvironment [127,128], supporting tumor growth, although these findings appear to relate to CD36's role as a lipid transporter [126]. Whether CD36 is involved in T1D pathogenesis remains to be seen. Galectin 3, another AGE binding scavenger receptor [129], is widely expressed immune cells where it can activate proinflammatory pathways including cytokine and chemokine release [130]. Encoded by LGALS3, there is some evidence to suggest LGALS3 is a T1D susceptibility gene [131] and this has been supported by a small number of in vitro and in vivo studies suggesting a role for galectin 3 in cytokine mediated β-cells apoptosis and survival [131–133]. More research into AGEs and scavenger receptor family is required to understand whether these receptors are involved in the modulation of immune activity in T1D and whether they have similar roles to RAGE in T1D development.

Despite AGE and RAGE interactions being studied for more than 20 years, most studies have focused on the influence of AGE-RAGE binding on pathological conditions. However, AGEs are produced under physiological conditions where their role is poorly understood and it is not clear whether varying AGE modifications can elicit different physiological responses via receptor signaling, such as via RAGE. Certainly, binding of AGEs to RAGE initiates intracellular signaling pathways leading to inflammation and oxidative stress which are important part of host–pathogen defense, but can also result in β-cell injury [101,106,108]. However, AGE ligation resulting in RAGE signaling is also implicated in many other inflammatory conditions including neurodegenerative conditions, rheumatoid arthritis, and inflammatory bowel disease [82,98,134,135]. The binding of AGEs to RAGE commonly activates the nuclear factor kappa B (NF-κB) inflammatory pathway and other transcription factors such as mitogen activated protein kinase (MAPK), and Janus kinase (JAK-STAT), increasing the production of proinflammatory cytokines (Figure 4) [136].

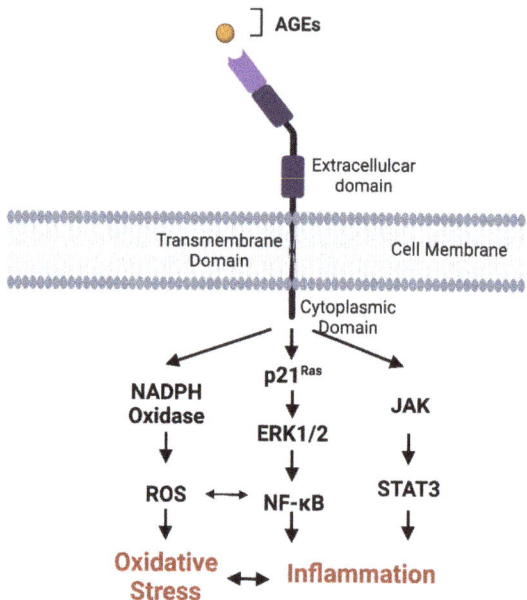

Figure 4. AGE-RAGE signaling. RAGE is composed of three extracellular domains, which include a V type ligand-binding domain and two C domains, one transmembrane domain and a cytoplasmic domain essential for signal transduction. RAGE ligands such as AGE bind to the V domain of RAGE on the cell membrane, leading to the initiation of inflammatory pathways such as JAK-STAT, NADPH Oxidase- NF-κB, p21^{Ras} and production of reactive oxygen species resulting in β-cell damage.

Circulating RAGE isoforms lacking the transmembrane domain, collectively termed soluble RAGE (sRAGE), are also present in all mammals (Figure 4). These are comprised of the endogenously secreted esRAGE and a cleaved isoform derived from membrane bound RAGE [137]. The function of sRAGE is not fully understood but is thought to have anti-inflammatory properties by competing with membrane bound RAGE for ligands [138,139]. Salonen et al. (2016) [140] found that sRAGE concentrations are reduced during seroconversion to positivity for islet autoantibodies in children who later progressed to T1D. Studies in children at high risk for developing T1D have also identified functional polymorphisms of the RAGE gene (*AGER*) which impact circulating sRAGE concentrations and significantly alter the risk for T1D development [106,141]. Lower plasma sRAGE concentrations in early life are also associated with a more severe presentation of T1D at diagnosis including diabetic ketoacidosis [142]. At the point of diagnosis and beyond, higher sRAGE concentrations are associated with the presence of microvascular and macrovascular complications and greater mortality in adults with T1D [143]. Taken together, these studies suggest that high sRAGE may be triggered by activation of the AGE-RAGE axis and act to counter chronic inflammation.

RAGE is also expressed by many of the immune cells involved in the pathogenesis of T1D such as dendritic cells, macrophages and T and B lymphocytes, and this appears to be linked to their function and activity. A reduction of RAGE expression on T cells significantly reduces proinflammatory cytokines such as IFN-γ responsible for islet inflammation [144] and influences T regulatory cell function [145]. Chen et al. (2008) [146] found that antagonism of RAGE with a small molecule inhibitor TTP488 reduced the destruction of islets transplanted into NOD mice with diabetes, delaying islet rejection. A study by Han et al. (2014) demonstrated that AGEs promote RAGE expression on CD4$^+$ T cells and differentiation to proinflammatory CD4$^+$ T cell subsets. This was prevented by the knockdown of RAGE [147]. These data suggest that RAGE signaling may alter T cell phenotype impacting autoimmunity and inflammation, as seen in T1D. Studies using human T cells cultured from peripheral blood mononuclear cells (PBMC) found that RAGE expression on CD4$^+$ and CD8$^+$ T cells in participants with normal blood glucose was higher in participants who progressed into T1D than those who did not. Culturing human CD8$^+$ T cells with and without RAGE ligands found that RAGE expression was significantly increased in T cells exposed to RAGE ligands [148]. These findings suggest that increased RAGE expression on T cells occurs prior to T1D onset [149] and that increased consumption of AGEs can enhance RAGE expression on T cells, modulating T cells behavior [146,148].

Although increased dietary AGEs consumption has been shown to be associated with β-cell injury and defective insulin secretion in mice via the AGE and RAGE pathway, the precise mechanisms in which dietary AGEs interact with RAGE remain to be elucidated. In mice, RAGE receptors are found to be expressed on the cell surface of APCs and CD4$^+$ and CD8$^+$ T cells. However, a study examining RAGE expression in human T cells found that RAGE is expressed exclusively intracellularly [148]. Therefore, more research is required to understand the interaction between dietary AGEs which are found extracellularly, and RAGE receptors which are expressed both on the cell surface and intracellularly depending on the cell type. Therapeutically, only a few studies examined pathways to block RAGE signaling in T1D. A recent study in NOD mice has clearly shown that increasing sRAGE through intraperitoneal administration of human recombinant sRAGE can reduce AGE burden, improve insulin expression and delay T1D onset via improvements in Treg function [145]. Another study by Zhang et al. (2020) examined the use of inhibitors to decrease the accumulation of other RAGE ligands such as High Mobility Group Box Protein -1 (HMGB-1), which was found to delay the onset of T1D in mouse models [150]. Indeed, activation of RAGE by binding HMGB-1 acts as an immune mediator to enhance autoimmune progression and diabetes onset in NOD mice [151]. These findings provide further evidence that interruptions in the dietary AGE-RAGE axis might be key in managing immunoinflammatory diseases such as T1D.

3. Conclusions

Although the role of AGEs and RAGE in T1D remains to be fully understood, there is clear evidence suggesting that this axis is involved in both the development and progression of T1D. AGEs interact with the immunological receptor RAGE to impact immune function and inflammation. Further, consumption of AGEs alters β-cells function and risk factors for T1D such as insulin sensitivity and obesity. Lowering of dietary AGE intake or interruption of AGE-RAGE binding reduces the incidence of T1D in murine models. Meanwhile, population-based studies have also identified that increases in circulating AGEs increases risk for T1D development in childhood and adolescence. Given that AGEs are regularly consumed as part of Western diets, as well as being made endogenously when sugar concentrations are elevated in the body, AGEs are important modifiable environmental risk factors for T1D. Hence, modifying dietary AGEs represents a simple and risk-free approach that should be further investigated in animal and clinical studies to examine the impacts on β-cell function, autoimmunity and T1D development.

Author Contributions: C.D.; writing—original draft preparation, R.O.W.; writing—review and editing, supervision, I.B.; writing—review and editing, C.C.; writing—review and editing, supervision, J.M.F.; writing—review and editing, supervision, funding acquisition, A.K.F.; writing—review and editing, supervision. All authors have read and agreed to the published version of the manuscript.

Funding: A.K.F. is supported by a UQ Research Support Fellowship. J.M.F. is supported by a Leadership Award from the National health and Medical Research Council of Australia (GNT 2010053). This work was also supported by Mater Foundation.

Institutional Review Board Statement: Not applicable.

Informed Consent Statement: Not applicable.

Data Availability Statement: Not applicable.

Conflicts of Interest: The authors declare no conflict of interest.

References

1. Mobasseri, M.; Shirmohammadi, M.; Amiri, T.; Vahed, N.; Hosseini Fard, H.; Ghojazadeh, M. Prevalence and incidence of type 1 diabetes in the world: A systematic review and meta-analysis. *Health Promot. Perspect.* **2020**, *10*, 98–115. [CrossRef]
2. Saberzadeh-Ardestani, B.; Karamzadeh, R.; Basiri, M.; Hajizadeh-Saffar, E.; Farhadi, A.; Shapiro, A.M.J.; Tahamtani, Y.; Baharvand, H. Type 1 Diabetes Mellitus: Cellular and Molecular Pathophysiology at a Glance. *Cell J.* **2018**, *20*, 294–301. [CrossRef]
3. DiMeglio, L.A.; Evans-Molina, C.; Oram, R.A. Type 1 diabetes. *Lancet* **2018**, *391*, 2449–2462. [CrossRef]
4. Leslie, R.D.; Evans-Molina, C.; Freund-Brown, J.; Buzzetti, R.; Dabelea, D.; Gillespie, K.M.; Goland, R.; Jones, A.G.; Kacher, M.; Phillips, L.S.; et al. Adult-Onset Type 1 Diabetes: Current Understanding and Challenges. *Diabetes Care* **2021**, *44*, 2449–2456. [CrossRef] [PubMed]
5. Herold, K.C.; Bundy, B.N.; Long, S.A.; Bluestone, J.A.; DiMeglio, L.A.; Dufort, M.J.; Gitelman, S.E.; Gottlieb, P.A.; Krischer, J.P.; Linsley, P.S.; et al. An Anti-CD3 Antibody, Teplizumab, in Relatives at Risk for Type 1 Diabetes. *N. Engl. J. Med.* **2019**, *381*, 603–613. [CrossRef]
6. Moran, A.; Bundy, B.; Becker, D.J.; DiMeglio, L.A.; Gitelman, S.E.; Goland, R.; Greenbaum, C.J.; Herold, K.C.; Marks, J.B.; Raskin, P.; et al. Interleukin-1 antagonism in type 1 diabetes of recent onset: Two multicentre, randomised, double-blind, placebo-controlled trials. *Lancet* **2013**, *381*, 1905–1915. [CrossRef]
7. Feutren, G.; Papoz, L.; Assan, R.; Vialettes, B.; Karsenty, G.; Vexiau, P.; Du Rostu, H.; Rodier, M.; Sirmai, J.; Lallemand, A.; et al. Cyclosporin increases the rate and length of remissions in insulin-dependent diabetes of recent onset: Results of a multicentre double-blind trial. *Lancet* **1986**, *2*, 119–124. [CrossRef]
8. Bone, R.N.; Evans-Molina, C. Combination Immunotherapy for Type 1 Diabetes. *Curr. Diabetes Rep.* **2017**, *17*, 50. [CrossRef]
9. Australian National Diabetes Audit. *Australian National Diabetes Audit—Australian Quality Clinical Audit 2019 Annual Report*; Australian Government Department of Health: Canberra, Australia, 2019.
10. Atkinson, M.A.; Eisenbarth, G.S.; Michels, A.W. Type 1 diabetes. *Lancet* **2014**, *383*, 69–82. [CrossRef]
11. Fousteri, G.; Ippolito, E.; Ahmed, R.; Hamad, A.R.A. Beta-cell Specific Autoantibodies: Are they Just an Indicator of Type 1 Diabetes? *Curr. Diabetes Rev.* **2017**, *13*, 322–329. [CrossRef]
12. Ilonen, J.; Lempainen, J.; Hammais, A.; Laine, A.P.; Harkonen, T.; Toppari, J.; Veijola, R.; Knip, M.; Finnish Pediatric Diabetes, R. Primary islet autoantibody at initial seroconversion and autoantibodies at diagnosis of type 1 diabetes as markers of disease heterogeneity. *Pediatr. Diabetes* **2018**, *19*, 284–292. [CrossRef] [PubMed]
13. Wang, J.; Miao, D.; Babu, S.; Yu, J.; Barker, J.; Klingensmith, G.; Rewers, M.; Eisenbarth, G.S.; Yu, L. Prevalence of autoantibody-negative diabetes is not rare at all ages and increases with older age and obesity. *J. Clin. Endocrinol. Metab.* **2007**, *92*, 88–92. [CrossRef]
14. Chiou, J.; Geusz, R.J.; Okino, M.-L.; Han, J.Y.; Miller, M.; Melton, R.; Beebe, E.; Benaglio, P.; Huang, S.; Korgaonkar, K.; et al. Interpreting type 1 diabetes risk with genetics and single-cell epigenomics. *Nature* **2021**, *594*, 398–402. [CrossRef] [PubMed]
15. Szablewski, L. Role of immune system in type 1 diabetes mellitus pathogenesis. *Int. Immunopharmacol.* **2014**, *22*, 182–191. [CrossRef] [PubMed]
16. Pugliese, A. Autoreactive T cells in type 1 diabetes. *J. Clin. Investig.* **2017**, *127*, 2881–2891. [CrossRef]
17. Hyttinen, V.; Kaprio, J.; Kinnunen, L.; Koskenvuo, M.; Tuomilehto, J. Genetic Liability of Type 1 Diabetes and the Onset Age Among 22,650 Young Finnish Twin Pairs: A Nationwide Follow-Up Study. *Diabetes* **2003**, *52*, 1052–1055. [CrossRef]
18. Redondo, M.J.; Jeffrey, J.; Fain, P.R.; Eisenbarth, G.S.; Orban, T. Concordance for Islet Autoimmunity among Monozygotic Twins. *N. Engl. J. Med.* **2008**, *359*, 2849–2850. [CrossRef]
19. Makino, S.; Kunimoto, K.; Muraoka, Y.; Mizushima, Y.; Katagiri, K.; Tochino, Y. Breeding of a non-obese, diabetic strain of mice. *Jikken Dobutsu* **1980**, *29*, 1–13. [CrossRef]
20. Chen, Y.G.; Mathews, C.E.; Driver, J.P. The Role of NOD Mice in Type 1 Diabetes Research: Lessons from the Past and Recommendations for the Future. *Front. Endocrinol.* **2018**, *9*, 51. [CrossRef]
21. Burrack, A.L.; Martinov, T.; Fife, B.T. T Cell-Mediated Beta Cell Destruction: Autoimmunity and Alloimmunity in the Context of Type 1 Diabetes. *Front. Endocrinol.* **2017**, *8*, 343. [CrossRef]
22. Xing, Y.; Hogquist, K.A. T-Cell Tolerance: Central and Peripheral. *Cold Spring Harb. Perspect. Biol.* **2012**, *4*, a006957. [CrossRef] [PubMed]
23. Jeker, L.T.; Bour-Jordan, H.; Bluestone, J.A. Breakdown in peripheral tolerance in type 1 diabetes in mice and humans. *Cold Spring Harb. Perspect. Med.* **2012**, *2*, a007807. [CrossRef] [PubMed]

24. Erdem, N.; Montero, E.; Roep, B.O. Breaking and restoring immune tolerance to pancreatic beta-cells in type 1 diabetes. *Curr. Opin. Endocrinol. Diabetes Obes.* **2021**, *28*, 397–403. [CrossRef] [PubMed]
25. Rewers, M.; Ludvigsson, J. Environmental risk factors for type 1 diabetes. *Lancet* **2016**, *387*, 2340–2348. [CrossRef]
26. Esposito, S.; Toni, G.; Tascini, G.; Santi, E.; Berioli, M.G.; Principi, N. Environmental Factors Associated with Type 1 Diabetes. *Front. Endocrinol.* **2019**, *10*, 592. [CrossRef]
27. Redondo, M.J.; Steck, A.K.; Pugliese, A. Genetics of type 1 diabetes. *Pediatr. Diabetes* **2018**, *19*, 346–353. [CrossRef] [PubMed]
28. Roep, B.O.; Thomaidou, S.; van Tienhoven, R.; Zaldumbide, A. Type 1 diabetes mellitus as a disease of the beta-cell (do not blame the immune system?). *Nat. Rev. Endocrinol.* **2021**, *17*, 150–161. [CrossRef]
29. Insel, R.A.; Dunne, J.L.; Atkinson, M.A.; Chiang, J.L.; Dabelea, D.; Gottlieb, P.A.; Greenbaum, C.J.; Herold, K.C.; Krischer, J.P.; Lernmark, A.; et al. Staging presymptomatic type 1 diabetes: A scientific statement of JDRF, the Endocrine Society, and the American Diabetes Association. *Diabetes Care* **2015**, *38*, 1964–1974. [CrossRef]
30. Katsarou, A.; Gudbjornsdottir, S.; Rawshani, A.; Dabelea, D.; Bonifacio, E.; Anderson, B.J.; Jacobsen, L.M.; Schatz, D.A.; Lernmark, A. Type 1 diabetes mellitus. *Nat. Rev. Dis. Prim.* **2017**, *3*, 17016. [CrossRef]
31. Claessens, L.A.; Wesselius, J.; van Lummel, M.; Laban, S.; Mulder, F.; Mul, D.; Nikolic, T.; Aanstoot, H.J.; Koeleman, B.P.C.; Roep, B.O. Clinical and genetic correlates of islet-autoimmune signatures in juvenile-onset type 1 diabetes. *Diabetologia* **2020**, *63*, 351–361. [CrossRef]
32. Pundziute-Lyckå, A.; Persson, L.A.; Cedermark, G.; Jansson-Roth, A.; Nilsson, U.; Westin, V.; Dahlquist, G. Diet, growth, and the risk for type 1 diabetes in childhood: A matched case-referent study. *Diabetes Care* **2004**, *27*, 2784–2789. [CrossRef] [PubMed]
33. Kibirige, M.; Metcalf, B.; Renuka, R.; Wilkin, T.J. Testing the Accelerator Hypothesis: The relationship between body mass and age at diagnosis of type 1 diabetes. *Diabetes Care* **2003**, *26*, 2865–2870. [CrossRef] [PubMed]
34. Knerr, I.; Wolf, J.; Reinehr, T.; Stachow, R.; Grabert, M.; Schober, E.; Rascher, W.; Holl, R.W. The 'accelerator hypothesis': Relationship between weight, height, body mass index and age at diagnosis in a large cohort of 9,248 German and Austrian children with type 1 diabetes mellitus. *Diabetologia* **2005**, *48*, 2501–2504. [CrossRef]
35. Nucci, A.M.; Virtanen, S.M.; Cuthbertson, D.; Ludvigsson, J.; Einberg, U.; Huot, C.; Castano, L.; Aschemeier, B.; Becker, D.J.; Knip, M.; et al. Growth and development of islet autoimmunity and type 1 diabetes in children genetically at risk. *Diabetologia* **2021**, *64*, 826–835. [CrossRef] [PubMed]
36. Ciężki, S.; Kurpiewska, E.; Bossowski, A.; Głowińska-Olszewska, B. Multi-Faceted Influence of Obesity on Type 1 Diabetes in Children—From Disease Pathogenesis to Complications. *Front. Endocrinol.* **2022**, *13*, 890833. [CrossRef]
37. Von Scholten, B.J.; Kreiner, F.F.; Gough, S.C.L.; von Herrath, M. Current and future therapies for type 1 diabetes. *Diabetologia* **2021**, *64*, 1037–1048. [CrossRef]
38. Holmes-Walker, D.J.; Abraham, M.B.; Chee, M.; Jones, T.W. Glycaemic outcomes in Australasian children and adults with type 1 diabetes: Failure to meet targets across the age spectrum. *Intern. Med. J.* **2022**. ahead of print. [CrossRef]
39. Abdul-Rasoul, M.; Habib, H.; Al-Khouly, M. 'The honeymoon phase' in children with type 1 diabetes mellitus: Frequency, duration, and influential factors. *Pediatr. Diabetes* **2006**, *7*, 101–107. [CrossRef]
40. Jansen, A.; Homo-Delarche, F.; Hooijkaas, H.; Leenen, P.J.; Dardenne, M.; Drexhage, H.A. Immunohistochemical Characterization of Monocytes-Macrophages and Dendritic Cells Involved in the Initiation of the Insulitis and β-Cell Destruction in NOD Mice. *Diabetes* **1994**, *43*, 667–675. [CrossRef]
41. Coppieters, K.T.; Dotta, F.; Amirian, N.; Campbell, P.D.; Kay, T.W.; Atkinson, M.A.; Roep, B.O.; von Herrath, M.G. Demonstration of islet-autoreactive CD8 T cells in insulitic lesions from recent onset and long-term type 1 diabetes patients. *J. Exp. Med.* **2012**, *209*, 51–60. [CrossRef]
42. In't Veld, P.; Lievens, D.; de Grijse, J.; Ling, Z.; van der Auwera, B.; Pipeleers-Marichal, M.; Gorus, F.; Pipeleers, D. Screening for insulitis in adult autoantibody-positive organ donors. *Diabetes* **2007**, *56*, 2400–2404. [CrossRef] [PubMed]
43. Campbell-Thompson, M.; Wasserfall, C.; Kaddis, J.; Albanese-O'Neill, A.; Staeva, T.; Nierras, C.; Moraski, J.; Rowe, P.; Gianani, R.; Eisenbarth, G.; et al. Network for Pancreatic Organ Donors with Diabetes (nPOD): Developing a tissue biobank for type 1 diabetes. *Diabetes/Metab. Res. Rev.* **2012**, *28*, 608–617. [CrossRef]
44. In't Veld, P. Insulitis in human type 1 diabetes: The quest for an elusive lesion. *Islets* **2011**, *3*, 131–138. [CrossRef]
45. Hutchings, P.; Rosen, H.; O'Reilly, L.; Simpson, E.; Gordon, S.; Cooke, A. Transfer of diabetes in mice prevented by blockade of adhesion-promoting receptor on macrophages. *Nature* **1990**, *348*, 639–642. [CrossRef] [PubMed]
46. Jun, H.S.; Yoon, C.S.; Zbytnuik, L.; van Rooijen, N.; Yoon, J.W. The role of macrophages in T cell-mediated autoimmune diabetes in nonobese diabetic mice. *J. Exp. Med.* **1999**, *189*, 347–358. [CrossRef]
47. Yang, L.J. Big mac attack: Does it play a direct role for monocytes/macrophages in type 1 diabetes? *Diabetes* **2008**, *57*, 2922–2923. [CrossRef]
48. Lehuen, A.; Diana, J.; Zaccone, P.; Cooke, A. Immune cell crosstalk in type 1 diabetes. *Nat. Rev. Immunol.* **2010**, *10*, 501–513. [CrossRef] [PubMed]
49. Hawiger, D.; Inaba, K.; Dorsett, Y.; Guo, M.; Mahnke, K.; Rivera, M.; Ravetch, J.V.; Steinman, R.M.; Nussenzweig, M.C. Dendritic cells induce peripheral T cell unresponsiveness under steady state conditions in vivo. *J. Exp. Med.* **2001**, *194*, 769–779. [CrossRef]
50. Probst, H.C.; Lagnel, J.; Kollias, G.; van den Broek, M. Inducible Transgenic Mice Reveal Resting Dendritic Cells as Potent Inducers of CD8+ T Cell Tolerance. *Immunity* **2003**, *18*, 713–720. [CrossRef]
51. Morel, P.A. Dendritic cell subsets in type 1 diabetes: Friend or foe? *Front. Immunol.* **2013**, *4*, 415. [CrossRef]

52. Ganguly, D.; Haak, S.; Sisirak, V.; Reizis, B. The role of dendritic cells in autoimmunity. *Nat. Rev. Immunol.* **2013**, *13*, 566–577. [CrossRef]
53. Creusot, R.J.; Postigo-Fernandez, J.; Teteloshvili, N. Altered Function of Antigen-Presenting Cells in Type 1 Diabetes: A Challenge for Antigen-Specific Immunotherapy? *Diabetes* **2018**, *67*, 1481–1494. [CrossRef]
54. Saxena, V.; Ondr, J.K.; Magnusen, A.F.; Munn, D.H.; Katz, J.D. The Countervailing Actions of Myeloid and Plasmacytoid Dendritic Cells Control Autoimmune Diabetes in the Nonobese Diabetic Mouse. *J. Immunol.* **2007**, *179*, 5041–5053. [CrossRef] [PubMed]
55. Uno, S.; Imagawa, A.; Okita, K.; Sayama, K.; Moriwaki, M.; Iwahashi, H.; Yamagata, K.; Tamura, S.; Matsuzawa, Y.; Hanafusa, T.; et al. Macrophages and dendritic cells infiltrating islets with or without beta cells produce tumour necrosis factor-α in patients with recent-onset type 1 diabetes. *Diabetologia* **2007**, *50*, 596–601. [CrossRef] [PubMed]
56. Chen, X.; Makala, L.H.; Jin, Y.; Hopkins, D.; Muir, A.; Garge, N.; Podolsky, R.H.; She, J.X. Type 1 diabetes patients have significantly lower frequency of plasmacytoid dendritic cells in the peripheral blood. *Clin. Immunol.* **2008**, *129*, 413–418. [CrossRef] [PubMed]
57. Vuckovic, S.; Withers, G.; Harris, M.; Khalil, D.; Gardiner, D.; Flesch, I.; Tepes, S.; Greer, R.; Cowley, D.; Cotterill, A.; et al. Decreased blood dendritic cell counts in type 1 diabetic children. *Clin. Immunol.* **2007**, *123*, 281–288. [CrossRef]
58. Wallberg, M.; Cooke, A. Immune mechanisms in type 1 diabetes. *Trends Immunol.* **2013**, *34*, 583–591. [CrossRef] [PubMed]
59. Haase, C.; Skak, K.; Michelsen, B.K.; Markholst, H. Local Activation of Dendritic Cells Leads to Insulitis and Development of Insulin-Dependent Diabetes in Transgenic Mice Expressing CD154 on the Pancreatic β-Cells. *Diabetes* **2004**, *53*, 2588–2595. [CrossRef] [PubMed]
60. Phillips, J.M.; Parish, N.M.; Raine, T.; Bland, C.; Sawyer, Y.; de La Pena, H.; Cooke, A. Type 1 diabetes development requires both CD4+ and CD8+ T cells and can be reversed by non-depleting antibodies targeting both T cell populations. *Rev. Diabet. Stud.* **2009**, *6*, 97–103. [CrossRef]
61. Clark, M.; Kroger, C.J.; Tisch, R.M. Type 1 Diabetes: A Chronic Anti-Self-Inflammatory Response. *Front. Immunol.* **2017**, *8*, 1898. [CrossRef]
62. Chervonsky, A.V.; Wang, Y.; Wong, F.S.; Visintin, I.; Flavell, R.A.; Janeway, C.A., Jr.; Matis, L.A. The role of Fas in autoimmune diabetes. *Cell* **1997**, *89*, 17–24. [CrossRef]
63. Chatenoud, L.; Thervet, E.; Primo, J.; Bach, J.F. Anti-CD3 antibody induces long-term remission of overt autoimmunity in nonobese diabetic mice. *Proc. Natl. Acad. Sci. USA* **1994**, *91*, 123–127. [CrossRef]
64. Rodriguez-Calvo, T.; Suwandi, J.S.; Amirian, N.; Zapardiel-Gonzalo, J.; Anquetil, F.; Sabouri, S.; Von Herrath, M.G. Heterogeneity and Lobularity of Pancreatic Pathology in Type 1 Diabetes during the Prediabetic Phase. *J. Histochem. Cytochem.* **2015**, *63*, 626–636. [CrossRef]
65. Itoh, N.; Hanafusa, T.; Miyazaki, A.; Miyagawa, J.; Yamagata, K.; Yamamoto, K.; Waguri, M.; Imagawa, A.; Tamura, S.; Inada, M.; et al. Mononuclear cell infiltration and its relation to the expression of major histocompatibility complex antigens and adhesion molecules in pancreas biopsy specimens from newly diagnosed insulin-dependent diabetes mellitus patients. *J. Clin. Investig.* **1993**, *92*, 2313–2322. [CrossRef]
66. Assalino, M.; Genevay, M.; Morel, P.; Demuylder-Mischler, S.; Toso, C.; Berney, T. Recurrence of type 1 diabetes after simultaneous pancreas-kidney transplantation in the absence of GAD and IA-2 autoantibodies. *Am. J. Transplant.* **2012**, *12*, 492–495. [CrossRef]
67. Williams, A.J.; Thrower, S.L.; Sequeiros, I.M.; Ward, A.; Bickerton, A.S.; Triay, J.M.; Callaway, M.P.; Dayan, C.M. Pancreatic volume is reduced in adult patients with recently diagnosed type 1 diabetes. *J. Clin. Endocrinol. Metab.* **2012**, *97*, E2109–E2113. [CrossRef] [PubMed]
68. Rodriguez-Calvo, T.; Ekwall, O.; Amirian, N.; Zapardiel-Gonzalo, J.; von Herrath, M.G. Increased immune cell infiltration of the exocrine pancreas: A possible contribution to the pathogenesis of type 1 diabetes. *Diabetes* **2014**, *63*, 3880–3890. [CrossRef]
69. Visperas, A.; Vignali, D.A. Are Regulatory T Cells Defective in Type 1 Diabetes and Can We Fix Them? *J. Immunol.* **2016**, *197*, 3762–3770. [CrossRef] [PubMed]
70. Hull, C.M.; Peakman, M.; Tree, T.I.M. Regulatory T cell dysfunction in type 1 diabetes: What's broken and how can we fix it? *Diabetologia* **2017**, *60*, 1839–1850. [CrossRef] [PubMed]
71. Grinberg-Bleyer, Y.; Baeyens, A.; You, S.; Elhage, R.; Fourcade, G.; Gregoire, S.; Cagnard, N.; Carpentier, W.; Tang, Q.; Bluestone, J.; et al. IL-2 reverses established type 1 diabetes in NOD mice by a local effect on pancreatic regulatory T cells. *J. Exp. Med.* **2010**, *207*, 1871–1878. [CrossRef] [PubMed]
72. Dwyer, C.J.; Ward, N.C.; Pugliese, A.; Malek, T.R. Promoting Immune Regulation in Type 1 Diabetes Using Low-Dose Interleukin-2. *Curr. Diabetes Rep.* **2016**, *16*, 46. [CrossRef]
73. Dong, S.; Hiam-Galvez, K.J.; Mowery, C.T.; Herold, K.C.; Gitelman, S.E.; Esensten, J.H.; Liu, W.; Lares, A.P.; Leinbach, A.S.; Lee, M.; et al. The effect of low-dose IL-2 and Treg adoptive cell therapy in patients with type 1 diabetes. *JCI Insight* **2021**, *6*, e147474. [CrossRef] [PubMed]
74. Long, S.A.; Rieck, M.; Sanda, S.; Bollyky, J.B.; Samuels, P.L.; Goland, R.; Ahmann, A.; Rabinovitch, A.; Aggarwal, S.; Phippard, D.; et al. Rapamycin/IL-2 combination therapy in patients with type 1 diabetes augments Tregs yet transiently impairs beta-cell function. *Diabetes* **2012**, *61*, 2340–2348. [CrossRef]
75. Gardner, G.; Fraker, C.A. Natural Killer Cells as Key Mediators in Type I Diabetes Immunopathology. *Front. Immunol.* **2021**, *12*, 722979. [CrossRef]

76. Stene, L.C.; Oikarinen, S.; Hyoty, H.; Barriga, K.J.; Norris, J.M.; Klingensmith, G.; Hutton, J.C.; Erlich, H.A.; Eisenbarth, G.S.; Rewers, M. Enterovirus infection and progression from islet autoimmunity to type 1 diabetes: The Diabetes and Autoimmunity Study in the Young (DAISY). *Diabetes* **2010**, *59*, 3174–3180. [CrossRef]
77. Lönnrot, M.; Salminen, K.; Knip, M.; Savola, K.; Kulmala, P.; Leinikki, P.; Hyypiä, T.; Akerblom, H.K.; Hyöty, H. Enterovirus RNA in serum is a risk factor for beta-cell autoimmunity and clinical type 1 diabetes: A prospective study. *J. Med. Virol.* **2000**, *61*, 214–220. [CrossRef]
78. Simonen-Tikka, M.L.; Pflueger, M.; Klemola, P.; Savolainen-Kopra, C.; Smura, T.; Hummel, S.; Kaijalainen, S.; Nuutila, K.; Natri, O.; Roivainen, M.; et al. Human enterovirus infections in children at increased risk for type 1 diabetes: The Babydiet study. *Diabetologia* **2011**, *54*, 2995–3002. [CrossRef] [PubMed]
79. Ho, J.; Rosolowsky, E.; Pacaud, D.; Huang, C.; Lemay, J.A.; Brockman, N.; Rath, M.; Doulla, M. Diabetic ketoacidosis at type 1 diabetes diagnosis in children during the COVID-19 pandemic. *Pediatr. Diabetes* **2021**, *22*, 552–557. [CrossRef]
80. Qeadan, F.; Tingey, B.; Egbert, J.; Pezzolesi, M.G.; Burge, M.R.; Peterson, K.A.; Honda, T. The associations between COVID-19 diagnosis, type 1 diabetes, and the risk of diabetic ketoacidosis: A nationwide cohort from the US using the Cerner Real-World Data. *PLoS ONE* **2022**, *17*, e0266809. [CrossRef]
81. Uribarri, J.; Woodruff, S.; Goodman, S.; Cai, W.; Chen, X.; Pyzik, R.; Yong, A.; Striker, G.E.; Vlassara, H. Advanced glycation end products in foods and a practical guide to their reduction in the diet. *J. Am. Diet. Assoc.* **2010**, *110*, 911–916.e12. [CrossRef] [PubMed]
82. Ramasamy, R.; Vannucci, S.J.; Yan, S.S.D.; Herold, K.; Yan, S.F.; Schmidt, A.M. Advanced glycation end products and RAGE: A common thread in aging, diabetes, neurodegeneration, and inflammation. *Glycobiology* **2005**, *15*, 16R–28R. [CrossRef] [PubMed]
83. Scheijen, J.; Clevers, E.; Engelen, L.; Dagnelie, P.C.; Brouns, F.; Stehouwer, C.D.A.; Schalkwijk, C.G. Analysis of advanced glycation endproducts in selected food items by ultra-performance liquid chromatography tandem mass spectrometry: Presentation of a dietary AGE database. *Food Chem.* **2016**, *190*, 1145–1150. [CrossRef] [PubMed]
84. Singh, V.P.; Bali, A.; Singh, N.; Jaggi, A.S. Advanced glycation end products and diabetic complications. *Korean J. Physiol. Pharmacol.* **2014**, *18*, 1–14. [CrossRef] [PubMed]
85. Poulsen, M.W.; Hedegaard, R.V.; Andersen, J.M.; de Courten, B.; Bugel, S.; Nielsen, J.; Skibsted, L.H.; Dragsted, L.O. Advanced glycation endproducts in food and their effects on health. *Food Chem. Toxicol.* **2013**, *60*, 10–37. [CrossRef]
86. Jud, P.; Sourij, H. Therapeutic options to reduce advanced glycation end products in patients with diabetes mellitus: A review. *Diabetes Res. Clin. Pract.* **2019**, *148*, 54–63. [CrossRef]
87. Sergi, D.; Boulestin, H.; Campbell, F.M.; Williams, L.M. The Role of Dietary Advanced Glycation End Products in Metabolic Dysfunction. *Mol. Nutr. Food Res.* **2021**, *65*, e1900934. [CrossRef]
88. Sharma, C.; Kaur, A.; Thind, S.S.; Singh, B.; Raina, S. Advanced glycation End-products (AGEs): An emerging concern for processed food industries. *J. Food Sci. Technol.* **2015**, *52*, 7561–7576. [CrossRef]
89. Chen, J.H.; Lin, X.; Bu, C.; Zhang, X. Role of advanced glycation end products in mobility and considerations in possible dietary and nutritional intervention strategies. *Nutr. Metab.* **2018**, *15*, 72. [CrossRef]
90. Huebschmann, A.G.; Regensteiner, J.G.; Vlassara, H.; Reusch, J.E. Diabetes and advanced glycoxidation end products. *Diabetes Care* **2006**, *29*, 1420–1432. [CrossRef] [PubMed]
91. Stirban, A.; Gawlowski, T.; Roden, M. Vascular effects of advanced glycation endproducts: Clinical effects and molecular mechanisms. *Mol. Metab.* **2014**, *3*, 94–108. [CrossRef]
92. Qu, W.; Yuan, X.; Zhao, J.; Zhang, Y.; Hu, J.; Wang, J.; Li, J. Dietary advanced glycation end products modify gut microbial composition and partially increase colon permeability in rats. *Mol. Nutr. Food Res.* **2017**, *61*, 1700118. [CrossRef]
93. Seiquer, I.; Rubio, L.A.; Peinado, M.J.; Delgado-Andrade, C.; Navarro, M.P. Maillard reaction products modulate gut microbiota composition in adolescents. *Mol. Nutr. Food Res.* **2014**, *58*, 1552–1560. [CrossRef]
94. Zhang, Z.; Li, D. Thermal processing of food reduces gut microbiota diversity of the host and triggers adaptation of the microbiota: Evidence from two vertebrates. *Microbiome* **2018**, *6*, 99. [CrossRef] [PubMed]
95. Marungruang, N.; Fåk, F.; Tareke, E. Heat-treated high-fat diet modifies gut microbiota and metabolic markers in apoe−/− mice. *Nutr. Metab.* **2016**, *13*, 22. [CrossRef]
96. Zhou, H.; Sun, L.; Zhang, S.; Zhao, X.; Gang, X.; Wang, G. Evaluating the Causal Role of Gut Microbiota in Type 1 Diabetes and Its Possible Pathogenic Mechanisms. *Front. Endocrinol.* **2020**, *11*, 125. [CrossRef] [PubMed]
97. Snelson, M.; Coughlan, M.T. Dietary Advanced Glycation End Products: Digestion, Metabolism and Modulation of Gut Microbial Ecology. *Nutrients* **2019**, *11*, 215. [CrossRef] [PubMed]
98. Forbes, J.M.; Cooper, M.E. Mechanisms of diabetic complications. *Physiol. Rev.* **2013**, *93*, 137–188. [CrossRef]
99. Bos, D.C.; de Ranitz-Greven, W.L.; de Valk, H.W. Advanced Glycation End Products, Measured as Skin Autofluorescence and Diabetes Complications: A Systematic Review. *Diabetes Technol. Ther.* **2011**, *13*, 773–779. [CrossRef]
100. Beyan, H.; Riese, H.; Hawa, M.I.; Beretta, G.; Davidson, H.W.; Hutton, J.C.; Burger, H.; Schlosser, M.; Snieder, H.; Boehm, B.O.; et al. Glycotoxin and autoantibodies are additive environmentally determined predictors of type 1 diabetes: A twin and population study. *Diabetes* **2012**, *61*, 1192–1198. [CrossRef]
101. Coughlan, M.T.; Yap, F.Y.; Tong, D.C.; Andrikopoulos, S.; Gasser, A.; Thallas-Bonke, V.; Webster, D.E.; Miyazaki, J.; Kay, T.W.; Slattery, R.M.; et al. Advanced glycation end products are direct modulators of beta-cell function. *Diabetes* **2011**, *60*, 2523–2532. [CrossRef]

102. Zhao, Z.; Zhao, C.; Zhang, X.H.; Zheng, F.; Cai, W.; Vlassara, H.; Ma, Z.A. Advanced glycation end products inhibit glucose-stimulated insulin secretion through nitric oxide-dependent inhibition of cytochrome c oxidase and adenosine triphosphate synthesis. *Endocrinology* **2009**, *150*, 2569–2576. [CrossRef]
103. Borg, D.J.; Yap, F.Y.T.; Keshvari, S.; Simmons, D.G.; Gallo, L.A.; Fotheringham, A.K.; Zhuang, A.; Slattery, R.M.; Hasnain, S.Z.; Coughlan, M.T.; et al. Perinatal exposure to high dietary advanced glycation end products in transgenic NOD8.3 mice leads to pancreatic beta cell dysfunction. *Islets* **2018**, *10*, 10–24. [CrossRef]
104. Peppa, M.; He, C.; Hattori, M.; McEvoy, R.; Zheng, F.; Vlassara, H. Fetal or neonatal low-glycotoxin environment prevents autoimmune diabetes in NOD mice. *Diabetes* **2003**, *52*, 1441–1448. [CrossRef] [PubMed]
105. Mericq, V.; Piccardo, C.; Cai, W.; Chen, X.; Zhu, L.; Striker, G.E.; Vlassara, H.; Uribarri, J. Maternally transmitted and food-derived glycotoxins: A factor preconditioning the young to diabetes? *Diabetes Care* **2010**, *33*, 2232–2237. [CrossRef] [PubMed]
106. Forbes, J.M.; Soderlund, J.; Yap, F.Y.; Knip, M.; Andrikopoulos, S.; Ilonen, J.; Simell, O.; Veijola, R.; Sourris, K.C.; Coughlan, M.T.; et al. Receptor for advanced glycation end-products (RAGE) provides a link between genetic susceptibility and environmental factors in type 1 diabetes. *Diabetologia* **2011**, *54*, 1032–1042. [CrossRef] [PubMed]
107. Forbes, J.M.; Sourris, K.C.; de Courten, M.P.; Dougherty, S.L.; Chand, V.; Lyons, J.G.; Bertovic, D.; Coughlan, M.T.; Schlaich, M.P.; Soldatos, G.; et al. Advanced glycation end products (AGEs) are cross-sectionally associated with insulin secretion in healthy subjects. *Amino Acids* **2014**, *46*, 321–326. [CrossRef]
108. Vlassara, H.; Uribarri, J. Advanced glycation end products (AGE) and diabetes: Cause, effect, or both? *Curr. Diabetes Rep.* **2014**, *14*, 453. [CrossRef]
109. Bhatt, H.B.; Smith, R.J. Fatty liver disease in diabetes mellitus. *Hepatobiliary Surg. Nutr.* **2015**, *4*, 101–108. [CrossRef]
110. Barros, B.S.V.; Santos, D.C.; Pizarro, M.H.; del Melo, L.G.N.; Gomes, M.B. Type 1 Diabetes and Non-Alcoholic Fatty Liver Disease: When Should We Be Concerned? A Nationwide Study in Brazil. *Nutrients* **2017**, *9*, 878. [CrossRef]
111. De Courten, B.; de Courten, M.P.; Soldatos, G.; Dougherty, S.L.; Straznicky, N.; Schlaich, M.; Sourris, K.C.; Chand, V.; Scheijen, J.L.; Kingwell, B.A.; et al. Diet low in advanced glycation end products increases insulin sensitivity in healthy overweight individuals: A double-blind, randomized, crossover trial. *Am. J. Clin. Nutr.* **2016**, *103*, 1426–1433. [CrossRef]
112. Vlassara, H.; Cai, W.; Tripp, E.; Pyzik, R.; Yee, K.; Goldberg, L.; Tansman, L.; Chen, X.; Mani, V.; Fayad, Z.A.; et al. Oral AGE restriction ameliorates insulin resistance in obese individuals with the metabolic syndrome: A randomised controlled trial. *Diabetologia* **2016**, *59*, 2181–2192. [CrossRef] [PubMed]
113. Harcourt, B.E.; Sourris, K.C.; Coughlan, M.T.; Walker, K.Z.; Dougherty, S.L.; Andrikopoulos, S.; Morley, A.L.; Thallas-Bonke, V.; Chand, V.; Penfold, S.A.; et al. Targeted reduction of advanced glycation improves renal function in obesity. *Kidney Int.* **2011**, *80*, 190–198. [CrossRef]
114. Leung, C.; Herath, C.B.; Jia, Z.; Goodwin, M.; Mak, K.Y.; Watt, M.J.; Forbes, J.M.; Angus, P.W. Dietary glycotoxins exacerbate progression of experimental fatty liver disease. *J. Hepatol.* **2014**, *60*, 832–838. [CrossRef]
115. Leung, C.; Herath, C.B.; Jia, Z.; Andrikopoulos, S.; Brown, B.E.; Davies, M.J.; Rivera, L.R.; Furness, J.B.; Forbes, J.M.; Angus, P.W. Dietary advanced glycation end-products aggravate non-alcoholic fatty liver disease. *World J. Gastroenterol.* **2016**, *22*, 8026–8040. [CrossRef]
116. Egana-Gorrono, L.; Lopez-Diez, R.; Yepuri, G.; Ramirez, L.S.; Reverdatto, S.; Gugger, P.F.; Shekhtman, A.; Ramasamy, R.; Schmidt, A.M. Receptor for Advanced Glycation End Products (RAGE) and Mechanisms and Therapeutic Opportunities in Diabetes and Cardiovascular Disease: Insights from Human Subjects and Animal Models. *Front. Cardiovasc. Med.* **2020**, *7*, 37. [CrossRef] [PubMed]
117. Chuah, Y.K.; Basir, R.; Talib, H.; Tie, T.H.; Nordin, N. Receptor for advanced glycation end products and its involvement in inflammatory diseases. *Int. J. Inflam.* **2013**, *2013*, 403460. [CrossRef]
118. Goh, S.Y.; Cooper, M.E. Clinical review: The role of advanced glycation end products in progression and complications of diabetes. *J. Clin. Endocrinol. Metab.* **2008**, *93*, 1143–1152. [CrossRef] [PubMed]
119. Goldin, A.; Beckman, J.A.; Schmidt, A.M.; Creager, M.A. Advanced glycation end products: Sparking the development of diabetic vascular injury. *Circulation* **2006**, *114*, 597–605. [CrossRef]
120. Xue, J.; Rai, V.; Singer, D.; Chabierski, S.; Xie, J.; Reverdatto, S.; Burz, D.S.; Schmidt, A.M.; Hoffmann, R.; Shekhtman, A. Advanced glycation end product recognition by the receptor for AGEs. *Structure* **2011**, *19*, 722–732. [CrossRef]
121. Ohgami, N.; Nagai, R.; Ikemoto, M.; Arai, H.; Miyazaki, A.; Hakamata, H.; Horiuchi, S.; Nakayama, H. CD36, serves as a receptor for advanced glycation endproducts (AGE). *J. Diabetes Complicat.* **2002**, *16*, 56–59. [CrossRef]
122. Horiuchi, S.; Sakamoto, Y.; Sakai, M. Scavenger receptors for oxidized and glycated proteins. *Amino Acids* **2003**, *25*, 283–292. [CrossRef] [PubMed]
123. Ohgami, N.; Nagai, R.; Miyazaki, A.; Ikemoto, M.; Arai, H.; Horiuchi, S.; Nakayama, H. Scavenger Receptor Class B Type I-mediated Reverse Cholesterol Transport Is Inhibited by Advanced Glycation End Products *. *J. Biol. Chem.* **2001**, *276*, 13348–13355. [CrossRef]
124. Ohgami, N.; Nagai, R.; Ikemoto, M.; Arai, H.; Kuniyasu, A.; Horiuchi, S.; Nakayama, H. CD36, a Member of the Class B Scavenger Receptor Family, as a Receptor for Advanced Glycation End Products *. *J. Biol. Chem.* **2001**, *276*, 3195–3202. [CrossRef] [PubMed]
125. Puchałowicz, K.; Rać, M.E. The Multifunctionality of CD36 in Diabetes Mellitus and Its Complications—Update in Pathogenesis, Treatment and Monitoring. *Cells* **2020**, *9*, 1877. [CrossRef]

126. Chen, Y.; Zhang, J.; Cui, W.; Silverstein, R.L. CD36, a signaling receptor and fatty acid transporter that regulates immune cell metabolism and fate. *J. Exp. Med.* **2022**, *219*, e20211314. [CrossRef] [PubMed]
127. Wang, H.; Franco, F.; Tsui, Y.-C.; Xie, X.; Trefny, M.P.; Zappasodi, R.; Mohmood, S.R.; Fernández-García, J.; Tsai, C.-H.; Schulze, I.; et al. CD36-mediated metabolic adaptation supports regulatory T cell survival and function in tumors. *Nat. Immunol.* **2020**, *21*, 298–308. [CrossRef]
128. Ma, X.; Xiao, L.; Liu, L.; Ye, L.; Su, P.; Bi, E.; Wang, Q.; Yang, M.; Qian, J.; Yi, Q. CD36-mediated ferroptosis dampens intratumoral CD8$^+$ T cell effector function and impairs their antitumor ability. *Cell Metab.* **2021**, *33*, 1001–1012.e5. [CrossRef]
129. Vlassara, H.; Li, Y.M.; Imani, F.; Wojciechowicz, D.; Yang, Z.; Liu, F.T.; Cerami, A. Identification of galectin-3 as a high-affinity binding protein for advanced glycation end products (AGE): A new member of the AGE-receptor complex. *Mol. Med.* **1995**, *1*, 634–646. [CrossRef]
130. Li, Y.; Li, T.; Zhou, Z.; Xiao, Y. Emerging roles of Galectin-3 in diabetes and diabetes complications: A snapshot. *Rev. Endocr. Metab. Disord.* **2022**, *23*, 569–577. [CrossRef]
131. Karlsen, A.E.; Størling, Z.M.; Sparre, T.; Larsen, M.R.; Mahmood, A.; Størling, J.; Roepstorff, P.; Wrzesinski, K.; Larsen, P.M.; Fey, S.; et al. Immune-mediated β-cell destruction in vitro and in vivo—A pivotal role for galectin-3. *Biochem. Biophys. Res. Commun.* **2006**, *344*, 406–415. [CrossRef]
132. Saksida, T.; Nikolic, I.; Vujicic, M.; Nilsson, U.J.; Leffler, H.; Lukic, M.L.; Stojanovic, I.; Stosic-Grujicic, S. Galectin-3 deficiency protects pancreatic islet cells from cytokine-triggered apoptosis in vitro. *J. Cell. Physiol.* **2013**, *228*, 1568–1576. [CrossRef] [PubMed]
133. Mensah-Brown, E.P.K.; Al Rabesi, Z.; Shahin, A.; Al Shamsi, M.; Arsenijevic, N.; Hsu, D.K.; Liu, F.T.; Lukic, M.L. Targeted disruption of the galectin-3 gene results in decreased susceptibility to multiple low dose streptozotocin-induced diabetes in mice. *Clin. Immunol.* **2009**, *130*, 83–88. [CrossRef] [PubMed]
134. Hudson, B.I.; Lippman, M.E. Targeting RAGE Signaling in Inflammatory Disease. *Annu. Rev. Med.* **2018**, *69*, 349–364. [CrossRef] [PubMed]
135. Dong, H.; Zhang, Y.; Huang, Y.; Deng, H. Pathophysiology of RAGE in inflammatory diseases. *Front. Immunol.* **2022**, *13*, 931473. [CrossRef] [PubMed]
136. Bongarzone, S.; Savickas, V.; Luzi, F.; Gee, A.D. Targeting the Receptor for Advanced Glycation Endproducts (RAGE): A Medicinal Chemistry Perspective. *J. Med. Chem.* **2017**, *60*, 7213–7232. [CrossRef]
137. Raucci, A.; Cugusi, S.; Antonelli, A.; Barabino, S.M.; Monti, L.; Bierhaus, A.; Reiss, K.; Saftig, P.; Bianchi, M.E. A soluble form of the receptor for advanced glycation endproducts (RAGE) is produced by proteolytic cleavage of the membrane-bound form by the sheddase a disintegrin and metalloprotease 10 (ADAM10). *FASEB J.* **2008**, *22*, 3716–3727. [CrossRef]
138. Ebert, H.; Lacruz, M.E.; Kluttig, A.; Simm, A.; Greiser, K.H.; Tiller, D.; Kartschmit, N.; Mikolajczyk, R. Advanced glycation end products and their ratio to soluble receptor are associated with limitations in physical functioning only in women: Results from the CARLA cohort. *BMC Geriatr.* **2019**, *19*, 299. [CrossRef]
139. Le Bagge, S.; Fotheringham, A.K.; Leung, S.S.; Forbes, J.M. Targeting the receptor for advanced glycation end products (RAGE) in type 1 diabetes. *Med. Res. Rev.* **2020**, *40*, 1200–1219. [CrossRef]
140. Salonen, K.M.; Ryhanen, S.J.; Forbes, J.M.; Harkonen, T.; Ilonen, J.; Simell, O.; Veijola, R.; Groop, P.H.; Knip, M. A drop in the circulating concentrations of soluble receptor for advanced glycation end products is associated with seroconversion to autoantibody positivity but not with subsequent progression to clinical disease in children en route to type 1 diabetes. *Diabetes Metab. Res. Rev.* **2017**, *33*, e2872. [CrossRef]
141. Salonen, K.M.; Ryhanen, S.J.; Forbes, J.M.; Harkonen, T.; Ilonen, J.; Laine, A.P.; Groop, P.H.; Knip, M.; Finnish Pediatric Diabetes, R. Circulating concentrations of soluble receptor for AGE are associated with age and AGER gene polymorphisms in children with newly diagnosed type 1 diabetes. *Diabetes Care* **2014**, *37*, 1975–1981. [CrossRef]
142. Salonen, K.M.; Ryhanen, S.J.; Forbes, J.M.; Borg, D.J.; Harkonen, T.; Ilonen, J.; Simell, O.; Veijola, R.; Groop, P.H.; Knip, M. Decrease in circulating concentrations of soluble receptors for advanced glycation end products at the time of seroconversion to autoantibody positivity in children with prediabetes. *Diabetes Care* **2015**, *38*, 665–670. [CrossRef]
143. Thomas, M.C.; Woodward, M.; Neal, B.; Li, Q.; Pickering, R.; Marre, M.; Williams, B.; Perkovic, V.; Cooper, M.E.; Zoungas, S.; et al. Relationship between levels of advanced glycation end products and their soluble receptor and adverse outcomes in adults with type 2 diabetes. *Diabetes Care* **2015**, *38*, 1891–1897. [CrossRef] [PubMed]
144. Moser, B.; Desai, D.D.; Downie, M.P.; Chen, Y.; Yan, S.F.; Herold, K.; Schmidt, A.M.; Clynes, R. Receptor for advanced glycation end products expression on T cells contributes to antigen-specific cellular expansion in vivo. *J. Immunol.* **2007**, *179*, 8051–8058. [CrossRef]
145. Leung, S.S.; Borg, D.J.; McCarthy, D.A.; Boursalian, T.E.; Cracraft, J.; Zhuang, A.; Fotheringham, A.K.; Flemming, N.; Watkins, T.; Miles, J.J.; et al. Soluble RAGE Prevents Type 1 Diabetes Expanding Functional Regulatory T Cells. *Diabetes* **2022**, *71*, 1994–2008. [CrossRef]
146. Chen, Y.; Akirav, E.M.; Chen, W.; Henegariu, O.; Moser, B.; Desai, D.; Shen, J.M.; Webster, J.C.; Andrews, R.C.; Mjalli, A.M.; et al. RAGE ligation affects T cell activation and controls T cell differentiation. *J. Immunol.* **2008**, *181*, 4272–4278. [CrossRef] [PubMed]
147. Han, X.Q.; Gong, Z.J.; Xu, S.Q.; Li, X.; Wang, L.K.; Wu, S.M.; Wu, J.H.; Yang, H.F. Advanced glycation end products promote differentiation of CD4$^+$ T helper cells toward pro-inflammatory response. *J. Huazhong Univ. Sci. Technol. Med. Sci.* **2014**, *34*, 10–17. [CrossRef] [PubMed]

148. Akirav, E.M.; Preston-Hurlburt, P.; Garyu, J.; Henegariu, O.; Clynes, R.; Schmidt, A.M.; Herold, K.C. RAGE expression in human T cells: A link between environmental factors and adaptive immune responses. *PLoS ONE* **2012**, *7*, e34698. [CrossRef] [PubMed]
149. Durning, S.P.; Preston-Hurlburt, P.; Clark, P.R.; Xu, D.; Herold, K.C.; Type 1 Diabetes TrialNet Study, G. The Receptor for Advanced Glycation Endproducts Drives T Cell Survival and Inflammation in Type 1 Diabetes Mellitus. *J. Immunol.* **2016**, *197*, 3076–3085. [CrossRef]
150. Zhang, J.; Chen, L.; Wang, F.; Zou, Y.; Li, J.; Luo, J.; Khan, F.; Sun, F.; Li, Y.; Liu, J.; et al. Extracellular HMGB1 exacerbates autoimmune progression and recurrence of type 1 diabetes by impairing regulatory T cell stability. *Diabetologia* **2020**, *63*, 987–1001. [CrossRef] [PubMed]
151. Han, J.; Zhong, J.; Wei, W.; Wang, Y.; Huang, Y.; Yang, P.; Purohit, S.; Dong, Z.; Wang, M.H.; She, J.X.; et al. Extracellular high-mobility group box 1 acts as an innate immune mediator to enhance autoimmune progression and diabetes onset in NOD mice. *Diabetes* **2008**, *57*, 2118–2127. [CrossRef]

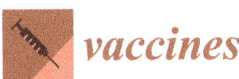

Review

Epigenetics in Tuberculosis: Immunomodulation of Host Immune Response

Avinash Khadela [1,†], Vivek P. Chavda [2,*,†], Humzah Postwala [3], Yesha Shah [3], Priya Mistry [3] and Vasso Apostolopoulos [4,5,*]

1. Department of Pharmacology, L. M. College of Pharmacy, Ahmedabad 380009, India
2. Department of Pharmaceutics and Pharmaceutical Technology, L. M. College of Pharmacy, Ahmedabad 380009, India
3. PharmD Section, L. M. College of Pharmacy, Ahmedabad 380009, India
4. Immunology and Translational Research Group, Institute for Health and Sport, Victoria University, Melbourne, VIC 3030, Australia
5. Immunology Program, Australian Institute for Musculoskeletal Science (AIMSS), Melbourne, VIC 3021, Australia
* Correspondence: vivek.chavda@lmcp.ac.in (V.P.C.); vasso.apostolopoulos@vu.edu.au (V.A.)
† These authors contributed equally to this work.

Abstract: Tuberculosis is a stern, difficult to treat chronic infection caused by acid-fast bacilli that tend to take a long time to be eradicated from the host's environment. It requires the action of both innate and adaptive immune systems by the host. There are various pattern recognition receptors present on immune cells, which recognize foreign pathogens or its product and trigger the immune response. The epigenetic modification plays a crucial role in triggering the susceptibility of the host towards the pathogen and activating the host's immune system against the invading pathogen. It alters the gene expression modifying the genetic material of the host's cell. Epigenetic modification such as histone acetylation, alteration in non-coding RNA, DNA methylation and alteration in miRNA has been studied for their influence on the pathophysiology of tuberculosis to control the spread of infection. Despite several studies being conducted, many gaps still exist. Herein, we discuss the immunopathophysiological mechanism of tuberculosis, the essentials of epigenetics and the recent encroachment of epigenetics in the field of tuberculosis and its influence on the outcome and pathophysiology of the infection.

Keywords: *Mycobacterium tuberculosis*; epigenetics; histone modification; DNA methylation; miRNAs

1. Introduction

Mycobacterium tuberculosis (Mtb) is a major worldwide concern for public health, being mainly a poverty-based disease that affects the most vulnerable in the population [1]. Approximately one third of the world's population are or have been infected by Mtb. Globally, infectious diseases still account for 25% of deaths, only surpassed by cardiovascular diseases [2]. The World Health Organization (WHO) reported that an estimated 8.6 million people contract Mtb annually, of which two thirds are males. The mortality of 1.3 million patients sees 320,000 cases related to concurrent HIV infection [3]. The current average annual incidence of smear positive Mtb stands at 84 per 100,000 cases annually in India [4]. There has been a decrease in the incidence of Mtb infections in the United States of America since 2010 by almost 2–3% [5]. Apart from this, Africa accounts for a quarter of newly diagnosed Mtb cases globally and for more than 25% of Mtb infection-related deaths. The main goal of pharmacological management of Mtb includes prevention of disease transmission and sterilization of the lesion [6]. The current treatment protocols for first line regimen remains with isoniazid, rifampicin, pyrazinamide and ethambutol, which are either used on their own or in combination [7]. As expected, Mtb bacilli have undergone several mutations, which are generally infrequent, although this leads to poorer responses when treated with single agents [8]. Thus, when a combination of drugs are used, it resolves the problem of resistance as well as enhances the efficacy of the drugs as they work via different mechanisms. For multidrug resistant infections, however, which do not respond to first line agents, a group of drugs defined as the second/third line agents are used which are more toxic, expensive and less efficacious when compared to first line agents [9]. Newer agents for the treatment of multi drug resistant Mtb infections include bedaquiline and delamanid [10]. Another approach to prevent the widespread infection of Mtb is the development of a vaccine derived from an attenuated strain of *M. bovis*, which has been in use since the 1930s [11]. The bacillus of Calmette and Guerin (BCG) vaccine acts by providing accelerated immune responses and thus reducing the spread of infection [12]. There are a number of issues that act as obstacles for the management of Mtb infections, for example, social stigma, marginalization, poor adherence to treatment due to prolonged duration [13,14]. In addition, immune impairment, for example, those with HIV infection, further increases risk of infection and concurrent infections.

Several newer strategies are currently under development to overcome the problems with the current standard of care. Interferon (IFN)α [15], IFNγ [16], imiquimod [17], interleukin (IL)-12 [18], granulocyte-monocyte colony stimulating factor (GM-CSF) [19], levamisole [20] are some agents that are under consideration as anti-Mtb treatments. Along with this, a vaccine derived from *M. vaccae*, which is a rapidly growing saprophytic mycobacterium, is also being evaluated as a novel approach against Mtb infections but has shown variable results thus far [21]. In an attempt to prevent the problem of treatment adherence, which has been one of the major reasons of relapse and development of resistance, the WHO has recommended a method of supervision known as 'directly observed treatment short course' since the 1990s, which has shown improved outcomes in terms of adherence to treatment and efficacy [22–24].

In recent times, personalised therapy (also called host directed therapy) for conditions such as Mtb are being developed. In order to develop the personalised host directed therapy, the understanding of epigenetic processes can play a distinguishing role [25]. Some recent studies have reported epigenetic changes such as histone modification, DNA methylation and miRNA mediated regulation brought through Mtb pathogen interaction with the host's cells. The role of various cytokines such as IFN-γ, IL-12 and TNF-α to induce acetylation and methylation on histone proteins can be explored to develop novel therapeutic strategies. The field of targeting epigenetic modifications known as epi-therapeutics is new and requires lot of work in order to develop successful therapy [26]. Herein, we present the immunopathophysiology of Mtb infection and the epigenetic modification brought by Mtb pathogen and recent in vitro and in vivo experiments, which can be explored further to develop successful therapies using epigenetics.

2. Immuno-Pathophysiology of *Mycobacterium tuberculosis*

Mycobacterium tuberculosis pathogen is predominantly present in the environment in the form of aerosol and it gains access into the body via the lungs through inhalation [27]. Its presentation to the host body depends on the virulence of the pathogen and the host's immune system [26]. This can be explained by its immune pathophysiological mechanism including both arms of the immune system, the innate and adaptive immune response. If the Mtb pathogen manages to invade the physical barrier, then it is presented to the innate immune system of the host. As such, invasion of Mtb leads to substantial changes in the host immune cells and activates the innate immune response as the first line of defense [28]. Various immune cells are involved as the response to infection; however, in the case of Mtb infection, the first cells to encounter the pathogen are macrophages [29]. Pathogens that enter the body express pathogen-associated molecular patterns, which have conserved motifs that serve as ligands for host pattern recognition receptors (PRR) including toll-like receptors (TLRs) and, in turn, gives rise to danger-associated molecular patterns. As such, these molecular patterns aid the immune system to elicit an innate immune response against the invading Mtb pathogen [30]. In addition, the pathogen has several ligands on its surface including mannose, lectin, surface protein A, cluster of differentiation (CD)14, which are recognized by PRRs [25]. The PRRs can be cataloged mainly into TLRs, c-type lectin receptors, nod-like receptors, retinoic acid inducible (RIG)-I like receptors, complement receptors (1, 3, 4), mannose receptor, scavenger receptor, CD14 and CD43 [31]. Of all the PRRs, TLR-1, -2, -4, -9, play an important role in the pathogenesis of the Mtb. TLR-1, -2, -4 are presented on both immune cells and non-immune cells whereas TLR-9 is presented only on immune cells. Furthermore, the inflammasome pathway is instigated by PRRs, which play an important role in innate immune mechanisms via the regulation of caspase-1 in response to pathogen associated molecular patterns and danger associated molecular patterns recognition by host cells [32]. Mtb also aggressively stirs up the assembly of pentraxin-3 (PTX-3), a 42 KDa soluble PRR involved in acute immune responses towards infection [33]. In adaptive immune responses, B and T cells (CD4+, CD8+, regulatory T (Treg)), NK cells, macrophages and dendritic cells are involved in Mtb infections. The recruitment of NK-cells, granulocytes and activated macrophages (via lysosomes and ROS) is important for killing the pathogen, and leads to the hallmark characteristic of Mtb formation of the granuloma [34,35]. In addition, Mtb primed immune cells secrete pro-inflammatory cytokines, IL-1, IL-6, IL-12, IL-18, IFNγ, and TNFα.

The excessive stimulation by IFNγ over time leads to the conversion of activated macrophages to epithelioid macrophages (long elongated nucleated cells). They surround the infection in the lungs and form the granuloma. Within the granuloma there are high levels of TNFα, which limit the infection [36], as well as central caseating necrosis, which is surrounded by epithelial macrophages, lymphocytes and fibroblasts (produce collagen around caseating necrosis). Further, the level of 1-alpha hydroxylase is upregulated at the site of granuloma, which leads to its calcification [35,37]. If Mtb remains within the granuloma, the infection is termed latent Mtb infection. When host immunity is compromised, it leads to the reactivation of Mtb, known as secondary tuberculosis [38]. This is mediated by type-4 delayed hypersensitivity reaction. Moreover, Tregs are present that suppress the mycobactericidal activity of immune cells with the help of IL-10, IL-35, TGFβ. Thus, the interaction between the Mtb pathogen and the host's immune cells contributes to the immune-pathogenesis of Mtb [26,39]. In addition, Mtb bacillus specifically exploits the moonlighting functions of PE proteins by utilizing immune signalling pathway, which subsequently helps in growth as proliferation of the pathogen inside the host. These PE6 proteins, by binding to the iron inside the cell, help progression of the disease via pathogenic proliferation and intracellular pathogenic survival. Vitamin D also plays a role in the pathogenesis of Mtb infections, as it leads to the formation of cathelicidins and defensins, which contribute to the destruction of the pathogen [40].

3. Tuberculosis and Epigenetic Regulations and Modifications

The epigenetic concepts were developed in the 1940s by CH Waddington, as a process influencing genetic outcomes without changing cell sequencing [41]. Epigenetic regulations include any alteration in gene expression due to chromosomal modifications without actually modifying the sequencing of nucleotides in the coding DNA [42]. The Mtb pathogen takes over and reprograms the host epigenome via histone modifications, DNA methylation and miRNA mediated regulation of genes as a self-protective mechanism [43,44]. These modifications play an important role in Mtb-induced host immunomodulation [26]. The tubercular bacilli induces various perturbations in the epigenetic regulations, specifically in those mediated by DNA methylation [45]. Using multiple cohorts, tissue types and transcriptomic analysis showed that epigenetic changes associated with Mtb induces oxidative stress. This leads to premature cellular ageing and induces senescence [45]. These induced changes by the bacteria are reversible and, as such, can be easily an effective target for therapeutics. IFNγ induces expression of HLA-DR α/β mRNA, which is inhibited by the Mtb-bacilli along with partial inhibition of CIITA expression in the Mtb infected macrophages without having any effect on the expression of IFN regulatory factor-

1 mRNA [46]. Epigenetic mechanisms regulate the transcriptional profile of immune system related genes contributing to the interaction between the host and the infectious agent [47]. More recently, it was reported that the sensitive Mtb strains lead to sufficient immune activation in the host to clear the infection but the resistant Mtb strains cause sub-optimal immune induction by enabling better intracellular survival of bacilli by over-expressing genes, inducing host lipid metabolism [48].

The immune cells which are predominantly involved in these modifications induced by Mtb pathogen include T cells and macrophages. Both T effector and T helper cells play important roles in the epigenetic pathology of Mtb. CD4 promotor is responsible for epigenetic repression of matured CD8+ T cells. In addition, Tregs are capable of inducing histone modifications as well as DNA methylation on various transcription factors including FOXP3. MHC II expression and subsequent CIITA role are highly influenced by epigenetic changes such as DNA methylation. Macrophages also play an important role in the pathogenesis of Mtb. These are sensitive to histone methylation-based epigenetic changes in the host cells.

3.1. Histone Modifications

Histone proteins widely known as chromatin remodeling proteins that are responsible for formation of the nucleosome octamer around the DNA after around 1.7 turns. These histone proteins are responsible for normal structural integrity of chromatin. Eight different classes of post-translational histone modifications with 60 sites for modifications are present [49]. These include proline isomerization, arginine deamination, lysine/arginine methylation, serine, glutamate poly-ADP ribosylation, threonine/tyrosine, ubiquitination, sumolylation and lysine acetylation [50]. All these modifications are covalent in nature and are guided by various enzymes such as kinases, phosphatase, histone deacetylase (HDAC), histone acetyl transferase (HAT), histone methyltransferases (HMTs) and histone demethylase (HDMs) [51].

3.1.1. Histone Methylation

Methylation occurs on lysine or arginine residues of the histones, and leads to activation or suppression of the genes, respectively. Methylation can take place in mono, di- or trimeric forms each having different consequences. Around 90% of methylation takes place at the cytosines of CpG sites in human somatic cells [52]. Methylation at CpG, due to which gene expression is silenced as a result of prevention of association of transcription or DNA binding factors to their respective binding sites by recruiting co-repressors in order to methylate CpG nucleotides, leads to chromatin modification into its repressor forms [53]. Rv1988 is a mycobacterial histone methyltransferase secretary protein which demethylates the amino acid arginine specifically at 42nd position in the histone H3, which has a profound effect on host gene transcription due to its capacity to localize with the chromatin in the host nucleus. This Rv1988 is known to repress gene expression by methylating histone H3 at R42 [54]. A similar finding has also been available for other mycobacterial proteins such as Rv2966c. This type of proteins loosens the host defense by decreasing the effect of genes with protective activity, thus acting as first line of attack during infection [51]. Another report showed the induction of H4K20me1 and its regulation of apoptosis and subsequent inflammation in assisting Mtb survival induced by histone methyl transferase SET8 [55]. The result of these methylation modifications depending on their nature, suppress gene expression, alter host histones via controlling of the cell signaling, etc. For instance, the downregulation of KDM6B gene induced by Mtb pathogen leads to hypermethylation of the host histone protein H3K27.

3.1.2. Histone Acetylation

Addition of an acetyl group to the lysine site leads to modifications in DNA expression. Any molecule that can mediate the addition of this acetyl group on the host proteins are termed as HATs. In this context, the Mtb antigenic proteins acts as HATs and induces acetylation changes not just on histones but also on non-histone proteins. NF-κB p65 is an example of non-histone acetylation modification. The inflammatory response against the Mtb is mediated by various host enzymes such as matrix metalloproteinase (MMP), a zinc-dependent endopeptidase that plays a crucial role in the development of cavitation. On acetylation of these MMP proteins, there is intracellular survival of Mtb bacilli in the host tissue. They are secreted by Mtb-infected monocytes and macrophages along with non-infected stromal cells. The epigenetic mechanisms act as important regulators of MMP activity in various non-infectious as well as infectious diseases including Mtb [56,57]. The implications of epigenetics in induction of MMP- 1/3, especially by histone acetylation associated with transcriptional activation, is investigated and demonstrated in a study. The class 1 HDAC expression is also suppressed by Mtb infection in macrophages [58]. HDACs are known to be negative regulators for the expression of genes [59]. Thus, MMP upregulation in Mtb infection leads to lung tissue damage and the HDAC and HATs activity is required for induction in expression of MMPs. This MMP-induced tissue breakdown is the most important contributor in immune pathophysiology as well as host epigenetic changes [58]. The observed changes in gene transcription during development are due to histone modifications such as methylation in the arginine residues of histone H3 [60].

Several HDACs, such as HDAC1, HDAC2, HDAC3 and sirtuins, catalyze histone deacetylation out of which HDAC3 predominantly causes deacetylation during Mtb infection [61]. The suppression of IL12B expression by Mtb via HDAC1 is also shown [62]. Host gene expression is suppressed by HDAC-induced deacetylation, whereas HAT-induced histone tail acetylation leads to chromatin activation by increasing spacings between the nucleosomes [63]. Other proteins, such as ESAT-6 and LpqH, inhibit MHC-II expression and antigen presentation by inducing histone modifications [64]. Mtb infections also inhibit various IFN-induced genes such as HLA-DR, CD64, CIITA trans-activator irrespective of normal JAK-STAT1 signaling cascade activation [65]. Similarly, another mycobacterial protein Rv3763 is responsible for histone hypoacetylation at CIITA promoter via suppressing INF-γ induced genes. The interaction of Rv2966c with the macrophage epigenome affects the non-CpG methylation at specific loci and is also known [66]. Thus, epigenetic modifications on histones requires proper homeostasis as it has a pivotal role for proper gene expression regulation. The mechanism of the consequences of Mtb-induced histone modifications are summarized in Figure 1.

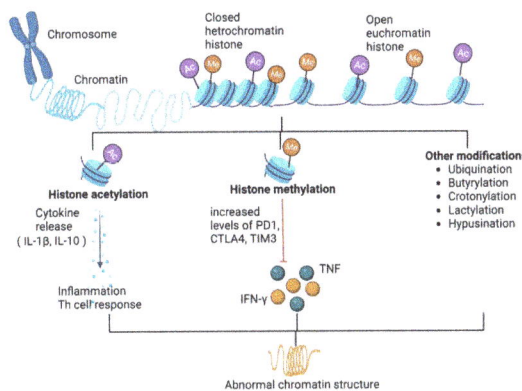

Figure 1. Consequences of *Mycobacterium tuberculosis* induced methylation, acetylation and other histone modifications in the host's immunity. Abbreviations: Ac: acetylation, Me: methylation, IL-1β: interleukin 1-beta, PD1: programmed cell death-1, CTLA4: cytotoxic T-lymphocyte–associated antigen 4, IFN-γ: interferon gamma, TIM3: T-cell immunoglobulin and mucin domain 3, TNF: tumor necrosis factor.

3.2. Alteration in Expression of Non-Coding RNAs

The proteins produced as a result of translational processes are dependent on the code sequences present on the RNA templates. However, after the sequencing of the entire mammalian genome and transcriptome was published, it was noted that some of the sequences of the RNA were not reflected in the coded proteins [67]. Thus, these were categorized as non-coding RNAs (nc-RNAs), also known as micro RNAs (miRNAs) [68]. miRNAs basically play a role in regulation of bacterial infections; thus, its dysregulation leads to various infectious diseases as well as immune disorders [69]. These nc-RNAs, approximately 22 nucleotides in length, have a considerable regulatory role in certain cellular mechanisms such as DNA methylation as well as histone modifications and other, around one-third of mammalian genes [70]. These miRNAs are basically endogenously acting gene silencers that repress gene expression at a translational level by targeting mRNA [71]. Important cellular pathways such as cell proliferation, angiogenesis, invasion is regulated by these miRNAs along with other complex epigenetic mechanisms such as dynamics of chromatin structures and genome organization in nucleus [72]. All these regulation of gene processes are a result of a combination of mature miRNAs and RNA-induced silencing complex [73]. miRNAs are also involved in regulation of the immune response against Mtb of dendritic cells (DCs). The role of miRNAs in patients with Mtb infections and TB patients was proved by a study showing overexpression of more than 59 miRNAs in TB patients' serum compared to healthy controls [74]. Moreover, after being infected by Mtb, host macrophages induce a particular modulation of miRNA [75]. During Mtb infection, miRNA mediates various signaling pathways as well as apoptosis and autophagy. For instance, miR-1178 and miR-708-5p when overexpressed, it negatively regulates TLR-4, resulting in inhibition of expression of proinflammatory mediators such as IFN-γ, IL-6, IL-1β and TNF-α [76,77]. miR-125a upregulation leads to negative regulation of NF-κB pathway via TRAF6, ultimately leading to blockage of proinflammatory cytokines [78]. miR-27b is triggered by the Mtb-induced TLR2/MyD88/NF-κB pathways, which further inhibits NF-κB and proinflammatory gene activity while increasing p53, thus positively regulating cellular apoptosis [79]. miR-381-3p mediates reduced CD1c expression and subsequent reduction of T-cell immune response in Mtb infected DCs [80]. Moreover, miR-99b is highly expressed in Mtb-infected DCs, which upregulate the expression of inflammatory mediators such as IL-6, 12 and 1β, as well as TNF-α, thus activating DCs to clear the phagocytic Mtb [81]. Other than these, miR-let-7f, miR-132, miR-26a, miR-20b, miR-155, miR-21, miR-146a are also important in regulation of cellular pathways, as briefly summarized in Figure 2. There are many host ncRNAs that are not yet discovered with unknown functions and regulatory networks due to their complexity, which still needs to be studied further [82].

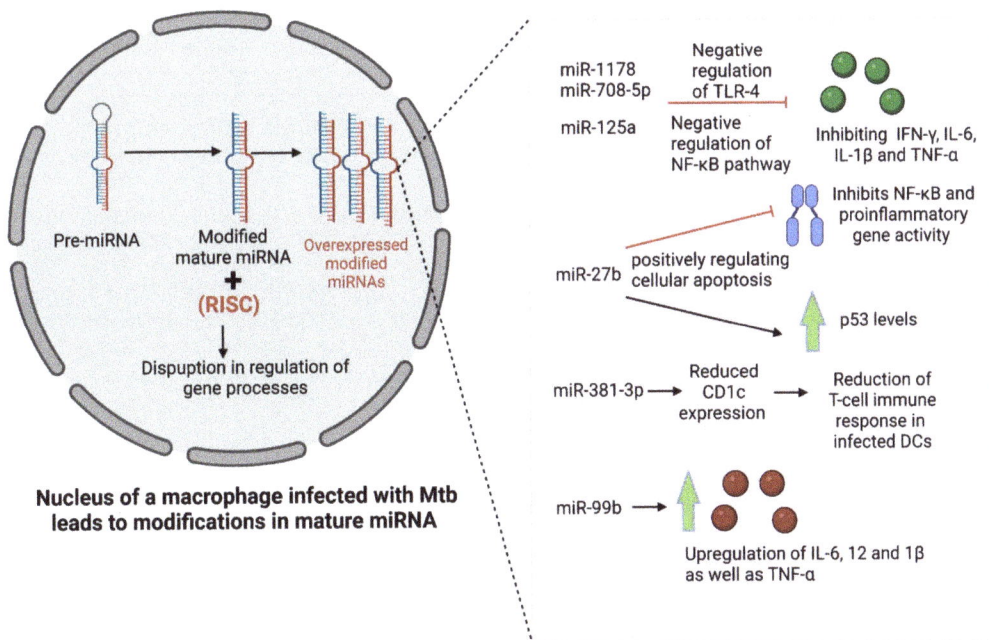

Figure 2. Mechanism of induction of changes due to Mtb infection-induced modifications in the miRNA. Abbreviations: miRNA: micro-RNAs, RISC: RNA-induced silencing complex, Mtb: mycobacteriaum TB, TLR: toll-like receptors, NF-KB: nuclear factor kappa B, IFN-γ: interferon gamma, IL: interleukin, CD1c: cluster of differentiation, DC: dendritic cells, TNF: tumor necrosis factor.

3.3. Alterations in DNA Methylation

DNA methylation takes place when Mtb induces the transfer of a methyl group from cytosine base (carbon 5 position) mediated by DNA methyltransferase enzymes to form 5-methylcytosine [83]. It also plays an important role in different cellular processes such as differentiation, development, reprogramming, as well as gene silencing that leads to induction of diseases including TB [84]. It was shown in a study that the methylation Mtb immunity-related genes are upregulated, which leads to suppression of immune response against Mtb, which indicated DNA methylation to be an important epigenetic target [85]. It was demonstrated that MamA, an adenine methyltransferase, is encoded by Rv3263 and responsible for all detectable methylation modification by a particular Mtb strain, H37Rv. The effects of these mycobacterial Rv proteins are summarized in Table 1

Table 1. Protein and their effects on respective epigenetic changes.

Protein	Epigenetic Target	Effect
Rv3423.1	Histone acetyl transferase	It leads to increase in no. of bacteria in host intracellular environment and their survival [86].
Rv2966c	DNA methylation (non CpG context)	It showed the ability to localize the host's cell nucleus and repression of specific genes [66].
Rv1988	Histone methyltransferase	It demethylates the amino acid arginine specifically at 42nd position in the histone H3, which has a profound effect on host gene transcription due to its capacity to localize with the chromatin in the host nucleus [54].
Rv3763	Histone acetyl transferase	It is responsible for histone hypoacetylation at CIITA promoter via suppressing IFN-γ induced genes [66].
Rv3263	DNA methylation	It is responsible for all detectable methylation modification by a particular Mtb strain, H37Rv [87].

Abbreviations: CIITA, Class II trans activator; IFN, interferon; Mtb, mycobacterium tuberculosis; Th1, helper T cells.

The contribution of methylation-mediated regulatory pathways in showing lineage specific characteristics seen in different strains of Mtb is proven [87]. Thus, the interference of Mtb with host epigenome as an aid to survival is very well known. A study report identifies over differentially methylated regions (DMRs) in Mtb infected macrophages. This proves the use of non-canonical strategies by Mtb bacilli to establish infection [88]. It was indicated in a study by genetic ontology analysis; the contribution to many immune-biological functions such as immune cell activation and regulation as well as cellular response to IFN-γ and cytotoxicity by DMR-associated genes [89]. This epigenetic modification is quite stable compared to the histone modification' thus, it is quite less reversible process leading to silencing of the gene expression for a much longer time. DNA methylation shows dynamic effects on the Mtb infected DCs. Significant changes in the DMRs majorly at low CpG density regions as well as in distal regulatory or enhancer regions after Mtb infection in DCs compared to uninfected cells [90]. Around 40% of miRNAs were differently expressed in Mtb-infected DCs [91]. Mtb-infected macrophages lead to significant methylation level alterations in inflammatory related genes showing quite a larger increase in the promoter region of IL-17 compared to other receptors in infected macrophages, as shown in Figure 3. Moreover, these methylation pattern changes depend on the type of Mtb strain as well as host genotype [92]. Early secreted antigen 6 (ESAT6) has a significant role in reducing IFN-γ induced methylation of histone H3K4 and acetylation of CIITA p1 locus histone. Furthermore, inhibition of type IV CIITA expression was found to be TLR-2-dependent; on the other hand, type I CIITA expression inhibition was TLR-2-independent, both mediated by ESAT6 [93]. Methylation was increased in Mtb-infected monocytes, which presented a reduced anti-inflammatory cytokine IL-10 secretion and an increased proinflammatory cytokine IL-12 secretion, which indicates impaired monocyte ability in regulating excess inflammation, which leads to lung injury [94]. Enhanced intracellular survival (Eis) protein secreted by Mtb leads to increased survival of infected macrophages by acetylation of histone proteins [95]. Thus, the susceptibility of the Mtb bacilli depends on the methylation status that varies in different ethnic groups [96].

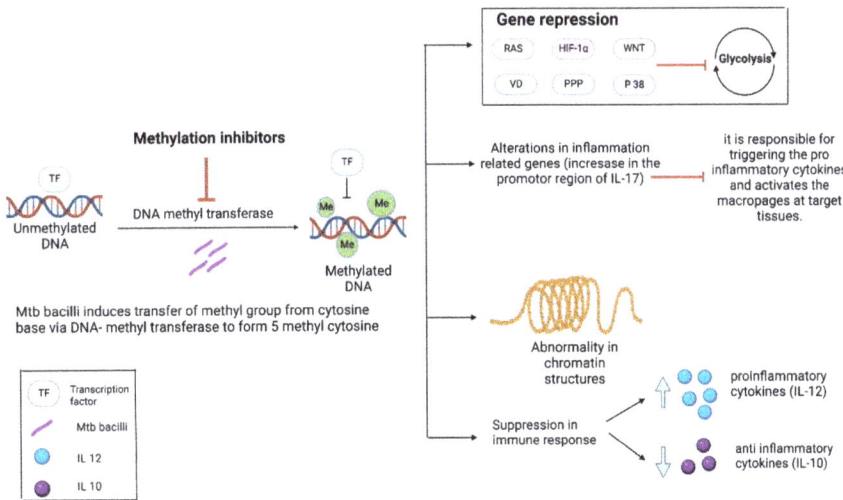

Figure 3. Induction of DNA-methylation by Mtb and its subsequent effect on the host immunity. Abbreviations: TF: Transcription factor, DNA: Deoxy ribonucleic acid, Me: Methylation, IL: Interleukin, RAS: Rat sarcoma virus, HIF: Hypoxia inducible factor, WNT: Wingless-related integration site, VD: Vitamin D, PPP: Pentose phosphate pathway.

4. Therapies Targeting Epigenetic Modifications for *Mycobacterium tuberculosis*

Targeting epigenetics works on the concept of targeting the host instead of the Mtb bacilli directly, also known as HDT (Table 2) [97].

Table 2. Targets affected by epigenetic modifications and therapeutic agents targeting those modifications.

Epigenetic Modifications	Targets Involved	Therapeutic Agents
Histone modifications	MMP IL-12b, IL-1β CIITA, HLA-DR, CD64 NF-κB JAK-STAT pathways	Nonspecific HDAC inhibitors: SAHA (vorinostat) Trichostatin A (TSA) Phenylbutyrate (PBA) HDAC6 specific: Tubustatin A MC2780 HDAC3 specific: RGFP966 Bromodomain inhibitors HAT inhibitor: Anacardiac acid
Alterations in expression of non-coding RNA	DCs TLR4 NF-κB CD1c	Antisense mRNA targeting agents: Phosphorothioate-modified antisense oligodeoxyribonucleotides (PS-ODNs) Phosphoryl guanidine oligo-2′-O-methylribonucleotides (2′-OMe PGOs) Phosphorothioate antisense oligonucleotides (PAOs)
Alteration in DNA methylation	IFN-γ Monocyte derived-DCs TLR2 IL-17, IL-12, IL-10	Methylation inhibitors: 5-Azacytidine Zebularine

Abbreviations: CIITA, Class II trans activator; CD, cluster of differentiation; DC, dendritic cells; HAT, histone acetyltransferases; HDAC, histone deacetylases; HLA, human leukocyte antigen; IFN, interferon; IL, interleukin; JAK-STAT, Janus kinase-signal transducer and activator of transcription; MMP, matrix metalloproteinase; NF-κB, nuclear factor kappa B; SAHA, suberoylandilide hydroxamic acid; TLR, toll-like receptors.

It has been reported that broad chemical inhibition of HDAC enhances anti-microbial response against Mtb by differentiating macrophages into a comparatively stronger bactericidal phenotype along with decreased secretion of inflammatory cytokines. A highly accepted in vivo model for inhibition of HDAC in M-marium-infected zebrafish embryos significantly reduces the mycobacterial burden, whereas selective class IIa inhibition leads to a prominent decrease in bacterial outgrowth [98]. HDAC inhibitors such as suberoylandilide hydroxamic acid (SAHA), marketed as vorinostat and trichostatin A (TSA), are looked forward to as they provide quite improved bacterial clearance by modulating the epigenetic modifications induced by Mtb. These show mixed effects as, along with resolving inflammation, they also impair microbicidal activities of macrophages by impairing its functions [99]. This is achieved by reducing the levels of reactive oxygen species (ROS) as well as nitric oxide (NO) in the exposed macrophages [100]. Another nonspecific HDAC inhibitor phenylbutyrate when used in combination with vitamin D acts as a dual targeted therapy against the host as well as the pathogen [97]. SAHA is also known to increase IL-1β levels and decrease IL-10 levels in host alveolar macrophages and monocyte-derived macrophages along with enhanced exhibition of IFN-γ and GM-CSF coproduction [101]. These older broad spectrum HDAC inhibitors have a quite wider site of action and targets several different HDACs. By contrast, another specific HDAC-6 inhibitor tubustatin was studied in mice and has been associated with improved resolution of bacteraemia, less organ dysfunction as well as modulated stress response by increasing monocyte and neutrophil counts and reversing lymphopenia [102,103]. It has more specific actions and has greater selectivity. As opposed to broad spectrum HDAC inhibitor, tubustatin enhances the macrophage generation of mitochondrial ROS, as a TLR-generated microbicidal response leading to increased intracellular microbial clearance [104,105]. Silencing as well as chemical inhibition of HDAC by these specific inhibitors induces expression of an orphan nuclear receptor, transcription factor Nur77. It is known to promote anti-inflammatory functions in macrophages by rewiring the tricarboxylic acid (TCA) cycle [106]. Deficiency of Nur77 is associated with increased functional occurrence of proinflammatory phenotype of macrophages, which leads to increased IL-6, 12 and IFN-γ production. Mtb modulates cytokine secretion to invade host defence. Thus, targeting HDACs by counteracting its transcriptional regulation can be quite useful therapeutically [107–109]. Along with the epigenetic modulations of HDAC inhibitors, various alternative functions of these agents also contribute to its bactericidal activity [110]. Enhanced anti-Mtb activity of macrophages is dependent on HDAC-6. Its expression is specifically maintained in monocyte-derived macrophages more importantly in patients with resistant Mtb infection. HDAC-6 is also required for maintaining acidic environment in Mtb containing phagosomes in infected macrophages. Thus, it acts as an important novel target for HDT against Mtb [111]. Tubustatin A and HDAC-6 inhibitor (MC2780) significantly inhibit Mtb growth by upregulation of TNFα, IL-12 and IFNγ as well as downregulation of IL-10 [112]. It recruits a greater number of macrophages, DCs and neutrophils, thus inducing delayed innate immune response. RGFP966 is an HDAC3 inhibitor that was also found to modulate pro-inflammatory macrophage secretion by Mtb infected macrophages by decreasing IL-6 and TNF secretion [113]. It induces NOS2, CASP1 as well as the M1 marker CD86. Along with vitamin D3, it leads to two fold induction in cAMP by inhibition of epigenetic mechanism of acetylation during Mtb infection, proving to be an important HDT in TB [97]. SIRT or sirtuins are NAD+ dependent HDACs, which are usually known for their implications on the pathologies of age-related disorders. Owing to the fact that these sirtuins share their targets with HDACs, their inhibitors can be explored for anti-inflammatory properties.The SIRT-1/2 specific inhibitor cambinol was shown to protect against endotoxic and toxic shock via inhibition via the production of pro-inflammatory cytokines in vitro. Thus, SIRT-1/2 might prove to have significant therapeutic potential in Mtb infection [114].

Anacardiac acid is an HAT inhibitor drug which produces isonicotinoylhydrazones on coupling with anti-TB drug isoniazid. These isonicotinoylhydrazones have shown potent inhibitory activity against Mtb [115]. Bromodomains are conserved structural motifs which are associated with chromatin modifying proteins such as HATs [116]. During infection or inflammation, bromodomain inhibitors provide specific targeting along with individual histone post translational modifications. These bromodomain and extra terminal domain family of proteins (BET) link histone acetylation status to the transcription. These drugs are predicted to downregulate systemic inflammation during severe infections by acting at CpG low promotors and allowing modulation of some most potent lipopolysaccharide (LPS) responses, leading to subsequent induction of IL-6, 12 and NO [117]. JQ1-BET (Bromodomain and Extra-Terminal domain), a specific inhibitor of bromodomain, suggests a possible targeted approach with these agents. Another systemic histone, I-BET, reduces the induction of various inflammatory cytokines such as IL-6, 1b, IFNβ following LPS stimulation via TLR4 and TNF-α by activated murine macrophages [118,119].

Glutamate synthase is an enzyme associated with the pathogenicity of Mtb by forming a poly-L glutamate cell wall structure. Thus, phosphorothioate-modified antisense oligodeoxyribonucleotides acting against the mRNA of this enzyme had been shown to reduce the amount of cell wall L-glutamate by 24% and 1.25 log reduction in Mtb growth [120]. A combination of three PS-ODNs, which are 5'-, 3'-hairpin-modified targeting mycolyl transferase transcripts, was each tested in Mtb and shown to reduce the transcription of target gene by 90% and also lead to an 8-fold increase in Mtb sensitivity to isoniazid [121]. Phosphoryl guanidine oligo-2'-O-methylribonucleotides (2'-OMe PGOs) is a novel antisense mRNA targeting molecule that has shown high biological activity by effective intracellular uptake as well as inhibition of target *ald* gene in the infected macrophages [122]. Another thiocationic lipid-based formulation of phosphorothioate antisense oligonucleotides (PAOs) has also shown in vitro efficacy against Mtb [123].

DNA-methylation inhibitor drugs are another class of compounds which target host epigenetics such as 5-azacytidine, which is a cytidine analogue with a nitrogen atom instead of C5 [124]. It is phosphorylated and gets incorporated into the DNA during the process of replication. The process of methylation is widely reduced as a result of irreversible DNMT1-aza linkage, which triggers enzyme degradation [125]. A phase Ib/IIa open label, non-randomized clinical trial (NCT03941496) is being conducted by Andrew DiNardo et al. by using injectable azacytidine in pulmonary TB. A total of 50 participants will be recruited and will be given SQ azacytidine for 25 days in a dose escalation fashion starting from 5 mg/m^2 up to a maximum of 75 mg/m^2 5 days for each dose. Overall incidence and severity of all adverse events as well as measurement of epigenetic mediated immune exhaustion were defined as primary outcomes of the study. The results of this ongoing trial are still in process. Zebularine, another methylation inhibitor drug, shows similar mechanism as azacytidine, where its diphosphate form reactivates the silenced genes after incorporating into the DNA leading to subsequent inhibition of DNA methylation. However, its effectiveness is yet to be proved in TB [126].

CRISPR-associated protein 9 (Cas9), when fused with an acetyltransferase, catalyses the target site acetylation of H3K27, which leads to transcriptional activation of target genes [127]. Apart from this, the CRISPR-Cas9 system, when fused with LSD-1, a histone demethylase, targets various regions of DNA that enhances the expression of a range of genes [128]. This technology has recently been studied, which may prove to be of great importance therapeutically. In this context, Cas9 epigenetic effectors could be used therapeutically as it would be capable to artificially install or remove various epigenetic changes and track the causal effects of the induced epigenetic modifications [129]. Various different drug molecules used in vivo and in vitro are currently being studied to determine whether any modulate the epigenome (Table 3).

Table 3. Summary of drugs affecting epigenetics in various in vivo and in vitro models of tuberculosis.

Target of the Therapy	Therapeutic Agent	Nature of STUDY	Results
HDAC non-specific inhibitors	Vorinostat Valproic acid	In vitro (H37Rv cultures)	Vorinostat and Valproic acid showed 1.5 and 2 log reduction in CFU, respectively. Both improved the efficacy of rifampicin against Mtb [130].
	Trichostatin A	In vivo (*M. marinum* infected zebrafish)	32% reduction of bacterial burden in pre-treated model [98].
	Phenylbutyrate with Vitamin D	In vivo (Humans)	Decline in concentrations of cytokines such as TNFα, CCL11/5, PDGF-β Increase in LC3 expression [131]
	Phenylbutyrate with Vitamin D	In vivo (Humans- RCT)	28.8% increase in rate of patients' culture conversion compared to placebo [132].
HDAC 6 inhibitors	Tubastatin A	In vivo (C57BL/6 mice model infected with Mtb)	6 log reduction in CFU after 14 days Upregulation of TNFα, IL-12, IFNγ and downregulation of IL-10 [112].
	Tubastatin A	In vitro (THP-1 cell line)	Inhibition of TNFα and IL-6 in the cell line [105].
Bromodomain inhibitor	CBP30	In vitro (heparinized human blood)	No effect on expression of TNFα [133].
HAT inhibitors	Isonicotinoylhydrazones derived from anacardic acid	In vitro (*M. smegmatis* mc2155 cells)	MIC of 4 µg/mL Synergistic actions with isoniazid [115].
DNA methylation inhibitors	Azacytidine	In vivo (Humans)	The trial is still ongoing (NCT03941496)

Abbreviations: CCL-11; C-C motif chemokine-11, CFU; colony forming units, DNA; Deoxyribose nucleic acid, HAT; Histone acetyl transferase, HDAC; Histone deacetylase, IFN-γ; interferon-γ, IL-12; interleukin-12, LC-3; microtubule associated protein light chain-3, MIC; minimum inhibitory concentration, Mtb; mycobacterium tuberculosis, PDGF-β; platelet derived growth factor-β, RCT; randomized control trial, TNF-α; tumour necrosis factor-α.

5. Way Forward

Epigenetic alterations such as histone modifications, alteration in expression of non-coding RNAs, alteration in DNA methylation and miRNA all are interlinked, which determine the disease outcome and pathology, collectively termed as epigenetic processes. The epigenetic changes induced in Mtb are reversible and can be easily rectified with the use of drug modulating epigenetic processes. Some recent successes have been obtained in the use of "epi-drugs" for epigenetic treatment in various cancers [134]. Although epigenetics has a key place in disease outcome and pathology, less research has been conducted as compared to the genomic studies.

The collective knowledge of epigenetic, genomic, proteomic and transcriptomic is required for Mtb-primed immune cells in order to expose the susceptibility of the Mtb pathogen and to target the novel mechanistic pathways and interaction in order to protect the host against the infection. Moreover, the relationships between enzymes such as MMP responsible for cavitation and epigenetic processes such as histone acetylation can be further explored. A recent study considered the effect of a classical anti-Mtb drug isoniazid on epigenetics via post-translational modifications such as iso-nicotinylation at histone sites by increasing the levels of isonicotinyl-CoA. These modifications carried out by isoniazid can lead to malignancies. Thus, through more epigenetic studies, many more mechanisms of such iatrogenic reactions to anti-TB drugs can be explained [135]. The Mtb pathogen also utilizes various epigenetic processes to proliferate in host, which can be targeted effectively as a therapeutic option.

HAT and HDAC are being studied for developing improved regimen and therapeutic alternatives for resistant Mtb cases. In one study, it was noted that over-expression in over 59 miRNAs was responsible for regulating TLR-4 and various pro-inflammatory cytokines. Around 90% of alteration in DNA methylation occurs at cytosine of CpG sites. Moreover, over 23,000 DMRs and also GO analysis had proven the role of non-canonical pathway and the effects of immune cells such as macrophages and DCs in disease induction, respectively, as we know that Mtb and its related products can modulate the epigenetic processes to establish the infection. As mentioned above, the mechanism of PE6 proteins in Mtb can be explored more in order to develop novel HDT strategies for Mtb [136]. Different methods such as pyrosequencing, whole genome bisulfite sequencing, expression of miRNA, chromatin immunoprecipitation and PCR can be studied further and understand of the epigenetic processes in Mtb pathogen. These studies on host epigenetics also explain the immunosuppressive states and their interaction with the Mtb pathogen and how innate and adaptive immunity works, which can help in development of next generation vaccines and various therapeutic regimens. Moreover, the blood analysis for the epigenetically modified products can provide an important tool for the diagnosis of the infection and can serve as a putative biomarker. The mechanisms of hypomethylating agents such as Azacytidine can be targeted on the methylation for Mtb, which leads to specific gene silencing [85]. However, the major issue with targeting epigenetics with agents such as azacytidine is their toxicity. Aza- or sulphur-containing drugs have an established toxicity profile and are known to be intolerable by a large population. Targeting other epigenetic modifications such as histone methylation or acetylation can be safer compared to the use of azacytidine. Thus, a novel epigenetic-targeted therapy ideally should overcome the shortcomings of the currently available treatment regimen for which a lot of other targets as well as agents acting on the existing targets are to be explored.

6. Conclusions

Several factors that influence the progression of Mtb infection in the host include environmental factors such as malnutrition, dense population, genetic factors, the host's immune status and the virulence of the Mtb pathogen. All of these components are interspersed and are challenging to determine causality for each. Hence, the study of the epigenetic processes becomes very important in order to understand the progression of the Mtb. There are various epigenetic processes such as histone modifications, alteration in expression of non-coding RNAs, alteration in DNA methylation and miRNA that can be explored, as they are ideal candidates for a therapeutic target owing to how the host environment induces epigenetic changes. They can also be used to monitor the progression of the disease or the efficacy of the therapy administered. Furthermore, 'how epigenetics' influences the activation of the latent Mtb infection and how it can be managed in an infected individuals could be the key to the complete eradication of the Mtb disease.

Author Contributions: A.K. and V.P.C. created the plot of the article. A.K., V.P.C., H.P., Y.S., P.M. and V.A. contributed to the writing of the article. V.P.C. and V.A. critically revised the article. All authors have read and agreed to the published version of the manuscript.

Funding: This research received no external funding.

Institutional Review Board Statement: Not applicable.

Informed Consent Statement: Not applicable.

Data Availability Statement: Not applicable.

Acknowledgments: VPC wants to dedicate this article for the 75th year celebration of L. M. College of pharmacy.

Conflicts of Interest: The authors declare no conflict of interest.

References

1. Nadjane Batista Lacerda, S.; de Abreu Temoteo, R.C.; Ribeiro Monteiro de Figueiredo, T.M.; Darliane Tavares de Luna, F.; Alves Nunes de Sousa, M.; de Abreu, L.L.; Luiz Affonso Fonseca, F. Individual and social vulnerabilities upon acquiring tuberculosis: A literature systematic review. *Int. Arch. Med.* **2014**, *7*, 35. [CrossRef] [PubMed]
2. WHO Report on Infectour Diseas. 20 August 1999. Available online: http://www.who.int/infectious-disease-report/ (accessed on 10 October 2022).
3. WHO. *Global Tuberculosis Report 2013*; World Health Organization: Geneva, Switzerland, 2013.
4. Chakraborty, A.K. Epidemiology of tuberculosis: Current status in India. *Indian J. Med. Res.* **2004**, *120*, 248–276. [PubMed]
5. Deutsch-Feldman, M.; Pratt, R.H.; Price, S.F.; Tsang, C.A.; Self, J.L. Tuberculosis—United States, 2020. *Morb. Mortal. Wkly. Rep.* **2021**, *70*, 409. [CrossRef]
6. Sotgiu, G.; Nahid, P.; Loddenkemper, R.; Abubakar, I.; Miravitlles, M.; Migliori, G.B. The ERS-endorsed official ATS/CDC/IDSA clinical practice guidelines on treatment of drug-susceptible tuberculosis. *Eur. Respir. J.* **2016**, *48*, 963–971. [CrossRef] [PubMed]
7. Schaberg, T.; Forssbohm, M.; Hauer, B.; Kirsten, D.; Kropp, R.; Loddenkemper, R.; Loytved, G.; Magdorf, K.; Rieder, H.L.; Sagebiel, D. Guidelines for Drug Treatment of Tuberculosis in Adults and Childhood. *Pneumologie* **2001**, *55*, 494–511. [CrossRef] [PubMed]
8. David, H.L. Probability distribution of drug-resistant mutants in unselected populations of Mycobacterium tuberculosis. *Appl. Microbiol.* **1970**, *20*, 810–814. [CrossRef]
9. Falzon, D.; Jaramillo, E.; Schünemann, H.; Arentz, M.; Bauer, M.; Bayona, J.; Blanc, L.; Caminero, J.; Daley, C.; Duncombe, C. WHO guidelines for the programmatic management of drug-resistant tuberculosis: 2011 update. *Eur. Respir. J.* **2011**, *38*, 516–528. [CrossRef]
10. Diacon, A.H.; Pym, A.; Grobusch, M.; Patientia, R.; Rustomjee, R.; Page-Shipp, L.; Pistorius, C.; Krause, R.; Bogoshi, M.; Churchyard, G.; et al. The Diarylquinoline TMC207 for Multidrug-Resistant Tuberculosis. *N. Engl. J. Med.* **2009**, *360*, 2397–2405. [CrossRef]
11. Frimodt-Moller, J.; Thomas, J.; Parthasarathy, R. Observations on the Protective Effect of Bcg Vaccination in a South Indian Rural Population. *Bull. World Health Organ.* **1964**, *30*, 545–574.
12. Young, D.B. Current tuberculosis vaccine development. *Clin. Infect. Dis.* **2000**, *30* (Suppl. 3), S254–S256. [CrossRef]
13. Van Hest, N.; Aldridge, R.; De Vries, G.; Sandgren, A.; Hauer, B.; Hayward, A.; de Oñate, W.A.; Haas, W.; Codecasa, L.; Caylà, J.J.E. Tuberculosis control in big cities and urban risk groups in the European Union: A consensus statement. *Eurosurveillance* **2014**, *19*, 20728. [CrossRef] [PubMed]
14. Hwang, L.Y.; Grimes, C.Z.; Beasley, R.P.; Graviss, E.A. Latent tuberculosis infections in hard-to-reach drug using population-detection, prevention and control. Tuberculosis (Edinburgh, Scotland). *Tuberculosis* **2009**, *89* (Suppl. 1), S41–S45. [CrossRef]
15. Giosuè, S.; Casarini, M.; Alemanno, L.; Galluccio, G.; Mattia, P.; Pedicelli, G.; Rebek, L.; Bisetti, A.; Ameglio, F. Effects of Aerosolized Interferon-α in Patients with Pulmonary Tuberculosis. *Am. J. Respir. Crit. Care Med.* **1998**, *158*, 1156–1162. [CrossRef] [PubMed]
16. Raad, I.; Hachem, R.; Leeds, N.; Sawaya, R.; Salem, Z.; Atweh, S. Use of adjunctive treatment with interferon-γ in an immunocompromised patient who had refractory multidrug-resistant tuberculosis of the brain. *Clin. Infect. Dis.* **1996**, *22*, 572–574. [CrossRef] [PubMed]
17. Arevalo, I.; Ward, B.; Miller, R.; Meng, T.-C.; Najar, E.; Alvarez, E.; Matlashewski, G.; Llanos-Cuentas, A. Successful treatment of drug-resistant cutaneous leishmaniasis in humans by use of imiquimod, an immunomodulator. *Clin. Infect. Dis.* **2001**, *33*, 1847–1851. [CrossRef] [PubMed]
18. Bermudez, L.E.; Petrofsky, M.; Wu, M.; Young, L.S. Clarithromycin Significantly Improves Interleukin-12-Mediated Anti-Mycobacterium aviumActivity and Abolishes Toxicity in Mice. *J. Infect. Dis.* **1998**, *178*, 896–899. [CrossRef]
19. Steward, W.P. Granulocyte and granulocyte-macrophage colony-stimulating factors. *Lancet* **1993**, *342*, 153–157. [CrossRef]
20. Singh, M.M.; Kumar, P.; Malaviya, A.N.; Kumar, R. Levamisole as an adjunct in the treatment of pulmonary tuberculosis. *Am. Rev. Respir. Dis.* **1981**, *123*, 277–279. [CrossRef]
21. Durban Immunotherapy Trial Group. Immunotherapy with Mycobacterium vaccae in patients with newly diagnosed pulmonary tuberculosis: A randomised controlled trial. *Lancet* **1999**, *354*, 116–119. [CrossRef]
22. Migliori, G.; Hopewell, P.; Blasi, F.; Spanevello, A.; Raviglione, M. Improving the TB case management: The International Standards for Tuberculosis Care. *Eur. Respir. Soc.* **2006**, *28*, 687–690. [CrossRef]
23. Parida, A.; Bairy, K.; Chogtu, B.; Magazine, R.; Vidyasagar, S. Comparison of directly observed treatment short course (DOTS) with self-administered therapy in pulmonary tuberculosis in Udupi District of Southern India. *J. Clin. Diagn. Res.* **2014**, *8*, HC29–HC31. [PubMed]
24. Frieden, T.R.; Sbarbaro, J.A. Promoting adherence to treatment for tuberculosis: The importance of direct observation. *Bull. World Health Organ.* **2007**, *85*, 407–409. [CrossRef] [PubMed]
25. Marimani, M.; Ahmad, A.; Duse, A. The role of epigenetics, bacterial and host factors in progression of Mycobacterium tuberculosis infection. *Tuberculosis* **2018**, *113*, 200–214. [CrossRef] [PubMed]
26. Kathirvel, M.; Mahadevan, S. The role of epigenetics in tuberculosis infection. *Epigenomics* **2016**, *8*, 537–549. [CrossRef] [PubMed]
27. Churchyard, G.; Kim, P.; Shah, N.S.; Rustomjee, R.; Gandhi, N.; Mathema, B.; Dowdy, D.; Kasmar, A.; Cardenas, V. What We Know About Tuberculosis Transmission: An Overview. *J. Infect. Dis.* **2017**, *216*, S629–S635. [CrossRef] [PubMed]

28. Lerner, T.R.; Borel, S.; Gutierrez, M.G. The innate immune response in human tuberculosis. *Cell. Microbiol.* **2015**, *17*, 1277–1285. [CrossRef] [PubMed]
29. Liu, C.H.; Liu, H.; Ge, B. Innate immunity in tuberculosis: Host defense vs. pathogen evasion. *Cell. Mol. Immunol.* **2017**, *14*, 963–975. [CrossRef]
30. Sepehri, Z.; Kiani, Z.; Kohan, F.; Ghavami, S. Toll-Like Receptor 4 as an Immune Receptor AgainstMycobacterium tuberculosis: A Systematic Review. *Lab. Med.* **2019**, *50*, 117–129. [CrossRef]
31. Mortaz, E.; Adcock, I.M.; Tabarsi, P.; Masjedi, M.R.; Mansouri, D.; Velayati, A.A.; Casanova, J.-L.; Barnes, P.J. Interaction of Pattern Recognition Receptors with Mycobacterium Tuberculosis. *J. Clin. Immunol.* **2015**, *35*, 1–10. [CrossRef]
32. Lai, R.P.J.; Meintjes, G.; Wilkinson, K.A.; Graham, C.M.; Marais, S.; Van der Plas, H.; Deffur, A.; Schutz, C.; Bloom, C.; Munagala, I.; et al. HIV–tuberculosis-associated immune reconstitution inflammatory syndrome is characterized by Toll-like receptor and inflammasome signalling. *Nat. Commun.* **2015**, *6*, 8451. [CrossRef]
33. Sheneef, A.; Hussein, M.T.; Mohamed, T.; Mahmoud, A.; Yousef, L.M.; A Alkady, O. Pentraxin 3 Genetic Variants and The Risk of Active Pulmonary Tuberculosis. *Egypt. J. Immunol.* **2017**, *24*, 21–27.
34. Mayer-Barber, K.D.; Barber, D.L. Innate and adaptive cellular immune responses to Mycobacterium tuberculosis infection. *Cold Spring Harb. Perspect. Med.* **2015**, *5*, a018424. [CrossRef] [PubMed]
35. De Martino, M.; Lodi, L.; Galli, L.; Chiappini, E. Immune response to Mycobacterium tuberculosis: A narrative review. *Front. Pediatr.* **2019**, *7*, 350. [CrossRef] [PubMed]
36. Upadhyay, S.; Mittal, E.; A Philips, J. Tuberculosis and the art of macrophage manipulation. *Pathog. Dis.* **2018**, *76*, fty037. [CrossRef]
37. Jasenosky, L.D.; Scriba, T.J.; Hanekom, W.A.; Goldfeld, A.E. T cells and adaptive immunity to Mycobacterium tuberculosis in humans. *Immunol. Rev.* **2015**, *264*, 74–87. [CrossRef]
38. Hunter, R.L. Tuberculosis as a three-act play: A new paradigm for the pathogenesis of pulmonary tuberculosis. *Tuberculosis* **2016**, *97*, 8–17. [CrossRef] [PubMed]
39. Rahman, S.; Rehn, A.; Rahman, J.; Andersson, J.; Svensson, M.; Brighenti, S. Pulmonary tuberculosis patients with a vitamin D deficiency demonstrate low local expression of the antimicrobial peptide LL-37 but enhanced FoxP3+ regulatory T cells and IgG-secreting cells. *Clin. Immunol.* **2015**, *156*, 85–97. [CrossRef] [PubMed]
40. Marin-Luevano, S.P.; Rodriguez-Carlos, A.; Jacobo-Delgado, Y.; Valdez-Miramontes, C.; Enciso-Moreno, J.A.; Rivas-Santiago, B. Steroid hormone modulates the production of cathelicidin and human β-defensins in lung epithelial cells and macrophages promoting Mycobacterium tuberculosis killing. *Tuberculosis* **2021**, *128*, 102080. [CrossRef]
41. Noble, D. Conrad Waddington and the origin of epigenetics. *J. Exp. Biol.* **2015**, *218*, 816–818. [CrossRef]
42. Bird, A. Perceptions of epigenetics. *Nature* **2007**, *447*, 396–398. [CrossRef] [PubMed]
43. Bhavsar, A.; Guttman, J.A.; Finlay, B.B. Manipulation of host-cell pathways by bacterial pathogens. *Nature* **2007**, *449*, 827–834. [CrossRef] [PubMed]
44. Ribet, D.; Cossart, P. Post-translational modifications in host cells during bacterial infection. *FEBS Lett.* **2010**, *584*, 2748–2758. [CrossRef] [PubMed]
45. Bobak, C.A.; Abhimanyu; Natarajan, H.; Gandhi, T.; Grimm, S.L.; Nishiguchi, T.; Koster, K.; Longlax, S.C.; Dlamini, Q.; Kahari, J.; et al. Increased DNA methylation, cellular senescence and premature epigenetic aging in guinea pigs and humans with tuberculosis. *Aging* **2022**, *14*, 2174–2193. [CrossRef] [PubMed]
46. Wang, Y.; Curry, H.M.; Zwilling, B.S.; Lafuse, W. Mycobacteria Inhibition of IFN-γ Induced HLA-DR Gene Expression by Up-Regulating Histone Deacetylation at the Promoter Region in Human THP-1 Monocytic Cells. *J. Immunol.* **2005**, *174*, 5687–5694. [CrossRef]
47. Fatima, S.; Kumari, A.; Agarwal, M.; Pahuja, I.; Yadav, V.; Dwivedi, V.P.; Bhaskar, A. Epigenetic code during mycobacterial infections: Therapeutic implications for tuberculosis. *FEBS J.* **2021**, *289*, 4172–4191. [CrossRef]
48. Koo, M.-S.; Subbian, S.; Kaplan, G. Strain specific transcriptional response in Mycobacterium tuberculosis infected macrophages. *Cell Commun. Signal.* **2012**, *10*, 2. [CrossRef]
49. Kouzarides, T. Chromatin modifications and their function. *Cell* **2007**, *128*, 693–705. [CrossRef]
50. Peterson, C.L.; Laniel, M.-A. Histones and histone modifications. *Curr. Biol.* **2004**, *14*, R546–R551. [CrossRef]
51. Bhutani, N.; Burns, D.M.; Blau, H.M. DNA Demethylation Dynamics. *Cell* **2011**, *146*, 866–872. [CrossRef]
52. Vymetalkova, V.; Vodicka, P.; Vodenkova, S.; Alonso, S.; Schneider-Stock, R. DNA methylation and chromatin modifiers in colorectal cancer. *Mol. Asp. Med.* **2019**, *69*, 73–92. [CrossRef]
53. Deaton, A.M.; Bird, A. CpG islands and the regulation of transcription. *Genes Dev.* **2011**, *25*, 1010–1022. [CrossRef] [PubMed]
54. Yaseen, I.; Kaur, P.; Nandicoori, V.; Khosla, S. Mycobacteria modulate host epigenetic machinery by Rv1988 methylation of a non-tail arginine of histone H3. *Nat. Commun.* **2015**, *6*, 8922. [CrossRef]
55. Singh, V.; Prakhar, P.; Rajmani, R.S.; Mahadik, K.; Borbora, S.M.; Balaji, K.N. Histone Methyltransferase SET8 Epigenetically Reprograms Host Immune Responses to Assist Mycobacterial Survival. *J. Infect. Dis.* **2017**, *216*, 477–488. [CrossRef] [PubMed]
56. Houghton, A.M. Matrix metalloproteinases in destructive lung disease. *Matrix Biol.* **2015**, *44*, 167–174. [CrossRef] [PubMed]
57. Loffek, S.; Schilling, O.; Franzke, C.-W. Biological role of matrix metalloproteinases: A critical balance. *Eur. Respir. J.* **2011**, *38*, 191–208. [CrossRef] [PubMed]

58. Moores, R.C.; Brilha, S.; Schutgens, F.; Elkington, P.T.; Friedland, J.S. Epigenetic Regulation of Matrix Metalloproteinase-1 and -3 Expression in Mycobacterium tuberculosis Infection. *Front. Immunol.* **2017**, *8*, 602. [CrossRef]
59. Aung, H.T.; Schroder, K.; Himes, S.R.; Brion, K.; Van Zuylen, W.; Trieu, A.; Suzuki, H.; Hayashizaki, Y.; Hume, D.A.; Sweet, M.J.J.T.F.J. LPS regulates proinflammatory gene expression in macrophages by altering histone deacetylase expression. *FASEB J.* **2006**, *20*, 1315–1327. [CrossRef]
60. Khosla, S.; Sharma, G.; Yaseen, I. Learning epigenetic regulation from mycobacteria. *Microb. Cell* **2016**, *3*, 92–94. [CrossRef]
61. Sengupta, S.; Nayak, B.; Meuli, M.; Sander, P.; Mishra, S.; Sonawane, A. Mycobacterium tuberculosis phosphoribosyltransferase promotes bacterial survival in macrophages by inducing histone hypermethylation in autophagy-related genes. *Front. Cell. Infect. Microbiol.* **2021**, *11*, 676456. [CrossRef]
62. Chandran, A.; Antony, C.; Jose, L.; Mundayoor, S.; Natarajan, K.; Kumar, R.A. Mycobacterium tuberculosis Infection Induces HDAC1-Mediated Suppression of IL-12B Gene Expression in Macrophages. *Front. Cell. Infect. Microbiol.* **2015**, *5*, 90. [CrossRef]
63. Shahbazian, M.D.; Grunstein, M. Functions of site-specific histone acetylation and deacetylation. *Annu. Rev. Biochem.* **2007**, *76*, 75–100. [CrossRef] [PubMed]
64. Kumar, D.; Nath, L.; Kamal, M.A.; Varshney, A.; Jain, A.; Singh, S.; Rao, K.V. Genome-wide Analysis of the Host Intracellular Network that Regulates Survival of Mycobacterium tuberculosis. *Cell* **2010**, *140*, 731–743. [CrossRef] [PubMed]
65. Almeida Da Silva, P.E.; Palomino, J.C. Molecular basis and mechanisms of drug resistance in Mycobacterium tuberculosis: Classical and new drugs. *J. Antimicrob. Chemother.* **2011**, *66*, 1417–1430. [CrossRef] [PubMed]
66. Sharma, G.; Upadhyay, S.; Srilalitha, M.; Nandicoori, V.K.; Khosla, S. The interaction of mycobacterial protein Rv2966c with host chromatin is mediated through non-CpG methylation and histone H3/H4 binding. *Nucleic Acids Res.* **2015**, *43*, 3922–3937. [CrossRef] [PubMed]
67. Borchert, G.M.; Lanier, W.; Davidson, B.L. RNA polymerase III transcribes human microRNAs. *Nat. Struct. Mol. Biol.* **2006**, *13*, 1097–1101. [CrossRef]
68. Sontheimer, E.J.; Carthew, R.W. Silence from within: Endogenous siRNAs and miRNAs. *Cell* **2005**, *122*, 9–12. [CrossRef]
69. Maudet, C.; Mano, M.; Eulalio, A. MicroRNAs in the interaction between host and bacterial pathogens. *FEBS Lett.* **2014**, *588*, 4140–4147. [CrossRef]
70. Bentwich, I.; Avniel, A.; Karov, Y.; Aharonov, R.; Gilad, S.; Barad, O.; Barzilai, A.; Einat, P.; Einav, U.; Meiri, E.; et al. Identification of hundreds of conserved and nonconserved human microRNAs. *Nat. Genet.* **2005**, *37*, 766–770. [CrossRef]
71. Lewis, B.P.; Burge, C.B.; Bartel, D.P. Conserved Seed Pairing, Often Flanked by Adenosines, Indicates that Thousands of Human Genes are MicroRNA Targets. *Cell* **2005**, *120*, 15–20. [CrossRef]
72. Hua, Z.; Lv, Q.; Ye, W.; Wong, C.-K.A.; Cai, G.; Gu, D.; Ji, Y.; Zhao, C.; Wang, J.; Yang, B.B.J.P.o. MiRNA-directed regulation of VEGF and other angiogenic factors under hypoxia. *PLoS ONE* **2006**, *1*, e116. [CrossRef]
73. Cheng, A.M.; Byrom, M.W.; Shelton, J.; Ford, L.P. Antisense inhibition of human miRNAs and indications for an involvement of miRNA in cell growth and apoptosis. *Nucleic Acids Res.* **2005**, *33*, 1290–1297. [CrossRef] [PubMed]
74. Pennini, M.E.; Liu, Y.; Yang, J.; Croniger, C.M.; Boom, W.H.; Harding, C.V. CCAAT/Enhancer-Binding Protein β and δ Binding to CIITA Promoters Is Associated with the Inhibition of CIITA Expression in Response to Mycobacterium tuberculosis 19-kDa Lipoprotein. *J. Immunol.* **2007**, *179*, 6910–6918. [CrossRef] [PubMed]
75. Sharbati, J.; Lewin, A.; Kutz-Lohroff, B.; Kamal, E.; Einspanier, R.; Sharbati, S. Integrated microRNA-mRNA-analysis of human monocyte derived macrophages upon Mycobacterium avium subsp. hominissuis infection. *PLoS ONE* **2011**, *6*, e20258. [CrossRef]
76. Shi, G.; Mao, G.; Xie, K.; Wu, D.; Wang, W. MiR-1178 regulates mycobacterial survival and inflammatory responses in Mycobacterium tuberculosis-infected macrophages partly via TLR4. *J. Cell. Biochem.* **2018**, *119*, 7449–7457. [CrossRef]
77. Li, W.; Zhang, Q. MicroRNA-708-5p regulates mycobacterial vitality and the secretion of inflammatory factors in Mycobacterium tuberculosis-infected macrophages by targeting TLR4. *Eur. Rev. Med. Pharmacol. Sci.* **2019**, *23*, 8028–8038.
78. Niu, W.; Sun, B.; Li, M.; Cui, J.; Huang, J.; Zhang, L. TLR-4/microRNA-125a/NF-κB signaling modulates the immune response to Mycobacterium tuberculosis infection. *Cell Cycle* **2018**, *17*, 1931–1945. [CrossRef] [PubMed]
79. Liang, S.; Song, Z.; Wu, Y.; Gao, Y.; Gao, M.; Liu, F.; Wang, F.; Zhang, Y. MicroRNA-27b Modulates Inflammatory Response and Apoptosis during Mycobacterium tuberculosis Infection. *J. Immunol.* **2018**, *200*, 3506–3518. [CrossRef]
80. Wen, Q.; Zhou, C.; Xiong, W.; Su, J.; He, J.; Zhang, S.; Du, X.; Liu, S.; Wang, J.; Ma, L. MiR-381-3p Regulates the Antigen-Presenting Capability of Dendritic Cells and Represses Antituberculosis Cellular Immune Responses by Targeting CD1c. *J. Immunol.* **2016**, *197*, 580–589. [CrossRef]
81. Singh, Y.; Kaul, V.; Mehra, A.; Chatterjee, S.; Tousif, S.; Dwivedi, V.P.; Suar, M.; Van Kaer, L.; Bishai, W.R.; Das, G. Mycobacterium tuberculosis Controls MicroRNA-99b (miR-99b) Expression in Infected Murine Dendritic Cells to Modulate Host Immunity. *J. Biol. Chem.* **2013**, *288*, 5056–5061. [CrossRef]
82. Wei, L.; Liu, K.; Jia, Q.; Zhang, H.; Bie, Q.; Zhang, B. The Roles of Host Noncoding RNAs in Mycobacterium tuberculosis Infection. *Front. Immunol.* **2021**, *12*, 664787. [CrossRef]
83. Skvortsova, K.; Stirzaker, C.; Taberlay, P. The DNA methylation landscape in cancer. *Essays Biochem.* **2019**, *63*, 797–811. [CrossRef] [PubMed]
84. Liu, R.; Wu, X.-m.; He, X.; Wang, R.-z.; Yin, X.-y.; Zhou, F.; Ji, M.-h.; Shen, J.-c.J.P.B. Contribution of DNA methyltransferases to spared nerve injury induced depression partially through epigenetically repressing Bdnf in hippocampus: Reversal by ketamine. *Pharmacol. Biochem. Behav.* **2021**, *200*, 173079. [CrossRef] [PubMed]

85. Dinardo, A.R.; Rajapakshe, K.; Nishiguchi, T.; Grimm, S.L.; Mtetwa, G.; Dlamini, Q.; Kahari, J.; Mahapatra, S.; Kay, A.W.; Maphalala, G.; et al. DNA hypermethylation during tuberculosis dampens host immune responsiveness. *J. Clin. Investig.* **2020**, *130*, 3113–3123. [CrossRef]
86. Jose, L.; Ramachandran, R.; Bhagavat, R.; Gomez, R.L.; Chandran, A.; Raghunandanan, S.; Omkumar, R.V.; Chandra, N.; Mundayoor, S.; Kumar, R.A.J.T.F.j. Hypothetical protein Rv3423. 1 of Mycobacterium tuberculosis is a histone acetyltransferase. *FEBS J.* **2016**, *283*, 265–281. [CrossRef] [PubMed]
87. Shell, S.S.; Prestwich, E.G.; Baek, S.-H.; Shah, R.R.; Sassetti, C.M.; Dedon, P.C.; Fortune, S.M. DNA Methylation Impacts Gene Expression and Ensures Hypoxic Survival of Mycobacterium tuberculosis. *PLoS Pathog.* **2013**, *9*, e1003419. [CrossRef]
88. Sharma, G.; Sowpati, D.T.; Singh, P.; Khan, M.Z.; Ganji, R.; Upadhyay, S.; Banerjee, S.; Nandicoori, V.K.; Khosla, S.J.S.r. Genome-wide non-CpG methylation of the host genome during M. tuberculosis infection. *Sci. Rep.* **2016**, *6*, 25006. [CrossRef]
89. Lyu, M.; Zhou, J.; Jiao, L.; Wang, Y.; Zhou, Y.; Lai, H.; Xu, W.; Ying, B. Deciphering a TB-related DNA methylation biomarker and constructing a TB diagnostic classifier. *Mol. Ther. Nucleic Acids* **2022**, *27*, 37–49. [CrossRef]
90. Yadav, V.; Dwivedi, V.P.; Bhattacharya, D.; Mittal, A.; Moodley, P.; Das, G.J.J.o.G.; Research, G. Understanding the host epigenetics in Mycobacterium tuberculosis infection. *J. Genet. Genome Res.* **2015**, *2*. [CrossRef]
91. Siddle, K.J.; Deschamps, M.; Tailleux, L.; Nédélec, Y.; Pothlichet, J.; Lugo-Villarino, G.; Libri, V.; Gicquel, B.; Neyrolles, O.; Laval, G.; et al. A genomic portrait of the genetic architecture and regulatory impact of microRNA expression in response to infection. *Genome Res.* **2014**, *24*, 850–859. [CrossRef]
92. Zheng, L.; Leung, E.T.; Wong, H.; Lui, C.Y.G.; Lee, N.; To, K.-F.; Choy, K.W.; Chan, R.C.; Ip, M. Unraveling methylation changes of host macrophages in Mycobacterium tuberculosis infection. *Tuberculosis* **2016**, *98*, 139–148. [CrossRef]
93. Kumar, P.; Agarwal, R.; Siddiqui, I.; Vora, H.; Das, G.; Sharma, P.J.I. ESAT6 differentially inhibits IFN-γ-inducible class II transactivator isoforms in both a TLR2-dependent and-independent manner. *Immunol. Cell Biol.* **2012**, *90*, 411–420. [CrossRef] [PubMed]
94. Frantz, F.G.; Castro, R.C.; Fontanari, C.; Bollela, V.R.; Zambuzi, F.A. DNA Methylation impairs monocyte function in tuberculosis leading to disease progression. *Am. Assoc. Immnol.* **2019**, *202* (Suppl. 1), 125.10.
95. Crossman, D.K. *Characterization of a Novel Acetyltransferase Found Only in Pathogenic Strains of Mycobacterium Tuberculosis*; The University of Alabama at Birmingham: Birmingham, AL, USA, 2007.
96. Andraos, C.; Koorsen, G.; Knight, J.C.; Bornman, L. Vitamin D receptor gene methylation is associated with ethnicity, tuberculosis, and TaqI polymorphism. *Hum. Immunol.* **2011**, *72*, 262–268. [CrossRef] [PubMed]
97. Campo-Patino, M.; Heater, S.; Simmons, J.; Peterson, G.; Stein, C.; Mayanja-Kizza, H.; Boom, W.; Hawn, T. Selective HDAC3 Inhibitor Restricts Mycobacterial Growth and Modulates Macrophage Immune Responses. *Am. Thorac. Soc.* **2019**, *199*, A4425. [CrossRef]
98. Moreira, J.D.; Koch, B.E.V.; van Veen, S.; Walburg, K.V.; Vrieling, F.; Guimarães, T.M.P.D.; Meijer, A.H.; Spaink, H.; Ottenhoff, T.H.M.; Haks, M.C.; et al. Functional Inhibition of Host Histone Deacetylases (HDACs) Enhances in vitro and in vivo Anti-mycobacterial Activity in Human Macrophages and in Zebrafish. *Front. Immunol.* **2020**, *11*, 36. [CrossRef] [PubMed]
99. Roger, T.; Lugrin, J.; LE Roy, D.; Goy, G.; Mombelli, M.; Koessler, T.; Ding, X.C.; Chanson, A.-L.; Reymond, M.K.; Miconnet, I.; et al. Histone deacetylase inhibitors impair innate immune responses to Toll-like receptor agonists and to infection. *Blood* **2011**, *117*, 1205–1217. [CrossRef] [PubMed]
100. Li, Y.; Liu, B.; Fukudome, E.Y.; Kochanek, A.R.; Finkelstein, R.A.; Chong, W.; Jin, G.; Lu, J.; Demoya, M.A.; Velmahos, G.C.; et al. Surviving lethal septic shock without fluid resuscitation in a rodent model. *Surgery* **2010**, *148*, 246–254. [CrossRef]
101. Cox, D.; Coleman, A.; Gogan, K.; Dunne, P.; Basdeo, S.; Keane, J. Vorinostat (SAHA) promotes innate and adaptive immunity to Mycobacterium tuberculosis. *Access Microbiol.* **2020**, *2*, 29. [CrossRef]
102. Cheng, X.; Liu, Z.; Liu, B.; Zhao, T.; Li, Y.; Alam, H.B. Selective histone deacetylase 6 inhibition prolongs survival in a lethal two-hit model. *J. Surg. Res.* **2015**, *197*, 39–44. [CrossRef]
103. Ariffin, J.K.; Das Gupta, K.; Kapetanovic, R.; Iyer, A.; Reid, R.C.; Fairlie, D.; Sweet, M.J. Histone Deacetylase Inhibitors Promote Mitochondrial Reactive Oxygen Species Production and Bacterial Clearance by Human Macrophages. *Antimicrob. Agents Chemother.* **2016**, *60*, 1521–1529. [CrossRef]
104. Falkenberg, K.J.; Johnstone, R.W. Histone deacetylases and their inhibitors in cancer, neurological diseases and immune disorders. *Nat. Rev. Drug Discov.* **2014**, *13*, 673–691. [CrossRef] [PubMed]
105. Vishwakarma, S.; Iyer, L.R.; Muley, M.; Singh, P.K.; Shastry, A.; Saxena, A.; Kulathingal, J.; Vijaykanth, G.; Raghul, J.; Rajesh, N.; et al. Tubastatin, a selective histone deacetylase 6 inhibitor shows anti-inflammatory and anti-rheumatic effects. *Int. Immunopharmacol.* **2013**, *16*, 72–78. [CrossRef] [PubMed]
106. Clocchiatti, A.; Di Giorgio, E.; Ingrao, S.; Meyer-Almes, F.; Tripodo, C.; Brancolini, C. Class IIa HDACs repressive activities on MEF2-depedent transcription are associated with poor prognosis of ER + breast tumors. *FASEB J.* **2013**, *27*, 942–954. [CrossRef]
107. Hamers, A.A.; Vos, M.; Rassam, F.; Marinković, G.; Kurakula, K.; van Gorp, P.J.; de Winther, M.P.; Gijbels, M.J.; de Waard, V.; de Vries, C.J. Bone Marrow–Specific Deficiency of Nuclear Receptor Nur77 Enhances Atherosclerosis. *Circ. Res.* **2012**, *110*, 428–438. [CrossRef] [PubMed]
108. Hanna, R.N.; Shaked, I.; Hubbeling, H.G.; Punt, J.A.; Wu, R.; Herrley, E.; Zaugg, C.; Pei, H.; Geissmann, F.; Ley, K.; et al. NR4A1 (Nur77) Deletion Polarizes Macrophages Toward an Inflammatory Phenotype and Increases Atherosclerosis. *Circ. Res.* **2012**, *110*, 416–427. [CrossRef]

109. Etna, M.P.; Giacomini, E.; Severa, M.; Coccia, E.M. Pro- and anti-inflammatory cytokines in tuberculosis: A two-edged sword in TB pathogenesis. *Semin. Immunol.* **2014**, *26*, 543–551. [CrossRef] [PubMed]
110. Grégoire, S.; Tremblay, A.M.; Xiao, L.; Yang, Q.; Ma, K.; Nie, J.; Mao, Z.; Wu, Z.; Giguère, V.; Yang, X.-J.J.J.o.B.C. Control of MEF2 transcriptional activity by coordinated phosphorylation and sumoylation. *J. Biol. Chem.* **2006**, *281*, 4423–4433. [CrossRef] [PubMed]
111. Zhang, F.; Yu, S.; Chai, Q.; Wang, J.; Wu, T.; Liu, R.; Liu, Y.; Liu, C.H.; Pang, Y. HDAC6 contributes to human resistance against Mycobacterium tuberculosis infection via mediating innate immune responses. *FASEB J.* **2021**, *35*, e22009. [CrossRef]
112. Wang, X.; Tang, X.; Zhou, Z.; Huang, Q. Histone deacetylase 6 inhibitor enhances resistance to Mycobacterium tuberculosis infection through innate and adaptive immunity in mice. *Pathog. Dis.* **2018**, *76*, fty064. [CrossRef]
113. Campo, M.; Heater, S.; Peterson, G.J.; Simmons, J.D.; Skerrett, S.J.; Mayanja-Kizza, H.; Stein, C.M.; Boom, W.H.; Hawn, T.R. HDAC3 inhibitor RGFP966 controls bacterial growth and modulates macrophage signaling during Mycobacterium tuberculosis infection. *Tuberculosis* **2021**, *127*, 102062. [CrossRef]
114. Lugrin, J.; Ciarlo, E.; Santos, A.; Grandmaison, G.; Dos Santos, I.; Le Roy, D.; Roger, T. The sirtuin inhibitor cambinol impairs MAPK signaling, inhibits inflammatory and innate immune responses and protects from septic shock. *Biochim. Biophys. Acta* **2013**, *1833*, 1498–1510. [CrossRef] [PubMed]
115. Swamy, B.N.; Suma, T.; Rao, G.V.; Reddy, G.C. Synthesis of isonicotinoylhydrazones from anacardic acid and their in vitro activity against Mycobacterium smegmatis. *Eur. J. Med. Chem.* **2007**, *42*, 420–424. [CrossRef] [PubMed]
116. Zeng, L.; Zhou, M.-M. Bromodomain: An acetyl-lysine binding domain. *FEBS Lett.* **2002**, *513*, 124–128. [CrossRef]
117. Smale, S.T.; Tarakhovsky, A.; Natoli, G. Chromatin Contributions to the Regulation of Innate Immunity. *Annu. Rev. Immunol.* **2014**, *32*, 489–511. [CrossRef]
118. Chan, C.H.; Fang, C.; Qiao, Y.; Yarilina, A.; Prinjha, R.K.; Ivashkiv, L.B. BET bromodomain inhibition suppresses transcriptional responses to cytokine-Jak-STAT signaling in a gene-specific manner in human monocytes. *Eur. J. Immunol.* **2015**, *45*, 287–297. [CrossRef] [PubMed]
119. Koenis, D.S.; Medzikovic, L.; van Loenen, P.B.; van Weeghel, M.; Huveneers, S.; Vos, M.; Gogh, I.J.E.-V.; Bossche, J.V.D.; Speijer, D.; Kim, Y.; et al. Nuclear Receptor Nur77 Limits the Macrophage Inflammatory Response through Transcriptional Reprogramming of Mitochondrial Metabolism. *Cell Rep.* **2018**, *24*, 2127–2140.e7. [CrossRef] [PubMed]
120. Harth, G.; Zamecnik, P.C.; Tang, J.-Y.; Tabatadze, D.; Horwitz, M.A. Treatment of Mycobacterium tuberculosis with antisense oligonucleotides to glutamine synthetase mRNA inhibits glutamine synthetase activity, formation of the poly-L-glutamate/glutamine cell wall structure, and bacterial replication. *Proc. Natl. Acad. Sci. USA* **2000**, *97*, 418–423. [CrossRef] [PubMed]
121. Harth, G.; Zamecnik, P.C.; Tabatadze, D.; Pierson, K.; Horwitz, M.A. Hairpin extensions enhance the efficacy of mycolyl transferase-specific antisense oligonucleotides targeting Mycobacterium tuberculosis. *Proc. Natl. Acad. Sci. USA* **2007**, *104*, 7199–7204. [CrossRef]
122. Skvortsova, Y.V.; Salina, E.G.; Burakova, E.A.; Bychenko, O.S.; Stetsenko, D.A.; Azhikina, T.L. A New Antisense Phosphoryl Guanidine Oligo-2'-O-Methylribonucleotide Penetrates Into Intracellular Mycobacteria and Suppresses Target Gene Expression. *Front. Pharmacol.* **2019**, *10*, 1049. [CrossRef]
123. Das, A.R.; Dattagupta, N.; Sridhar, C.N.; Wu, W.-K. A novel thiocationic liposomal formulation of antisense oligonucleotides with activity against Mycobacterium tuberculosis. *Scand. J. Infect. Dis.* **2003**, *35*, 168–174. [CrossRef] [PubMed]
124. Kaminskas, E.; Farrell, A.T.; Wang, Y.-C.; Sridhara, R.; Pazdur, R. FDA Drug Approval Summary: Azacitidine (5-azacytidine, Vidaza™) for Injectable Suspension. *Oncologist* **2005**, *10*, 176–182. [CrossRef] [PubMed]
125. Momparler, R.L. Pharmacology of 5-Aza-2'-deoxycytidine (decitabine). In *Seminars in Hematology*; Elsevier: Amsterdam, The Netherlands, 2015.
126. Cheng, J.C.; Matsen, C.; Gonzales, F.A.; Ye, W.; Greer, S.; Marquez, V.E.; Jones, P.A.; Selker, E.U. Inhibition of DNA Methylation and Reactivation of Silenced Genes by Zebularine. *JNCI J. Natl. Cancer Inst.* **2003**, *95*, 399–409. [CrossRef] [PubMed]
127. Hilton, I.B.; D'Ippolito, A.M.; Vockley, C.M.; Thakore, P.I.; Crawford, G.E.; Reddy, T.E.; Gersbach, C.A. Epigenome editing by a CRISPR-Cas9-based acetyltransferase activates genes from promoters and enhancers. *Nat. Biotechnol.* **2015**, *33*, 510–517. [CrossRef] [PubMed]
128. Kearns, N.; Pham, H.; Tabak, B.; Genga, R.M.; Silverstein, N.J.; Garber, M.; Maehr, R. Functional annotation of native enhancers with a Cas9–histone demethylase fusion. *Nat. Methods* **2015**, *12*, 401–403. [CrossRef] [PubMed]
129. Hsu, P.D.; Lander, E.S.; Zhang, F. Development and Applications of CRISPR-Cas9 for Genome Engineering. *Cell* **2014**, *157*, 1262–1278. [CrossRef] [PubMed]
130. Rao, M.; Valentini, D.; Zumla, A.; Maeurer, M. Evaluation of the efficacy of valproic acid and suberoylanilide hydroxamic acid (vorinostat) in enhancing the effects of first-line tuberculosis drugs against intracellular Mycobacterium tuberculosis. *Int. J. Infect. Dis.* **2018**, *69*, 78–84. [CrossRef] [PubMed]
131. Rekha, R.S.; Mily, A.; Sultana, T.; Haq, A.; Ahmed, S.; Kamal, S.M.M.; Van Schadewijk, A.; Hiemstra, P.S.; Gudmundsson, G.H.; Agerberth, B.; et al. Immune responses in the treatment of drug-sensitive pulmonary tuberculosis with phenylbutyrate and vitamin D3 as host directed therapy. *BMC Infect. Dis.* **2018**, *18*, 303. [CrossRef]

132. Mily, A.; Rekha, R.S.; Kamal, S.M.M.; Arifuzzaman, A.S.M.; Rahim, Z.; Khan, L.; Haq, A.; Zaman, K.; Bergman, P.; Brighenti, S.; et al. Significant Effects of Oral Phenylbutyrate and Vitamin D3 Adjunctive Therapy in Pulmonary Tuberculosis: A Randomized Controlled Trial. *PLoS ONE* **2015**, *10*, e0138340. [CrossRef]
133. Hammitzsch, A.; Tallant, C.; Fedorov, O.; O'Mahony, A.; Brennan, P.E.; Hay, D.A.; Martinez, F.O.; Al-Mossawi, M.H.; de Wit, J.; Vecellio, M.; et al. CBP30, a selective CBP/p300 bromodomain inhibitor, suppresses human Th17 responses. *Proc. Natl. Acad. Sci. USA* **2015**, *112*, 10768–10773. [CrossRef]
134. Gauba, K.; Gupta, S.; Shekhawat, J.; Sharma, P.; Yadav, D.; Banerjee, M. Immunomodulation by epigenome alterations in Mycobacterium tuberculosis infection. *Tuberculosis* **2021**, *128*, 102077. [CrossRef]
135. Jiang, Y.; Li, Y.; Liu, C.; Zhang, L.; Lv, D.; Weng, Y.; Cheng, Z.; Chen, X.; Zhan, J.; Zhang, H. Isonicotinylation is a histone mark induced by the anti-tuberculosis first-line drug isoniazid. *Nat. Commun.* **2021**, *12*, 5548. [CrossRef] [PubMed]
136. Sharma, N.; Shariq, M.; Quadir, N.; Singh, J.; Sheikh, J.A.; Hasnain, S.E.; Ehtesham, N.Z. Mycobacterium tuberculosis Protein PE6 (Rv0335c), a Novel TLR4 Agonist, Evokes an Inflammatory Response and Modulates the Cell Death Pathways in Macrophages to Enhance Intracellular Survival. *Front. Immunol.* **2021**, *12*, 696491. [CrossRef] [PubMed]

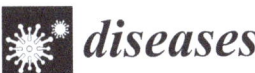

Case Report

The Role of Novel Motorized Spiral Enteroscopy in the Diagnosis of Cecal Tumors

Amir Selimagic [1,*], Ada Dozic [2] and Azra Husic-Selimovic [1]

1. Department of Gastroenterohepatology, General Hospital "Prim. dr. Abdulah Nakas", 71 000 Sarajevo, Bosnia and Herzegovina
2. Department of Internal Medicine, General Hospital "Prim. dr. Abdulah Nakas", 71 000 Sarajevo, Bosnia and Herzegovina
* Correspondence: amir.selimagic@obs.ba; Tel.: +387-33-285-100; Fax: +387-33-285-370

Abstract: Small bowel and ileocecal diseases remain a diagnostic and therapeutic challenge, despite the introduction of various modalities for deep enteroscopy. Novel Motorized Spiral Enteroscopy is an innovative technology that uses an overtube with a raised spiral at the distal end to pleat the small intestine. It consumes less time and meets both the diagnostic and therapeutic needs of small bowel diseases. The objective of this article is to highlight the possibility of using NMSE as an alternative technique when a target lesion is inaccessible during conventional colonoscopy or cecal intubation cannot be achieved. We report the case of a 61-year-old man who presented with pain in the right lower abdominal segment, diarrhea, and rapid weight loss for more than 3 months. An initial ultrasound showed a suspicious liver metastasis. Computerized tomography scans showed an extensive ileocecal tumor mass with liver metastasis. The colonoscopy was unsuccessful and incomplete due to dolichocolon and intestinal tortuosity. Later, endoscopy was performed using a Novel Motorized Spiral Enteroscope in a retrograde approach, passing the scope through the anus and colon up to the ileocecal segment, where a tumor biopsy was performed and adenocarcinoma was pathohistologically confirmed.

Keywords: motorized spiral enteroscopy; small bowel disease; gastrointestinal tumor

Citation: Selimagic, A.; Dozic, A.; Husic-Selimovic, A. The Role of Novel Motorized Spiral Enteroscopy in the Diagnosis of Cecal Tumors. *Diseases* **2022**, *10*, 79. https://doi.org/10.3390/diseases10040079

Academic Editors: Vasso Apostolopoulos, Jack Feehan and Vivek P. Chavda

Received: 27 August 2022
Accepted: 2 October 2022
Published: 4 October 2022

Publisher's Note: MDPI stays neutral with regard to jurisdictional claims in published maps and institutional affiliations.

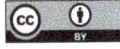

Copyright: © 2022 by the authors. Licensee MDPI, Basel, Switzerland. This article is an open access article distributed under the terms and conditions of the Creative Commons Attribution (CC BY) license (https://creativecommons.org/licenses/by/4.0/).

1. Introduction

The role of endoscopy in the diagnosis and treatment of gastrointestinal disorders has become irreplaceable in the past decades. Even though new endoscopic modalities have been developed, distant parts of the gastrointestinal system, especially the small bowel, remain inaccessible by endoscopic methods in some cases. In 2001, video capsule endoscopy was presented as an innovative technology that enabled examination of the entire small bowel but with a significant drawback regarding the impossibility of performing therapeutic interventions [1]. Further development of deep enteroscopy was made with the introduction of double-balloon (DBE) endoscopy, and later on, single balloon endoscopy (SBE) with the push and pull technique [1,2]. However, these techniques also have certain limitations, such as long procedure duration, and, in some cases, inefficiency in achieving a complete examination of the small bowel [3–5]. Spiral enteroscopy is a technique that uses a spiral tube at the bottom end of the endoscope allowing diagnostic and therapeutic access to obscure parts of the digestive tract. It was used for the first time in 2008. However, it has been found to be a time-consuming and complex procedure since it requires two operators and a manual rotation [6–8].

Novel Motorized Spiral Enteroscopy (NMSE) is a new technology with an incorporated motor adjacent to the endoscope. The spiral enteroscope control unit regulates the direction and speed of rotation of the spiral segment (Figure 1) [8,9]. In addition, it is performed by a single operator.

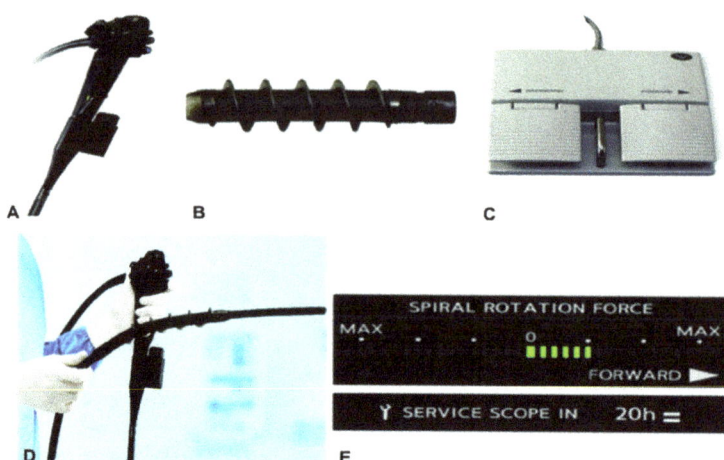

Figure 1. (**A**) Integrated motor in motorized spiral enteroscope. (**B**) Power spiral tube. (**C**) Foot switch with forward and backward pedals. (**D**) Power spiral enteroscope. (**E**) Force gauge on power spiral control unit for visual indication of the rotational direction. Pictures courtesy of Olympus Corp, Tokyo, Japan.

In 2016, Neuhaus et al. [10] reported the first clinical use of this procedure for the treatment of angiodysplasias in the jejunum of a 48-year-old patient with iron-deficiency anemia. Since then, NMSE has become the focus of research as a potential solution for the limitations of currently available device-assisted enteroscopy techniques. This technique is considered effective and safe and allows for performing both diagnostic and therapeutic interventions on the small bowel. It also has a shorter duration compared to other deep enteroscopy modalities [11]. The most common indications for NMSE include obscure gastrointestinal bleeding and suspected inflammatory bowel disease. In addition, it is used for therapeutic interventions such as polypectomy, hemostasis, or stricture dilatation [6].

Since this is a newly introduced diagnostic procedure that is used only in a small number of facilities, the available literature on this topic is very limited. In addition to the small intestine, the use of this device via the retrograde route can be of great importance in the diagnosis of ileocecal diseases when the target lesions are difficult to access with conventional colonoscopy. According to the literature, 1.6–16.7% of all colonoscopies are found to be unsuccessful due to failure to achieve cecal intubation [12–14]. The most frequent causes of incomplete colonoscopy are stenosis or inadequate bowel cleansing, previous abdominal or pelvic surgery, female sex, older age, low body mass index, and diverticulosis [12,15,16]. In addition, an abnormally long, tortuous colon is considered a significant factor that may result in a failed cecal intubation [17]. In 4.3% of patients who underwent incomplete colonoscopy, an advanced tumor was missed [12,18]. This finding highlights the significance of the visualization of the entire colon during the examination. Therefore, NMSE could be a promising and effective alternative technique to achieve the visualization of the entire colon and access to target lesions. Here, we report the case of a patient with a tumor of the terminal ileum and caecum who was not a candidate for biopsy via colonoscopy due to dolichocolon.

2. Case Presentation

A 61-year-old man presented to the hospital with a history of pain in the right groin area, a change in his bowel habits with frequent mushy stools, and unintentional weight loss. These symptoms started about 3 months prior to admission. He was a professional driver with a history of type 2 diabetes mellitus and arterial hypertension who did not consume alcohol or tobacco. No family history of cancer or other inherited medical conditions were reported. Physical examination revealed mild pain to palpations in the right upper and lower quadrants of the abdomen. There were no other abnormal findings during the examination.

The initial evaluation included laboratory tests, which revealed elevated tumor markers CEA 3410 μg/L (upper reference limit 3.4 μg/L) and CA 19-9 292 U/mL (upper reference limit 25 U/mL), whereas AFP was normal (1.23 kU/L; upper reference limit 5.8 kU/L). The other laboratory findings were normal.

The initial abdominal ultrasound verified changes in the liver parenchyma suspected of metastatic lesions. The abdomen and pelvis CT scans showed multiple focal nodal areas of the liver parenchyma highly suspicious for liver metastases. In the area of the caecum, there was an infiltrative thickening of the wall of the terminal ileum area with associated luminal narrowing, reactive changes of perivisceral adipose tissue, and reactive lymphadenopathy (Figure 2). The proximal endoscopy findings were normal.

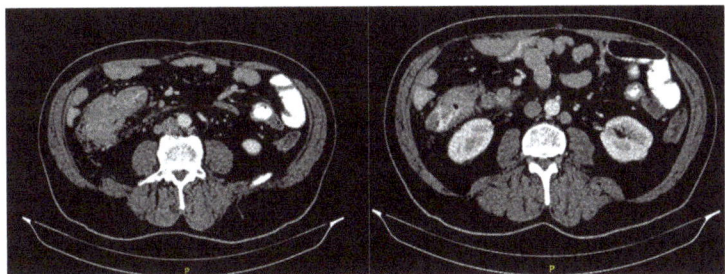

Figure 2. Abdominal CT scan showing tumor mass.

Colonoscopy was incomplete since it was performed only up to hepatic flexure. Further progression to CT-verified cecal infiltration was unsuccessful due to an abnormally long, large intestine (dolichocolon) and malignant rotation of the intestine. NMSE was performed in a retrograde approach in order to reach the ileocecal infiltration. A spiral enteroscope was used to examine the colon because of the abnormal tortuosity of the intestine due to a tumor of the ileocecal segment as well as dolichocolon. A series of light movements of the spiral enteroscope enabled passing through the lumen of the large bowel and reaching a region with circular infiltration that almost completely obstructed the lumen (Figure 3).

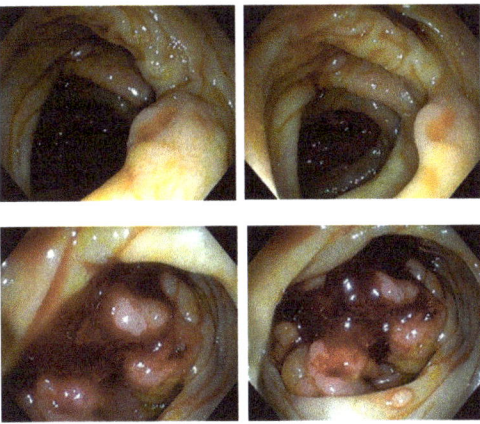

Figure 3. Endoscopic picture of cecal region tumor by Novel Motorised Spiral Enteroscope.

Six biopsies were taken and adenocarcinoma was pathohistologically confirmed (Figure 4). The patient was presented to a multidisciplinary team to decide on further treatment.

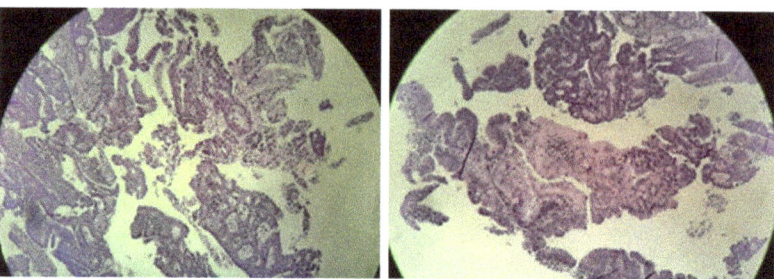

Figure 4. Microscopic images of cecal adenocarcinoma.

3. Discussion

The small bowel and ileocecal segment diseases accompanied by pathological intestinal tortuosity have always been a significant drawback for endoscopists. In the last two decades, with the introduction of DBE in 2001 and SBE in 2006, enteroscopic examination has significantly improved [1,19–21]. Video capsule endoscopy was found to be useful for the visualization of the entire small bowel. However, it does not allow the performing of therapeutic interventions and biopsies, which represents a significant limitation of this procedure [22]. The NMSE is a revolutionary endoscopic tool for the diagnosis and therapy of distant areas of the gastrointestinal tract that are inaccessible by proximal and distal endoscopy. Therefore, it is extremely useful for examination and interventions in the deep parts of the small bowel [23]. In this case, NMSE enabled a complete visualization of the colon and reached the ileocecal infiltration quickly and efficiently by "pleating" the abnormally long, tortuous colon. In addition, this technique allowed the performing of control movements of the endoscope and provided a more stable position for obtaining representative biopsies compared to the conventional colonoscope.

The available literature mainly deals with the usage of this procedure for the diagnosis and treatment of small bowel diseases since it has been primarily developed for that purpose. However, some authors have reported the benefits of using this technique in cases when conventional colonoscopy is unsuccessful.

In a recent study, the authors reported about 36 patients who had previously undergone incomplete diagnostic and/or therapeutic colonoscopies due to dolichocolon [12]. The cecal intubation rate was 100% and the median cecal intubation time was 10 min (range 4–30). The diagnostic yield was 64%, and neoplastic lesions were found in 23 patients. No adverse events were noted. They concluded that NMSE is an effective alternative for diagnostic and therapeutic colonoscopy in patients with dolichocolon. To the best of our knowledge, our case represents the first use of this device after an incomplete colonoscopy due to dolichocolon in our country and region.

Beyna et al. [24] evaluated the efficacy and safety of NMSE for diagnostic colonoscopy in 30 patients. Diverticulosis was the most common finding (43.3%) and the average procedure time was 20.8 min (range 11.4–55.3). No severe adverse events occurred. According to these results, NMSE is also considered safe and feasible for diagnostic colonoscopy.

In other studies, this procedure was mainly performed using anterograde and/or retrograde approaches in patients with gastrointestinal bleeding and unrevealing proximal and distal endoscopy and in cases when small bowel disease was suspected [25,26]. Prasad et al. [6] reported a case series of 14 patients in whom NMSE was performed in anterograde, retrograde, or both approaches, and the most common findings were strictures or ulcers of the jejunum and ileum. Ramchandani et al. [27] reported about 61 patients who underwent NMSE due to symptomatic small bowel disease. Total enteroscopy was performed in 60.6% of patients, for whom 29.5%, both anterograde and retrograde approaches were used. Singh et al. [28] evaluated 54 patients for small-bowel disease using NMSE. They have also used this technique in both anterograde and retrograde approaches. The retrograde approach was performed when the anterograde approach was contraindicated and in patients with previous imaging findings that showed suspected lesions within 150 cm of the ileocecal valve [28]. The average duration of a procedure performed in a retrograde approach was 35 min in a study by Ramchandi et al. and 90 min in a study by Prasad et al. [6,27].

Since NMSE is a new technology, data are lacking on its efficacy and safety in comparison with other endoscopic modalities. According to the literature, cecal intubation was achieved in 88–95% using DBE [29–31], 100% using short DBE [32], 93–100% for SBE [33–35], and 92% for manually driven spiral overtube-assisted colonoscopy [36]. The diagnostic yield of DBE was 68.1% [1,37] and for SBE, it was 47 to 60% [38–40]. The diagnostic and therapeutic yields of the NMSE were 80% and 86.7%, respectively [23].

In addition, recent research has shown that spiral enteroscopy could be an effective solution for ERCP in patients with altered gastrointestinal anatomy (after gastric and duodenal resection) and it could significantly shorten the time required to perform the procedure [41].

So far, rare adverse events associated with NMSE have been reported, including acute pancreatitis, perforations, and erosive lesions of the esophageal mucosa [24]. No adverse events were encountered in our case as well as in other recent studies and case reports [12,24,27]. However, Prasad et al. reported major adverse events, which included hypothermia (3 out of 14 patients) and pancreatitis (1 out of 14 patients) [6].

In this report, we aimed to highlight the possibility of performing NMSE in patients after unsuccessful conventional diagnostic or therapeutic colonoscopy, especially in patients with dolichocolon and suspected ileocecal disease. As already understood, failure to achieve cecal intubation during the examination of the colon increases the risk of missing a lesion, especially neoplasms in the inaccessible parts of the bowel. Therefore, the visualization of the entire colon is necessary and when it cannot be achieved during conventional colonoscopy, NMSE should be performed as a safe and effective alternative technique. It could be considered an alternative technique in patients who have undergone incomplete colonoscopy due to different causes, mainly in patients with a long, tortuous colon, presence of angulation or fixation of bowel loops, as well as adhesions due to previous surgeries. In these cases, NMSE is effective because it enables the straightening of the loops by pleating the bowel. This mechanism allows for the deeper advancement of the endoscope through the colon and provides a more stable position for the device while performing polypectomies and biopsies compared to a conventional colonoscope. This technique should not be applied in cases where strictures of the bowel are present and cause severe narrowing of the intestinal lumen. In these cases, if increased resistance is detected, spiral rotation is stopped automatically to avoid perforation. In addition, the larger caliber of the spiral overtube and the rigidity of the attachment segment can increase the risk of perforation.

Additional studies with a larger number of patients are needed to examine the safety and efficacy of NMSE and to compare this new technology with conventional colonoscopy and balloon-associated enteroscopy.

4. Conclusions

The NMSE is a procedure that enables both diagnostic and therapeutic interventions for small bowel diseases. However, this case report highlights the possibility of using this innovative tool as an alternative technique when the target lesion is difficult to access during conventional colonoscopy. Its advantages include a simplified technique performed by a single operator, a shorter time of examination, and the ability to perform both diagnostic and therapeutic interventions.

Author Contributions: Conceptualization, A.S.; methodology, A.S.; writing—original draft preparation, A.S. and A.D.; writing—review and editing, A.H.-S. All authors have read and agreed to the published version of the manuscript.

Funding: This research received no external funding.

Institutional Review Board Statement: The study was conducted in accordance with the Declaration of Helsinki.

Informed Consent Statement: Informed consent was obtained from the patient involved in the study.

Data Availability Statement: Not applicable.

Conflicts of Interest: The authors declare no conflict of interest.

References

1. Nehme, F.; Goyal, H.; Perisetti, A.; Tharian, B.; Sharma, N.; Tham, T.C.; Chhabra, R. The Evolution of Device-Assisted Enteroscopy: From Sonde Enteroscopy to Motorized Spiral Enteroscopy. *Front. Med.* **2021**, *8*, 792668. [CrossRef] [PubMed]
2. Schneider, M.; Höllerich, J.; Beyna, T. Device-assisted enteroscopy: A review of available techniques and upcoming new technologies. *World J. Gastroenterol.* **2019**, *25*, 3538–3545. [CrossRef] [PubMed]
3. Tsujikawa, T.; Saitoh, Y.; Andoh, A.; Imaeda, H.; Hata, K.; Minematsu, H.; Senoh, K.; Hayafuji, K.; Ogawa, A.; Nakahara, T.; et al. Novel single-balloon enteroscopy for diagnosis and treatment of the small intestine: Preliminary experiences. *Endoscopy* **2007**, *40*, 11–15. [CrossRef]
4. Yamamoto, H.; Sekine, Y.; Sato, Y.; Higashizawa, T.; Miyata, T.; Iino, S.; Ido, K.; Sugano, K. Total enteroscopy with a nonsurgical steerable double-balloon method. *Gastrointest. Endosc.* **2001**, *53*, 216–220. [CrossRef]
5. Hartmann, D.; Eickhoff, A.; Tamm, R.; Riemann, J.F. Balloon-assisted enteroscopy using a single-balloon technique. *Endoscopy* **2007**, *39*, E276. [CrossRef]
6. Prasad, M.; Prasad, V.M.; Sangameswaran, A.; Verghese, S.C.; Murthy, V.; Prasad, M.; Shanker, G.K.; Koppal, S. A spiraling journey into the small bowel: A case series of novel motorized power spiral enteroscopies. *VideoGIE* **2020**, *5*, 591–596. [CrossRef]
7. Ramchandani, M.; Reddy, D.N.; Gupta, R.; Lakhtakia, S.; Tandan, M.; Darisetty, S.; Rao, G.V. Spiral enteroscopy: A preliminary experience in Asian population. *J. Gastroenterol. Hepatol.* **2010**, *25*, 1754–1757. [CrossRef] [PubMed]
8. Akerman, P.A. Spiral enteroscopy versus double-balloon enteroscopy: Choosing the right tool for the job. *Gastrointest. Endosc.* **2013**, *77*, 252–254. [CrossRef]
9. Beyna, T.; Arvanitakis, M.; Schneider, M.; Hoellerich, J.; Deviere, J.; Neuhaus, H. 47 first prospective clinical trial on total motorized spiral enteroscopy (tmset). *Gastrointest. Endosc.* **2019**, *89*, AB48. [CrossRef]
10. Neuhaus, H.H.; Beyna, T.T.; Schneider, M.; Devière, J. Novel motorized spiral enteroscopy: First clinical case. *VideoGIE* **2016**, *1*, 32–33. [CrossRef] [PubMed]
11. Akerman, P.A.; Demarco, D.C.; Pangtay, J.; Pangtay-Chio, I. Tu1556 A Novel Motorized Spiral Enteroscope Can Advance Rapidly, Safely and Deeply Into the Small Bowel. *Gastrointest. Endosc.* **2011**, *73*, AB446. [CrossRef]
12. Al-Toma, A.; Hergelink, D.O.; van Noorden, J.T.; Koornstra, J.J. Prospective evaluation of the Motorized Spiral Enteroscope for previous incomplete colonoscopy. *Endosc. Int. Open* **2022**, *10*, E1112–E1117. [CrossRef]
13. Shah, H.A.; Paszat, L.F.; Saskin, R.; Stukel, T.; Rabeneck, L. Factors Associated With Incomplete Colonoscopy: A Population-Based Study. *Gastroenterology* **2007**, *132*, 2297–2303. [CrossRef]
14. Loffeld, R.J.L.F.; van der Putten, A.B.M.M. The Completion Rate of Colonoscopy in Normal Daily Practice: Factors Associated with Failure. *Digestion* **2009**, *80*, 267–270. [CrossRef]
15. Rex, D.K.; Schoenfeld, P.S.; Cohen, J.; Pike, I.M.; Adler, D.G.; Fennerty, M.B.; Lieb, J.G., 2nd; Park, W.G.; Rizk, M.K.; Sawhney, M.S.; et al. Quality indicators for colonoscopy. *Gastrointest. Endosc.* **2015**, *81*, 31–53. [CrossRef]
16. Anderson, J.C.; Gonzalez, J.D.; Messina, C.R.; Pollack, B.J. Factors that predict incomplete colonoscopy: Thinner is not always better. *Am. J. Gastroenterol.* **2000**, *95*, 2784–2787. [CrossRef]
17. Rex, D.K. Achieving cecal intubation in the very difficult colon. *Gastrointest. Endosc.* **2008**, *67*, 938–944. [CrossRef]
18. Neerincx, M.; Droste, J.S.T.S.; Mulder, C.J.J.; Räkers, M.; Bartelsman, J.F.W.M.; Loffeld, R.J.; Tuynman, H.A.R.E.; Brohet, R.M.; van der Hulst, R.W.M. Colonic work-up after incomplete colonoscopy: Significant new findings during follow-up. *Endoscopy* **2010**, *42*, 730–735. [CrossRef]
19. Yamamoto, H.; Ogata, H.; Matsumoto, T.; Ohmiya, N.; Ohtsuka, K.; Watanabe, K.; Yano, T.; Matsui, T.; Higuchi, K.; Nakamura, T.; et al. Clinical Practice Guideline for Enteroscopy. *Dig. Endosc.* **2017**, *29*, 519–546. [CrossRef]
20. Khashab, M.A.; Pasha, S.F.; Muthusamy, V.R.; Acosta, R.D.; Bruining, D.H.; Chandrasekhara, V.; Chathadi, K.V.; Eloubeidi, M.A.; Fanelli, R.D.; Faulx, A.L.; et al. The role of deep enteroscopy in the management of small-bowel disorders. *Gastrointest. Endosc.* **2015**, *82*, 600–607. [CrossRef]
21. Rahmi, G.; Samaha, E.; Vahedi, K.; Ponchon, T.; Fumex, F.; Filoche, B.; Gay, G.; Delvaux, M.; Lorenceau-Savale, C.; Malamut, G.; et al. Multicenter comparison of double-balloon enteroscopy and spiral enteroscopy. *J. Gastroenterol. Hepatol.* **2013**, *28*, 992–998. [CrossRef]
22. Iddan, G.; Meron, G.; Glukhovsky, A.; Swain, P. Wireless capsule endoscopy. *Nature* **2000**, *405*, 417. [CrossRef]
23. Beyna, T.; Arvanitakis, M.; Schneider, M.; Gerges, C.; Hoellerich, J.; Devière, J.; Neuhaus, H. Total motorized spiral enteroscopy: First prospective clinical feasibility trial. *Gastrointest. Endosc.* **2021**, *93*, 1362–1370. [CrossRef]

24. Beyna, T.; Schneider, M.; Pullmann, D.; Gerges, C.; Kandler, J.; Neuhaus, H. Motorized spiral colonoscopy: A first single-center feasibility trial. *Endoscopy* **2017**, *50*, 518–523. [CrossRef]
25. Mans, L.; Arvanitakis, M.; Neuhaus, H.; Devière, J. Motorised spiral enteroscopy for occult bleeding. *Dig. Dis.* **2018**, *36*, 325–327. [CrossRef]
26. Tang, R.S.Y.; Wong, M.T.L.; Lai, J.C.T.; Chiu, P.W.Y. Total enteroscopy by antegrade motorized spiral enteroscopy under conscious sedation for acute overt obscure gastrointestinal bleeding. *Endoscopy* **2020**, *52*, E251–E252. [CrossRef]
27. Ramchandani, M.; Rughwani, H.; Inavolu, P.; Singh, A.P.; Tevethia, H.V.; Jagtap, N.; Sekaran, A.; Kanakagiri, H.; Darishetty, S.; Reddy, D.N. Diagnostic yield and therapeutic impact of novel motorized spiral enteroscopy in small-bowel disorders: A single-center, real-world experience from a tertiary care hospital (with video). *Gastrointest. Endosc.* **2020**, *93*, 616–626. [CrossRef]
28. Singh, P.; Singla, V.; Bopanna, S.; Shawl, M.R.; Garg, P.; Agrawal, J.; Arya, A.; Mittal, V.; Bhargava, R.; Madan, K. Safety and efficacy of the novel motorized power spiral enteroscopy: A single-center experience. *DEN Open* **2022**, *3*, e148. [CrossRef]
29. Suzuki, T.; Matsushima, M.; Tsukune, Y.; Fujisawa, M.; Yazaki, T.; Uchida, T.; Gocyo, S.; Okita, I.; Shirakura, K.; Sasao, K.; et al. Double-balloon endoscopy versus magnet-imaging enhanced colonoscopy for difficult colonoscopies, a randomized study. *Endoscopy* **2012**, *44*, 38–42. [CrossRef]
30. Pasha, S.F.; Harrison, M.E.; Das, A.; Corrado, C.M.; Arnell, K.N.; Leighton, J.A. Utility of double-balloon colonoscopy for completion of colon examination after incomplete colonoscopy with conventional colonoscope. *Gastrointest. Endosc.* **2007**, *65*, 848–853. [CrossRef]
31. Moreels, T.G.; Macken, E.J.; Roth, B.; Van Outryve, M.J.; Pelckmans, P.A. Cecal intubation rate with the double-balloon endoscope after incomplete conventional colonoscopy: A study in 45 patients. *J. Gastroenterol. Hepatol.* **2010**, *25*, 80–83. [CrossRef] [PubMed]
32. Hotta, K.; Katsuki, S.; Ohata, K.; Abe, T.; Endo, M.; Shimatani, M.; Nagaya, T.; Kusaka, T.; Matsuda, T.; Uraoka, T.; et al. A multicenter, prospective trial of total colonoscopy using a short double-balloon endoscope in patients with previous incomplete colonoscopy. *Gastrointest. Endosc.* **2012**, *75*, 813–818. [CrossRef] [PubMed]
33. Teshima, C.W.; Aktas, H.; Haringsma, J.; Kuipers, E.J.; Mensink, P.B. Single-balloon-assisted colonoscopy in patients with previously failed colonoscopy. *Gastrointest. Endosc.* **2010**, *71*, 1319–1323. [CrossRef] [PubMed]
34. Dzeletovic, I.; Harrison, M.E.; Pasha, S.F.; Crowell, M.D.; Decker, G.A.; Gurudu, S.R.; Leighton, J.A. Comparison of Single- Versus Double-Balloon Assisted-Colonoscopy for Colon Examination After Previous Incomplete Standard Colonoscopy. *Dig. Dis. Sci.* **2012**, *57*, 2680–2686. [CrossRef]
35. Keswani, R.N. Single-balloon colonoscopy versus repeat standard colonoscopy for previous incomplete colonoscopy: A randomized, controlled trial. *Gastrointest. Endosc.* **2011**, *73*, 507–512. [CrossRef] [PubMed]
36. Schembre, D.B.; Ross, A.S.; Gluck, M.N.; Brandabur, J.J.; McCormick, S.E.; Lin, O.S. Spiral overtube–assisted colonoscopy after incomplete colonoscopy in the redundant colon. *Gastrointest. Endosc.* **2011**, *73*, 515–519. [CrossRef] [PubMed]
37. Xin, L.; Liao, Z.; Jiang, Y.-P.; Li, Z.-S. Indications, detectability, positive findings, total enteroscopy, and complications of diagnostic double-balloon endoscopy: A systematic review of data over the first decade of use. *Gastrointest. Endosc.* **2011**, *74*, 563–570. [CrossRef]
38. Lenz, P.; Domagk, D. Double- vs. single-balloon vs. spiral enteroscopy. *Best Pract. Res. Clin. Gastroenterol.* **2012**, *26*, 303–313. [CrossRef]
39. Takano, N.; Yamada, A.; Watabe, H.; Togo, G.; Yamaji, Y.; Yoshida, H.; Kawabe, T.; Omata, M.; Koike, K. Single-balloon versus double-balloon endoscopy for achieving total enteroscopy: A randomized, controlled trial. *Gastrointest. Endosc.* **2011**, *73*, 734–739. [CrossRef]
40. Khashab, M.A.; Lennon, A.M.; Dunbar, K.B.; Singh, V.K.; Chandrasekhara, V.; Giday, S.; Canto, M.I.; Buscaglia, J.M.; Kapoor, S.; Shin, E.J.; et al. A comparative evaluation of single-balloon enteroscopy and spiral enteroscopy for patients with mid-gut disorders. *Gastrointest. Endosc.* **2010**, *72*, 766–772. [CrossRef]
41. Beyna, T.; Schneider, M.; Höllerich, J.; Neuhaus, H. Motorized spiral enteroscopy–assisted ERCP after Roux-en-Y reconstructive surgery and bilioenteric anastomosis: First clinical case. *VideoGIE* **2020**, *5*, 311–313. [CrossRef] [PubMed]

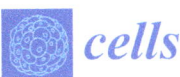

Article

COVID-19 Pathology in the Lung, Kidney, Heart and Brain: The Different Roles of T-Cells, Macrophages, and Microthrombosis

Tino Emanuele Poloni [1,2,*,†], Matteo Moretti [3,†], Valentina Medici [1], Elvira Turturici [1], Giacomo Belli [3], Elena Cavriani [3], Silvia Damiana Visonà [3], Michele Rossi [4], Valentina Fantini [5], Riccardo Rocco Ferrari [5], Arenn Faye Carlos [1], Stella Gagliardi [6], Livio Tronconi [3,7], Antonio Guaita [1,4,5] and Mauro Ceroni [1,6]

1. Department of Neurology and Neuropathology, Golgi-Cenci Foundation, Abbiategrasso, 20081 Milan, Italy
2. Department of Rehabilitation, ASP Golgi-Redaelli, Abbiategrasso, 20081 Milan, Italy
3. Department of Public Health, Experimental and Forensic Medicine, University of Pavia, 27100 Pavia, Italy
4. Unit of Biostatistics, Golgi-Cenci Foundation, Abbiategrasso, 20081 Milan, Italy
5. Laboratory of Neurobiology and Neurogenetic, Golgi-Cenci Foundation, Abbiategrasso, 20081 Milan, Italy
6. Unit of Molecular Biology and Transcriptomics IRCCS Mondino Foundation, 27100 Pavia, Italy
7. Department of Forensic Medicine, IRCCS Mondino Foundation, 27100 Pavia, Italy
* Correspondence: e.poloni@golgicenci.it; Tel.: +39-029466409; Fax: +39-0294608148
† These authors contributed equally to this work.

Abstract: Here, we aim to describe COVID-19 pathology across different tissues to clarify the disease's pathophysiology. Lungs, kidneys, hearts, and brains from nine COVID-19 autopsies were compared by using antibodies against SARS-CoV-2, macrophages-microglia, T-lymphocytes, B-lymphocytes, and activated platelets. Alzheimer's Disease pathology was also assessed. PCR techniques were used to verify the presence of viral RNA. COVID-19 cases had a short clinical course (0–32 days) and their mean age was 77.4 y/o. Hypoxic changes and inflammatory infiltrates were present across all tissues. The lymphocytic component in the lungs and kidneys was predominant over that of other tissues ($p < 0.001$), with a significantly greater presence of T-lymphocytes in the lungs ($p = 0.020$), which showed the greatest presence of viral antigens. The heart showed scant SARS-CoV-2 traces in the endothelium–endocardium, foci of activated macrophages, and rare lymphocytes. The brain showed scarce SARS-CoV-2 traces, prominent microglial activation, and rare lymphocytes. The pons exhibited the highest microglial activation ($p = 0.017$). Microthrombosis was significantly higher in COVID-19 lungs ($p = 0.023$) compared with controls. The most characteristic pathological features of COVID-19 were an abundance of T-lymphocytes and microthrombosis in the lung and relevant microglial hyperactivation in the brainstem. This study suggests that the long-term sequelae of COVID-19 derive from persistent inflammation, rather than persistent viral replication.

Keywords: COVID-19; SARS-CoV-2; lung; kidney; heart; brain; inflammation; elderly; neuropathology

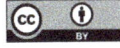

1. Introduction

Coronaviruses (CoVs) are enveloped, positive-sense, single-stranded RNA viruses. They are characterized by frequent genomic recombination, high prevalence, and wide distribution, and they typically infect the respiratory and digestive tracts of several animal species, as well as humans. In certain geographical areas, the close interface between humans and animals facilitates zoonotic transmissions, resulting in the emergence of new human CoVs [1]. Common human CoVs include two alpha-CoVs (HCoV-229E and HCoV-NL63) and two beta-CoVs (HCoV-OC43 and HCoV-HKU1) which cause mild, self-limiting upper-respiratory-tract infections [2]. Contrarily, SARS-CoV and MERS-CoV are two highly pathogenic beta-CoVs, which have been identified as the etiologic agents of SARS (severe acute respiratory syndrome) and MERS (middle east respiratory syndrome) outbreaks in 2002 and 2012, respectively. In autumn 2019, an outbreak of severe pneumonia of unidentified etiology was reported in Wuhan, Hubei Province, China. On 9 January 2020, China announced the identification of a novel beta-CoV as the etiologic agent of the outbreak. The virus was subsequently named SARS-CoV-2 by the International Committee on Taxonomy of Viruses. It causes a systemic disease identified as coronavirus 2019 disease (COVID-19). The mortality rates due to SARS-CoV (9.6%) and MERS-CoV (34.3%) are significantly higher than that of SARS-CoV-2 infection (4.4%), but the latter is more easily transmittable, which explains its rapid spread and the massive number of cases worldwide [3]. SARS-CoV-2 represents a "perfect pandemic virus", surpassing SARS-CoV and MERS-CoV in terms of infected people, geographical expansion, and deaths [4]. On 1 March 2020, COVID-19 was declared a pandemic by the World Health Organization (WHO) and remains to this day a global threat to public health (WHO-March 2020). By August 2022, there had been 589,680,368 confirmed cases of COVID-19, with 6,436,519 deaths reported to the WHO (https://covid19.who.int/ accessed on 20 August 2022). Although the respiratory system is undoubtedly the main target of SARS-CoV-2, the infection is characterized by a broad spectrum of clinical manifestations denoting a multiple-organ disease, which has been confirmed by pathologic studies [5–8]. The involvement of different organs and extent of the lesions can be considered reliable prognostic factors for adverse outcomes in COVID-19 patients and for the development of post-acute COVID-19 syndrome [9]. Indeed, post-acute COVID-19 syndrome, divided into subacute or ongoing symptomatic COVID-19 (4–12 weeks after disease onset) and chronic or post-COVID syndrome (beyond 12 weeks), may affect the lungs, kidneys, heart, and brain with variable severity [9]. Pulmonary outcomes range from a chronic cough to respiratory insufficiency due to fibrosis [10], renal dysfunction may persist and lead to chronic kidney disease [11], heart complications include arrhythmias and heart failure [10,12], and the so-called "brain fog" affects cognitive functions after the acute phase of the disease [13].

Damage to the lungs is typically marked by diffuse alveolar damage (DAD) of variable degrees and stages (acute–proliferative–fibrotic), with edema and hyaline membrane formation, cytopathic features, and hyperplasia of type-2 pneumocytes, and the presence of SARS-CoV-2 antigens, accompanied by macrophage and lymphocyte infiltration, organizing pneumonia, and frequent superimposed bacterial infection. Moreover, vascular damage is often described with the formation of microthrombi and thrombi, hemorrhagic infarctions, and pulmonary thrombo-embolism [3,14–24]. DAD is a key pathophysiological mechanism of lung damage in SARS-CoV-2 infection that is present in 88% of cases; however, it is not pathognomonic for COVID-19. Indeed, DAD with prominent hyaline membrane formation is also very frequent in SARS-CoV (98%) and influenza A/H1N1 (90% in the 2009 pandemic). On the other hand, micro-thrombotic disease has been reported with a similarly high prevalence among COVID-19 (57%) and SARS (58%) cases, while it is lower for H1N1 (24%) flu cases [25].

At the kidney level, the main histological findings are acute tubular injury, inflammatory infiltrates, and microvascular occlusion of glomerular and peritubular capillaries, frequently accompanied by arteriolosclerosis and glomerular degeneration (pre-existing chronic renal disease). Transmission electron microscopy has revealed the presence of viral particles in the tubular epithelium and podocytes [8,22,23,26,27].

Regarding the heart, the most common findings are pericarditis and myocarditis with inflammatory foci associated with myocyte injury and fibrosis that may also reflect a pre-existing disease [15,16,21,23,28–30]. In the heart, there are only scarce molecular traces of SARS-CoV-2 [31], while macrophage infiltration is predominant with a low number of lymphocytes [32]. Other authors have reported a predominance of thrombosis and micro-thrombosis leading to ischemic injury [30,33].

From a neuropathologic standpoint, a wide range of changes are observed. In almost all postmortem evaluations, brain congestion, edema, and neuronal loss caused by severe hypoxic phenomena due to pulmonary and heart complications have been observed. Moreover, inflammatory processes are frequently described, including acute disseminated encephalomyelitis (ADEM)-like features and different patterns of immune-induced meningoencephalitis with meningeal, perivascular, or parenchymal lympho-monocytic infiltrates, while the presence of SARS-CoV-2 in the brain remains controversial. Microglial activation with microglial nodules is often detected. In this regard, it should be considered that the elderly population is the most affected by the severe form of COVID-19, and many patients had pre-existing neurocognitive disorders; thus, brain inflammation changes and consequent neurological manifestations may be greatly influenced by the presence of microglial "priming" due to neurodegeneration [34–44]. Vascular injuries of either the ischemic or hemorrhagic type are also reported, including macroscopic and microscopic lesions caused by clotting alterations and/or endotheliitis [35,37,40–42,45–47].

Although the liver is one of the most important immunological organs in the body and alterations in liver parameters are frequently reported in COVID-19, especially in severe cases, the pathological findings are non-specific and the impairment of liver function does not appear clinically relevant in SARS-CoV-2 infection [48–50].

Many assume the presence of active viral replication, not only in the lungs, but also in other organs [51–53], probably depending on the differential expression of angiotensin-converting enzyme 2 (ACE-2) receptors and TMPRSS-2 transmembrane protease, which are the main cellular factors involved in viral entry [54]. COVID-19 induces multi-organ damage, the pathological aspects of which are essential for understanding the pathophysiology of the acute disease, as well as its long-term manifestations. Nonetheless, comparative studies between the various organs involved are still lacking. The aims of this work are: (1) to describe how the above-mentioned organs are involved and how SARS-CoV-2 spreads and persists throughout the organism; (2) to compare the inflammatory infiltrates of the lungs, the organ massively affected by the viral invasion, with those of the kidneys, heart, and brain, which are non-primary targets for the virus; (3) to emphasize the pathological features specific for SARS-CoV-2 infection through a comparison between COVID-19 and non-COVID lungs, and between COVID-19 brains with and without neurodegenerative burden (i.e., Alzheimer's disease—AD pathology) and non-COVID brains with and without AD pathology; and (4) to investigate the role of microthrombosis.

2. Materials & Methods

2.1. Study Design, Setting, Participants, and Clinical Data

This is an observational study based on a cross-sectional analysis of clinical and pathological data from COVID-19 cases. The study comprises patients from elderly care units who died during the first tumultuous pandemic peak. Most of them were not hospitalized, and the availability of blood tests is scant; thus, the information obtained through a retrospective review of medical records is limited to clinical data. COVID-19 cases were subjected to forensic autopsies, ordered by the Prosecutor. Human autopsy samples were harvested and provided by the Unit of Legal Medicine and Forensic Sciences (Department of Public Health, Experimental and Forensic Medicine, University of Pavia, Pavia, Italy). All consecutive COVID-19 autopsies performed between 17 April and 4 June 2020 were considered for this study. The inclusion criteria were: (1) SARS-CoV-2 infection (Delta-variant) confirmed by a positive pharyngeal swab and (2) continuous refrigeration of the cadaver at 4 °C leading to the time of autopsy with adequate tissue preservation for histological multi-organ comparison, including the brain. Of the 15 COVID-19 autopsies performed, 9 were selected, while 6 were excluded for inadequate preservation of the brain tissue. Owing to the presence of cognitive disturbances in over half of the cases, and the fact that these disturbances worsened during COVID-19, we chose to also evaluate the presence of AD neuropathology. In addition, 10 matched controls were studied: for lung comparison, 5 cases with non-COVID pneumonia were selected from the Unit of Legal Medicine, while, for neuropathological comparison, 5 non-COVID brains were selected from the Abbiategrasso Brain Bank (ABB) at the Golgi-Cenci Foundation (Abbiategrasso, Milan, Italy), including 3 cases with AD pathology and 2 with no AD pathology. A retrospective review of medical charts was performed by two forensic medical doctors, a geriatrician, and a neurologist in order to ascertain the clinical history of the selected cases. The patients were clinically defined for the presence or absence of comorbidities, dementia, delirium, and sepsis. The DSM-5 criteria were used to define the mental state and identify any pre-existing cognitive dysfunction, namely major neurocognitive disorder (major-NCD) to indicate dementia and mild-NCD to designate mild cognitive impairment (MCI). Sepsis was considered a severe bacterial superinfection with at least one positive blood culture.

2.2. Autopsies and Sampling of the Organs

All autopsies were conducted respecting all the recommendations for forensic autopsy in SARS-CoV-2 infected cadavers [55]. All tissue samples were harvested and processed as previously described [34,56]. Briefly, the sampling protocol for pathological examination included 1 section per each pulmonary lobe; 5 heart sections from a mid-horizontal slice (anterior and posterior right ventricle, septum, left ventricle, and 1 epicardial coronary); and 1 section from each kidney, including the cortex and medulla (The Royal College of Pathologists 2020) [57]. For the neuropathological characterization, a total of 7 sections were considered: frontal, temporal, parietal, and occipital lobes; hippocampus–entorhinal cortex; pons; and the cerebellum. Before fixation, a small portion from the fronto-basal region was frozen for quantitative Reverse-Transcription–PCR (qRT-PCR) and droplet digital PCR (ddPCR) analysis in order to detect viral RNA [58]. The liver, hypophysis, thyroid, spleen, adrenal glands, uterus, or prostate, besides the brain, lungs, heart, and kidneys, were also included in the routine histopathological examination. Upon Hematoxylin–Eosin (H&E) staining, we did not observe any peculiar features that could be related to COVID-19. Moreover, the subjects of the present study did not show any clinical signs related to a possible liver failure or impairment. Therefore, despite the liver being one of the most important organs of the body, we chose to perform the study on the brain, lungs, heart, and kidneys, for which the clinical picture and the routinary H&E staining provided the most interesting results.

In accordance with Italian Law, this research was performed on small portions of biological samples routinely taken during autopsies that had already been examined for diagnostic and/or forensic purposes. The subjects of the study were kept anonymous. The reference law is the authorization n9/2016 of the guarantor of privacy, then replaced by Regulation (EU) 2016/679 of the European Parliament and of the Council. The ABB autopsy and sampling protocol [59] were approved by the Ethics Committee of the University of Pavia on 6 October 2009 (Committee report 3/2009).

2.3. Histology and Immunohistochemistry

All sections were compared for morphology using Hematoxylin–Eosin (H&E) staining. Alzheimer's Disease (AD) severity was assessed on sections immunostained with antibodies against beta-amyloid (4G8, monoclonal antibody, BioLegend San Diego, CA, USA; 1:1000) and phospho-tau (AT8, monoclonal antibody, clone MN1020, Thermo Fisher Scientific Waltham, MA, USA; 1:200) and defined according to Montine's scheme (low-intermediate–high AD pathology) [60].

To assess SARS-CoV-2 presence, inflammatory infiltrates, and microthrombi, the following anatomical regions were considered: inferior left lung lobe, right kidney, left heart ventricle, frontal lobe (gray–white matter) for the forebrain, and pons for the hindbrain. Antibodies against the following antigens were used: SARS-CoV-2 nucleocapsid (monoclonal antibody, clone B46F, and Invitrogen Waltham, MA USA; 1:100), CD68 (monocytes and activated macrophages: polyclonal antibody and Invitrogen; 1:500—brain microglia:monoclonal antibody clone KP1, and Dako Santa Clara, CA 95051 United States; 1:100), CD3 (T-lymphocytes: monoclonal antibody, clone SP7, and Invitrogen; 1:200—brain: monoclonal antibody, clone F7.2.38, and Dako; 1:50), CD20 (B-lymphocytes: polyclonal antibody and Invitrogen; 1:300—brain: monoclonal antibody, clone L26, and Dako; 1:100), CD42b (activated platelets: monoclonal antibody, clone 42C01, and Invitrogen; 1:100), and GFAP (astrocytes: polyclonal antibody, and Dako Z0334; 1:1000).

The most affected sections were chosen among all of the anatomical regions; successively, low magnification (4×) was used to explore the slide and higher magnifications

(10–20×) to investigate the morphological aspects. For each representative slide, 5 areas of 4.7 mm^2 were evaluated (the 4 corners and the center). In order to characterize the infiltrate, the most affected area was selected for scoring. To grade the reactions, comparable semi-quantitative 4-point scoring systems (0–3) were used. To quantify the presence of lymphocytes and monocyte–macrophages in the different infiltrates of the various tissues, we effectively applied the method described by Matschke and colleagues based on cell counts: 0/4.7 mm^2 = 0, none; 1–9/4.7 mm^2 = 1, mild; 10–49/4.7 mm^2 = 2, moderate; and >49/4.7 mm^2 = 3, severe [35]. To evaluate the activation of brain microglia, we applied the 0–3 scoring method already consolidated in our laboratory [34]. To quantify the microthrombi, the thrombosed capillaries were counted (0/4.7 mm^2 = 0, none; 1/4.7 mm^2 = 1, mild; 2/4.7 mm^2 = 2, moderate; and ≥3/4.7 mm^2 = 3, severe). Scores of 0–1 (none-mild) were considered not relevant in all tissues and reactions, while scores of 2–3 represented a moderate to severe pathological alteration. Two neurologists with expertise in neuropathology and two pathologists blinded to the clinical history performed the pathological assessment. Whenever discrepancies between the gradings emerged, the area was reassessed together until an agreement was reached.

2.4. Statistical Analysis

All statistical analyses were conducted using R (version 4.2.1; R Core Team; R Foundation, Released 2021, Vienna, Austria). *p*-values of < 0.05 were considered significant. Given the ordinal nature of the scores and the low number of cases, a nonparametric statistical test was used. The T and B lymphocyte sum was considered as a further variable. Friedman's test with Durbin–Conover pairwise comparison was used to compare the different tissues within subjects (R package PMCMR). Score differences between the cases and controls for each organ were compared using the Mann–Whitney U test.

3. Results
3.1. General and Clinical Characteristics

The demographic and clinical features of the study participants are shown in Table 1. The nine COVID-19 patients (four females and five males) died 0 to 32 days after diagnosis (mean: 10 days). At death, their mean age was 77.4 (range: 29–94), and the mean post mortem interval was 7 days (range: 3–13). All subjects, except for patient COV2 (a previously healthy young man), had several comorbidities of varying severity, including pulmonary diseases, hypertension, diabetes, obesity, and cancer. None of them had severe heart failure. Six had a history of NCD (four major-NCD and two mild-NCD), five of whom had a clinical course complicated by delirium (three as the first COVID-19 symptom). The other three were cognitively normal. All cases developed severe lymphopenia and typical symptoms (fever–cough–dyspnea), except for the COV2 case, who was asymptomatic and died from hemorrhagic shock due to accidental trauma. Three had sepsis before death and only one was treated in an intensive care unit; however, none of them underwent orotracheal intubation (Table 1). The five cases with non-COVID pneumonia (from the Institute of Legal Medicine) and the five non-COVID ABB controls were matched for age and comorbidities. These subjects died of either of the following: pneumonia–pulmonary failure, heart failure, cachexia due to terminal dementia, or cancer.

Table 1. General and clinical information.

Code	PMD (Days/Hours)	General and Clinical Features					
		Sex	Age (y/o)	Anamnesis; Cause of Death	NCD	DEL	SEP
COV2	7 d	M	29	NR; hemorrhagic shock	no	no	no
COV4	5 d	M	67	Obesity, HTN, and CVD; CIP and respiratory failure	no	no	yes

Table 1. Cont.

Code	PMD (Days/Hours)	Sex	Age (y/o)	Anamnesis; Cause of Death	NCD	DEL	SEP
COV6	11 d	F	90	HTN and COPD; respiratory failure	no	no	no
COV3	7 d	M	87	T2D and CVD; respiratory failure	Mild (VCI)	Hyper/Hypo (early onset)	no
COV10	7 d	M	81	AF and paraparesis (previous GBS); respiratory failure	Mild (VCI)	Hypo (late onset)	yes
COV1	7 d	F	74	NR; respiratory failure	Major (AD)	Hyper (early onset)	no
COV5	3 d	F	94	T2D, HTN, CVD, and AF; multiorgan failure	Major (AD + VaD)	Hypo (early onset)	yes
COV8	13 d	F	83	HTN; respiratory failure	Major (AD)	no	no
COV9	6 d	M	92	HTN and cerebrovascular disease; respiratory failure	Major (AD + VaD)	Hyper/Hypo (late onset)	no
L1	4 d	F	76	AF; multiorgan failure 7 days after head trauma	no	no	no
L2	5 d	M	92	HTN CVD, and cerebrovascular disease; respiratory failure	Major (VaD)	Hypo (late onset)	no
L3	6 d	F	60	CVD; multiorgan failure 3 days after head trauma	no	no	no
L4	4 d	M	62	HTN; respiratory failure	no	no	yes
L5	8 d	M	74	HTN and COPD; multiorgan failure 10 days after intestinal perforation	Major (AD + VaD)	Hypo (late onset)	yes
B1	3 h	M	79	T2D; liver cancer	no	no	no
B2	8 h	M	79	HTN, CVD, and cerebrovascular disease; cachexia	Mild (VCI) and hemiparesis	no	no
B3	16 h	F	83	HTN, CVD, and cerebrovascular disease; CHF	Major (AD + VaD)	no	no
B4	15 h	F	85	CVD and cerebrovascular disease; CHF	Major (AD + VaD)	Hyper (prev. ep)	no
B5	15 h	F	89	HTN, COPD, and cerebrovascular disease; cachexia	Major (AD)	Hyper (prev. ep)	no

Note: COVID-19 cases are labeled as 'COV', control cases are identified as 'B' (Brain Bank) for brain and L (lung control) for lungs; PMD was measured in days (d) or hours (h). Abbreviations (in alphabetical order): AD, Alzheimer's disease; AF, atrial fibrillation; CHF, chronic heart failure; COPD, chronic obstructive pulmonary disease; CVD, cardiovascular disease; DEL, delirium; GBS, Guillain Barre Syndrome; HTN, hypertension; n/a, not available; NCD, neurocognitive disorder; NR, nothing relevant in medical history; PMD, post mortem delay; prev. ep., previous episode; SEP, sepsis; T2D, type 2 diabetes; VaD, vascular dementia; VCI, mild vascular cognitive impairment.

3.2. Pathological Findings in COVID-19 Cases

The general and specific pathological findings of the COVID-19 cases are summarized in Table 2, and their most representative histological details are displayed in Figure 1.

The lung samples showed: (1) severe capillary congestion, edema, and DAD with cytopathic alterations in type-2 pneumocytes; (2) SARS-CoV-2 positivity in alveolar pneumocytes of five cases, ubiquitous alveolar macrophages, interstitial pneumonia with fibrosis and moderate to severe inflammatory septal infiltrates (mainly T-lymphocytes, present in all cases), and frequent superimposed bacterial infection; and (3) microthrombi and frequent clots inside the vessels in seven cases.

Findings from the kidneys included: (1) congestion and acute glomerular alterations in three cases; (2) SARS-CoV-2 positivity in the tubular epithelium and the capillary endothelium in three cases, and moderate to severe inflammatory infiltrates (T-lymphocytes and B-lymphocytes in the majority of cases, while macrophages were quite rare in all but one case); and (3) microthrombi and clots in two cases.

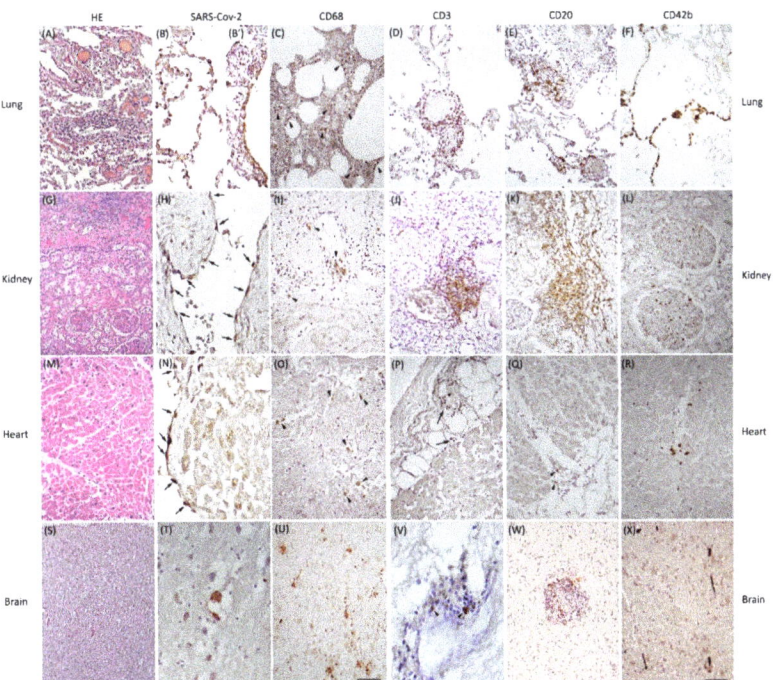

Figure 1. Pathological features of COVID-19. In the lung, H&E revealed severe congestion, diffuse alveolar damage, and interstitial pneumonia presenting as septal infiltrate shown in the middle of the image (**A**); SARS-CoV-2 positivity is evident in alveolar pneumocytes showing cytopathic features (**B**) and in the bronchiolar ciliated epithelium (**B'**); diffuse interstitial macrophages detected by CD68 antibody (**C**, arrowheads); T-lymphocyte (**D**) and B-lymphocyte (**E**) infiltrates are revealed by CD3 and CD20 reactions, respectively; CD42b marks several microthrombi in capillary and interstitial vessels characterized by a "rosary crown" feature (**F**). In the kidney, H&E labeled acute glomerular alterations in the lower part of the image and inflammatory infiltrates at the top (**G**); SARS-CoV-2 immunoreactivity detectable in some vascular endothelial cells (**H**, arrows); occasional foci of macrophages detected by the CD68 antibody (**I**, arrowheads); as in the lung, T-lymphocyte (**J**) and B-lymphocyte (**K**) infiltrates are revealed by CD3 and CD20 reactions, respectively; occasional microthrombi in the glomerular capillary are marked by CD42b antibody (**L**). In the heart, H&E stained parenchymal dissociation and myocyte vacuolization in the upper part of the image (**M**); rare SARS-CoV-2 traces observed in the endocardium (**N**, arrows); occasional foci of interstitial macrophages labeled by the CD68 antibody (**O**, arrowheads), rare subepicardial T-lymphocyte (**P**, arrows) and B-lymphocyte (**Q**, arrowheads) infiltrates revealed by CD3 and CD20 reactions in the upper and lower parts of the images, respectively; CD42b antibody marks focal and sporadic capillary microthrombi (**R**). In the brain, H&E revealed diffuse neuronal loss and cortical edema characterized by spongiosis (**S**); very rare SARS-CoV-2-positive cells detected in the pons (**T**); amoeboid microglial cells and several microglial nodules identified by the CD68 antibody, mainly in the brainstem (**U**); rare T and B lymphocytes are observed in the perivascular spaces (**V**) and in some nodules (**W**); frequent capillary microthrombi are observed in the brainstem (**X**). Scale bars: 230 μm (**S**); 162 μm (**G**); 140 μm (**C,U**); 75 μm (**A,E,F,K,M,P,W**); 64 μm (**D,I,O,Q,R,X**); 60 μm (**J**); 52 μm (**L**); 44 μm (**B'**); 39 μm (**B**); and 30 μm (**H,N,V,T**).

Table 2. Pathological data. *Acute alterations*: AE, acute emphysema; AGA, acute glomerular alterations; AH, alveolar hemorrhage; BS, bacterial superimposition; C, congestion; DAD, diffuse alveolar damage; E, edema; HA, hypoxic alterations (congestion, edema, spongiosis, and neuronal loss); IF, inflammatory foci; MA, myocyte alterations (parenchymal dissociation and/or wavy fibers); MV, myocyte vacuolization; RA, reactive astrocytes. *Chronic alterations*: A, anthracosis; AD, Alzheimer's disease; AS, atherosclerosis; CE, chronic emphysema; CH, cardiomyocyte hypertrophy; F, fibrosis; GS, glomerulosclerosis; SVD, small-vessel disease. *Markers*: AP and BL activated platelets (CD42b) and B-lymphocytes (CD20); M, macrophage/microglia (CD68); TL, T-lymphocytes (CD3); VA, viral (SARS-CoV-2) antigen; Vd, viral droplet digital polymerase chain reaction (ddPCR); Vr, viral real-time polymerase chain reaction (RT-PCR). n/a, not available; +, present; -, absent. -, COVID-19 cases are labeled as 'COV', control cases are identified as 'B' (Brain Bank) for brain and L (lung control) for lungs.

	General Pathological Features				Specific Pathological Features																										
	Lung (Acute; chronic findings)	Kidney (Acute; chronic findings)	Heart (Acute; chronic findings)	Brain (Acute; chronic findings)	Lung						Kidney						Heart						Brain-Frontal Lobe							Brain-Pons		
CASE					M	TL	BL	AP	VA		M	TL	BL	AP	VA		M	TL	BL	AP	VA		M	TL	BL	AP	VA	Vr	Vd	M	TL	BL	AP	VA
COV2	Mild C, AE, interstitial-subpleural IF; F, CE, A	Severe C	MA	HA; no AD, no SVD, mild gliosis-RA					+						-						-						-	n/a	n/a					-
COV4	Severe C, interstitial-subpleural AH, AE, E, DAD, BS, IF; CE, A	Severe C, cortical-medullary IF; GS	MV, BS, MA, Subepicardial IF; F, CH	HA; no AD, SVD, mild gliosis					-						-						-						-	-	-					-
COV6	AE, E, interstitial IF; F, A	Cortical IF; F	Mild C	HA; low AD, mild gliosis					-						-						-						-	-	-					-
COV3	Severe C, AE, DAD, interstitial IF; AS, CE, A	Severe C, AGA, cortical-medullary IF; F, AS, GS	MV, MA; F, AS	HA; low AD, SVD, mild gliosis					+						-						+						-	-	+					+
COV10	Severe C, AE, BS, interstitial IF; AS	Severe C, AGA; F	MA, interstitial-subepicardial IF; F	HA; no AD, SVD, perivascular gliosis					+						-						-						-	-	+					-
COV1	C, AE, AH, E, DAD, BS, interstitial IF; F, CE	Cortical IF; F, GS	MA, BS; F	HA; high AD, perivascular gliosis					+						+						-						-	-	-					-
COV5	Severe C, AH, AE, E, DAD, BS, interstitial IF; A, CE	Severe C, cortical-IF, AGA, GS	MV, MA, subepicardial IF; F, CH	HA; intermediate AD, SVD, mild gliosis-RA					+						+						-						-	-	+					-

Table 2. *Cont.*

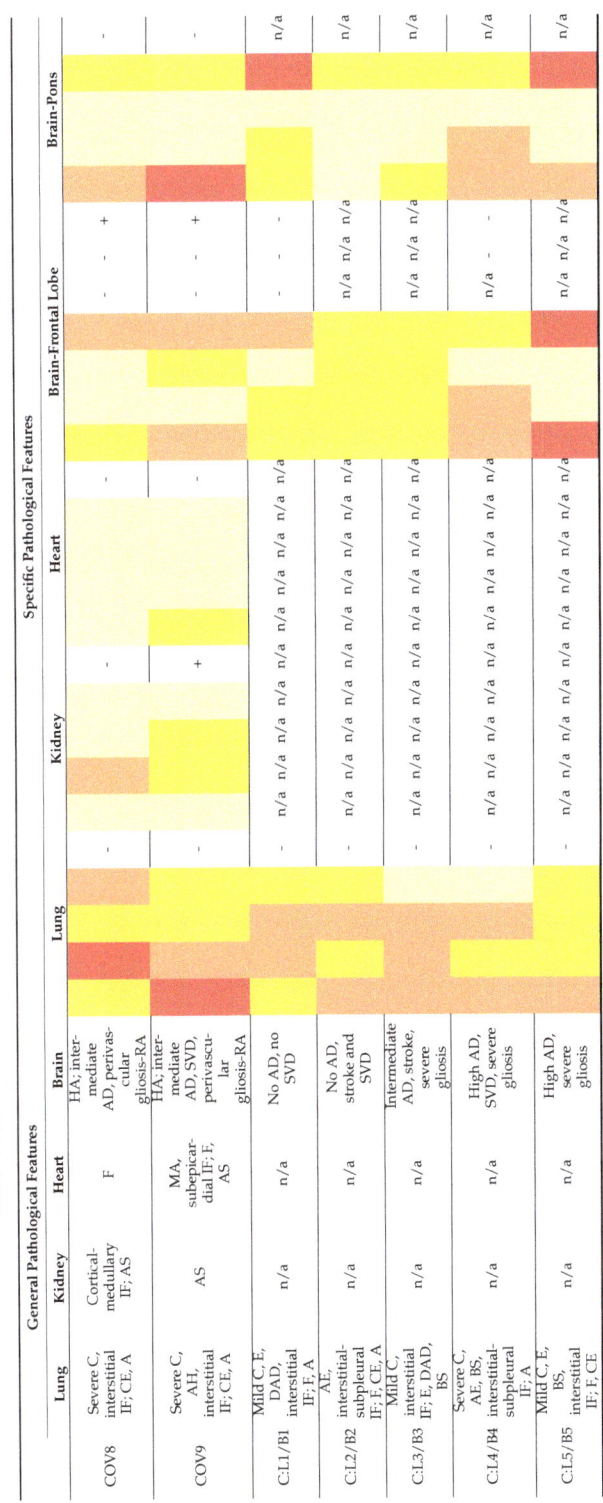

The heart samples revealed: (1) hypoxic myocytic injuries; (2) sporadic SARS-CoV-2 traces in the endothelial and endocardial cells of one case, perivascular–parenchymal inflammatory infiltrates (prominent only in two cases) characterized by predominant macrophages with no evidence of T-lymphocytes and rare B-lymphocytes; and (3) relevant microthrombi in only one case.

The neuropathological hallmarks were: (1) diffuse cortical edema due to extreme hypoxia with cortical swelling, spongiosis, and severe neuronal rarefaction in the cerebral cortex and hippocampus; (2) very limited traces of SARS-CoV-2 antigens in pontine neurons of one case, perivascular and parenchymal inflammatory infiltrates characterized by the enhancement of CD68-positive amoeboid cells (activated microglia), which are more abundant in the pons (all cases) than in the frontal cortex, with a tendency to nodular aggregation and neuronophagia, and very scant B–T lymphocytes as vascular cuffing or inside few nodules; and (3) frequent microthrombi in the frontal lobe (eight cases) and pons (six cases) with rare ischemic rarefaction of the surrounding tissue.

Although all COVID-19 subjects had a positive pharyngeal swab, none of them expressed positivity for SARS-CoV-2 RNA in the brain using qRT-PCR. Nonetheless, traces of viral RNA were detected in the frontal lobe of almost all cases through ddPCR, a more sensitive technique.

Apart from COV2, all of the other cases had pre-existing or age-related pathologies. The lungs frequently showed emphysema, dystelectasis, and anthracosis. The kidneys showed glomerulosclerosis and arteriolosclerosis. The heart samples presented with myocardiosclerosis, lipofuscin deposits, and fatty infiltrates. The brain samples showed different degrees of atrophy and AD pathology (six cases showing cortical neuritic plaques associated with microglial activation and astrogliosis with reactive astrocytes), and small-vessel disease (SVD), including enlarged perivascular spaces, arteriolosclerosis, myelin loss, hemosiderin leakage, and microbleeds (five cases).

3.3. Pathological Findings in Control Non-COVID Cases (n = Five Lungs; n = Five Brains)

The lungs of non-COVID cases showed congestion, edema, and DAD with septal lympho-monocytic infiltrates associated with intra-alveolar fibrinopurulent exudates consisting of neutrophils and macrophages (similar to COVID-19 cases with superimposed bacterial infection). The control brains presented both AD pathology and vascular diseases (SVD and cerebral infarcts). Similar to the COVID-19 cases with AD, the three controls affected by AD showed severe astrogliosis and cortical microglial nodules with a distribution resembling that of neuritic plaques.

3.4. Comparison of Pathological Findings

The presence of T-B lymphocytes as a whole (sum of scores) was similar in the lungs and kidneys (Figure 2A; Table 3), albeit with a significantly greater presence of T lymphocytes in the lungs ($p = 0.020$; Figure 2B). The lymphocyte component within the inflammatory infiltrates of lungs and kidneys was clearly predominant over that of other tissues ($p < 0.001$; Figure 2A; Tables 2 and 3), as well as the presence of the viral antigen, particularly in the type-2 pneumocytes and bronchiolar epithelial cells (Figure 1B,B'). The heart had relevant inflammatory foci in only two cases, characterized by the presence of macrophages (Figure 1O), the substantial absence of lymphocytes, and very rare SARS-CoV-2 traces in the endothelium–endocardium (Figure 1N).

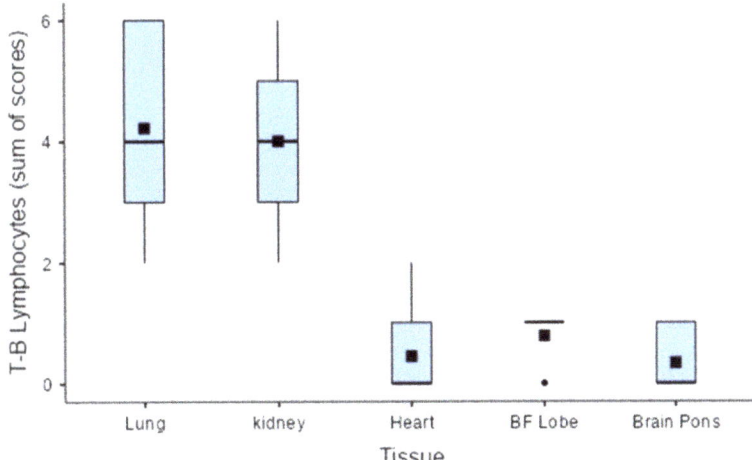
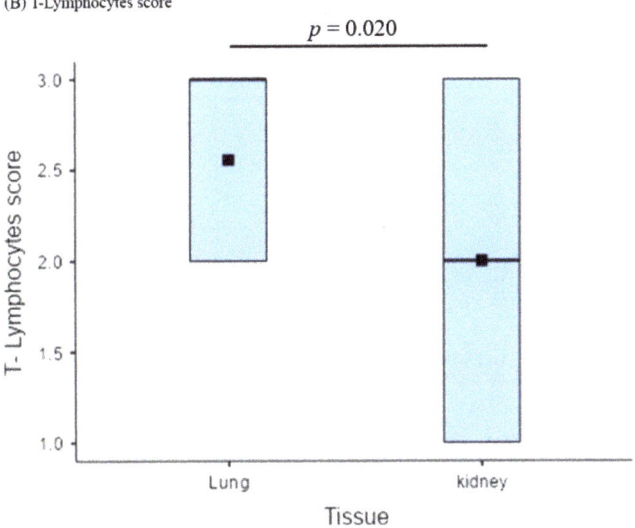

Figure 2. Lymphocytic infiltrates. (**A**) Box plot comparing the sum of the B and T lymphocyte scores across lungs, kidneys, heart, brain frontal lobe (BF), and pons (BP); the lymphocyte component within the inflammatory infiltrates of lungs and kidneys was clearly predominant over that of other tissues ($p < 0.001$); (**B**) box plot showing a comparison between T lymphocyte scores in the lungs and in the kidneys; The presence of T-B lymphocytes as a whole (sum of scores) was similar in the lungs and kidneys, albeit with a significantly greater presence of T lymphocytes in the lungs ($p = 0.020$).

Comparing lung T-B lymphocytes between COVID-19 cases and controls, there was no significant difference (Figure 3A); nonetheless, the T-component was considerably more represented in COVID-19 pneumonia (Figure 1D) ($p = 0.010$; Figure 3B).

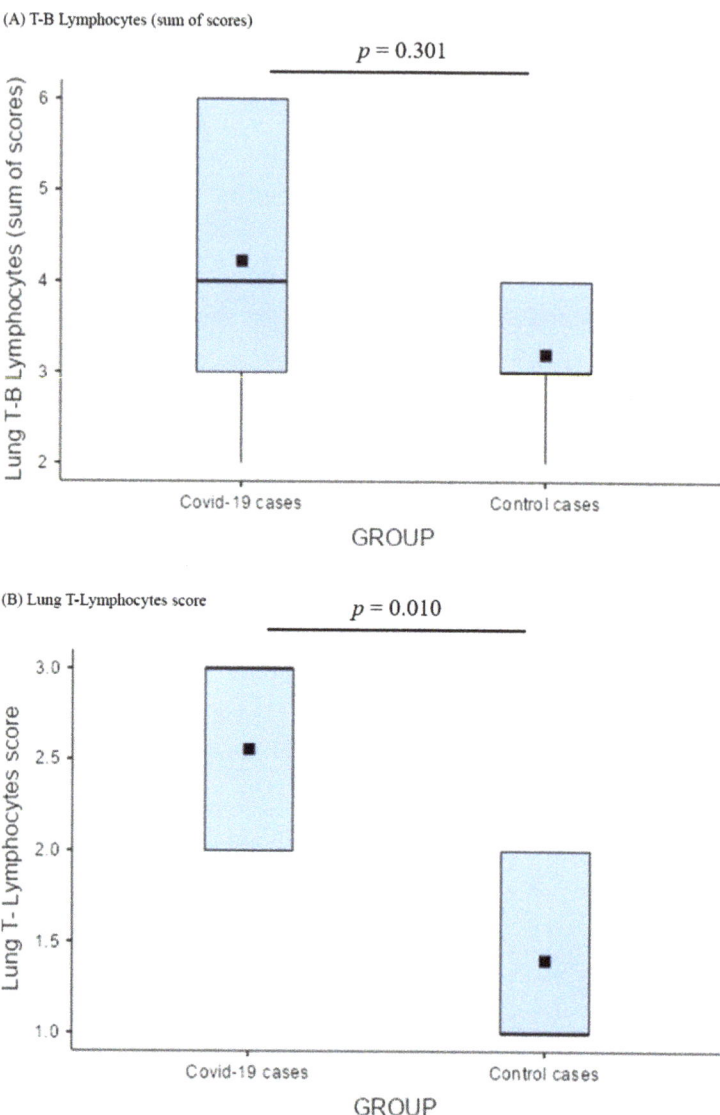

Figure 3. Comparison of lymphocytic infiltrates among the lungs of cases and controls. (**A**) Box plot describing the comparison between the lung B–T lymphocyte of COVID-19 cases versus control cases; lung T-B lymphocytes (sum of scores) did not show any significant difference; (**B**) lung T lymphocyte score comparison among COVID-19 cases and control cases according to a box plot demonstrated that the T-component was considerably more represented in COVID-19 pneumonia ($p = 0.010$).

As for the brain, the preponderance of microglial activation (innate immunity) over the lymphocytic response (adaptive immunity) was distinct. In the frontal lobe, this phenomenon did not differ between COVID-19 cases and controls; these two groups showed similar levels of microglial activation, probably reflecting an inflammatory boost related to the presence of neurodegeneration (Figure 4A). On the other hand, the significantly greater microglial activation in the pons of COVID-19 cases (Figure 4B), associated with traces of viral antigen (Figure 1T), emerged as a specific topographical phenomenon within the brain

(p = 0.017; Figure 4B). Microthrombosis assumed a clinico-pathological relevance only in the lungs, with a significant prevalence of pulmonary microthrombi in COVID-19 cases (Figure 5; p = 0.023) in comparison with non-COVID pneumonia.

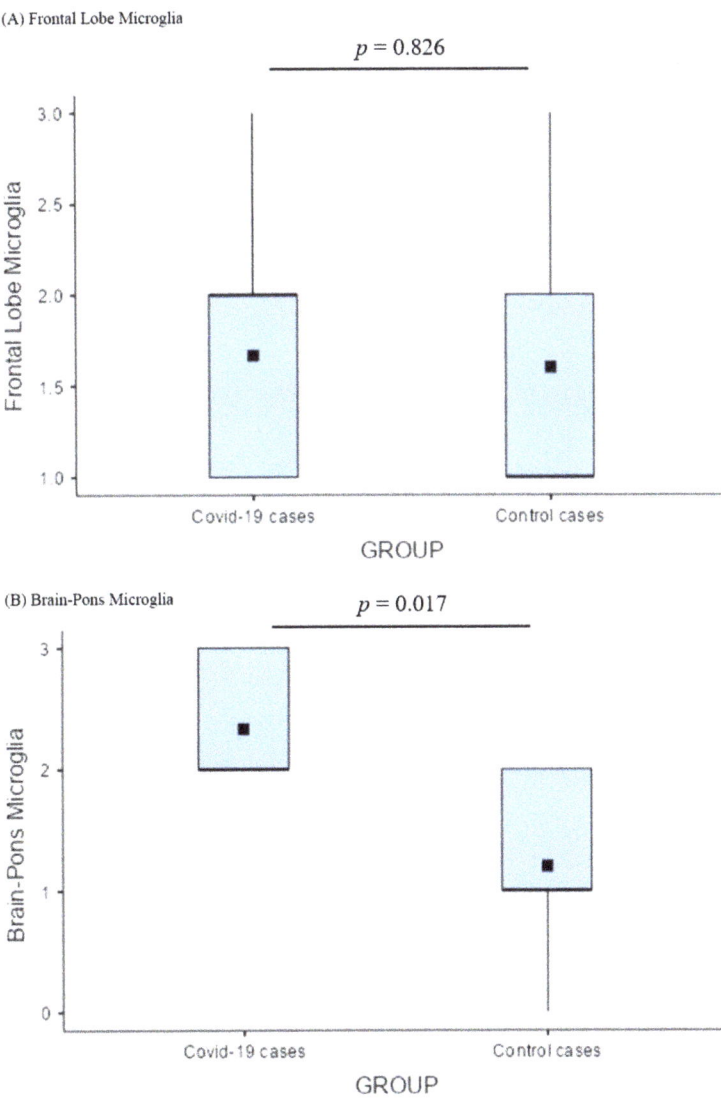

Figure 4. Comparison of microglial activation between the brains of cases and controls. (**A**) In the frontal lobe, microglial activation (innate immunity) did not differ between COVID-19 cases and controls; (**B**) Comparison of pontine microglia between COVID-19 cases and control cases by a box plot showed a significantly greater microglial activation in the pons of COVID-19 cases (p = 0.017).

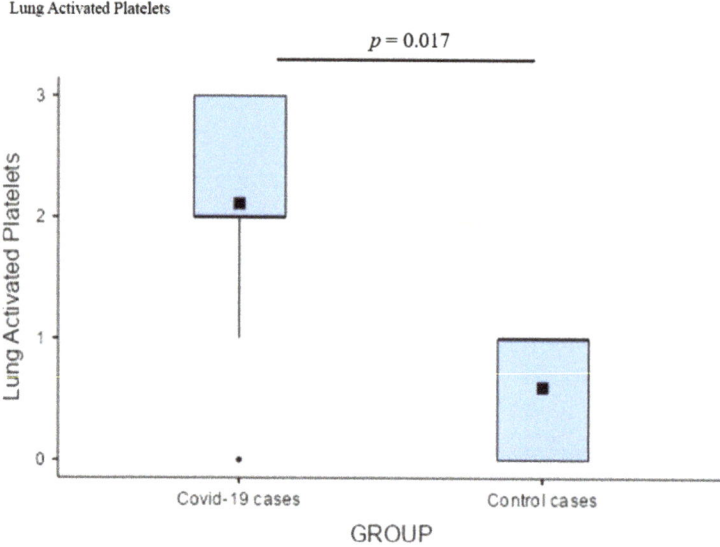

Figure 5. Box plot comparing activated platelets between the lungs of cases and controls demonstrating a predominance of pulmonary microthrombi in COVID-19 cases ($p = 0.023$).

Table 3. Summary of statistical analyses.

	χ^2	p-Value
Friedman rank sum test	31.8	<0.001
Pairwise comparisons (Durbin–Conover)	t	p-value
Sum of T-B Lymphocytes Lungs vs. Kidneys	0.438	0.665
Sum of T-B Lymphocytes Lungs vs. Heart	10.506	<0.001
Sum of T-B Lymphocytes Lungs vs. Brain frontal lobe	8.536	<0.001
Sum of T-B Lymphocytes Lungs vs. Brain pons	11.162	<0.001
Sum of T-B Lymphocytes Kidneys vs. Heart	10.068	<0.001
Sum of T-B Lymphocytes Kidneys vs. Brain frontal lobe	8.098	<0.001
Sum of T-B Lymphocytes Kidneys vs. Brain frontal pons	10.725	<0.001

4. Discussion

Due to its intrinsic characteristics, SARS-CoV-2 infection is accompanied from the earliest stages by an extreme cytokine outpouring. This so-called "cytokine storm" is a form of severe inflammatory response syndrome due to a hyperactivation of the innate immune system with dysregulated and excessive production of pro-inflammatory cytokines, including IL-6, IL-1, IFN, and TNF-alpha [61]. This type of reaction is specifically related to highly pathogenic beta-CoVs and is frequently observed among patients affected by severe COVID-19. Our results confirm that inflammatory and immune-mediated alterations augment the direct cytopathic damage induced by the virus, causing epithelial and endothelial damage, vascular leakage, and dampening of the T-cell response, accompanied by the overactivation of cells from the macrophage lineage. Hence, the severe form of COVID-19 is a multi-organ disease characterized by a combination of viral invasion, lympho-monocytic infiltration, and clotting alterations with mixed detrimental effects due to acute cytopathic injury, inflammation, microthrombosis, and chronic suffering leading to fibrosis. Further detrimental effects are induced by lung failure causing severe hypoxia in all tissues. The main results to discuss are summarized in the following points. (A) SARS-CoV-2 antigens: both pulmonary and renal tissues present capsid antigens, respectively, in the bronchial epithelia and alveolar pneumocytes, as well as in the tubular epithelial and capillary endothelial cells, but the organ with the heaviest burden of viral antigens is the lung, while their presence is negligible in the heart (rare endothelial cells of one case) and brain (rare pontine neurons of one case), with no evidence of active viral replication; (B) inflammatory infiltrates: lymphocytic presence is most prominent in pulmonary and renal tissues, while the heart and brain display very scant lymphocytes with a clear predominance of the monocyte–macrophage–microglia compartment; (C) comparison between COVID-19 and other types of pneumonia: T-lymphocytes were significantly more represented in the lungs infected by SARS-CoV-2; (D) comparison between COVID-19 and control brains: in the frontal cortex of COVID-19 cases, there was a slight and non-significant microglial boosting that was probably related to pre-existing neurodegeneration (AD pathology), rather than to COVID-19, while microglial hyperactivation was significantly higher in the pons of COVID-19 cases, showing several microglial nodules that appeared to be specifically related to SARS-CoV-2 infection; (E) microthrombosis: while it is a frequent finding across all organs, it appears to represent a specific COVID-19 feature only in the lungs.

This research work has some limitations: (1) the low number of cases of mainly elderly people, who happen to constitute the most affected population, thus representing an interesting standpoint; (2) the study comprised patients from elderly care units who died during the first tumultuous pandemic peak, most of whom were not hospitalized; thus, the serum and blood parameters measured before death were not available in most cases, and the determination of a correlation between blood parameters and pathological changes was not possible; (3) the lack of RNA samples from all tissues apart from the frontal lobe, as most tissue samples from the autopsy were immediately formalin-fixed and paraffin-embedded for safety reasons, making subsequent RNA extraction very difficult in terms of quality and quantity; (4) the predominance of superimposed bacterial infection in the control lungs, making them "not pure" controls for viral pneumonia; however, superimposed bacterial infection was also very frequent in SARS-CoV-2 pneumonia. The strength of this research is the focus on histological differences between organs and tissues of clinically well-documented COVID-19 cases, along with the comparison with lungs and brains from non-COVID matched controls to estimate the specific role of SARS-CoV-2 in determining the pathological changes. Furthermore, we developed a method for histological assessment that considered large areas of tissue to select the most affected zones of an individual organ, which were used for scoring. This approach was proven effective in characterizing and comparing the inflammatory infiltrates.

4.1. SARS-CoV-2 Antigens

The parallel comparison between organs confirmed that each tissue interacted differently with SARS-CoV-2, showing interesting similarities and differences. As previously observed by us and other authors [22,24,30], SARS-CoV-2 replicates predominantly, and persists for longer periods, in the alveolar and bronchial epithelium (five cases), where it induces severe cytopathic effects (atypia and death of type-2 pneumocytes). These findings correlate with the abundance of ACE2, TMPRSS2 serine threonine transmembrane protease, and basagin (CD147), which are expressed not only in the alveolar epithelia, but also in the bronchial epithelia. CD147 is now being recognized as a secondary docking site that may increase SARS-CoV-2 virulence and tropism for the upper airways compared with SARS-CoV [62,63].

Similarly, but to a lesser degree, the kidneys showed occasional viral antigens inside the tubular epithelial and capillary endothelial cells. The presence of viral particles in the tubular epithelium has also been reported in other studies [27,64] and may contribute to renal damage. Acute tubular injury is, in fact, often observed in severe COVID-19, and the cause is likely multifactorial; it may result from hypoxia, vascular dysfunctions, severe inflammation, and cytokine release syndrome, along with renal viral tropism, and its consequent direct cytopathic effect on tubular epithelial cells [27,65]. In renal tissues, the co-expression of ACE2 receptors and TMPRSS2 protease has been reported [66–68]. This information, coupled with our results, suggests that some viral replication may also take place in the kidneys.

In the heart, SARS-CoV-2 positivity was found only in the endocardium and endothelium of a single case. Even though many have found the presence of ACE2 and TMPRSS2 to be consistent in the heart (especially in people with heart comorbidities), our results suggest that myocardial damage is not imputable to direct viral assault. The virus probably penetrates the heart, but the lack of cytopathic findings and the viral antigen negativity, observed by us as well as by others [31], indicates that the virus does not replicate within the heart, despite the presence of ACE-2 receptors that are, however, mainly expressed by endothelial cells. Further studies are required to elucidate the biological reasons for the absence of active viral replication in the myocardium. It is possible that multiple alternative causes concur with the cardiac damage, among which, invariably, are generalized hypoxia, inflammatory damage, and microangiopathy [20,33].

From a neuropathological standpoint, our data suggest that SARS-CoV-2 slightly penetrates the brain, but does not actively replicate within it. In the brain tissue, ACE2 and TMPRSS2 are very scarcely present [54,69]. Indeed, our results demonstrate very limited traces of viral proteins in a cluster of neurons located in the pons of a single case. The antigen positivity likely results from virions or viral particles ascending from the respiratory and pharyngeal mucosa through the lower cranial nerves. This hypothesis is in line with the findings reported by Matschke et al. [35], who identified SARS-CoV-2 in the lower cranial nerves. SARS-CoV-2 may also be present in the brain through the direct infection of endothelial cells that have a receptor structure favoring direct infection by the virus. Indeed, some authors have reported the sporadic presence of viral antigens within the brain endothelia [45,53,70] and the possible occurrence of endotheliitis [41,42,71]. In our study, viral RNA was detected in minimal quantities in almost all brains using ddPCR, which is a very sensitive method capable of amplifying fragments of the viral genome originating from the blood [58].

Our data suggest that SARS-CoV-2 causes an acute infection with progressive "cleaning" of the virus from the affected tissues. In particular, the virus was not detectable in four out of nine of the COVID-19 lungs, while a significant inflammatory infiltrate persisted in all cases. Along with other studies [54,72], our data indicate that, similar to SARS-CoV and MERS-CoV, SARS-CoV-2 does not produce a persistent infection. Eventually, the virus is cleared from the tissues it infects; nonetheless, the consequences of the disease may last longer, resulting in persistent symptoms lasting weeks to months after the acute phase. Hence, an accurate analysis of the inflammatory phenomena that accompany SARS-CoV-2 infection is important.

4.2. Inflammatory Infiltrates

Examining the inflammatory infiltrates more closely, it is evident how the lymphocytic component is essentially more prominent in the lungs, less prevalent, but still relevant, in the kidneys, and negligible, if not absent, in the heart and brain (Figure 2A). In particular, the sum of lymphocytes showed the highest scores in the pulmonary and renal tissues, where it tended to be superimposable (Figure 2A). Although the lungs and kidneys seemed to behave similarly, the lungs actively reacted to the massive viral invasion and replication, which was not so evident in the renal tissue. Indeed, T-lymphocytes were significantly more prominent inside the pulmonary infiltrates (Figure 2B). This was probably a specific adaptive immune response against the intense viral replication, as demonstrated by the presence of the highest T-lymphocyte scores in association with the abiding positivity for SARS-CoV-2 (Table 2).

Contrarily, the heart and brain, which were less directly affected by the infection, displayed a scant lymphocytic presence, and the preponderance of macrophages and microglial cells, respectively, as a non-specific immune response (innate immunity) to antigenic perturbation and immune-complex formation. In the heart samples, we observed moderate macrophage infiltration in two cases (Table 2). Such findings confirm the possibility of a macrophagic inflammatory response in the heart that has also been reported by others [32]. It is not yet clear whether this finding may represent a pathophysiological basis for the occasional reported cases of myocarditis and/or pericarditis in the literature [73–75]. Overall, pathological reports regarding the heart have yielded inconsistent results, and the mechanism of myocardial injury is probably multifactorial.

4.3. Comparison between COVID-19 and Other Types of Pneumonia

It is noteworthy that COVID-19 and non-COVID types of pneumonia share the same pathology with congestion, edema, DAD with septal lympho-monocytic infiltrates, and intra-alveolar exudate. A number of scientific articles have recently been published regarding the pulmonary features of COVID-19, describing several clinical, radiologic, and autopsy findings that closely resemble those seen in SARS and MERS cases, and also in other types of viral pneumonia, such as H1N1 flu cases [25]. These observations are consistent with ours; in particular, DAD emerges as a common key pathophysiological mechanism. Such findings suggest that the pathophysiology of alveolar damage in SARS-CoV-2 infection is the same as that of other known causes of acute respiratory distress syndrome (ARDS). Nonetheless, our results outline the prominent T-lymphocyte response precisely in the site of the greatest viral replication. Indeed, even with a similar inflammatory infiltrate (sum of B and T lymphocytes not significantly different; Figure 3A), a significantly greater presence of T lymphocytes was observed in COVID-19 lungs compared with the control ones (Figure 3B). The relevant presence of T lymphocytes underlines the role of these cells in the specific response where viral replication is particularly active. We can assume that such a response may be common to other types of pneumonia with purely viral etiology.

4.4. Comparison between COVID-19 and Control Brains

In the analysis of the central nervous system, we focused on the frontal lobe and the pons, which are two important areas of the forebrain and hindbrain, respectively. Brain pathology is characterized by the hyperactivation of microglia that exhibit amoeboid morphology and phagocytic properties, which have also been described by others [37,76]. In turn, microglial amoeboid cells tend to agglomerate into micronodules. When comparing the frontal lobe of people with COVID-19 with that of matched controls, we found similar features (Figure 4A). It should be considered that they were almost always elderly people with cognitive problems affected by some degree of pre-existing vascular or degenerative pathologies that, per se, induced cortical hypoxia and inflammatory changes. Indeed, we have already reported that, in those cases with dementia, the distribution of the inflammatory nodules closely paralleled that of amyloid plaques, regardless of SARS-CoV-2 infection [34]. Instead, regardless of the cognitive state, microglial hyperactivation was significantly more intense in the pontine structures of COVID-19 cases compared with controls (Figure 4B). This phenomenon, also observed by others [35,76], appears to be specific to the "COVID-19 encephalopathy" and may be activated by viral debris and isolated virions originating from the tracheobronchial and oropharyngeal mucosa through the lower cranial nerves [35]. Moreover, microglial activation in the brain is probably enhanced by infection-induced cytokine release and blood–brain barrier damage due to immune complex formation [76]. The topography of inflammatory lesions during SARS-CoV-2 infection represents the neuropathological basis of "COVID-19 encephalopathy", which clinically presents as behavioral changes, lethargy, vegetative and autonomic dysfunctions, and absence of hypoxic drive [34,76,77].

The overall impact triggered by hypoxia and inflammation may accelerate neurodegeneration, causing the so-called "brain fog" occurring after the acute phase of the disease [13]. These phenomena may be enhanced in the elderly by the presence of a pre-existing degenerative burden, which causes microglial priming that, in turn, results in a more intense inflammatory response, favored by "immunological senescence" (lowered adaptive immunity with lower lymphocytic specific response) and "inflammaging" (age-related hyperactivation of innate immunity leading to an excessive non-specific inflammatory reaction) [78–80]. Furthermore, transcriptomics studies conducted by us and others confirm the pivotal role of hypoxia and persistent microglial activation in the brain, by demonstrating transcriptional changes in the genes involved in the hypoxic response and the modulation of several microglial functions, including migration and phagocytic induction [58,81]. Where there was no active viral replication, a non-specific macrophage–microglial response predominated, which, in elderly subjects, can be favored by the neurodegenerative load, hence demonstrating the importance of a comparison that included patients with AD (the most common neurodegenerative disease).

Although several authors have proposed theories regarding a possible neurotropism of SARS-CoV-2 and its possible persistence in the CNS causing long-term consequences [51,53,82], in our cases, the brain showed scant lymphocytic infiltration and very limited traces of SARS-CoV-2 antigens with no associated evidence of viral replication and encephalitis. The pathological features we have shown are quite different from those of viral encephalitis caused by neurotropic viruses [83], in which the presence of abundant viral antigens, abundant lymphocyte infiltrate, and direct cytopathic effects are observed, as well as that occurring in the lung. From these observations and literature analysis, it is inferred that SARS-CoV-2 is probably not a neurotropic virus and, importantly, there is no evidence proving its persistence within the brain after acute infection, at least in most cases.

4.5. Microthrombosis

Regarding the occurrence of thrombosis and microthrombosis, it should be considered that these phenomena, due to both clotting and endothelial alterations, are described in more than half of COVID-19, SARS, and MERS cases, while they are fairly less common in pneumonia caused by A/H1N1. Such findings suggest that thrombotic complications may be more specifically correlated with beta-CoVs than flu viruses [25,84,85]. In our study, we did not observe gross abnormalities, thrombosis of the large vessels, or infarcts; these phenomena have been reported by others [86–88] and are probably related to a protracted clinical course, which was not the case in our series. Nonetheless, we noted frequent microthrombosis in all organs. In particular, this phenomenon was significantly more prominent in COVID-19 lungs compared with control lungs (Figure 5) affected by non-COVID pneumonia. This confirms that microthrombosis is an event specific to SARS-CoV-2 infection. The pathology of such a phenomenon may be explained by Virchow's triad: (1) the endothelial dysfunction and endothelial damage due to viral tropism and endotheliitis [7]; (2) the hypercoagulability state and increased blood viscosity due to the release of damage-associated molecular patterns (DAMPS) and to the higher load of cytokines, immunoglobulins, and immune complexes traveling within the blood [89,90]; and (3) the prolonged stasis that may result from immobilization during hospitalization. Microthrombosis in the lungs is an event specific to SARS-CoV-2 pneumonia and contributes to the clinical severity, lung failure, and mortality.

Our results confirm that thrombosis inside small pulmonary vessels (Figure 1F) is a COVID-specific phenomenon. The same cannot be stated for the small vessels of the brain, in which microthrombi are present both in cases and in controls, and are probably more related to prolonged agony, co-morbidities, and post-mortem phenomena, rather than to SARS-CoV-2 infection. Indeed, the only young case (COV2) with rapid death and no concomitant pathologies had little or no presence of microthrombi in all organs, suggesting a possible contribution of agony length, age, and co-morbidities to platelet aggregation inside small vessels.

5. Conclusions

We can conclude that: (1) viral replication appears to be active and have a direct pathogenetic role in the lungs and, to a lesser degree, in the kidneys; (2) the type of infiltrate depends on the relationship that the virus establishes with the tissue; in particular, the more active viral replication is, the more T-lymphocytes are present, while a macrophage–microglial response predominates where there is no evidence of active viral replication; and (3) the most specific COVID-19 pathological features consist of an abundance of T-lymphocytes and microthrombosis at the pulmonary level, and relevant microglial hyperactivation in the brainstem.

A careful examination of the pathological pictures present in the various tissues is the basis for understanding acute and long-term symptoms. Overall, our findings suggest that tissue damage in the lungs and kidneys may be caused by a direct viral cytopathic effect along with inflammation-mediated mechanisms. On the other hand, the heart and brain may be damaged mainly by an abnormal and persistent inflammation. Additionally, pre-existing pathologies (e.g., neurodegeneration) and COVID-19's clinical course (e.g., presence of critical illness, hemodynamic instability, hypoxia, and sepsis) affect the clinicopathological pictures. The presence of sequelae across all organs appears to be the result of a combination of the aforementioned factors. It is probable that a complete recovery from COVID-19 requires the termination of both viral infection and the associated inflammation, which can take many months.

The biologically detrimental effects of SARS-CoV-2 infection and related inflammatory changes are at least partially reversible. A deeper understanding of these phenomena is important to improve the management of COVID-19 patients, also after the acute phase. During the post-acute phase of the disease, rehabilitative interventions, such as physical activity, cognitive training, and psychosocial support, should be provided as soon as possible to restore previous functional performances.

Author Contributions: Conceptualization, T.E.P., M.M. and M.C.; Data curation, T.E.P., M.M., V.M., E.T., G.B., E.C., S.D.V., M.R., V.F., R.R.F. and S.G.; Formal analysis, T.E.P., M.M., E.T., M.R., V.F., R.R.F. and A.F.C.; Investigation, T.E.P., M.M., V.M., E.T., G.B., E.C., S.D.V., A.F.C., S.G. and M.C.; Methodology, T.E.P., M.M., V.M., G.B., E.C., S.D.V., M.R. and M.C.; Resources, V.F., R.R.F. and S.G.; Visualization, M.R. and R.R.F.; Writing—original draft, T.E.P., M.M., V.M., E.T., R.R.F. and A.F.C.; Writing—review and editing, L.T., A.G. and M.C. All authors have read and agreed to the published version of the manuscript.

Funding: This study was supported by Fondo di Beneficenza Intesa Sanpaolo (Italy). Project code: B/2020/0045.

Institutional Review Board Statement: The study procedures were in accordance with the principles outlined in the Declaration of Helsinki of 1964 and the following amendments. In accordance with Italian Law, this research was performed on small portions of biological samples routinely taken during autopsies that had already been examined for diagnostic and/or forensic purposes. The subjects of the study were kept anonymous. The reference law is the authorization n9/2016 of the guarantor of privacy, then replaced by Regulation (EU) 2016/679 of the European Parliament and of the Council. In line with our institution's Human Research Ethics Committee, the ABB performs its activities following the ethical standards of the BNE Code of Conduct. The ABB autopsy and sampling protocol were approved by the Ethics Committee of the University of Pavia on 6 October 2009 (Committee report 3/2009).

Informed Consent Statement: Informed consent was obtained from all subjects belonging to the ABB.

Data Availability Statement: The dataset of this research has been deposited in the official computer archive of the Golgi-Cenci Foundation, and it is available upon request.

Acknowledgments: We are grateful to our brain donors, who are generously contributing to research. We are grateful to Arcangelo Ceretti, Mauro Colombo, Federica Zagari, Xhulja Profka. and to "Federazione Alzheimer Italia" for their precious work in the Brain Bank project.

Conflicts of Interest: The authors declare that the research was conducted in the absence of any commercial or financial relationships that could be construed as a potential conflict of interest.

References

1. Wu, D.; Wu, T.; Liu, Q.; Yang, Z. The SARS-CoV-2 outbreak: What we know. *Int. J. Infect. Dis.* **2020**, *94*, 44–48. [CrossRef]
2. Corman, V.M.; Muth, D.; Niemeyer, D.; Drosten, C. Hosts and Sources of Endemic Human Coronaviruses. *Adv. Virus Res.* **2018**, *100*, 163–188.

3. Zhu, Z.; Lian, X.; Su, X.; Wu, W.; Marraro, G.A.; Zeng, Y. From SARS and MERS to COVID-19: A brief summary and comparison of severe acute respiratory infections caused by three highly pathogenic human coronaviruses. *Respir. Res.* **2020**, *21*, 224. [CrossRef]
4. Hu, B.; Guo, H.; Zhou, P.; Shi, Z.L. Characteristics of SARS-CoV-2 and COVID-19. *Nat. Rev. Microbiol.* **2021**, *19*, 141–154. [CrossRef]
5. Deshmukh, V.; Motwani, R.; Kumar, A.; Kumari, C.; Raza, K. Histopathological observations in COVID-19: A systematic review. *J. Clin. Pathol.* **2021**, *74*, 76–83. [CrossRef] [PubMed]
6. Caramaschi, S.; Kapp, M.E.; Miller, S.E.; Eisenberg, R.; Johnson, J.; Epperly, G.; Maiorana, A.; Silvestri, G.; Giannico, G.A. Histopathological findings and clinicopathologic correlation in COVID-19: A systematic review. *Mod. Pathol.* **2021**, *34*, 1614–1633. [CrossRef] [PubMed]
7. Wong, D.W.L.; Klinkhammer, B.M.; Djudjaj, S.; Villwock, S.; Timm, M.C.; Buhl, E.M.; Wucherpfennig, S.; Cacchi, C.; Braunschweig, T.; Knüchel-Clarke, R.; et al. Multisystemic cellular tropism of SARS-CoV-2 in autopsies of COVID-19 patients. *Cells* **2021**, *10*, 1900. [CrossRef] [PubMed]
8. Menter, T.; Haslbauer, J.D.; Nienhold, R.; Savic, S.; Hopfer, H.; Deigendesch, N.; Frank, S.; Turek, D.; Willi, N.; Pargger, H.; et al. Postmortem examination of COVID-19 patients reveals diffuse alveolar damage with severe capillary congestion and variegated findings in lungs and other organs suggesting vascular dysfunction. *Histopathology* **2020**, *77*, 198–209. [CrossRef] [PubMed]
9. Nalbandian, A.; Sehgal, K.; Gupta, A.; Madhavan, M.V.; McGroder, C.; Stevens, J.S.; Cook, J.R.; Nordvig, A.S.; Shalev, D.; Sehrawat, T.S.; et al. Post-acute COVID-19 syndrome. *Nat. Med.* **2021**, *27*, 601–615. [CrossRef] [PubMed]
10. Ahmad, M.S.; Shaik, R.A.; Ahmad, R.K.; Yusuf, M.; Khan, M.; Almutairi, A.B.; Alghuyaythat, W.K.Z.; Almutairi, S.B. "LONG COVID": An insight. *Eur. Rev. Med. Pharmacol. Sci.* **2021**, *25*, 5561–5577. [PubMed]
11. Yende, S.; Parikh, C.R. Long COVID and kidney disease. *Nat. Rev. Nephrol.* **2021**, *17*, 792–793. [CrossRef]
12. Raveendran, A.V.; Jayadevan, R.; Sashidharan, S. Long COVID: An overview. *Diabetes Metab. Syndr. Clin. Res. Rev.* **2021**, *15*, 869–875. [CrossRef]
13. Hampshire, A.; Trender, W.; Chamberlain, S.R.; Jolly, A.E.; Grant, J.E.; Patrick, F.; Mazibuko, N.; Williams, S.C.R.; Barnby, J.M.; Hellyer, P.; et al. Cognitive deficits in people who have recovered from COVID-19. *eClinicalMedicine* **2021**, *39*, 101044. [CrossRef]
14. Vasquez-Bonilla, W.O.; Orozco, R.; Argueta, V.; Sierra, M.; Zambrano, L.I.; Muñoz-Lara, F.; López-Molina, D.S.; Arteaga-Livias, K.; Grimes, Z.; Bryce, C.; et al. A review of the main histopathological findings in coronavirus disease 2019. *Hum. Pathol.* **2020**, *105*, 74–83. [CrossRef]
15. Falasca, L.; Nardacci, R.; Colombo, D.; Lalle, E.; Di Caro, A.; Nicastri, E.; Antinori, A.; Petrosillo, N.; Marchioni, L.; Biava, G.; et al. Postmortem Findings in Italian Patients with COVID-19: A Descriptive Full Autopsy Study of Cases with and without Comorbidities. *J. Infect. Dis.* **2020**, *222*, 1807–1815. [CrossRef]
16. Fox, S.E.; Akmatbekov, A.; Harbert, J.L.; Li, G.; Quincy Brown, J.; Vander Heide, R.S. Pulmonary and cardiac pathology in African American patients with COVID-19: An autopsy series from New Orleans. *Lancet Respir. Med.* **2020**, *8*, 681–686. [CrossRef]
17. Grosse, C.; Grosse, A.; Salzer, H.J.F.; Dünser, M.W.; Motz, R.; Langer, R. Analysis of cardiopulmonary findings in COVID-19 fatalities: High incidence of pulmonary artery thrombi and acute suppurative bronchopneumonia. *Cardiovasc. Pathol.* **2020**, *49*, 107263. [CrossRef]
18. Edler, C.; Schröder, A.S.; Aepfelbacher, M.; Fitzek, A.; Heinemann, A.; Heinrich, F.; Klein, A.; Langenwalder, F.; Lütgehetmann, M.; Meißner, K.; et al. Dying with SARS-CoV-2 infection—An autopsy study of the first consecutive 80 cases in Hamburg, Germany. *Int. J. Leg. Med.* **2020**, *134*, 1275–1284. [CrossRef]
19. Borczuk, A.C.; Salvatore, S.P.; Seshan, S.V.; Patel, S.S.; Bussel, J.B.; Mostyka, M.; Elsoukkary, S.; He, B.; DEL Vecchio, C.; Fortarezza, F.; et al. COVID-19 pulmonary pathology: A multi-institutional autopsy cohort from Italy and New York City. *Mod. Pathol.* **2020**, *33*, 2156–2168. [CrossRef]
20. Romanova, E.S.; Vasilyev, V.V.; Startseva, G.; Karev, V.; Rybakova, M.G.; Platonov, P.G. Cause of death based on systematic post-mortem studies in patients with positive SARS-CoV-2 tissue PCR during the COVID-19 pandemic. *J. Intern. Med.* **2021**, *290*, 655–665. [CrossRef]
21. Schaller, T.; Hirschbühl, K.; Burkhardt, K.; Braun, G.; Trepel, M.; Märkl, B.; Claus, R. Postmortem Examination of Patients with COVID-19. *JAMA* **2020**, *323*, 2518–2520. [CrossRef]
22. Bradley, B.T.; Maioli, H.; Johnston, R.; Chaudhry, I.; Fink, S.L.; Xu, H.; Najafian, B.; Deutsch, G.; Lacy, J.M.; Williams, T.; et al. Histopathology and ultrastructural findings of fatal COVID-19 infections in Washington State: A case series. *Lancet* **2020**, *396*, 320–332. [CrossRef]
23. Duarte-Neto, A.N.; Monteiro, R.; Da Silva, L.F.F.; Malheiros, D.M.A.C.; De Oliveira, E.P.; Theodoro-Filho, J.; Pinho, J.R.R.; Gomes-Gouvêa, M.S.; Salles, A.P.M.; De Oliveira, I.R.S.; et al. Pulmonary and systemic involvement in COVID-19 patients assessed with ultrasound-guided minimally invasive autopsy. *Histopathology* **2020**, *77*, 186–197. [CrossRef]
24. Elsoukkary, S.S.; Mostyka, M.; Dillard, A.; Berman, D.R.; Ma, L.X.; Chadburn, A.; Yantiss, R.K.; Jessurun, J.; Seshan, S.V.; Borczuk, A.C.; et al. Autopsy Findings in 32 Patients with COVID-19: A Single-Institution Experience. *Pathobiology* **2021**, *88*, 56–68. [CrossRef]
25. Hariri, L.P.; North, C.M.; Shih, A.R.; Israel, R.A.; Maley, J.H.; Villalba, J.A.; Vinarsky, V.; Rubin, J.; Okin, D.A.; Sclafani, A.; et al. Lung Histopathology in Coronavirus Disease 2019 as Compared With Severe Acute Respiratory Syndrome and H1N1 Influenza: A Systematic Review. *Chest* **2021**, *159*, 73–84. [CrossRef]

26. Santoriello, D.; Khairallah, P.; Bomback, A.S.; Xu, K.; Kudose, S.; Batal, I.; Barasch, J.; Radhakrishnan, J.; D'Agati, V.; Markowitz, G. Postmortem Kidney Pathology Findings in Patients with COVID-19. *J. Am. Soc. Nephrol.* **2020**, *31*, 2158–2167. [CrossRef]
27. Su, H.; Yang, M.; Wan, C.; Yi, L.-X.; Tang, F.; Zhu, H.-Y.; Yi, F.; Yang, H.-C.; Fogo, A.B.; Nie, X.; et al. Renal histopathological analysis of 26 postmortem findings of patients with COVID-19 in China. *Kidney Int.* **2020**, *98*, 219–227. [CrossRef]
28. Lindner, D.; Fitzek, A.; Bräuninger, H.; Aleshcheva, G.; Edler, C.; Meissner, K.; Scherschel, K.; Kirchhof, P.; Escher, F.; Schultheiss, H.-P.; et al. Association of Cardiac Infection with SARS-CoV-2 in Confirmed COVID-19 Autopsy Cases. *JAMA Cardiol.* **2020**, *5*, 1281–1285. [CrossRef]
29. Schurink, B.; Roos, E.; Radonic, T.; Barbe, E.; Bouman, C.S.C.; de Boer, H.H.; de Bree, G.J.; Bulle, E.B.; Aronica, E.M.; Florquin, S.; et al. Viral presence and immunopathology in patients with lethal COVID-19: A prospective autopsy cohort study. *Lancet Microbe* **2020**, *1*, e290–e299. [CrossRef]
30. Hanley, B.; Naresh, K.N.; Roufosse, C.; Nicholson, A.G.; Weir, J.; Cooke, G.S.; Thursz, M.; Manousou, P.; Corbett, R.; Goldin, R.; et al. Articles Histopathological findings and viral tropism in UK patients with severe fatal COVID-19: A post-mortem study. *Lancet Microbe* **2020**, *1*, e245–e253. [CrossRef]
31. Dal Ferro, M.; Bussani, R.; Paldino, A.; Nuzzi, V.; Collesi, C.; Zentilin, L.; Schneider, E.; Correa, R.; Silvestri, F.; Zacchigna, S.; et al. SARS-CoV-2, myocardial injury and inflammation: Insights from a large clinical and autopsy study. *Clin. Res. Cardiol.* **2021**, *110*, 1822–1831. [CrossRef] [PubMed]
32. Basso, C.; Leone, O.; Rizzo, S.; De Gaspari, M.; Van Der Wal, A.C.; Aubry, M.-C.; Bois, M.C.; Lin, P.T.; Maleszewski, J.J.; Stone, J.R. Pathological features of COVID-19-associated myocardial injury: A multicentre cardiovascular pathology study. *Eur. Heart J.* **2020**, *41*, 3827–3835. [CrossRef] [PubMed]
33. Sang, C.J.; Burkett, A.; Heindl, B.; Litovsky, S.H.; Prabhu, S.D.; Benson, P.V.; Rajapreyar, I. Cardiac pathology in COVID-19: A single center autopsy experience. *Cardiovasc. Pathol.* **2021**, *54*, 107370. [CrossRef] [PubMed]
34. Poloni, T.E.; Medici, V.; Moretti, M.; Visonà, S.D.; Cirrincione, A.; Carlos, A.F.; Davin, A.; Gagliardi, S.; Pansarasa, O.; Cereda, C.; et al. COVID-19-related neuropathology and microglial activation in elderly with and without dementia. *Brain Pathol.* **2021**, *31*, 12997. [CrossRef]
35. Matschke, J.; Lütgehetmann, M.; Hagel, C.; Sperhake, J.P.; Schröder, A.S.; Edler, C.; Mushumba, H.; Fitzek, A.; Allweiss, L.; Dandri, M.; et al. Neuropathology of patients with COVID-19 in Germany: A post-mortem case series. *Lancet Neurol.* **2020**, *19*, 919–929. [CrossRef]
36. Von Weyhern, C.H.; Kaufmann, I.; Neff, F.; Kremer, M. Early evidence of pronounced brain involvement in fatal COVID-19 outcomes. *Lancet* **2020**, *395*, e109. [CrossRef]
37. Al-Dalahmah, O.; Thakur, K.T.; Nordvig, A.S.; Prust, M.L.; Roth, W.; Lignelli, A.; Uhlemann, A.-C.; Miller, E.H.; Kunnath-Velayudhan, S.; del Portillo, A.; et al. Neuronophagia and microglial nodules in a SARS-CoV-2 patient with cerebellar hemorrhage. *Acta Neuropathol. Commun.* **2020**, *8*, 147. [CrossRef]
38. Al-Sarraj, S.; Troakes, C.; Hanley, B.; Osborn, M.; Richardson, M.P.; Hotopf, M.; Bullmore, E.; Everall, I.P. Invited Review: The spectrum of neuropathology in COVID-19. *Neuropathol. Appl. Neurobiol.* **2021**, *47*, 3–16. [CrossRef]
39. Deigendesch, N.; Sironi, L.; Kutza, M.; Wischnewski, S.; Fuchs, V.; Hench, J.; Frank, A.; Nienhold, R.; Mertz, K.D.; Cathomas, G.; et al. Correlates of critical illness-related encephalopathy predominate postmortem COVID-19 neuropathology. *Acta Neuropathol.* **2020**, *140*, 583–586. [CrossRef]
40. Jaunmuktane, Z.; Mahadeva, U.; Green, A.; Sekhawat, V.; Barrett, N.A.; Childs, L.; Shankar-Hari, M.; Thom, M.; Jäger, H.R.; Brandner, S. Microvascular injury and hypoxic damage: Emerging neuropathological signatures in COVID-19. *Acta Neuropathol.* **2020**, *140*, 397–400. [CrossRef]
41. Kirschenbaum, D.; Imbach, L.L.; Rushing, E.J.; Frauenknecht, K.B.M.; Gascho, D.; Ineichen, B.V.; Keller, E.; Kohler, S.; Lichtblau, M.; Reimann, R.R.; et al. Intracerebral endotheliitis and microbleeds are neuropathological features of COVID-19. *Neuropathol. Appl. Neurobiol.* **2021**, *47*, 454–459. [CrossRef]
42. Lee, M.-H.; Perl, D.P.; Nair, G.; Li, W.; Maric, D.; Murray, H.; Dodd, S.J.; Koretsky, A.P.; Watts, J.A.; Cheung, V.; et al. Microvascular Injury in the Brains of Patients with COVID-19. *N. Engl. J. Med.* **2021**, *384*, 481–483. [CrossRef]
43. Reichard, R.R.; Kashani, K.B.; Boire, N.A.; Constantopoulos, E.; Guo, Y.; Lucchinetti, C.F. Neuropathology of COVID-19: A spectrum of vascular and acute disseminated encephalomyelitis (ADEM)-like pathology. *Acta Neuropathol.* **2020**, *140*, 1–6. [CrossRef]
44. Solomon, I.H.; Normandin, E.; Bhattacharyya, S.; Mukerji, S.S.; Keller, K.; Ali, A.S.; Adams, G.; Hornick, J.L.; Padera, R.F., Jr.; Sabeti, P. Neuropathological Features of COVID-19. *N. Engl. J. Med.* **2020**, *383*, 989–992. [CrossRef]
45. Bryce, C.; Grimes, Z.; Pujadas, E.; Ahuja, S.; Beth Beasley, M.; Albrecht, R.; Hernandez, T.; Stock, A.; Zhao, Z.; Al Rasheed, M.; et al. Pathophysiology of SARS-CoV-2: Targeting of endothelial cells renders a complex disease with thrombotic microangiopathy and aberrant immune response. The Mount Sinai COVID-19 autopsy experience. *Mod. Pathol.* **2021**, *34*, 1456–1467. [CrossRef]
46. Kantonen, J.; Mahzabin, S.; Mäyränpää, M.I.; Tynninen, O.; Paetau, A.; Andersson, N.; Sajantila, A.; Vapalahti, O.; Carpén, O.; Kekäläinen, E.; et al. Neuropathologic features of four autopsied COVID-19 patients. *Brain Pathol.* **2020**, *30*, 1012–1016. [CrossRef]
47. Meinhardt, J.; Radke, J.; Dittmayer, C.; Franz, J.; Thomas, C.; Mothes, R.; Laue, M.; Schneider, J.; Brünink, S.; Greuel, S.; et al. Olfactory transmucosal SARS-CoV-2 invasion as a port of central nervous system entry in individuals with COVID-19. *Nat. Neurosci.* **2021**, *24*, 168–175. [CrossRef]

48. Zhang, Y.; Zheng, L.; Liu, L.; Zhao, M.; Xiao, J.; Zhao, Q. Liver impairment in COVID-19 patients: A retrospective analysis of 115 cases from a single centre in Wuhan city, China. *Liver Int.* **2020**, *40*, 2095–2103. [CrossRef]
49. Başkıran, A.; Akbulut, S.; Şahin, T.T.; Tunçer, A.; Kaplan, K.; Bayındır, Y.; Yılmaz, S. Coronavirus Precautions: Experience of High Volume Liver Transplant Institute. *Turk. J. Gastroenterol.* **2022**, *33*, 145–152. [CrossRef]
50. Sahin, T.T.; Akbulut, S.; Yilmaz, S. COVID-19 pandemic: Its impact on liver disease and liver transplantation. *World J. Gastroenterol.* **2020**, *26*, 2987–2999. [CrossRef]
51. Yachou, Y.; El Idrissi, A.; Belapasov, V.; Ait Benali, S. Neuroinvasion, neurotropic, and neuroinflammatory events of SARS-CoV-2: Understanding the neurological manifestations in COVID-19 patients. *Neurol. Sci.* **2020**, *41*, 2657–2669. [CrossRef] [PubMed]
52. Guo, T.; Fan, Y.; Chen, M.; Wu, X.; Zhang, L.; He, T.; Wang, H.; Wan, J.; Wang, X.; Lu, Z. Cardiovascular Implications of Fatal Outcomes of Patients with Coronavirus Disease 2019 (COVID-19). *JAMA Cardiol.* **2020**, *5*, 811–818. [CrossRef]
53. Baig, A.M.; Khaleeq, A.; Ali, U.; Syeda, H. Evidence of the COVID-19 Virus Targeting the CNS: Tissue Distribution, Host-Virus Interaction, and Proposed Neurotropic Mechanisms. *ACS Chem. Neurosci.* **2020**, *11*, 995–998. [CrossRef]
54. Iadecola, C.; Anrather, J.; Kamel, H. Effects of COVID-19 on the Nervous System. *Cell* **2020**, *183*, 16–27.e1. [CrossRef]
55. Moretti, M.; Malhotra, A.; Visonà, S.D.; Finley, S.J.; Osculati, A.M.M.; Javan, G.T. The roles of medical examiners in the COVID-19 era: A comparison between the United States and Italy. *Forensic Sci. Med. Pathol.* **2021**, *17*, 262–270. [CrossRef]
56. Moretti, M.; Belli, G.; Morini, L.; Monti, M.C.; Osculati, A.M.M.; Visonà, S.D. Drug abuse-related neuroinflammation in human postmortem brains: An immunohistochemical approach. *J. Neuropathol. Exp. Neurol.* **2019**, *78*, 1059–1065. [CrossRef]
57. Osborn, M.; Lucas, S.; Stewart, R.; Swift, B.; Youd, E. Briefing on COVID-19. Autopsy practice relating to possible cases of COVID-19 (2019-nCov, novel coronavirus from China 2019/2020). The Royal College of Pathologists. 2020. Available online: https://www.rcpath.org/uploads/assets/d5e28baf-5789-4b0f-acecfe370eee6223/fe8fa85a-f004-4a0c-81ee4b2b9cd12cbf/Briefing-on-COVID-19-autopsy-Feb-2020.pdf (accessed on 3 May 2020).
58. Gagliardi, S.; Poloni, E.T.; Pandini, C.; Garofalo, M.; Dragoni, F.; Medici, V.; Davin, A.; Visonà, S.D.; Moretti, M.; Sproviero, D.; et al. Detection of SARS-CoV-2 genome and whole transcriptome sequencing in frontal cortex of COVID-19 patients. *Brain Behav. Immun.* **2021**, *97*, 13–21. [CrossRef]
59. Poloni, T.E.; Medici, V.; Carlos, A.F.; Davin, A.; Ceretti, A.; Mangieri, M.; Cassini, P.; Vaccaro, R.; Zaccaria, D.; Abbondanza, S.; et al. Abbiategrasso Brain Bank Protocol for Collecting, Processing and Characterizing Aging Brains. *J. Vis. Exp.* **2020**, *2020*, e60296. [CrossRef]
60. Montine, T.J.; Phelps, C.H.; Beach, T.G.; Bigio, E.H.; Cairns, N.J.; Dickson, D.W.; Duyckaerts, C.; Frosch, M.P.; Masliah, E.; Mirra, S.S.; et al. National Institute on Aging-Alzheimer's Association guidelines for the neuropathologic assessment of Alzheimer's disease: A practical approach. *Acta Neuropathol.* **2012**, *123*, 1–11. [CrossRef]
61. Ragab, D.; Salah Eldin, H.; Taeimah, M.; Khattab, R.; Salem, R. The COVID-19 Cytokine Storm; What We Know So Far. *Front. Immunol.* **2020**, *11*, 1446. [CrossRef]
62. Zhang, Y.; Tang, L.V. Overview of Targets and Potential Drugs of SARS-CoV-2 According to the Viral Replication. *J. Proteome Res.* **2021**, *20*, 49–59. [CrossRef] [PubMed]
63. Wang, K.; Chen, W.; Zhang, Z.; Deng, Y.; Lian, J.-Q.; Du, P.; Wei, D.; Zhang, Y.; Sun, X.-X.; Gong, L.; et al. CD147-spike protein is a novel route for SARS-CoV-2 infection to host cells. *Signal Transduct. Target. Ther.* **2020**, *5*, 283. [CrossRef]
64. Farkash, E.A.; Wilson, A.M.; Jentzen, J.M. Ultrastructural Evidence for Direct Renal Infection with SARS-CoV-2. *JASN* **2020**, *31*, 1683–1687. [CrossRef] [PubMed]
65. Lynch, M.R.; Tang, J. COVID-19 and Kidney Injury. *Rhode Isl. Med. J.* **2020**, *103*, 24–28.
66. Pan, X.W.; Xu, D.; Zhang, H.; Zhou, W.; Wang, L.H.; Cui, X.G. Identification of a potential mechanism of acute kidney injury during the COVID-19 outbreak: A study based on single-cell transcriptome analysis. *Intensive Care Med.* **2020**, *46*, 1114–1116. [CrossRef]
67. Hassanein, M.; Radhakrishnan, Y.; Sedor, J.; Vachharajani, T.; Vachharajani, V.T.; Augustine, J.; Demirjian, S.; Thomas, G. COVID-19 and the kidney. *Clevel. Clin. J. Med.* **2020**, *87*, 619–631. [CrossRef]
68. Mizuiri, S. ACE and ACE2 in kidney disease. *World J. Nephrol.* **2015**, *4*, 74–82. [CrossRef]
69. Liu, J.; Li, Y.; Liu, Q.; Yao, Q.; Wang, X.; Zhang, H.; Chen, R.; Ren, L.; Min, J.; Deng, F.; et al. SARS-CoV-2 cell tropism and multiorgan infection. *Cell Discov.* **2021**, *7*, 17. [CrossRef]
70. Beyerstedt, S.; Barbosa Casaro, E.; Bevilaqua Rangel, É. COVID-19: Angiotensin-converting enzyme 2 (ACE2) expression and tissue susceptibility to SARS-CoV-2 infection. *Eur. J. Clin. Microbiol. Infect. Dis.* **2021**, *40*, 905–919. [CrossRef]
71. Varga, Z.; Flammer, A.J.; Steiger, P.; Haberecker, M.; Andermatt, R.; Zinkernagel, A.S.; Mehra, M.R.; Schuepbach, R.A.; Ruschitzka, F.; Moch, H. Endothelial cell infection and endotheliitis in COVID-19. *Lancet* **2020**, *395*, 1417–1418. [CrossRef]
72. Boldrini, M.; Canoll, P.D.; Klein, R.S. How COVID-19 Affects the Brain. *JAMA Psychiatry* **2021**, *78*, 682–683. [CrossRef]
73. Paul, J.F.; Charles, P.; Richaud, C.; Caussin, C.; Diakov, C. Myocarditis revealing COVID-19 infection in a young patient. *Eur. Heart J. Cardiovasc. Imaging* **2020**, *21*, 776. [CrossRef]
74. Mele, D.; Flamigni, F.; Rapezzi, C.; Ferrari, R. Myocarditis in COVID-19 patients: Current problems. *Intern. Emerg. Med.* **2021**, *16*, 1123–1129. [CrossRef]
75. Kumar, R.; Kumar, J.; Daly, C.; Edroos, S.A. Acute pericarditis as a primary presentation of COVID-19. *BMJ Case Rep.* **2020**, *13*, e237617. [CrossRef]

76. Lee, M.H.; Perl, D.P.; Steiner, J.; Pasternack, N.; Li, W.; Maric, D.; Safavi, F.; Horkayne-Szakaly, I.; Jones, R.; Stram, M.N.; et al. Neurovascular injury with complement activation and inflammation in COVID-19. *Brain* **2022**, *145*, 2555–2568. [CrossRef]
77. Poloni, T.E.; Carlos, A.F.; Cairati, M.; Cutaia, C.; Medici, V.; Marelli, E.; Ferrari, D.; Galli, A.; Bognetti, P.; Davin, A.; et al. Prevalence and prognostic value of Delirium as the initial presentation of COVID-19 in the elderly with dementia: An Italian retrospective study. *eClinicalMedicine* **2020**, *26*, 100490. [CrossRef]
78. Akbar, A.N.; Gilroy, D.W. Aging immunity may exacerbate COVID-19. *Science. Am. Assoc. Adv. Sci.* **2020**, *369*, 256–257.
79. Mueller, A.L.; Mcnamara, M.S.; Sinclair, D.A. Why does COVID-19 disproportionately affect older people? *Aging* **2020**, *12*, 9959–9981. [CrossRef] [PubMed]
80. Salimi, S.; Hamlyn, J.M.; Le Couteur, D. COVID-19 and Crosstalk with the Hallmarks of Aging. *J. Gerontol. Ser. A Biol. Sci. Med. Sci.* **2020**, *75*, e34–e41. [CrossRef] [PubMed]
81. Fullard, J.F.; Lee, H.-C.; Voloudakis, G.; Suo, S.; Javidfar, B.; Shao, Z.; Peter, C.; Zhang, W.; Jiang, S.; Corvelo, A.; et al. Single-nucleus transcriptome analysis of human brain immune response in patients with severe COVID-19. *Genome Med.* **2021**, *13*, 118. [CrossRef] [PubMed]
82. Dong, M.; Zhang, J.; Ma, X.; Tan, J.; Chen, L.; Liu, S.; Xin, Y.; Zhuang, L. ACE2, TMPRSS2 distribution and extrapulmonary organ injury in patients with COVID-19. *Biomed. Pharmacother.* **2020**, *131*, 110678. [CrossRef]
83. Ludlow, M.; Kortekaas, J.; Herden, C.; Hoffmann, B.; Tappe, D.; Trebst, C.; Griffin, D.E.; Brindle, H.; Solomon, T.; Brown, A.S.; et al. Neurotropic virus infections as the cause of immediate and delayed neuropathology. *Acta Neuropathol.* **2016**, *131*, 159–184.
84. Ackermann, M.; Verleden, S.E.; Kuehnel, M.; Haverich, A.; Welte, T.; Laenger, F.; Vanstapel, A.; Werlein, C.; Stark, H.; Tzankov, A.; et al. Pulmonary Vascular Endothelialitis, Thrombosis, and Angiogenesis in COVID-19. *N. Engl. J. Med.* **2020**, *383*, 120–128. [CrossRef]
85. McFadyen, J.D.; Stevens, H.; Peter, K. The Emerging Threat of (Micro)Thrombosis in COVID-19 and Its Therapeutic Implications. *Circ. Res.* **2020**, *127*, 571–587. [CrossRef]
86. Pisano, T.J.; Hakkinen, I.; Rybinnik, I. Large Vessel Occlusion Secondary to COVID-19 Hypercoagulability in a Young Patient: A Case Report and Literature Review. *J. Stroke Cerebrovasc. Dis.* **2020**, *29*, 105307. [CrossRef]
87. Baram, A.; Kakamad, F.H.; Abdullah, H.M.; Mohammed-Saeed, D.H.; Hussein, D.A.; Mohammed, S.H.; Abdulrahman, B.B.; Mirza, A.J.; Abdulla, B.A.; Rahim, H.M.; et al. Large vessel thrombosis in patient with COVID-19, a case series. *Ann. Med. Surg.* **2020**, *60*, 526–530. [CrossRef]
88. Avila, J.; Long, B.; Holladay, D.; Gottlieb, M. Thrombotic complications of COVID-19. *Am. J. Emerg. Med.* **2021**, *39*, 213–218. [CrossRef]
89. Iba, T.; Levy, J.H.; Levi, M.; Thachil, J. Coagulopathy in COVID-19. *J. Thromb. Haemost.* **2020**, *18*, 2103–2109. [CrossRef]
90. Soy, M.; Keser, G.; Atagündüz, P.; Tabak, F.; Atagündüz, I.; Kayhan, S. Cytokine storm in COVID-19: Pathogenesis and overview of anti-inflammatory agents used in treatment. *Clin. Rheumatol.* **2020**, *39*, 2085–2094. [CrossRef]

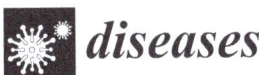

Review

Thromboembolic Events in Patients with Inflammatory Bowel Disease: A Comprehensive Overview

Dhir Gala [1,*], Taylor Newsome [1], Nicole Roberson [1], Soo Min Lee [1], Marvel Thekkanal [1], Mili Shah [1], Vikash Kumar [2], Praneeth Bandaru [3] and Vijay Gayam [3]

[1] American University of the Caribbean School of Medicine, 1 University Drive at Jordan Dr, Cupecoy, Sint Maarten, The Netherlands
[2] Department of Internal Medicine, The Brooklyn Hospital Center, 121 DeKalb Ave, Brooklyn, NY 11201, USA
[3] Department of Gastroenterology, The Brooklyn Hospital Center, 121 DeKalb Ave, Brooklyn, NY 11201, USA
* Correspondence: dhirgala@gmail.com

Abstract: Inflammatory bowel disease (IBD), Crohn's disease and ulcerative colitis are chronic inflammatory disorders of the intestines. The underlying inflammation activates the coagulation cascade leading to an increased risk of developing arterial and venous thromboembolic events such as deep vein thrombosis and pulmonary embolism. Patients with IBD are at a 2–3-fold increased risk of developing thromboembolism. This risk increases in patients with active IBD disease, flare-ups, surgery, steroid treatment, and hospitalization. These complications are associated with significant morbidity and mortality making them important in clinical practice. Clinicians should consider the increased risk of thromboembolic events in patients with IBD and manage them with appropriate prophylaxis based on the risk. In this review, we discuss the literature associated with the pathophysiology of thromboembolism in patients with IBD, summarize the studies describing the various thromboembolic events, and the management of thromboembolism in patients with IBD.

Keywords: inflammatory bowel disease; thromboembolism; Crohn's disease; ulcerative colitis; deep vein thrombosis; pulmonary embolism

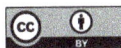

1. Introduction

Inflammatory Bowel Disease (IBD) is characterized by chronic inflammation of the intestines resulting from an interplay between environmental and genetic factors. The two main types of IBD are Crohn's disease and ulcerative colitis. While Crohn's disease and ulcerative colitis both present with many of the same symptoms, including persistent diarrhea, abdominal pain, weight loss, and fatigue, they differ in that Crohn's disease may affect any part of the digestive tract, whereas ulcerative colitis specifically affects the large intestine [1]. The prevalence of IBD is highest in Europe and North America with the prevalence of IBD in North America exceeding 0.3%. However, the incidence of IBD is beginning to stabilize in these regions and increase in other newly industrialized areas, such as Brazil and Taiwan, as they are becoming more Westernized [2]. In the USA, the incidence of Crohn's disease is higher in African Americans and whites, while ulcerative colitis is more common in Mexican Americans. Additionally, African Americans have a higher incidence of sequelae, such as IBD-associated arthritis ($p = 0.004$), and ophthalmological manifestations, such as uveitis ($p = 0.028$) from Crohn's disease than whites [3]. The most common age for onset of IBD is 20–30 years old, but those with Crohn's disease have a mean age of diagnosis that is 5–10 years earlier than those with ulcerative colitis [4].

IBD presentation is very general and may overlap with other syndromes or diseases, such as irritable bowel syndrome. Common symptoms include diarrhea (with or without blood), constipation (especially with ulcerative colitis), painful bowel movements, abdominal pain (right lower quadrant for Crohn's and periumbilical for ulcerative colitis), as well as nausea and vomiting [5]. Several environmental factors play a role in IBD, including smoking [6] and diet, with a Western diet, associated with low fiber, high sugar, and fatty foods, contributing to an increase in IBD incidence [7]. Additionally, the hygiene hypothesis posits that when children are raised in a highly hygienic environment, they are not exposed to organisms that help build the immune system. Therefore, this environment leads to an underdeveloped immune system which may result in IBD later in life, as this may be caused by an inappropriately large immune response to the contents of the intestines. Indeed, in many underdeveloped nations where children are exposed to intestinal helminths, the incidence of IBD is much lower than in countries where children are exposed to very hygienic environments that lack exposure to intestinal helminths [8].

Many complications are associated with IBD including many extraintestinal manifestations [9]. These complications include musculoskeletal system, dermatologic and oral systems, hepatopancreatobiliary system, ocular system, metabolic system, and renal system complications [9]. Joints, skin, and eyes are most commonly affected with manifestations such as peripheral arthritis, episcleritis, or erythema nodosum [10]. While it is important to keep in mind common complications of IBD, rare complications are also important to note. One rare complication associated with IBD is thrombosis.

2. Thrombosis

Thrombosis is the result of the coagulation cascade in which a fibrin clot forms in a vein or artery. Thrombosis is a normal response to endothelial injury and contributes to the healing response; however, thrombosis can also lead to myocardial infarction, pulmonary embolism (PE), and deep vein thrombosis (DVT), among other conditions [11]. The coagulation pathway has four main events: vessel constriction to limit blood flow to the site of injury, platelet activation to form the initial platelet plug, formation of the fibrin clot, and fibrinolysis to remove the clot as wound healing is completed. Any defects in the clotting cascade can lead to abnormal blood clots in the body leading to various pathologies [12]. The cascade is initiated by both the intrinsic (internal stimuli) and extrinsic (external stimuli/trauma) pathways. Both pathways converge on Factor X and continue through the cascade to ultimately form thrombin which provides positive feedback to continue clot formation [13]. Thrombin also converts fibrinogen to fibrin which forms the cross-linked fibrin clot, the end product of the cascade [12]. Many of the factors in the cascade are serine proteases, which can be inactivated by anticoagulants, such as antithrombin, a serpin that irreversibly inactivates serine proteases, which targets Factor Xa and thrombin. Heparin, an anticoagulant used to treat venous thrombosis stimulates antithrombin activity and thus accelerates the inactivation of various clotting factors [12].

While coagulation is part of a normal response to endothelial injury, various factors can predispose someone to venous thrombosis, which are described in Virchow's Triad: endothelial injury, stasis, and a hypercoagulable state [14]. Endothelial injury, resulting from smoking, chronic hypertension, or atherosclerosis, creates turbulent blood flow leading to thrombosis in the area of damage. Stasis of blood, common in bedridden patients, can interfere with the interaction between natural anticoagulant molecules and surface proteins leading to a thrombus. Lastly, a hypercoagulable state, seen in pregnancy, oral contraceptive use, and cancer, can also lead to resistance to natural anticoagulant molecules causing thrombus formation. Thus, these three factors can lead to abnormal thrombosis caused by various disease processes which also puts these patients at risk for thromboembolism and other complications [14,15].

3. Pathophysiology and Risk Factors for Thrombosis
3.1. Introduction

The underlying mechanism for disease in IBD is chronic inflammation. Research is not yet conclusive of whether the altered gut microbiota is a cause or effect of the inflammation leading to IBD; however, it is known to play a role in the pathophysiology of disease. The decreased diversity of intestinal bacteria species and decreased quantity of anti-inflammatory bacteria *Faecalibacterium prausnitzii* are known predictive factors [16].

The intestinal microbiota is located within the endothelial cells and normally enhances mucus secretion for digestion and promote fiber fermentation. Alteration of the microbiota, therefore, disrupts natural digestion processes and promotes inflammation via endothelial damage [17]. The pathophysiology of inflammation leading to IBD can be caused by genetic or biological factors combined with a self-immune response (Figure 1). Increased inflammation furthermore initiates the coagulation cascade leading to a higher risk of thrombosis.

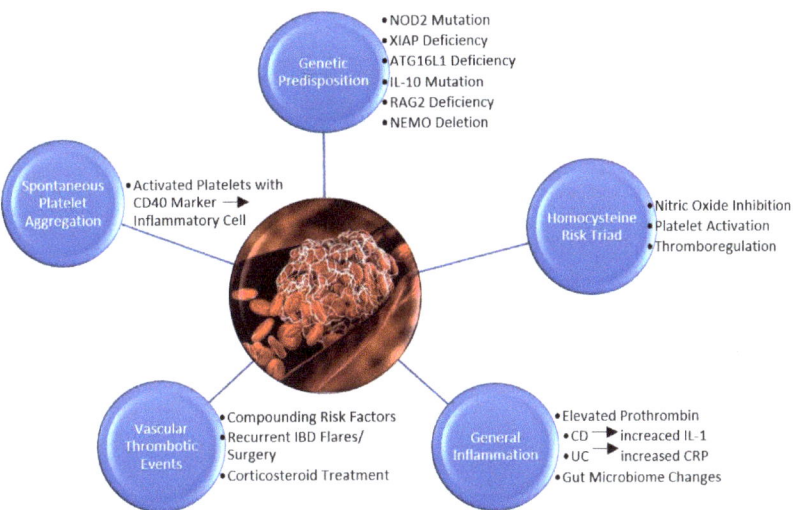

Figure 1. Summary of risk factors contributing to thrombosis in IBD.

3.2. Genetic Predisposition

A recent study used mouse models to test genetic mutations associated with IBD to include nucleotide-binding oligomerization domain-containing protein 2 (NOD2), ATG16L1, recombination activating gene 2 (RAG2), interleukin 10 (IL-10) receptor deficiency, and nuclear factor kappa beta (NF-κB) essential modulator (NEMO) [18]. NOD2 negatively regulates toll-like receptors to inhibit the NF-κB signaling for immune response and anti-inflammatory release of IL-10 [19,20]. Mutations in NOD2 thus lead to decreased immune regulation and increased intestinal inflammation. NOD2 mutations are also associated with decreased anti-inflammatory *Faecalibacterium* and increased infectious *Escherichia* species in the microbiota further leading to inflammation [21–23]. Studies suggest that NOD2 mutations lead to defective bacterial phagocytosis resulting in a heightened immune response necessary to compensate [24]. It is further hypothesized that NOD2 is involved in antimicrobial peptide (AMP) expression and production in secretory Paneth cells of the small intestines. Defects in Paneth cells eliminate one of the major immunomodulating elements in the small intestines and lead to increased intestinal inflammation [25]. Homozygous mutations of NOD2 are, therefore, associated with a 20-fold increased risk for Crohn's Disease [26]. Later studies have identified X-linked inhibitor of apoptosis (XIAP) deficiencies to be early indicators of IBD due to NOD2's dependency on XIAP to complete an immune response [27,28]. Although most research focuses on IBD in adults, genome wide association studies (GWAS) support IL-10 receptor mutations are correlated with pediatric IBD and neonatal onset IBD. The mutation inhibits IL-10 from regulating tumor necrosis factor (TNF-α), thus promoting a pro-inflammatory state in infants and children [29].

ATG16L1 deficiencies lead to inflammation through a similar mechanism. Defective ATG16L1 genes decrease microbial autophagy and require the immune response to heighten in compensation [30]. Gene deficiency is also associated with decreased antimicrobial activity and expression of cell defensin proteins HD5 and HD6 of Paneth cells [31]. The mutation furthermore is associated with an increase in *Bacteriodes fragilis* in the microbiota. *B. fragilisis* is naturally a commensal bacteria that are commonly decreased in the microbiota of patients with IBD. In the T300A variant of ATG16L1 mutations, however, *B. fragilis* is increased in the microbiota but is pro-inflammatory by inhibiting T-lymphocyte development [32]. ATG16L1 deficiencies thus result in intestinal inflammation associated with IBD. Khan et al. concluded that a RAG2 deficiency in mice also leads to chronic colitis indicative of IBD [33]. RAG2 deficiencies prevent correct VDJ recombination of lymphocytes. The deficiency thus inhibits the maturation of B and T cells and results in the overactivation of cytokine and chemokine response. The induced cytokine storm causes a domino effect of immune cell activation which triggers inflammatory factors. Some of the inflammatory induced factors include interferon gamma (INF-γ), TNF, IL-1, IL-6, IL-17, IL-18, and Janus kinase signal transduction and activator of transcription (JAK-STAT3) [34]. Cytokine storm activation, therefore, causes systemic inflammation correlated with IBD. NF-κB, although normally part of the pro-inflammatory pathway, may have protective factors for intestinal epithelial cells. Indeed, a study on mice with conditionally ablated NEMO, essential for NF-κB activation, developed intestinal inflammation leading to epithelial cell apoptosis and translocation of microbes into the mucosa [35].

3.3. Inflammation's Role in Thrombosis

Biological factors leading to IBD include a variety of elements causing increased inflammation which is a known initiator of the coagulation cascade. A study in 1995 concluded patients with Crohn's Disease and Ulcerative Colitis often have increased thrombin levels leading to thrombosis. The study used prothrombin fragments 1 and 2 (F1 + 2) and thrombin–antithrombin III complex (TAT) as markers to identify thrombin. The increased thrombin is due to the release of TNF and IL-1 inflammatory response initiating tissue factor (TF) to begin the coagulation cascade. The anticoagulation activity of endothelial thrombin and protein C is suppressed simultaneously. The study revealed Crohn's Disease was correlated with coagulation initiated by increased IL-1 levels, whereas Ulcerative Colitis was correlated with increased levels of C-reactive protein (CRP) [36]. CRP initiates the inflammatory response through IL-6 and IL-8 activation [37]. Thompson et al. validated the correlation between inflammatory-induced coagulation and IBD by reporting a decreased frequency of IBD in patients with Hemophilia or Von Willebrand Disease. Such patients have a deficiency of von Willebrand factor and factors VIII and XI of the coagulation cascade resulting in decreased thrombosis [38].

Another factor that leads to an increased risk of thrombosis in IBD includes changes in the gut microbiome which activates an inflammatory response and initiates coagulation. The use of antibiotics, specifically metronidazole, fluoroquinolones, and quinolones, is reported to have a strong association with the development of Crohn's Disease. A study reported, furthermore, that antibiotic use in the first year of life leads to an increased risk of developing IBD as a child [39].

3.4. Homocysteine Risk Triad

Further reports indicate an increase in the amino acid homocysteine also induces an inflammatory response in patients with disorders such as IBD, systemic lupus, rheumatoid arthritis, and multiple sclerosis. A leading cause of hyperhomocysteinemia is folate and vitamin B deficiency. Folate and vitamin B are cofactors required for the catabolism of homocysteine and vitamin deficiencies thus result in increased serum and mucosal homocysteine levels [40]. Inflammatory-induced malabsorption in the intestines and dietary restrictions used to treat IBD lead to a strong correlation with hyperhomocysteinemia. The mechanism of homocysteine-induced intestinal endothelial cell inflammation is due to vascular cell adhesion protein-1 (VCAM-1) upregulation, monocyte chemoattractant protein-1 (MCP-1) production, and p38 phosphorylation [41,42].

Homocysteine is known to cause inflammation through alternative mechanisms as well. Increased homocysteine inhibits nitric oxide (NO), thus inhibiting vasodilation. NO production is inhibited through increased production of reactive nitrogen and oxygen species [43,44] and a deficiency of common methyl donor s-adenosyl-methionine (SAM) preventing DNA methylation [45]. Increased homocysteine also inhibits thromboregulation factors by inhibiting protein C and thrombomodulin through the reduction of disulfide bonds on an epidermal growth factor domain [46]. A reduction of antithrombin activity is another mechanism of thromboregulation inhibition [47]. Increased homocysteine further leads to thrombosis through platelet activation due to an increase in factor V [48], thromboxane A2 [49,50], a three-fold increase in arachidonic acid peroxidation product 8-iso-prostaglandin F2α, [51] increasing TF, a cofactor for coagulation factor VII, and mRNA synthesis [52].

3.5. Venous Thrombotic Events

Studies of East Asian and Mediterranean populations concluded that women with IBD have an increased risk of venous thromboembolism (VTE) due to compounding risk factors such as hormone replacement therapy, oral contraceptives, and pregnancy. Oral contraceptives containing estrogen lead to increased production of coagulation factors, increasing VTE three to six-fold [53]. Pregnancy increased the risk of VTE in women five- to six-fold by simultaneously increasing fibrinogen production and decreasing the anticoagulant protein S [54].

Two studies of Asian populations, East Asia and Korea, concluded patients with IBD have a two-fold risk of VTE [55,56]. Asian populations have a significantly lower incidence of VTE in comparison to Western nations; the increased prevalence in patients with IBD, therefore, shows a strong correlation. The Korean study indicates a 27-fold risk of VTE during hospitalizations associated with IBD flares. Additionally, they noted a 40-fold risk of VTE during the postoperative stages of IBD-related bowel resection [56]. The study in East Asia indicated that 54% of patients with IBD and VTE had a surgical history [55]. The intestinal area attacked by IBD is more sensitive to inflammatory response due to the immense commensal bacterial population. Alteration of the gut microbiome due to chronic stress, surgery, or IBD attacks leads to inflammation and activation of the coagulation cascade leading to thrombosis. Furthermore, one of the primary treatments of IBD is corticosteroids which induce coagulation through an increase in factors VII, VIII, and IX [57]. Indeed, a study reported an approximately five-fold increase in the risk of VTE in patients receiving corticosteroid therapy for IBD [58].

3.6. Spontaneous Platelet Aggregation

Uniquely, studies indicate platelets are 30% more likely to spontaneously aggregate in patients with IBD regardless of disease severity and clinical activity [59]. In patients with IBD, platelets circulate in an activated state identified by P-selectin, GP53, β-thromboglobulin, and CD40 ligand (CD40L) markers [60,61]. The activated platelet markers in Crohn's Disease are more prevalent in capillaries indicative of platelet concentration and eventual thrombosis in the intestinal microcirculation [62].

Due to the presence of CD40L on activated platelets in patients with IBD, their platelets themselves are considered inflammatory cells [63]. The CD40L positive platelets can adhere to mucosal microvascular endothelium in the intestines to initiate an inflammatory response [64]. The mechanism of platelet inflammatory response is through upregulation of VCAM-1 and intercellular adhesion molecule-1 (ICAM-1) to secrete IL-8 and attract neutrophils. The platelets also attract monocytes and memory T-cells via chemokine RANTES [65]. In addition to containing CD40L surface markers, the activated platelets also express CD40 surface markers to activate platelets and recruit T-cells during intestinal inflammatory responses [64].

4. Thromboembolic Events in Patients with IBD

4.1. Introduction

Patients with IBD are at an increased risk for arterial and venous thromboembolic events (Figure 2). The most common ones are VTE and PE. Arterial thromboembolism (ATE) is less common than VTE in patients with IBD. However, numerous case reports and case series have reported ATE in patients with IBD. ATE may involve thrombosis and/or occlusion of the cerebral [66,67], splanchnic [68], carotid [69], coronary [70], aorta [71], renal, and upper and lower extremity [72] arteries. Incidence is more common after interventional procedures, however, can occur spontaneously.

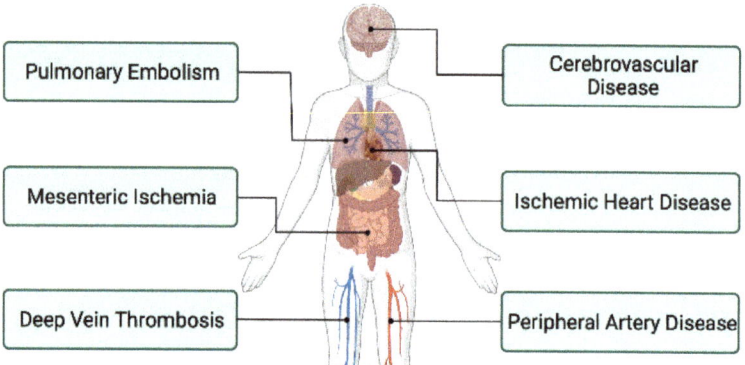

Figure 2. Arterial and venous thrombosis associated with IBD.

4.2. Deep Vein Thrombosis and Pulmonary Embolism

Over the past decade, multiple studies have focused on defining the association of IBD with the risk of VTE and have discussed the epidemiological and clinical features of VTEs in patients with IBD [73,74].

Various studies have looked at the incidence and risk of VTE in patients with IBD compared to the general population [75–78]. A few studies have compared the risk of VTE between hospitalized patients with IBD to patients without IBD [79–81]. Additionally, studies were done on more selective populations such as the risk of VTE in pregnant females with IBD [82] and the risk of VTE in postoperative patients with IBD [83]. Lastly, one study evaluated the risk of recurrent DVTs in adult patients with IBD [84] (Table 1).

Table 1. Summary of studies reporting the risk of VTE in patients with IBD.

Author (Year)	Findings
Yuhara (2013) [85]	This study found an RR of 2.2 (95% CI 1.83–2.65) when comparing the risk of VTE among subjects with and without IBD with similar results after adjusting for obesity and smoking.
Fumery (2014) [73]	The overall risk of VTE in an IBD population was increased by 96% in this study compared to the general population, (RR = 1.96, 95% CI = 1.67–2.30) with no statistical difference between UC and CD subgroups.
Papay (2013) [86]	This study found that 90% of VTE's were DVT's and PE's among patients with IBD.

Table 1. Cont.

Author (Year)	Findings
Bernstein (2007) [75]	VTE occurrence among hospitalized patients with IBD was significantly higher compared to hospitalized patients without IBD (IRR: 4.5 (UC) and 9.6 (CD)).
Novacek (2010) [84]	The probability of recurrence of VTE 5 years after cessation of anticoagulant medication was elevated among patients with IBD in comparison to patients without IBD (33.4%; 95% confidence interval [CI]: 21.8–45.0 vs. 21.7%; 95% CI: 18.8–24.6; $p = 0.01$).
Grainge (2010) [78]	This study found an RR of 3.0 (CI 1.7–6.3) when comparing VTE occurrence in hospitalized patients with IBD to those without.
Nguyen (2008) [80]	This study reported a significantly higher risk of VTE in patients with IBD discharges compared to non-IBD discharges. (OR 1.85 for UC and OR 1.48 for CD). Additionally, VTE was associated with increased mortality, longer hospital stays (by an average of 5 days) and a higher healthcare cost ($47,515 vs. $21,499) (OR 2.5)

In two meta-analyses that analyzed the overall risk of VTEs, DVT, and PE, it was found that there is an approximately 2-fold increased risk for VTEs in patients with IBD. [73,85]. The first study reported an approximately two-fold significantly increased risk of VTE in patients with IBC compared to the general population (RR = 2.20; 95% CI 1.83–2.65) [85]. Similarly, another meta-analysis study reported that patients with IBD were at a significantly increased risk for developing VTE compared to the general population (RR = 1.96; 95% CI: 1.67–2.30) with no difference between UC and CD [73].

A study by Papay et al. evaluated a total of 2811 patients with IBD reporting the incidence and prevalence of VTE and other related clinical features in this cohort [86]. This study reported an incidence and prevalence of all VTEs to be 6.3/1000 person-years and 5.6% (157/2811), respectively. The most commonly reported VTE included DVT and/or PE (about 90%). The other rare locations of VTE reported were the portal, the superior mesenteric, the splenic, the internal jugular, and the cerebral veins. Additionally, there was no significant difference in the frequency of all VTEs when comparing patients with CD to patients with UC. However, patients with CD had a higher prevalence and incidence of DVT and/or PE [86].

VTEs occur at a younger age in patients with IBD compared to the general population. Bernstein et al. analyzed data from hospitalized patients with and without IBD and found that hospitalized patients with IBD had a higher risk of VTE, DVT, and/or PE than those in the general population [79]. In patients younger than 40 years old, the most noticeable difference was observed. The incidence ratio rate for VTE was 4.5 for patients with UC and 9/6 for patients with CD compared to those in the general population. [79].

Patients with IBD are at a greater risk of morbidity and mortality from thromboembolic complications compared to the general population [87]. There is an increased risk of developing postoperative VTE in patients with IBD [88]. Indeed, a national study reported an increased risk of postoperative DVT and PE in patients with IBD undergoing intestinal (OR = 2.03; 95% CI, 1.52–2.70) or non-intestinal surgery (OR = 4.45; 95% CI, 1.72–11.49) [89].

Patients with IBD have a significantly higher risk for recurrent VTE compared to the general population. Indeed, a study reported the recurrence of thromboembolic events to be about 10–13% in patients with IBD [90]. Novacek et al. compared the risk of recurrent VTE in patients with and without IBD 5 years post discontinuation of anticoagulants reporting a statistically significant higher risk in patients with IBD (hazard ratio = 2.5; 95% CI: 1.4–4.2; $p = 0.001$) [84]. Additionally, a study found IBD to be an independent risk factor for recurrent VTE with a relative risk of 2.5 after controlling for activity status [84]. Similarly, another study reported an incidence of recurrent VTE to be 25% in patients with IBD. Additionally, the majority of the VTE was found to be the same type as DVT or PE and in the same location as the first episode [86].

The frequency of thromboembolic events is higher in patients with active IBD and correlates directly with the extent and severity of the diseases. Additionally, most thromboembolic events occur in the absence of provoking factors [42,90,91]. A study found that 74% of first-time VTE was unproved in patients with IBD [84]. Additionally, IBD complicated by stenosis, abscess or fistulas, use of corticosteroids, and recent hospitalizations for IBD flares were all associated with increased risk for VTEs [80].

Solem et al. reported that 80% of patients with IBD (both CD and UC) had active disease at the time of VTE. Additionally, 76% of the UC patients had concurrent pancolitis and 79% of CD patients had concurrent colonic involvement [91]. In contrast to the above, Talbot et al. found that VTEs occurred when the disease was in remission in almost 30% of patients and that peripheral VTEs occurred spontaneously in 77% of patients [90].

Studies have found hospitalizations associated with IBD flares to have significantly increased the risk of VTE. Grainge et al. reported a threefold increased relative risk of VTE in hospitalized patients with IBD compared to controls [78]. Similarly, Nguyen and Sam reported a significantly higher risk of VTE in patients with IBD (OR 1.85 for UC and OR 1.48 for CD). Additionally, they found VTE was associated with increased mortality, longer hospital stays a higher healthcare cost (OR 2.5) [80]. Indeed, other studies have confirmed the higher risk of VTE in all hospitalized patients with IBD secondary to non-flare-up, flare-up, or surgery [92].

4.3. Peripheral Artery Disease

The literature has mixed evidence for the risk of peripheral artery disease (PAD) associated with IBD. Two meta-analyses with two studies each reported no significant increase in the risk of PAD in patients with IBD [73,93]. On the contrary, Lin et al. reported a significantly increased risk of PAD in patients with IBD after adjusting for age, sex, and comorbidities (HR 1.24). Additionally, the risk for PAD was highest in patients with more than two annual IBD-related medical hospitalizations (HR 27.5) [94]. These findings suggest an association of disease severity with the risk of PAD.

Kirchgesner et al. reported a significantly higher risk of PAD in patients with IBD compared with the general population (SIR 1.27). Interestingly, they found a significant increase in the risk in patients with CD (SIR 1.65) but not with UC (SIR 1.07) [95]. Additionally, they noted that the risk was highest in patients with CD who were younger than 35 (SIR 3.04). Indeed, this risk decreased with increasing age, eventually, becoming non-significant in patients older than 75 years [95], suggesting an association between age and risk of PAD.

4.4. Cerebrovascular

While IBD manifests as an inflammatory disease in the colon, it can also be accompanied by disorders outside of the colon, including nervous system manifestations, such as cerebrovascular disease [96]. Many studies have investigated the link between IBD and cerebrovascular disease, with the majority detailing that those with IBD have an increased risk of cerebrovascular disease; however, there are some differences between those with ulcerative colitis and those with Crohn's disease [97,98]. While 33% of patients with IBD have extraintestinal manifestations, cerebrovascular disease is reported in only 3% of patients with IBD; however, it is still an important consideration, as some therapies may increase the risk of neurologic manifestations [99].

In a population-based cohort study analyzing 20,795 patients with IBD matched to 199,978 controls, Kristensen et al. aimed to identify differences between disease activity (IBD overall, persistent IBD, and IBD in remission) and risk of MI, stroke, and cardiovascular death. The study found that IBD overall and persistent IBD (persistent use of medications or hospitalizations throughout the study period) were associated with an increased risk for stroke (RR 1.15, 95% CI 1.04–1.27 and RR 1.55, 95% CI 1.18–2.04, respectively), while IBD in remission (no use of medication or hospitalizations throughout the study period) had a similar relative risk compared to controls [100]. Several meta-analyses and systematic reviews have also shown similar conclusions, especially when related to female patients [93,101].

A population study using the University of Manitoba IBD Epidemiology Database analyzed 8060 patients with IBD compared to a matched cohort of 80,489 controls. The study found that only patients with Crohn's disease were at an increased risk (1.32, 95% CI 1.05–1.66) for cerebrovascular disease [98]. A population-based nested case-control study within a cohort of 8054 patients with Crohn's disease matched to 161,078 patients without Crohn's disease analyzed the odds of ischemic stroke associated with Crohn's disease. It found that younger patients (less than 50 years old) with Crohn's disease had an increased risk of ischemic stroke compared to controls (OR 2.93, 95% CI 1.44–5.98) [97]. Therefore, there is evidence for a link between Crohn's disease specifically and cerebrovascular disease.

4.5. Ischemic Heart Disease

Chronic inflammation, which can be found in those with inflammatory bowel disease, can lead to cardiovascular disease, specifically ischemic heart disease and heart failure, by contributing to the pathogenesis of atherosclerosis and the risk of thrombotic events [102]. Several studies have noted an increased risk of ischemic heart disease in those with inflammatory bowel disease [98,100,103]; however, some studies only see this increased risk in some IBD populations with other characteristics, suggesting that there may be secondary risk factors that are contributory [103] (Table 2).

Table 2. Summary of studies reporting the risk of ischemic heart disease in patients with IBD.

Author	Findings
Kristensen (2013) [100]	Patients with IBD with flares or persistent disease had an increased risk (RR 1.17, 95% CI 1.05–1.31) of myocardial infarction compared to control patients. Patients with IBD with flares or persistent disease had an elevated risk (RR 1.35, 95% CI 1.25–1.45) of cardiovascular death compared to control patients. In patients with ongoing IBD flares this study reported an increased risk of myocardial infarction (RR 1.49, 95% CI 1.16–1.93) when compared to control patients. In patients with persistent IBD this study reported an elevated risk of myocardial infarction (RR 2.05, 95% CI 1.58–2.65) when compared to control patients.
Ha (2009) [103]	This study found that patients with IBD overall did not have an elevated risk of ischemic heart disease compared to controls but found that women over 40 years of age with IBD had a higher risk of myocardial infarction (HR = 1.6, $p = 0.003$) with similar risk between Crohn's disease and ulcerative.
Yarur (2011) [104]	The incidence of coronary artery disease was significantly elevated in patients with IBD (HR 4.08, CI 2.49–6.70) compared to control patients even after adjusting for concurrent risk factors.

In a cohort study of 20,795 patients with IBD, Kristensen et al. investigated the risk of myocardial infarction, stroke, and cardiovascular death. The patients with IBD were matched by age and sex to 199,978 controls. The study analyzed patients with IBD overall, those with flares or persistent IBD (defined as those with continued corticosteroid prescriptions or IBD hospitalizations during the study period), and those in remission (discontinued use of medications or no hospitalizations during the study period). It found that, overall, those with IBD had an increased risk of myocardial infarction (RR 1.17, 95% CI 1.05–1.31) and cardiovascular death (RR 1.35, 95% CI 1.25–1.45). The relative risks increased for myocardial infarction when considering flares (1.49, 95% CI 1.16–1.93) and persistent IBD (2.05, 95% CI 1.58–2.65). Additionally, in remission periods compared to controls, the relative risk of myocardial infarction and cardiovascular death was similar, suggesting that the severity of the disease played a role in the risk of ischemic heart disease [100].

Another longitudinal cohort study analyzed coronary artery disease in 356 patients with IBD matched to 712 controls. This study also found an increased incidence of coronary artery disease in those with patients with IBD compared to the control group. The unadjusted hazard ratio was 2.85 (95% CI 1.82–4.46) for developing coronary artery disease in the patients with IBD group. It also concluded that the patients with IBD in the study had a lower burden of other risk factors (hypertension, diabetes, dyslipidemia, and obesity, $p < 0.01$ for all risk factors), and thus IBD was a large contributing factor in the development of coronary artery disease in these patients with the adjusted hazard ratio considering these factors being 4.08 (95% CI 2.49–6.70) [104].

A study of 17,487 patients with IBD and 69,948 healthy controls found that patients with IBD overall did not have an increased risk of ischemic heart disease compared to controls but found that women over 40 years old with IBD had a higher risk of myocardial infarction (HR = 1.6, $p = 0.003$) with the risks between Crohn's disease and ulcerative colitis being similar. This study concluded that not all patients with IBD were at an increased risk of ischemic heart disease, but that certain groups who suffer from IBD may be [103].

Ultimately, there is evidence of an increased risk of ischemic heart disease for those with IBD [98,100,103]. However, not all studies have made this conclusion, so more studies and meta-analyses should be done to continue to assess this relationship. IBD in some specific groups or the presence of other risk factors may lead to greater risk than IBD alone [103].

4.6. Mesenteric Ischemia

Of all the thromboembolic events studied with IBD, ATE is less studied than VTE, and mesenteric ischemia is one of the least recognized complications [105]. However, several emerging studies have linked IBD to mesenteric ischemia.

Patients with IBD and/or chronic constipation were compared to control individuals without these conditions in a population-based case-control study nested in a cohort study to analyze the incidence and risk of intestinal ischemia in these populations. It was found that those with IBD have a higher odds ratio of ischemic colitis (4.2 95% CI 0.5–38.4), but no association was found with acute mesenteric ischemia [106]. A cross-sectional study analyzed the Nationwide Inpatient Sample database to compare hospitalized patients discharged with a diagnosis of IBD to hospitalized patients discharged without this diagnosis (control). It reported an adjusted odds ratio of 3.4 (95% CI 2.9–4.0) for an association of IBD with mesenteric ischemia. With a smaller CI in this study, a stronger connection was found between IBD and mesenteric ischemia in this study [81].

An additional study found mesenteric infarction to be a cause of abdominal pain in patients with ulcerative colitis, thus stressing the importance of including mesenteric ischemia in a differential diagnosis for patients with IBD presenting with abdominal pain. This study outlined four cases of patients with ulcerative colitis and abdominal pain who also were diagnosed with mesenteric colitis. One patient presented with abdominal pain before being diagnosed with ulcerative colitis, two presented with the pain at the time of diagnosis, and one presented after diagnosis [68]. Two additional case reports outline patients presenting with abdominal pain. In both cases, the patients were diagnosed with Crohn's disease and were also found to have mesenteric atherosclerosis with mesenteric artery thrombosis in one patient [107] and a thrombus in the superior mesenteric artery in the second patient [105]. Thus, this complication should be considered when patients with IBD present with abdominal pain.

5. Treatment for IBD and Its Effect on Thromboembolic Risk

The main objective of the treatment of IBD is to reduce symptoms and maintain remission [108,109]. Various factors must be considered to tailor the treatment for individual patients. Before initiating treatment, appropriate medication is determined by activity, distribution, severity (mild, moderate, severe, and fulminant), and response to previous treatment [110–113]. For induction of remission for mild to moderate active ulcerative colitis

(UC), 5-ASA (5-aminosalicylic acid) or mesalamine has been the drug of choice [108,114,115]. Corticosteroids have been used for moderate to severe UC or patients who have failed the therapy with 5-ASA [109,110,114,116]. In the case of steroid-dependent ulcerative colitis, azathioprine and mercaptopurine be effective [114,117,118]. Biologics (e.g., Infliximab) is considered in patients who failed corticosteroids and/or immunomodulators [116,119,120]. With an increased risk of thromboembolism in patients with IBD, the risk of VTE needs to be considered with the treatment of IBD.

In patients with IBD, platelets are activated and form aggregate [114]. An increasing number of abnormal platelet function contributing to the inflammation and pathophysiology of IBD have been reported [115–117]. Abnormal platelet function is observed through an increased level of chemokine RANTES in patient IBD [118,119]. With the activation of the platelets, it has been found to increase the risk of thromboembolism [90]. To induce and maintain remission in mild to moderate UC, 5-ASA is used as the first line of treatment [120]. 5-ASA has been shown to lower the levels of RANTES in the plasma of patients with IBD compared to control group without IBD [119]. 5-ASA inhibits platelet activation and might reduce thromboembolism; however, there is no specific study assessing the risk of VTE among the patients using 5-ASA. In a small study with a group of 26 patients, 5-ASA inhibited the platelet activation by thrombin ($p \leq 0.02$) [121]. Additionally, a randomized controlled trial assessing the safety and efficacy of 5-ASA on 206 patients with the active UC did not report any VTE complications [122]. Although more studies of 5-ASA on the risk are needed, it suggests that 5-ASA may reduce the risk of VTE in patients with IBD.

Hypercoagulation has been observed in patients using corticosteroids or adrenocorticotrophic hormone (ACTH) [123]. A case-control study with 38,765 patients with VTE reported that the use of systemic glucocorticoids has the greatest risk of VTE (Incidence rate ratio (IRR) 2.31; 95% CI, 2.18–2.45) and corresponds to 11 VTE cases per 1000 new users of the medication each year [124]. A study by Higgins et al. analyzed that 335 VTE cases were found within 12 months among the 15,100 patients with IBD. It reported that the absolute rate of VTE was 2.25% (296 of 13,165) for corticosteroid therapy. Patients taking the corticosteroids were at risk of developing VTE five times more than those who were treated with only biologics [58]. These studies suggest that there is a higher risk of VTE with the use of corticosteroids.

There has not been a reported incidence of thromboembolism with immunomodulatory therapy. In a study of 3391 Spanish patients with IBD, there is no report of VTE with the use of azathioprine and mercaptopurine after a median follow-up of 44 months [125]. In a prospective study looking at the tolerability of thiopurines, after the median follow-up of 32 months, no VTE events were reported from the analysis of 253 patients [126]. Similarly, a VTE event was not reported from the examination of 174 patients with Crohn's disease in the study of tolerability of methotrexate after thiopurine therapy [127]. These studies indicate that there may be no potential risk of VTE with immunomodulators.

Tumor necrosis factor (TNF) is a pro-inflammatory cytokine that has been known to activate coagulation [128,129]. Therefore, infliximab may reduce the risk of VTE. Anti-TNF therapy, administered in 452 hospitalizations out of 1048 hospitalizations, was associated with significantly lowering the risk of thromboembolism (OR = 0.201; 95% CI 0.041–0.994; p = 0.049) [130]. In a prospective study, 78 out of 103 patients with IBD that have responded to infliximab therapy have shown no increased risk for thrombosis. During the study, patients on infliximab did not develop VTE, while one patient who stopped infliximab and received corticosteroid treatment developed VTE in 1-year follow-up [131]. In another prospective study, it is suggested that infliximab may reduce the risk of VTE in patients with IBD [132]. Clot lysis profiles of patients on infliximab have been reported to decrease or normalize [131,132]. As a result, infliximab may be an effective treatment in reducing the risk of thromboembolism.

6. Treatment Recommendations for IBD to Reduce Risk

About 50% of VTE events arise from hospitalization, trauma, and surgery [133]. The risk of VTE increases with factors such as hospital admission, surgery, cancer, and IBD [134,135]. To lower the risk, lower molecular weighted heparin is generally recommended as prophylaxis to hospitalized patients with and without IBD [136,137].

At the time of active IBD, patients are at risk of developing VTE [90]. In a cohort study, the risk of VTE is reported to be higher compared to the time when the disease is inactive [78]. Additionally, there is an increased risk of recurrence in patients with IBD [84]. Although the risk of thrombosis increases with outpatient flares, the absolute risk is low [78]. VTE prophylaxis is not recommended during IBD flare in patients with no history of VTE [138]. However, thromboprophylaxis is recommended for moderate to severe IBD flares with a history of VTE [139].

Among patients with IBD, hospitalization increases the risk of VTE. It has been reported that VTE-associated mortality in patients with IBD is greater compared to patients without IBD [80]. With this risk in patients with IBD, pharmacological thromboprophylaxis is recommended when patients are admitted to the hospital [140]. In a study, the use of low-molecular-weight heparin dalteparin had reduced the thromboembolic events by 45% (Relative risk, 0.55; 95% CI, 0.38 to 0.80; $p = 0.0015$) compared to a placebo group [141]. A meta-analysis showed that heparin and low-molecular-weight heparin used for patients hospitalized with IBD flare up has no difference in adverse effects when compared to controls [142]. Thromboprophylaxis treatment during hospitalization is also associated with a reduced risk of VTE after discharge [92]. Additionally, heparin has been shown to have anti-inflammatory effects and tissue repair properties [143]. More evidence is needed, but studies have proposed some benefits of thromboprophylaxis.

While temporal trends of COVID-19 cases in patients with IBD across 73 countries parallel the epidemiological pattern of COVID-19 in the general population [144], it is important to note the immunosuppressive nature of the drugs used in IBD treatment in patients with concurrent IBD and COVID-19 infection [145]. Although many patients with IBD are prescribed immunosuppressants, which can negatively affect their response to a COVID-19 infection, it is recommended that they continue the therapy if they have no symptoms and are not infected by COVID-19. For patients with IBD who test positive for COVID-19 and have symptoms, the recommendation is to withhold IBD therapy until they recover [146]. Additional prophylactic anticoagulation therapy is recommended to discharged patients with positive COVID-19 as COVID-19 is associated with a hypercoagulable state and thus predisposes the patient to venous thromboembolism [147].

7. Conclusions

Thromboembolic events are associated with a substantial increase in mortality and morbidity. The inflammatory response in patients with IBD leads to a hypercoagulable state significantly increasing the risk of thromboembolic events. Several factors associated with IBD increase the risk of thromboembolic events such as the severity of disease, hospitalization, surgery, and corticosteroids. A thorough history must be conducted to assess the individual patients' risk of thromboembolism.

Guidelines indicate the use of thromboembolic events prophylaxis for all patients hospitalized with IBD flare up if no contraindication is present. For the prophylaxis of thromboembolic events, either heparin or low molecular weight heparin should be considered. However, it is unclear whether thromboembolic events prophylaxis should continue after discharge or not especially in patients with active disease. Future studies need to consider a risk-based model to assess the benefit and risk of thromboembolic events prophylaxis amongst patients with the highest risk. The risk assessment should be based on patients' demographic information, medical history, medications, and family history. Lastly, further guidelines are required for the management of ambulatory patients with active IBD disease as these patients are at a high risk of developing thromboembolic events.

Future studies need to focus on the type of anticoagulation and duration in patients who develop thromboembolic complications secondary to IBD.

Additionally, the pathophysiology of thromboembolic events in patients with IBD needs to be further investigated. A better understanding of the pathophysiology may allow for the recognition or development of biomarkers to sensitively assess the risk of VTE and guide management.

Although guidelines recommend the use of thromboembolic prophylaxis in patients admitted for IBD flare up, it is not widely used due to concerns about bleeding with anticoagulation and the lack of awareness of the increased risk of thromboembolic complications. We hope to increase clinician recognition of thromboembolic events in patients with IBD.

Author Contributions: D.G. conceptualized the idea. D.G., T.N., N.R., S.M.L., M.T., M.S., V.K., P.B. and V.G. collected the data and wrote the original draft of the manuscript. D.G., V.K., P.B. and V.G. reviewed and edited the manuscript. All authors have read and agreed to the published version of the manuscript.

Funding: This research received no external funding.

Conflicts of Interest: The authors declare no conflict of interest.

References

1. Fakhoury, M.; Negrulj, R.; Mooranian, A.; Al-Salami, H. Inflammatory bowel disease: Clinical aspects and treatments. *J. Inflamm. Res.* **2014**, *7*, 113–120. [CrossRef] [PubMed]
2. Ng, S.C.; Shi, H.Y.; Hamidi, N.; Underwood, F.E.; Tang, W.; Benchimol, E.I.; Panaccione, R.; Ghosh, S.; Wu, J.C.Y.; Chan, F.K.L.; et al. Worldwide incidence and prevalence of inflammatory bowel disease in the 21st century: A systematic review of population-based studies. *Lancet* **2017**, *390*, 2769–2778. [CrossRef]
3. Basu, D.; Lopez, I.; Kulkarni, A.; Sellin, J.H. Impact of race and ethnicity on inflammatory bowel disease. *Am. J. Gastroenterol.* **2005**, *100*, 2254–2261. [CrossRef] [PubMed]
4. Cosnes, J.; Gower-Rousseau, C.; Seksik, P.; Cortot, A. Epidemiology and natural history of inflammatory bowel diseases. *Gastroenterology* **2011**, *140*, 1785–1794. [CrossRef] [PubMed]
5. Yu, Y.R.; Rodriguez, J.R. Clinical presentation of Crohn's, ulcerative colitis, and indeterminate colitis: Symptoms, extraintestinal manifestations, and disease phenotypes. *Semin. Pediatr. Surg.* **2017**, *26*, 349–355. [CrossRef] [PubMed]
6. Harries, A.D.; Baird, A.; Rhodes, J. Non-smoking: A feature of ulcerative colitis. *Br. Med. J. Clin. Res. Ed.* **1982**, *284*, 706. [CrossRef]
7. Amre, D.K.; D'Souza, S.; Morgan, K.; Seidman, G.; Lambrette, P.; Grimard, G.; Israel, D.; Mack, D.; Ghadirian, P.; Deslandres, C.; et al. Imbalances in dietary consumption of fatty acids, vegetables, and fruits are associated with risk for Crohn's disease in children. *Am. J. Gastroenterol.* **2007**, *102*, 2016–2025. [CrossRef]
8. Weinstock, J.V.; Elliott, D.E. Helminths and the IBD hygiene hypothesis. *Inflamm. Bowel Dis.* **2009**, *15*, 128–133. [CrossRef]
9. Levine, J.S.; Burakoff, R. Extraintestinal manifestations of inflammatory bowel disease. *Gastroenterol. Hepatol.* **2011**, *7*, 235–241.
10. Rogler, G.; Singh, A.; Kavanaugh, A.; Rubin, D.T. Extraintestinal Manifestations of Inflammatory Bowel Disease: Current Concepts, Treatment, and Implications for Disease Management. *Gastroenterology* **2021**, *161*, 1118–1132. [CrossRef]
11. Grover, S.P.; Mackman, N. Intrinsic Pathway of Coagulation and Thrombosis. *Arterioscler. Thromb. Vasc. Biol.* **2019**, *39*, 331–338. [CrossRef] [PubMed]
12. Palta, S.; Saroa, R.; Palta, A. Overview of the coagulation system. *Indian J. Anaesth.* **2014**, *58*, 515–523. [CrossRef] [PubMed]
13. Bombeli, T.; Spahn, D.R. Updates in perioperative coagulation: Physiology and management of thromboembolism and haemorrhage. *Br. J. Anaesth.* **2004**, *93*, 275–287. [CrossRef] [PubMed]
14. Kumar, D.R.; Hanlin, E.; Glurich, I.; Mazza, J.J.; Yale, S.H. Virchow's contribution to the understanding of thrombosis and cellular biology. *Clin. Med. Res.* **2010**, *8*, 168–172. [CrossRef]
15. Brotman, D.J.; Deitcher, S.R.; Lip, G.Y.; Matzdorff, A.C. Virchow's triad revisited. *South Med. J.* **2004**, *97*, 213–214. [CrossRef]
16. Glassner, K.L.; Abraham, B.P.; Quigley, E.M.M. The microbiome and inflammatory bowel disease. *J. Allergy Clin. Immunol.* **2020**, *145*, 16–27. [CrossRef]
17. Valdes, A.M.; Walter, J.; Segal, E.; Spector, T.D. Role of the gut microbiota in nutrition and health. *BMJ* **2018**, *361*, k2179. [CrossRef]
18. Khan, I.; Ullah, N.; Zha, L.; Bai, Y.; Khan, A.; Zhao, T.; Che, T.; Zhang, C. Alteration of Gut Microbiota in Inflammatory Bowel Disease (IBD): Cause or Consequence? IBD Treatment Targeting the Gut Microbiome. *Pathogens* **2019**, *8*, 126. [CrossRef]
19. Ogura, Y.; Inohara, N.; Benito, A.; Chen, F.F.; Yamaoka, S.; Nunez, G. Nod2, a Nod1/Apaf-1 family member that is restricted to monocytes and activates NF-kappaB. *J. Biol. Chem.* **2001**, *276*, 4812–4818. [CrossRef]
20. Swidsinski, A.; Ladhoff, A.; Pernthaler, A.; Swidsinski, S.; Loening-Baucke, V.; Ortner, M.; Weber, J.; Hoffmann, U.; Schreiber, S.; Dietel, M.; et al. Mucosal flora in inflammatory bowel disease. *Gastroenterology* **2002**, *122*, 44–54. [CrossRef]
21. Al Nabhani, Z.; Dietrich, G.; Hugot, J.P.; Barreau, F. Nod2: The intestinal gate keeper. *PLoS Pathog.* **2017**, *13*, e1006177. [CrossRef] [PubMed]

22. Rehman, A.; Sina, C.; Gavrilova, O.; Hasler, R.; Ott, S.; Baines, J.F.; Schreiber, S.; Rosenstiel, P. Nod2 is essential for temporal development of intestinal microbial communities. *Gut* **2011**, *60*, 1354–1362. [CrossRef] [PubMed]
23. Li, E.; Hamm, C.M.; Gulati, A.S.; Sartor, R.B.; Chen, H.; Wu, X.; Zhang, T.; Rohlf, F.J.; Zhu, W.; Gu, C.; et al. Inflammatory bowel diseases phenotype, C. difficile and NOD2 genotype are associated with shifts in human ileum associated microbial composition. *PLoS ONE* **2012**, *7*, e26284. [CrossRef] [PubMed]
24. Watanabe, T.; Kitani, A.; Murray, P.J.; Strober, W. NOD2 is a negative regulator of Toll-like receptor 2-mediated T helper type 1 responses. *Nat. Immunol.* **2004**, *5*, 800–808. [CrossRef] [PubMed]
25. Wehkamp, J.; Salzman, N.H.; Porter, E.; Nuding, S.; Weichenthal, M.; Petras, R.E.; Shen, B.; Schaeffeler, E.; Schwab, M.; Linzmeier, R.; et al. Reduced Paneth cell alpha-defensins in ileal Crohn's disease. *Proc. Natl. Acad. Sci. USA* **2005**, *102*, 18129–18134. [CrossRef]
26. Hugot, J.P.; Chamaillard, M.; Zouali, H.; Lesage, S.; Cezard, J.P.; Belaiche, J.; Almer, S.; Tysk, C.; O'Morain, C.A.; Gassull, M.; et al. Association of NOD2 leucine-rich repeat variants with susceptibility to Crohn's disease. *Nature* **2001**, *411*, 599–603. [CrossRef]
27. Speckmann, C.; Ehl, S. XIAP deficiency is a mendelian cause of late-onset IBD. *Gut* **2014**, *63*, 1031–1032. [CrossRef]
28. Uhlig, H.H. Monogenic diseases associated with intestinal inflammation: Implications for the understanding of inflammatory bowel disease. *Gut* **2013**, *62*, 1795–1805. [CrossRef]
29. Shim, J.O.; Hwang, S.; Yang, H.R.; Moon, J.S.; Chang, J.Y.; Ko, J.S.; Park, S.S.; Kang, G.H.; Kim, W.S.; Seo, J.K. Interleukin-10 receptor mutations in children with neonatal-onset Crohn's disease and intractable ulcerating enterocolitis. *Eur. J. Gastroenterol. Hepatol.* **2013**, *25*, 1235–1240. [CrossRef]
30. Cadwell, K.; Liu, J.Y.; Brown, S.L.; Miyoshi, H.; Loh, J.; Lennerz, J.K.; Kishi, C.; Kc, W.; Carrero, J.A.; Hunt, S.; et al. A key role for autophagy and the autophagy gene Atg16l1 in mouse and human intestinal Paneth cells. *Nature* **2008**, *456*, 259–263. [CrossRef]
31. Gunther, C.; Martini, E.; Wittkopf, N.; Amann, K.; Weigmann, B.; Neumann, H.; Waldner, M.J.; Hedrick, S.M.; Tenzer, S.; Neurath, M.F.; et al. Caspase-8 regulates TNF-alpha-induced epithelial necroptosis and terminal ileitis. *Nature* **2011**, *477*, 335–339. [CrossRef] [PubMed]
32. Chu, H.; Khosravi, A.; Kusumawardhani, I.P.; Kwon, A.H.; Vasconcelos, A.C.; Cunha, L.D.; Mayer, A.E.; Shen, Y.; Wu, W.L.; Kambal, A.; et al. Gene-microbiota interactions contribute to the pathogenesis of inflammatory bowel disease. *Science* **2016**, *352*, 1116–1120. [CrossRef] [PubMed]
33. Ward, J.M.; Anver, M.R.; Haines, D.C.; Melhorn, J.M.; Gorelick, P.; Yan, L.; Fox, J.G. Inflammatory large bowel disease in immunodeficient mice naturally infected with Helicobacter hepaticus. *Lab. Anim. Sci.* **1996**, *46*, 15–20. [PubMed]
34. Fajgenbaum, D.C.; June, C.H. Cytokine Storm. *N. Engl. J. Med.* **2020**, *383*, 2255–2273. [CrossRef] [PubMed]
35. Nenci, A.; Becker, C.; Wullaert, A.; Gareus, R.; van Loo, G.; Danese, S.; Huth, M.; Nikolaev, A.; Neufert, C.; Madison, B.; et al. Epithelial NEMO links innate immunity to chronic intestinal inflammation. *Nature* **2007**, *446*, 557–561. [CrossRef] [PubMed]
36. Chamouard, P.; Grunebaum, L.; Wiesel, M.L.; Frey, P.L.; Wittersheim, C.; Sapin, R.; Baumann, R.; Cazenave, J.P. Prothrombin fragment 1 + 2 and thrombin-antithrombin III complex as markers of activation of blood coagulation in inflammatory bowel diseases. *Eur. J. Gastroenterol. Hepatol.* **1995**, *7*, 1183–1188. [CrossRef] [PubMed]
37. Bisoendial, R.J.; Kastelein, J.J.; Levels, J.H.; Zwaginga, J.J.; van den Bogaard, B.; Reitsma, P.H.; Meijers, J.C.; Hartman, D.; Levi, M.; Stroes, E.S. Activation of inflammation and coagulation after infusion of C-reactive protein in humans. *Circ. Res.* **2005**, *96*, 714–716. [CrossRef]
38. Thompson, N.P.; Wakefield, A.J.; Pounder, R.E. Inherited disorders of coagulation appear to protect against inflammatory bowel disease. *Gastroenterology* **1995**, *108*, 1011–1015. [CrossRef]
39. Kronman, M.P.; Zaoutis, T.E.; Haynes, K.; Feng, R.; Coffin, S.E. Antibiotic exposure and IBD development among children: A population-based cohort study. *Pediatrics* **2012**, *130*, e794–e803. [CrossRef]
40. Bhatia, P.; Singh, N. Homocysteine excess: Delineating the possible mechanism of neurotoxicity and depression. *Fundam. Clin. Pharmacol.* **2015**, *29*, 522–528. [CrossRef]
41. Danese, S.; Sgambato, A.; Papa, A.; Scaldaferri, F.; Pola, R.; Sans, M.; Lovecchio, M.; Gasbarrini, G.; Cittadini, A.; Gasbarrini, A. Homocysteine triggers mucosal microvascular activation in inflammatory bowel disease. *Am. J. Gastroenterol.* **2005**, *100*, 886–895. [CrossRef]
42. Danese, S.; Papa, A.; Saibeni, S.; Repici, A.; Malesci, A.; Vecchi, M. Inflammation and coagulation in inflammatory bowel disease: The clot thickens. *Am. J. Gastroenterol.* **2007**, *102*, 174–186. [CrossRef] [PubMed]
43. Topal, G.; Brunet, A.; Millanvoye, E.; Boucher, J.L.; Rendu, F.; Devynck, M.A.; David-Dufilho, M. Homocysteine induces oxidative stress by uncoupling of NO synthase activity through reduction of tetrahydrobiopterin. *Free Radic. Biol. Med.* **2004**, *36*, 1532–1541. [CrossRef] [PubMed]
44. Undas, A.; Brozek, J.; Szczeklik, A. Homocysteine and thrombosis: From basic science to clinical evidence. *Thromb. Haemost.* **2005**, *94*, 907–915. [CrossRef]
45. Ingrosso, D.; Cimmino, A.; Perna, A.F.; Masella, L.; De Santo, N.G.; De Bonis, M.L.; Vacca, M.; D'Esposito, M.; D'Urso, M.; Galletti, P.; et al. Folate treatment and unbalanced methylation and changes of allelic expression induced by hyperhomocysteinaemia in patients with uraemia. *Lancet* **2003**, *361*, 1693–1699. [CrossRef]
46. Lentz, S.R.; Sadler, J.E. Inhibition of thrombomodulin surface expression and protein C activation by the thrombogenic agent homocysteine. *J. Clin. Investig.* **1991**, *88*, 1906–1914. [CrossRef] [PubMed]
47. Giannini, M.J.; Coleman, M.; Innerfield, I. Letter: Antithrombin activity in homocystinuria. *Lancet* **1975**, *1*, 1094. [CrossRef]

48. Lentz, S.R.; Sobey, C.G.; Piegors, D.J.; Bhopatkar, M.Y.; Faraci, F.M.; Malinow, M.R.; Heistad, D.D. Vascular dysfunction in monkeys with diet-induced hyperhomocyst(e)inemia. *J. Clin. Investig.* **1996**, *98*, 24–29. [CrossRef] [PubMed]
49. Di Minno, G.; Davi, G.; Margaglione, M.; Cirillo, F.; Grandone, E.; Ciabattoni, G.; Catalano, I.; Strisciuglio, P.; Andria, G.; Patrono, C.; et al. Abnormally high thromboxane biosynthesis in homozygous homocystinuria. Evidence for platelet involvement and probucol-sensitive mechanism. *J. Clin. Investig.* **1993**, *92*, 1400–1406. [CrossRef]
50. Coppola, A.; Davi, G.; De Stefano, V.; Mancini, F.P.; Cerbone, A.M.; Di Minno, G. Homocysteine, coagulation, platelet function, and thrombosis. *Semin. Thromb. Hemost.* **2000**, *26*, 243–254. [CrossRef]
51. Davi, G.; Di Minno, G.; Coppola, A.; Andria, G.; Cerbone, A.M.; Madonna, P.; Tufano, A.; Falco, A.; Marchesani, P.; Ciabattoni, G.; et al. Oxidative stress and platelet activation in homozygous homocystinuria. *Circulation* **2001**, *104*, 1124–1128. [CrossRef] [PubMed]
52. Fryer, R.H.; Wilson, B.D.; Gubler, D.B.; Fitzgerald, L.A.; Rodgers, G.M. Homocysteine, a risk factor for premature vascular disease and thrombosis, induces tissue factor activity in endothelial cells. *Arterioscler. Thromb.* **1993**, *13*, 1327–1333. [CrossRef] [PubMed]
53. Stegeman, B.H.; de Bastos, M.; Rosendaal, F.R.; van Hylckama Vlieg, A.; Helmerhorst, F.M.; Stijnen, T.; Dekkers, O.M. Different combined oral contraceptives and the risk of venous thrombosis: Systematic review and network meta-analysis. *BMJ* **2013**, *347*, f5298. [CrossRef] [PubMed]
54. Melis, F.; Vandenbrouke, J.P.; Buller, H.R.; Colly, L.P.; Bloemenkamp, K.W. Estimates of risk of venous thrombosis during pregnancy and puerperium are not influenced by diagnostic suspicion and referral basis. *Am. J. Obs. Gynecol.* **2004**, *191*, 825–829. [CrossRef]
55. Weng, M.T.; Park, S.H.; Matsuoka, K.; Tung, C.C.; Lee, J.Y.; Chang, C.H.; Yang, S.K.; Watanabe, M.; Wong, J.M.; Wei, S.C. Incidence and Risk Factor Analysis of Thromboembolic Events in East Asian Patients with Inflammatory Bowel Disease, a Multinational Collaborative Study. *Inflamm. Bowel Dis.* **2018**, *24*, 1791–1800. [CrossRef]
56. Heo, C.M.; Kim, T.J.; Kim, E.R.; Hong, S.N.; Chang, D.K.; Yang, M.; Kim, S.; Kim, Y.H. Risk of venous thromboembolism in Asian patients with inflammatory bowel disease: A nationwide cohort study. *Sci. Rep.* **2021**, *11*, 2025. [CrossRef]
57. van Zaane, B.; Nur, E.; Squizzato, A.; Gerdes, V.E.; Buller, H.R.; Dekkers, O.M.; Brandjes, D.P. Systematic review on the effect of glucocorticoid use on procoagulant, anti-coagulant and fibrinolytic factors. *J. Thromb. Haemost.* **2010**, *8*, 2483–2493. [CrossRef] [PubMed]
58. Higgins, P.D.; Skup, M.; Mulani, P.M.; Lin, J.; Chao, J. Increased risk of venous thromboembolic events with corticosteroid vs. biologic therapy for inflammatory bowel disease. *Clin. Gastroenterol. Hepatol.* **2015**, *13*, 316–321. [CrossRef] [PubMed]
59. Webberley, M.J.; Hart, M.T.; Melikian, V. Thromboembolism in inflammatory bowel disease: Role of platelets. *Gut* **1993**, *34*, 247–251. [CrossRef]
60. van Wersch, J.W.; Houben, P.; Rijken, J. Platelet count, platelet function, coagulation activity and fibrinolysis in the acute phase of inflammatory bowel disease. *J. Clin. Chem. Clin. Biochem.* **1990**, *28*, 513–517. [CrossRef]
61. Danese, S.; Fiocchi, C. Platelet activation and the CD40/CD40 ligand pathway: Mechanisms and implications for human disease. *Crit. Rev. Immunol.* **2005**, *25*, 103–121. [CrossRef] [PubMed]
62. Collins, C.E.; Rampton, D.S.; Rogers, J.; Williams, N.S. Platelet aggregation and neutrophil sequestration in the mesenteric circulation in inflammatory bowel disease. *Eur. J. Gastroenterol. Hepatol.* **1997**, *9*, 1213–1217. [PubMed]
63. Klinger, M.H. Platelets and inflammation. *Anat. Embryol.* **1997**, *196*, 1–11. [CrossRef] [PubMed]
64. Danese, S.; de la Motte, C.; Sturm, A.; Vogel, J.D.; West, G.A.; Strong, S.A.; Katz, J.A.; Fiocchi, C. Platelets trigger a CD40-dependent inflammatory response in the microvasculature of inflammatory bowel disease patients. *Gastroenterology* **2003**, *124*, 1249–1264. [CrossRef]
65. Power, C.A.; Clemetson, J.M.; Clemetson, K.J.; Wells, T.N. Chemokine and chemokine receptor mRNA expression in human platelets. *Cytokine* **1995**, *7*, 479–482. [CrossRef] [PubMed]
66. Katsanos, A.H.; Kosmidou, M.; Giannopoulos, S.; Katsanos, K.H.; Tsivgoulis, G.; Kyritsis, A.P.; Tsianos, E.V. Cerebral arterial infarction in inflammatory bowel diseases. *Eur. J. Intern. Med.* **2014**, *25*, 37–44. [CrossRef] [PubMed]
67. Schneiderman, J.H.; Sharpe, J.A.; Sutton, D.M. Cerebral and retinal vascular complications of inflammatory bowel disease. *Ann. Neurol.* **1979**, *5*, 331–337. [CrossRef] [PubMed]
68. Irving, P.M.; Alstead, E.M.; Greaves, R.R.; Feakins, R.M.; Pollok, R.C.; Rampton, D.S. Acute mesenteric infarction: An important cause of abdominal pain in ulcerative colitis. *Eur. J. Gastroenterol. Hepatol.* **2005**, *17*, 1429–1432. [CrossRef] [PubMed]
69. Prior, A.; Strang, F.A.; Whorwell, P.J. Internal carotid artery occlusion in association with Crohn's disease. *Dig. Dis. Sci.* **1987**, *32*, 1047–1050. [CrossRef]
70. Mutlu, B.; Ermeydan, C.M.; Enc, F.; Fotbolcu, H.; Demirkol, O.; Bayrak, F.; Basaran, Y. Acute myocardial infarction in a young woman with severe ulcerative colitis. *Int. J. Cardiol.* **2002**, *83*, 183–185. [CrossRef]
71. Novacek, G.; Haumer, M.; Schima, W.; Muller, C.; Miehsler, W.; Polterauer, P.; Vogelsang, H. Aortic mural thrombi in patients with inflammatory bowel disease: Report of two cases and review of the literature. *Inflamm. Bowel Dis.* **2004**, *10*, 430–435. [CrossRef] [PubMed]
72. Haumer, M.; Teml, A.; Dirisamer, A.; Vogelsang, H.; Koppensteiner, R.; Novacek, G. Severe ulcerative colitis complicated by an arterial thrombus in the brachiocephalic trunk. *Inflamm. Bowel Dis.* **2007**, *13*, 937–938. [CrossRef] [PubMed]

73. Fumery, M.; Xiaocang, C.; Dauchet, L.; Gower-Rousseau, C.; Peyrin-Biroulet, L.; Colombel, J.F. Thromboembolic events and cardiovascular mortality in inflammatory bowel diseases: A meta-analysis of observational studies. *J. Crohns Colitis* **2014**, *8*, 469–479. [CrossRef] [PubMed]
74. Murthy, S.K.; Nguyen, G.C. Venous thromboembolism in inflammatory bowel disease: An epidemiological review. *Am. J. Gastroenterol.* **2011**, *106*, 713–718. [CrossRef] [PubMed]
75. Bernstein, C.N.; Blanchard, J.F.; Houston, D.S.; Wajda, A. The incidence of deep venous thrombosis and pulmonary embolism among patients with inflammatory bowel disease: A population-based cohort study. *Thromb. Haemost.* **2001**, *85*, 430–434.
76. Huerta, C.; Johansson, S.; Wallander, M.A.; Rodriguez, L.A.G. Risk factors and short-term mortality of venous thromboembolism diagnosed in the primary care setting in the United Kingdom. *Arch. Intern. Med.* **2007**, *167*, 935–943. [CrossRef]
77. Kappelman, M.D.; Horvath-Puho, E.; Sandler, R.S.; Rubin, D.T.; Ullman, T.A.; Pedersen, L.; Baron, J.A.; Sorensen, H.T. Thromboembolic risk among Danish children and adults with inflammatory bowel diseases: A population-based nationwide study. *Gut* **2011**, *60*, 937–943. [CrossRef]
78. Grainge, M.J.; West, J.; Card, T.R. Venous thromboembolism during active disease and remission in inflammatory bowel disease: A cohort study. *Lancet* **2010**, *375*, 657–663. [CrossRef]
79. Bernstein, C.N.; Nabalamba, A. Hospitalization-based major comorbidity of inflammatory bowel disease in Canada. *Can. J. Gastroenterol.* **2007**, *21*, 507–511. [CrossRef]
80. Nguyen, G.C.; Sam, J. Rising prevalence of venous thromboembolism and its impact on mortality among hospitalized inflammatory bowel disease patients. *Am. J. Gastroenterol.* **2008**, *103*, 2272–2280. [CrossRef]
81. Sridhar, A.R.; Parasa, S.; Navaneethan, U.; Crowell, M.D.; Olden, K. Comprehensive study of cardiovascular morbidity in hospitalized inflammatory bowel disease patients. *J. Crohns Colitis* **2011**, *5*, 287–294. [CrossRef] [PubMed]
82. Nguyen, G.C.; Boudreau, H.; Harris, M.L.; Maxwell, C.V. Outcomes of obstetric hospitalizations among women with inflammatory bowel disease in the United States. *Clin. Gastroenterol. Hepatol.* **2009**, *7*, 329–334. [CrossRef] [PubMed]
83. Wallaert, J.B.; De Martino, R.R.; Marsicovetere, P.S.; Goodney, P.P.; Finlayson, S.R.; Murray, J.J.; Holubar, S.D. Venous thromboembolism after surgery for inflammatory bowel disease: Are there modifiable risk factors? Data from ACS NSQIP. *Dis. Colon Rectum* **2012**, *55*, 1138–1144. [CrossRef] [PubMed]
84. Novacek, G.; Weltermann, A.; Sobala, A.; Tilg, H.; Petritsch, W.; Reinisch, W.; Mayer, A.; Haas, T.; Kaser, A.; Feichtenschlager, T.; et al. Inflammatory bowel disease is a risk factor for recurrent venous thromboembolism. *Gastroenterology* **2010**, *139*, 779–787.e771. [CrossRef] [PubMed]
85. Yuhara, H.; Steinmaus, C.; Corley, D.; Koike, J.; Igarashi, M.; Suzuki, T.; Mine, T. Meta-analysis: The risk of venous thromboembolism in patients with inflammatory bowel disease. *Aliment. Pharmacol. Ther.* **2013**, *37*, 953–962. [CrossRef]
86. Papay, P.; Miehsler, W.; Tilg, H.; Petritsch, W.; Reinisch, W.; Mayer, A.; Haas, T.; Kaser, A.; Feichtenschlager, T.; Fuchssteiner, H.; et al. Clinical presentation of venous thromboembolism in inflammatory bowel disease. *J. Crohns Colitis* **2013**, *7*, 723–729. [CrossRef]
87. Duricova, D.; Pedersen, N.; Elkjaer, M.; Gamborg, M.; Munkholm, P.; Jess, T. Overall and cause-specific mortality in Crohn's disease: A meta-analysis of population-based studies. *Inflamm. Bowel Dis.* **2010**, *16*, 347–353. [CrossRef]
88. O'Connor, O.J.; Cahill, R.A.; Kirwan, W.O.; Redmond, H.P. The incidence of postoperative venous thrombosis among patients with ulcerative colitis. *Ir. J. Med. Sci.* **2005**, *174*, 20–22. [CrossRef]
89. Merrill, A.; Millham, F. Increased risk of postoperative deep vein thrombosis and pulmonary embolism in patients with inflammatory bowel disease: A study of National Surgical Quality Improvement Program patients. *Arch. Surg.* **2012**, *147*, 120–124. [CrossRef]
90. Talbot, R.W.; Heppell, J.; Dozois, R.R.; Beart, R.W., Jr. Vascular complications of inflammatory bowel disease. *Mayo. Clin. Proc.* **1986**, *61*, 140–145. [CrossRef]
91. Solem, C.A.; Loftus, E.V.; Tremaine, W.J.; Sandborn, W.J. Venous thromboembolism in inflammatory bowel disease. *Am. J. Gastroenterol.* **2004**, *99*, 97–101. [CrossRef] [PubMed]
92. Ananthakrishnan, A.N.; Cagan, A.; Gainer, V.S.; Cheng, S.C.; Cai, T.; Scoville, E.; Konijeti, G.G.; Szolovits, P.; Shaw, S.Y.; Churchill, S.; et al. Thromboprophylaxis is associated with reduced post-hospitalization venous thromboembolic events in patients with inflammatory bowel diseases. *Clin. Gastroenterol. Hepatol.* **2014**, *12*, 1905–1910. [CrossRef] [PubMed]
93. Singh, S.; Singh, H.; Loftus, E.V., Jr.; Pardi, D.S. Risk of cerebrovascular accidents and ischemic heart disease in patients with inflammatory bowel disease: A systematic review and meta-analysis. *Clin. Gastroenterol. Hepatol.* **2014**, *12*, 382–393.e1. [CrossRef] [PubMed]
94. Lin, T.Y.; Chen, Y.G.; Lin, C.L.; Huang, W.S.; Kao, C.H. Inflammatory Bowel Disease Increases the Risk of Peripheral Arterial Disease: A Nationwide Cohort Study. *Medicine* **2015**, *94*, e2381. [CrossRef] [PubMed]
95. Kirchgesner, J.; Beaugerie, L.; Carrat, F.; Andersen, N.N.; Jess, T.; Schwarzinger, M.; BERENICE Study Group. Increased risk of acute arterial events in young patients and severely active IBD: A nationwide French cohort study. *Gut* **2018**, *67*, 1261–1268. [CrossRef]
96. Scheid, R.; Teich, N. Neurologic manifestations of ulcerative colitis. *Eur. J. Neurol.* **2007**, *14*, 483–493. [CrossRef]
97. Andersohn, F.; Waring, M.; Garbe, E. Risk of ischemic stroke in patients with Crohn's disease: A population-based nested case-control study. *Inflamm. Bowel Dis.* **2010**, *16*, 1387–1392. [CrossRef]

98. Bernstein, C.N.; Wajda, A.; Blanchard, J.F. The incidence of arterial thromboembolic diseases in inflammatory bowel disease: A population-based study. *Clin. Gastroenterol. Hepatol.* **2008**, *6*, 41–45. [CrossRef]
99. Casella, G.; Tontini, G.E.; Bassotti, G.; Pastorelli, L.; Villanacci, V.; Spina, L.; Baldini, V.; Vecchi, M. Neurological disorders and inflammatory bowel diseases. *World J. Gastroenterol.* **2014**, *20*, 8764–8782. [CrossRef]
100. Kristensen, S.L.; Ahlehoff, O.; Lindhardsen, J.; Erichsen, R.; Jensen, G.V.; Torp-Pedersen, C.; Nielsen, O.H.; Gislason, G.H.; Hansen, P.R. Disease activity in inflammatory bowel disease is associated with increased risk of myocardial infarction, stroke and cardiovascular death–a Danish nationwide cohort study. *PLoS ONE* **2013**, *8*, e56944. [CrossRef]
101. Xiao, Z.; Pei, Z.; Yuan, M.; Li, X.; Chen, S.; Xu, L. Risk of Stroke in Patients with Inflammatory Bowel Disease: A Systematic Review and Meta-analysis. *J. Stroke Cerebrovasc. Dis.* **2015**, *24*, 2774–2780. [CrossRef] [PubMed]
102. Wu, P.; Jia, F.; Zhang, B.; Zhang, P. Risk of cardiovascular disease in inflammatory bowel disease. *Exp. Ther. Med.* **2017**, *13*, 395–400. [CrossRef] [PubMed]
103. Ha, C.; Magowan, S.; Accortt, N.A.; Chen, J.; Stone, C.D. Risk of arterial thrombotic events in inflammatory bowel disease. *Am. J. Gastroenterol.* **2009**, *104*, 1445–1451. [CrossRef]
104. Yarur, A.J.; Deshpande, A.R.; Pechman, D.M.; Tamariz, L.; Abreu, M.T.; Sussman, D.A. Inflammatory bowel disease is associated with an increased incidence of cardiovascular events. *Am. J. Gastroenterol.* **2011**, *106*, 741–747. [CrossRef] [PubMed]
105. Nicolaides, S.; Vasudevan, A.; Langenberg, D.V. Inflammatory bowel disease and superior mesenteric artery thromboembolism. *Intest. Res.* **2020**, *18*, 130–133. [CrossRef] [PubMed]
106. Huerta, C.; Rivero, E.; Montoro, M.A.; Garcia-Rodriguez, L.A. Risk factors for intestinal ischaemia among patients registered in a UK primary care database: A nested case-control study. *Aliment. Pharmacol. Ther.* **2011**, *33*, 969–978. [CrossRef]
107. Qu, C.; Cao, J.; Liu, K.; Tan, B.; Zhu, C.; Li, K.; Qu, L. Crohn's Disease Complicated With Extensive Thrombosis of Limbs and Mesenteric Arteries: A Case Report and Literature Review. *Ann. Vasc. Surg.* **2019**, *58*, 382.e15–382.e19. [CrossRef]
108. Ng, S.C.; Kamm, M.A. Therapeutic strategies for the management of ulcerative colitis. *Inflamm. Bowel Dis.* **2009**, *15*, 935–950. [CrossRef]
109. Kozuch, P.L.; Hanauer, S.B. Treatment of inflammatory bowel disease: A review of medical therapy. *World J. Gastroenterol.* **2008**, *14*, 354–377. [CrossRef]
110. Travis, S.P.; Stange, E.F.; Lemann, M.; Oresland, T.; Bemelman, W.A.; Chowers, Y.; Colombel, J.F.; D'Haens, G.; Ghosh, S.; Marteau, P.; et al. European evidence-based Consensus on the management of ulcerative colitis: Current management. *J. Crohns Colitis* **2008**, *2*, 24–62. [CrossRef]
111. Kuhbacher, T.; Folsch, U.R. Practical guidelines for the treatment of inflammatory bowel disease. *World J. Gastroenterol.* **2007**, *13*, 1149–1155. [CrossRef] [PubMed]
112. Stange, E.F.; Travis, S.P.; Vermeire, S.; Reinisch, W.; Geboes, K.; Barakauskiene, A.; Feakins, R.; Flejou, J.F.; Herfarth, H.; Hommes, D.W.; et al. European evidence-based Consensus on the diagnosis and management of ulcerative colitis: Definitions and diagnosis. *J. Crohns Colitis* **2008**, *2*, 1–23. [CrossRef] [PubMed]
113. Kornbluth, A.; Sachar, D.B.; Practice Parameters Committee of the American College of G. Ulcerative colitis practice guidelines in adults (update): American College of Gastroenterology, Practice Parameters Committee. *Am. J. Gastroenterol.* **2004**, *99*, 1371–1385. [CrossRef] [PubMed]
114. Collins, C.E.; Cahill, M.R.; Newland, A.C.; Rampton, D.S. Platelets circulate in an activated state in inflammatory bowel disease. *Gastroenterology* **1994**, *106*, 840–845. [CrossRef]
115. Collins, C.E.; Rampton, D.S. Platelet dysfunction: A new dimension in inflammatory bowel disease. *Gut* **1995**, *36*, 5–8. [CrossRef]
116. Andoh, A.; Yoshida, T.; Yagi, Y.; Bamba, S.; Hata, K.; Tsujikawa, T.; Kitoh, K.; Sasaki, M.; Fujiyama, Y. Increased aggregation response of platelets in patients with inflammatory bowel disease. *J. Gastroenterol.* **2006**, *41*, 47–54. [CrossRef]
117. Yan, S.L.; Russell, J.; Harris, N.R.; Senchenkova, E.Y.; Yildirim, A.; Granger, D.N. Platelet abnormalities during colonic inflammation. *Inflamm. Bowel Dis.* **2013**, *19*, 1245–1253. [CrossRef]
118. Schurmann, G.M.; Bishop, A.E.; Facer, P.; Vecchio, M.; Lee, J.C.; Rampton, D.S.; Polak, J.M. Increased expression of cell adhesion molecule P-selectin in active inflammatory bowel disease. *Gut* **1995**, *36*, 411–418. [CrossRef]
119. Fagerstam, J.P.; Whiss, P.A.; Strom, M.; Andersson, R.G. Expression of platelet P-selectin and detection of soluble P-selectin, NPY and RANTES in patients with inflammatory bowel disease. *Inflamm. Res.* **2000**, *49*, 466–472. [CrossRef]
120. Hanauer, S.B. Inflammatory bowel disease. *N. Engl. J. Med.* **1996**, *334*, 841–848. [CrossRef]
121. Carty, E.; MacEy, M.; Rampton, D.S. Inhibition of platelet activation by 5-aminosalicylic acid in inflammatory bowel disease. *Aliment. Pharmacol. Ther.* **2000**, *14*, 1169–1179. [CrossRef] [PubMed]
122. Flourie, B.; Hagege, H.; Tucat, G.; Maetz, D.; Hebuterne, X.; Kuyvenhoven, J.P.; Tan, T.G.; Pierik, M.J.; Masclee, A.A.; Dewit, O.; et al. Randomised clinical trial: Once- vs. twice-daily prolonged-release mesalazine for active ulcerative colitis. *Aliment. Pharmacol. Ther.* **2013**, *37*, 767–775. [CrossRef] [PubMed]
123. Ozsoylu, S.; Strauss, H.S.; Diamond, L.K. Effects of corticosteroids on coagulation of the blood. *Nature* **1962**, *195*, 1214–1215. [CrossRef] [PubMed]
124. Johannesdottir, S.A.; Horvath-Puho, E.; Dekkers, O.M.; Cannegieter, S.C.; Jorgensen, J.O.; Ehrenstein, V.; Vandenbroucke, J.P.; Pedersen, L.; Sorensen, H.T. Use of glucocorticoids and risk of venous thromboembolism: A nationwide population-based case-control study. *JAMA Intern. Med.* **2013**, *173*, 743–752. [CrossRef] [PubMed]

125. Chaparro, M.; Ordas, I.; Cabre, E.; Garcia-Sanchez, V.; Bastida, G.; Penalva, M.; Gomollon, F.; Garcia-Planella, E.; Merino, O.; Gutierrez, A.; et al. Safety of thiopurine therapy in inflammatory bowel disease: Long-term follow-up study of 3931 patients. *Inflamm. Bowel Dis.* **2013**, *19*, 1404–1410. [CrossRef]
126. Macaluso, F.S.; Renna, S.; Maida, M.; Dimarco, M.; Sapienza, C.; Affronti, M.; Orlando, E.; Rizzuto, G.; Orlando, R.; Ventimiglia, M.; et al. Tolerability profile of thiopurines in inflammatory bowel disease: A prospective experience. *Scand J. Gastroenterol.* **2017**, *52*, 981–987. [CrossRef]
127. Seinen, M.L.; Ponsioen, C.Y.; de Boer, N.K.; Oldenburg, B.; Bouma, G.; Mulder, C.J.; van Bodegraven, A.A. Sustained clinical benefit and tolerability of methotrexate monotherapy after thiopurine therapy in patients with Crohn's disease. *Clin. Gastroenterol. Hepatol.* **2013**, *11*, 667–672. [CrossRef]
128. van der Poll, T.; Buller, H.R.; ten Cate, H.; Wortel, C.H.; Bauer, K.A.; van Deventer, S.J.; Hack, C.E.; Sauerwein, H.P.; Rosenberg, R.D.; ten Cate, J.W. Activation of coagulation after administration of tumor necrosis factor to normal subjects. *N. Engl. J. Med.* **1990**, *322*, 1622–1627. [CrossRef]
129. Page, M.J.; Bester, J.; Pretorius, E. The inflammatory effects of TNF-alpha and complement component 3 on coagulation. *Sci. Rep.* **2018**, *8*, 1812. [CrossRef]
130. deFonseka, A.M.; Tuskey, A.; Conaway, M.R.; Behm, B.W. Antitumor Necrosis Factor-alpha Therapy Is Associated With Reduced Risk of Thromboembolic Events in Hospitalized Patients With Inflammatory Bowel Disease. *J. Clin. Gastroenterol.* **2016**, *50*, 578–583. [CrossRef]
131. Bollen, L.; Vande Casteele, N.; Peeters, M.; Bessonov, K.; Van Steen, K.; Rutgeerts, P.; Ferrante, M.; Hoylaerts, M.F.; Vermeire, S.; Gils, A. Short-term effect of infliximab is reflected in the clot lysis profile of patients with inflammatory bowel disease: A prospective study. *Inflamm. Bowel Dis.* **2015**, *21*, 570–578. [CrossRef] [PubMed]
132. Detrez, I.; Thomas, D.; Van Steen, K.; Ballet, V.; Peeters, M.; Hoylaerts, M.F.; Van Assche, G.; Vermeire, S.; Ferrante, M.; Gils, A. Successful Infliximab Treatment is Associated With Reversal of Clotting Abnormalities in Inflammatory Bowel Disease Patients. *J. Clin. Gastroenterol.* **2020**, *54*, 819–825. [CrossRef] [PubMed]
133. Virani, S.S.; Alonso, A.; Benjamin, E.J.; Bittencourt, M.S.; Callaway, C.W.; Carson, A.P.; Chamberlain, A.M.; Chang, A.R.; Cheng, S.; Delling, F.N.; et al. Heart Disease and Stroke Statistics-2020 Update: A Report From the American Heart Association. *Circulation* **2020**, *141*, e139–e596. [CrossRef]
134. Heit, J.A. Venous thromboembolism epidemiology: Implications for prevention and management. *Semin. Thromb. Hemost.* **2002**, *28* (Suppl. 2), 3–13. [CrossRef]
135. Heit, J.A.; Silverstein, M.D.; Mohr, D.N.; Petterson, T.M.; O'Fallon, W.M.; Melton, L.J., 3rd. Risk factors for deep vein thrombosis and pulmonary embolism: A population-based case-control study. *Arch. Intern. Med.* **2000**, *160*, 809–815. [CrossRef] [PubMed]
136. Schunemann, H.J.; Cushman, M.; Burnett, A.E.; Kahn, S.R.; Beyer-Westendorf, J.; Spencer, F.A.; Rezende, S.M.; Zakai, N.A.; Bauer, K.A.; Dentali, F.; et al. American Society of Hematology 2018 guidelines for management of venous thromboembolism: Prophylaxis for hospitalized and nonhospitalized medical patients. *Blood Adv.* **2018**, *2*, 3198–3225. [CrossRef]
137. Geerts, W.H.; Bergqvist, D.; Pineo, G.F.; Heit, J.A.; Samama, C.M.; Lassen, M.R.; Colwell, C.W. Prevention of venous thromboembolism: American College of Chest Physicians Evidence-Based Clinical Practice Guidelines (8th Edition). *Chest* **2008**, *133*, 381S–453S. [CrossRef] [PubMed]
138. Nguyen, G.C.; Sharma, S. Feasibility of venous thromboembolism prophylaxis during inflammatory bowel disease flares in the outpatient setting: A decision analysis. *Inflamm. Bowel Dis.* **2013**, *19*, 2182–2189. [CrossRef] [PubMed]
139. Nguyen, G.C.; Bernstein, C.N.; Bitton, A.; Chan, A.K.; Griffiths, A.M.; Leontiadis, G.I.; Geerts, W.; Bressler, B.; Butzner, J.D.; Carrier, M.; et al. Consensus statements on the risk, prevention, and treatment of venous thromboembolism in inflammatory bowel disease: Canadian Association of Gastroenterology. *Gastroenterology* **2014**, *146*, 835–848.e836. [CrossRef] [PubMed]
140. Ra, G.; Thanabalan, R.; Ratneswaran, S.; Nguyen, G.C. Predictors and safety of venous thromboembolism prophylaxis among hospitalized inflammatory bowel disease patients. *J. Crohns Colitis* **2013**, *7*, e479–e485. [CrossRef] [PubMed]
141. Leizorovicz, A.; Cohen, A.T.; Turpie, A.G.; Olsson, C.G.; Vaitkus, P.T.; Goldhaber, S.Z.; Group, P.M.T.S. Randomized, placebo-controlled trial of dalteparin for the prevention of venous thromboembolism in acutely ill medical patients. *Circulation* **2004**, *110*, 874–879. [CrossRef] [PubMed]
142. Shen, J.; Ran, Z.H.; Tong, J.L.; Xiao, S.D. Meta-analysis: The utility and safety of heparin in the treatment of active ulcerative colitis. *Aliment. Pharmacol. Ther.* **2007**, *26*, 653–663. [CrossRef] [PubMed]
143. Michell, N.P.; Lalor, P.; Langman, M.J. Heparin therapy for ulcerative colitis? Effects and mechanisms. *Eur. J. Gastroenterol. Hepatol.* **2001**, *13*, 449–456. [CrossRef] [PubMed]
144. Kaplan, G.G.; Underwood, F.E.; Coward, S.; Agrawal, M.; Ungaro, R.C.; Brenner, E.J.; Gearry, R.B.; Kissous-Hunt, M.; Lewis, J.D.; Ng, S.C.; et al. The Multiple Waves of COVID-19 in Patients With Inflammatory Bowel Disease: A Temporal Trend Analysis. *Inflamm. Bowel Dis.* **2022**, izab339. [CrossRef] [PubMed]
145. Anikhindi, S.A.; Kumar, A.; Arora, A. COVID-19 in patients with inflammatory bowel disease. *Expert Rev. Gastroenterol. Hepatol.* **2020**, *14*, 1187–1193. [CrossRef]

146. Siegel, C.A.; Christensen, B.; Kornbluth, A.; Rosh, J.R.; Kappelman, M.D.; Ungaro, R.C.; Johnson, D.F.; Chapman, S.; Wohl, D.A.; Mantzaris, G.J. Guidance for Restarting Inflammatory Bowel Disease Therapy in Patients Who Withheld Immunosuppressant Medications During COVID-19. *J. Crohns Colitis* **2020**, *14*, S769–S773. [CrossRef]
147. Din, S.; Kent, A.; Pollok, R.C.; Meade, S.; Kennedy, N.A.; Arnott, I.; Beattie, R.M.; Chua, F.; Cooney, R.; Dart, R.J.; et al. Adaptations to the British Society of Gastroenterology guidelines on the management of acute severe UC in the context of the COVID-19 pandemic: A RAND appropriateness panel. *Gut* **2020**, *69*, 1769–1777. [CrossRef]

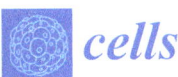

Review

Macrophages, Chronic Inflammation, and Insulin Resistance

He Li [1], Ya Meng [1], Shuwang He [2], Xiaochuan Tan [1], Yujia Zhang [1], Xiuli Zhang [1], Lulu Wang [3,*,†] and Wensheng Zheng [1,*,†]

1. Beijing City Key Laboratory of Drug Delivery Technology and Novel Formulation, Institute of Materia Medica, Chinese Academy of Medical Sciences & Peking Union Medical College, Beijing 100050, China
2. Shandong DYNE Marine Biopharmaceutical Co., Ltd., Rongcheng 264300, China
3. Institute of Medicinal Biotechnology, Chinese Academy of Medical Science and Peking Union Medical College, Beijing 100050, China
* Correspondence: wanglulu@imm.ac.cn (L.W.); zhengwensheng@imm.ac.cn (W.Z.); Tel.: +86-010-63165233 (W.Z.)
† Current address: No.1 Xian Nong Tan Street, Beijing 100050, China.

Abstract: The prevalence of obesity has reached alarming levels, which is considered a major risk factor for several metabolic diseases, including type 2 diabetes (T2D), non-alcoholic fatty liver, atherosclerosis, and ischemic cardiovascular disease. Obesity-induced chronic, low-grade inflammation may lead to insulin resistance, and it is well-recognized that macrophages play a major role in such inflammation. In the current review, the molecular mechanisms underlying macrophages, low-grade tissue inflammation, insulin resistance, and T2D are described. Also, the role of macrophages in obesity-induced insulin resistance is presented, and therapeutic drugs and recent advances targeting macrophages for the treatment of T2D are introduced.

Keywords: obesity; macrophages; chronic inflammation; insulin resistance; molecular mechanism

1. Introduction

The incidence of obesity is widespread in both developing and developed countries [1]. It is estimated that 57.8% of the global adult population will be overweight or obese by 2030 [2]. Obesity does not only affect adults, as the incidence of overweight and obesity in children has also risen sharply in recent years [3]. Obesity has a significant impact on the physiological functions of the human body and increases the risk of many metabolic diseases, including type 2 diabetes (T2D) [4,5], non-alcoholic fatty liver [6–8], atherosclerosis [9,10], cardiovascular disease [5], musculoskeletal diseases [11], and cancer [12–14]. This affects the quality of life of these patients and increases medical care costs.

Among them, obesity is closely related to the development of insulin resistance. Insulin target organs, such as adipose tissue, skeletal muscle, and liver, are affected by obesity at the morphological, functional, and molecular levels [15]. As one of the causes of T2D [16,17], insulin resistance is a pathological condition in which cells fail to respond normally to insulin stimulation [18]. Obesity causes various changes in adipose tissue, including metabolic and endocrine functions, such as the increased release of fatty acids, hormones, and proinflammatory molecules [19]. Lipid accumulation in skeletal muscle is associated with insulin resistance and markedly impairs glucose disposal function of skeletal muscle [20–23]. Insulin resistance induced by obesity in the liver characterized by impairment in the ability of insulin to inhibit glucose output, finally resulting in gluconeogenesis [24]. In response to high blood glucose levels, β-cells promote insulin production and lead to hyperinsulinemia [25]. Therefore, insulin resistance is often accompanied by hyperglycemia and hyperinsulinemia [26], until β-cells cannot maintain a compensatory increase in insulin, eventually leading to T2D [27].

Many molecular mechanisms have been proposed between obesity, insulin resistance, and T2D, including endoplasmic reticulum stress, oxidative stress, lipid homeostasis dysregulation, mitochondrial dysfunction, and hypoxia [28], but the molecular link is not fully understood. This review focuses on the chronic inflammation induced by obesity as a possible contributor to insulin resistance [29]. In obesity, changes in the polarization state of macrophages in the adipose tissue, liver, and muscle were detected [30], and the interactions between macrophages and insulin target organs may influence both metabolism and inflammation [31].

This review focuses on the molecular mechanisms between macrophages, chronic inflammation, insulin resistance, and T2D. We discuss the polarization, distribution, and accumulation of macrophages in insulin target organs such as adipose tissue, skeletal muscle, and liver, and summarize the relationship between macrophages and insulin resistance, as well as therapeutic drugs and recent advances targeting macrophages for the treatment of T2D.

2. Classification of Macrophages

Macrophages are a type of phagocyte and antigen-presenting cell, which can secrete trophic factors, immune mediators, and effectors, phagocytose pathogens, or cell debris, as well as process antigen and present antigen on the cell surface [32,33]. Diversity and plasticity are hallmarks of macrophages [34]. Two recognized subtypes of macrophages are classically activated M1 macrophages and alternately activated M2 macrophages [35,36] that represent two extremes of a dynamic changing state of macrophage activation [37]. M1 macrophages could be induced by IFN-γ, TNF-α, GM-CSF, and lipopolysaccharide (LPS) [38], while M2 macrophages are stimulated with IL-4 or IL-13 [37,39]. M1 macrophages are involved in promoting Th1 response, possessing strong microbicidal and tumoricidal activity mainly by the secretion of cytokines that inhibit the proliferation and damage of contiguous tissue, including TNF-α, IL6, IL-12, IL-23, nitric oxide, reactive oxygen, and inducible nitric oxide synthase (iNOS) [40,41]. M2 macrophages release arginase-1, IL-10, ornithine, and polyamines, and promote Th2 response, proliferation, tissue repair, immune tolerance, and tumor progression [42–45]. The M2 macrophages can be divided into four subdivisions based on the stimuli and induced transcriptional changes: alternatively activated macrophages activated by IL-4 or IL-13 (M2a), type 2 macrophages stimulated by immune complexes and LPS (M2b), deactivated macrophages activated by glucocorticoids or IL-10 (M2c), and M2-like macrophages activated by adenosines or IL-6 (M2d) [46,47]. M2 macrophages use oxidative metabolism to fulfill their functions, while M1 macrophages obtain energy through glycolysis, which favors the production of the proinflammatory cytokine IL-1β and nitric oxide [48].

It has also been pointed out that the use of M1 and M2 to classify macrophages is too polarized; the phenotype of macrophages is determined by many stimulating factors and cannot be generalized by limited subtypes [34]. New subtypes of macrophages different from M1 and M2 are constantly being discovered. Jaitin et al. found a new Trem2+ lipid-associated macrophage (LAM) subset after high-fat diet (HFD), which is the most strongly expanded immune cell subset of adipose tissue in the state of obesity. Trem2+ LAMs facilitate the processing and degradation of lipids by highly expressing fatty acids transporters Cd36, fatty acid binding proteins 4 and 5 (Fabp4, Fabp5), lipoprotein lipase (Lpl) and lysosomal acid lipase (Lipa). Jaitin et al. also discovered that Trem2 expression is an important factor in the prevention of adipose tissue dysfunction and metabolic disorders in obesity and that loss of Trem2 aggravates WAT hypertrophy in response to HFD feeding [49]. Moreover, Trem2+ macrophages are found in the plaque of mice with both early and advanced atherosclerotic lesions [50]. One study reported that Trem2+ macrophages express high levels of Trem2, Cd9, Spp1, and cathepsins (Ctsb, Ctsd and Ctsz), which is associated with lipid metabolic processes and lesion calcification while downregulating pro-inflammatory genes, and further finding that macrophage Trem2 negatively correlates with plaque stability [51].

Instead of fixed states, M1/M2 polarization is a dynamic process that can be reversed under physiological and pathological conditions [52]. A variety of signaling molecules and transcription factors are involved in regulating the polarization of macrophages, including PPAR, KLF, IRF, STAT, NF-κB, and HIF families. IRF/STAT signaling is a major pathway in modulating macrophage polarization. IFN-γ and LPS stimulated IRF/STAT signaling activates M1 phenotype via STAT1, IL-4, and IL-13, while M2 phenotype is activated via STAT6 [53]. It is also influenced by local microenvironmental conditions such as hypoxia [54] and diseases such as obesity, which are discussed in this article.

Macrophages can also be classified based on their locations and functions. Tissue-resident macrophages are different from monocytes that come from the bone marrow and circulate in the blood [55]. Different tissues have specialized tissue-resident macrophages, including Kupffer cells in the liver, adipose tissue macrophages (ATMs) in the adipose tissue, alveolar macrophages in the lung, red pulp and marginal zone macrophages in the spleen, and microglia in the brain. Kupffer cells and ATMs are the two major metabolic tissue macrophages [56]. ATMs in murine have been characterized as F4/80$^+$, CD11b$^+$, CD206$^+$, and CD301$^+$ cells, while human ATMs are characteristically CD14$^+$/CD16$^-$ and express markers CD68, CD163, CD204, and CD206. It has been established that ATMs in humans barely express markers for M1 and M2 classification, such as iNOS and arginase-1 [57]. Further, the KCs in mice are typically characterized by F4/80^{hi}, CD11b^{int}, CD68$^+$ cells. Additionally, T-cell immunoglobulin, mucin domain containing 4 (Tim4), and C-type lectin domain family 4 member F (Clec4F) have been described as surface markers specific to KCs [58,59]. The murine monocytes infiltrating the liver, on the other hand, are characterized as CD11b$^+$, Cx3cr1$^+$, Ly6c$^+$, CCR2. When KCs are depleted or tissues are injured or inflamed, monocytes become significant contributors to the liver macrophage pool [59]. KCs in humans lack distinctive markers and have often been characterized by their expression of CD68 and CD14. Recently study have shown that humans KCs also express MARCO, CD163, and Tim4 [60]. There is less understanding of the markers for monocytes in the human liver, but include CCR2, Cx3cr1, SA100A2, and CD14 [60].

3. Macrophage- and Obesity-Induced Insulin Resistance

Macrophages in insulin target the organs, including adipose tissue, liver, and muscle, that play a central role in inflammation and insulin resistance [61]. In the obese state, macrophages infiltrate the target organ, are activated to the M1 polarization state and produce abundant inflammatory cytokines, which negatively affect the transmission of insulin signals and increase the development of chronic inflammation, as well as insulin resistance [62–64].

3.1. Adipose Tissue and ATMs

Adipose tissue is a reservoir of fatty acids during fasting. When glucose levels have returned to normal after meals, free fatty acids (FFAs) are released into the circulation by adipose tissue and used by other tissues as an energy source [65]. They are also the main site of inflammation in the obese state, and the accumulation of ATMs is the key factor in modulating inflammation [66]. Compared to subcutaneous adipose tissue, VAT plays a critical role in insulin resistance, and the content of ATMs in VAT is also higher than that of subcutaneous adipose tissue [67]. The ATM pool in lean mice originates from yolk-sac progenitors and self-renews by proliferation [68,69]. Eventually, these resident ATMs are replaced by bone-marrow-derived macrophages, likely from monocytes [70]. Three major ATM populations have been described in lean mice. Primitive adipose tissue is populated by LYVE1$^+$ ATMs, which are closely associated with vasculature [71,72]. Further investigations identified one or two CD63$^+$ monocyte-derived ATM subpopulations based on differential expression of MHCII, CD11c, and CX3CR1 [49,73,74]. The separation of the two monocyte-derived ATMs remains unclear, and CD11c expression can be attributed to either.

ATMs are mainly in the M2 polarization state in the lean state [75]. Preventing the ability of macrophages from transitioning to the M2 state leads to accelerated weight gain and glucose intolerance in mice [76,77]. M2 macrophages can maintain insulin sensitivity and glucose homeostasis by secreting factors such as IL-10, IL-1, and catecholamines to regulate lipid metabolism, block inflammation response, and increase insulin sensitivity [78–80]. Although conflicting evidence suggests that M2 macrophages do not contribute to adipocyte metabolism or adaptive thermogenesis via the production of catecholamines [81], evidence also shows that macrophages in adipose tissue are capable of taking up and degrading catecholamines released by neurons and that this system could be improved by obesity and aging, resulting in a decreased response to cold stress and starvation [82,83].

One of the hallmarks of obesity-related chronic inflammation is the accumulation of ATMs [19]. Macrophages account for approximately 10% of white adipose tissue (WAT) in lean mice and humans compared to nearly 40% in obese humans and over 50% in extremely obese, leptin-deficient mice [19,84]. Preventing the accumulation of ATMs during obesity can inhibit the development of inflammation and insulin resistance [85]. Past studies believed that these macrophages were derived from peripheral blood mononuclear cells. However, recent studies have shown that the significant increase in ATMs in the early stage of obesity is mainly due to in situ macrophage proliferation, and migrating monocytes favor the accumulating of ATMs in the relatively late stages of obesity [86]. ATMs in obese mice are mainly in the M1 state, which can produce a large number of proinflammatory cytokines to influence the chronic inflammation state. The mechanism of obesity leading to changes in the polarization status of ATMs has not been fully explained, and its influencing factors may be multiple. Lumeng et al. had found that the M1 macrophages present in the inflammatory aggregates of adipose tissue originate from circulating monocytes, instead of being directly converted from M2 to M1 polarization state [87]. Expansion of adipose tissue may lead to adipocyte hypertrophy and hyperplasia, then releasing signal molecules such as MCP-1 and other inflammatory cytokines and chemokines, attracting a large number of bone marrow-derived monocytes to enter adipose tissue and subsequently differentiate into macrophages [19,88]. In addition, the chronic inflammation induced by obesity not only leads to the accumulation of macrophages, but also impairs the macrophage egress [89].

There are also differences in the distribution of macrophages in adipose tissue between lean and obese states: macrophages are evenly distributed throughout the adipose tissue in the lean state; while in the obese state, macrophages mainly appear in ring-like structures around dying adipocytes, known as crown-like structures (CLSs), to phagocytose the cells and continuously release proinflammatory cytokines [90]. Dying adipocytes display engulfment signals, inducing phagocytic cells to migrate to the site of cell death [85]. HFD-feeding increases the number of CLSs and the expression of proinflammatory cytokines [88]. Furthermore, Hill et al. found that obese adipose tissue contains multiple distinct ATMs populations, with Ly6c+ ATMs located outside the CLSs and are adipogenic. By inducing genes involved in cholesterol and lipid biosynthesis, Ly6c ATMs restore normal adipose physiology after adoptive transfer. The lipid-rich CD9+ ATMs located within the CLSs are responsible for the inflammatory signature of obese adipose tissue. In lean mice, adoptive transfer of CD9+ ATMs induces obesity-associated inflammation [73]. In contrast to CD9− ATMs, CD9+ ATMs express higher levels of CD16 and CD206 and are enriched for transcription factors AP-1 and NF-κB with associated genes such as Ccl2, Il1a, Il18, and Tnf [73]. The aforementioned Trem2+ lipid-associated macrophages are also recognized as the main expanded immune cell subsct in adipose tissue during obesity [49].

3.2. Liver and Kupffer Cells

The liver is the largest solid organ in the body [91]. It plays an indispensable role in neutralizing and eliminating toxic substances and regulating metabolism [92,93]. In response to postprandial hyperglycemia, the liver converts excess glucose into glycogen, and during fasting, the liver maintains blood glucose levels through glucose production [93]. Among all organs, the liver has the largest proportion of macrophages, with about 20–35% of hepatic non-parenchymal cells and 80–90% of tissue macrophages in the host [94].

The two macrophage populations in the liver include Kupffer cells and monocyte-derived macrophages. During obesity, Kupffer cells are activated to the M1 state, which attracts inflammatory monocytes into the liver and promotes their differentiation into monocyte-derived macrophages [95,96], resulting in an increased proportion of macrophages in the liver [97]. Monocyte-derived macrophages and inflammatory-activated Kupffer cells contribute to obesity-induced hepatic inflammation and insulin resistance. On the other side, the anti-inflammatory activation of Kupffer cells could reduce obesity-induced insulin resistance [98]. Monocyte-derived macrophages are smaller than Kupffer cells in mice [99], and the number of monocyte-derived macrophages is six-fold higher in HFD feeding mice compared to lean mice, while the number of Kupffer cells is similar between the two groups [100]. Correspondingly, Kupffer cells and monocyte-derived macrophages are essential for maintaining the homeostasis of the liver and whole body [101].

Chronic inflammation is known to induce insulin resistance in the liver [102,103]. Kupffer cells play a major role in liver insulin resistance induced by HFD feeding through producing various inflammatory mediators, including TNF-α, IL-6, IL-1β, prostaglandins, and reactive oxygen species, which play vital roles in promoting the development of insulin resistance [104–108]. Intravenous infusion of clodronate can selectively deplete Kupffer cells without affecting ATMs, which is found to enhance insulin signaling and hepatic insulin sensitivity significantly in the case of an HFD; it could also reduce adipose tissue weight without affecting body weight, liver weight, or steatosis [104]. After treatment with $GdCl_3$, a specific inhibitor of Kupffer cells, phagocytosis, and other functions of Kupffer cells were inhibited, and whole-body glucose tolerance was increased in mice [107]. Moreover, lipid accumulation in the liver caused by increased fatty acid absorption, increased liver synthesis, or reduced fatty acid oxidation in obesity can be used to predict T2D [103,109], and lipid metabolisms induced by macrophages-derived cytokines lead to lipotoxicity, which in turn causes liver inflammation and insulin resistance [110].

3.3. Muscle and Macrophages

Muscle mass is an important determinant of glucose tolerance, as less muscle mass has been associated with greater insulin resistance [111,112]. Increased blood glucose levels after meals induce insulin secretion, in which case the skeletal muscle is stimulated to absorb glucose, and approximately 60% of ingested glucose is taken up by skeletal muscle [113–115]. Insulin resistance in skeletal muscle is manifested by a decrease in insulin-stimulated glucose uptake, associated with impaired insulin signaling, glucose transport, oxidative phosphorylation, and glycogen synthesis [22].

Insulin resistance in skeletal muscle is caused by impaired insulin signaling and many post-receptor intracellular defects including impaired glucose transport, glucose phosphorylation, and reduced glucose oxidation and glycogen synthesis. Macrophage recruitment into skeletal muscle tissue is also involved in promoting insulin resistance [23,85,116]. Macrophages in skeletal muscle display phenotypic diversity and can switch between an M1 and M2 phenotype in response to changes in the specific environment. For example, macrophages are polarized to M1 phenotype in response to circulating FFAs, leading to release of pro-inflammatory cytokines [117]. Macrophage content in skeletal muscle correlates negatively and dynamically with insulin sensitivity [117,118]. The number of $CD68^+$ macrophages in the skeletal muscle of obese non-diabetic subjects is increased compared to lean subjects [117]. Studies have also found that HFD increases the $CD11b^+$ $F4/80^+$ macrophage numbers in muscle compared to lean mice [19,119]. During obesity, macrophages alter the inflammatory state of muscle cells by secreting cytokines and chemokines [117]. The chronic inflammatory condition impairs lipogenesis and lipolysis of adipose tissue, resulting in increased circulating FFAs and triggering ectopic fat deposition in skeletal muscle [114,120], and inflammatory cytokines secreted from macrophages induce lipolysis and lead to increased levels of lipid metabolisms, which is highly correlated with skeletal muscle insulin resistance [121] (Figure 1).

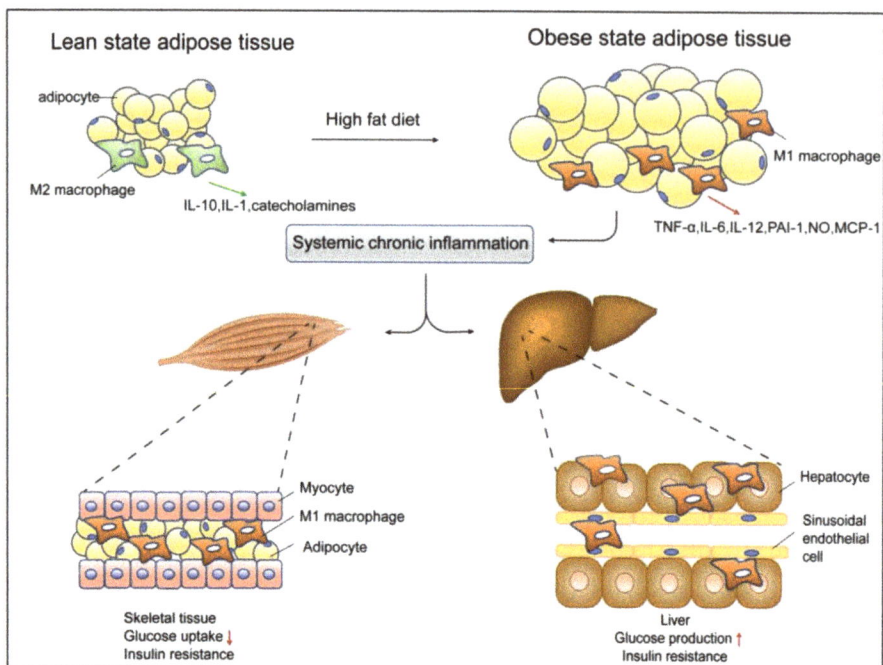

Figure 1. Obesity induces macrophage infiltration and insulin resistance in adipose tissue, liver, and skeletal muscle. In the lean state, tissue-resident M2 macrophages in adipose tissue secrete anti-inflammatory factors such as IL-1 and IL-10 to maintain an insulin-sensitive environment. During obesity, increased levels of nutrients result in adipocyte hypertrophy and apoptosis. Proinflammatory mediators result in M2 macrophage polarization into the M1 state, which triggers adipose tissue chronic inflammation. Other metabolic tissues, including skeletal muscle and liver, are also influenced by increased cytokine production and macrophage recruitment, resulting in lower glucose uptake in skeletal muscle and higher glucose production in the liver, fueling the insulin resistance state further.

3.4. Pancreas and Macrophages

Macrophages are constitutively present within islets under normal physiological conditions, where they play important roles in pancreas development and pancreas homeostasis. Macrophages are present during mouse embryonic development. In op/op mice lacking macrophages in the pancreas, it was found that these mice had less β-cell mass than normal mice during embryonic development and after birth, indicating that pancreas macrophages are necessary for increasing β-cell mass [122]. The mechanism by which macrophages support pancreas development is unclear, but may be related to cytokine production by macrophages, as low concentrations of IL-1β can stimulate β-cell proliferation [123]. Islet-resident macrophages also exert protective effects and contribute to the maintenance of islet homeostasis. Islet-resident macrophages express arginase I, CD206, and IL-10, etc., which are similar to M2 macrophages.

Numerous studies have revealed that macrophage infiltration in islets is increased in T2DM, C57BL/6 mice fed HFD, and db/db mice [124], and islet-resident macrophages content generally correlates with the degree of β-cell dysfunction [124,125]. High glucose could induce the secretion of chemokines from islets, which promoted monocyte and neutrophil migration. It is possible that the T2D milieu may induce chemokine production and promote macrophage infiltration into pancreas. Islets contain two subpopulations of macrophages: CD11b$^+$Ly-6C$^+$ monocytes/macrophages and CD11b$^+$Ly-6C$^-$ macrophages [126]. Islet-resident macrophages were mostly CD11b$^+$Ly-6C$^-$ cells, which exhibit an M2 phenotype in basal conditions. Compared to control db/+ and KKTa mice, fractions of these M2-type cells were not altered in db/db or KKAy mice. However, the number of CD11b$^+$Ly$^-$6C$^+$ macrophages was significantly increased in the T2D models. These cells express inflammatory cytokines, such as IL-1β and TNF-α, and exhibit an M1-type phenotype, which may indicate that macrophage polarity appears to be shifted towards M1 in T2D islets.

4. Mechanism of Inflammation and Insulin Resistance

Several inflammatory signaling pathways are implicated in inhibiting insulin functions, which can link inflammation to insulin resistance. JNK, IKK/NF-κB, JAK/STAT, and other pathways play major roles in forming chronic inflammation [127–131]. Inflammatory signaling is activated by several mechanisms, including the release of endogenous factors such as saturated fatty acids and heat shock proteins known as danger- or damage-associated molecular patterns (DAMPs), which are recognized by pattern recognition receptors (PRRs), and activate inflammation processes as well as inflammatory factors in the absence of exogenous factors such as pathogens [132]. DAMPs are produced largely by cellular stress, tissue damage, and inflammation [133]. PRRs include several types, such as Toll-like receptors (TLRs), RIG-I-like RNA helicases (RLHs), NOD-like receptors (NLRs), and AIM2-like receptors (ALRs) [134]. The PRRs can also recognize pathogen-associated molecular patterns (PAMPs) on pathogens and biological allergens, including LPS, peptidoglycan, and bacterial DNA [135,136].

4.1. JNK Pathway

Hotamisligil et al. found that the mRNA and protein levels of TNF-α in adipose tissue are increased under insulin resistance and obesity, and insulin sensitivity is improved after neutralizing TNF-α [66,137]. Further studies found that TNF-α is an adipose tissue-derived proinflammatory cytokine that is involved in obesity-induced insulin resistance [19]. Helped by TNFR-1, TNF-α plays an important role in activating and recruiting the immune cells to propagate inflammation. At that time, TNF-α was recognized to derive from adipocytes in obesity, and Xu et al. found that the WAT stromal vascular fraction (SVF) also secretes TNF-α [138]. Moreover, Taeye et al. revealed that macrophages are the main sources of TNF-α in the obese WAT [139], transplanted TNF-α deficient mice with TNF-α-sufficient or TNF-α-deficient bone marrow and found that macrophage-derived TNF-α contributes to inflammation development and insulin resistance in diet-induced obesity [139]. TNF-α knockout obese mice have improved insulin sensitivity compared to the control group [140]. The studies further found downstream signaling at the TNF-α-induced kinase levels. TNF-α induces a dual kinase system, including JNK kinases and IKK complex [141]. In the case of insulin resistance, JNK-1 and IKK signals are upregulated in adipose tissue [138], skeletal muscle [142], and liver [143]. JNK have JNK-1 and JNK-2 subsets, and JNK-1 plays a key role in the development of insulin resistance in adipose tissue and muscle [144]. JNK can be activated by TNF-α, IL-1β, and ultraviolet light [145]. JNK pathway is involved in impaired insulin signaling by causing the serine phosphorylation of insulin receptor substrate 1 (IRS-1), which reduces the tyrosine phosphorylation of IRS-1, thereby reducing PI3K and AKT signaling [146,147].

New research has found that proinflammatory molecule leukotriene B4 (LTB4) also induces insulin resistance through the JNK pathway [148]. LTB4 is a neutrophil chemotactic agent produced by arachidonic acid metabolism [149,150]. It is secreted by both immune cells, such as macrophages and eosinophils, and primary tissue cells, such as adipocytes, hepatocytes, myocytes, and endothelial cells [148]. LTB4 levels increase and play key roles in obesity-induced insulin resistance through the G protein-coupled receptor BLT-1, which is distributed mainly on immune cells and primary metabolite cells [148]. When primary tissue cells produce LTB4, it causes macrophages chemotaxis and migration into tissues, and macrophages secrete more LTB4 and act on primary tissue cells in a positive feedback loop, further inducing chronic tissue inflammation [148]. LTB4 treatment could stimulate

JNK activity and enhance IRS-1 serine phosphorylation, impairing insulin sensitivity in target cells [148]. Treatment of adipocytes and hepatocytes with LTB4 in vitro induces insulin resistance, and knockout of BLT-1 can improve adipose tissue inflammation and insulin sensitivity in obese mice [148].

4.2. IKK/NF-κB Pathway

In addition to the JNK signaling pathway, insulin resistance is also closely related to NF-κB activation, which is induced by TNF-α [116]. NF-κB is a transcription factor of Rel family proteins and is involved in inflammation and immune responses. IκB retains NF-κB in an inhibitory cytoplasmic complex at a steady-state, and IKK phosphorylation could phosphorylate IκBα under inflammation, which separates and degrades IκBα from NF-κB [151], allowing free NF-κB to translocate to the nucleus and interact with related DNA response elements binding, which induces transactivation of inflammatory genes such as TNF-α, IL-1β, and IL-6, further contributing to insulin resistance [152]. IKK2 is a central coordinator of inflammatory responses to activate NF-κB. Yuan et al. first showed the importance of NF-κB signaling in metabolic disorders, in that IKK2 heterozygous-deletion mice have improved glucose tolerance and reduced basal glucose and insulin values in HFD feeding compared with control [153]. Chiang et al. found that HFD feeding increases NF-κB activation in mice, which leads to an increased level of IKKε in hepatocytes and adipocytes, and IKKε knockout mice are protected from HFD-induced obesity and chronic inflammation [154].

IL-1β participates in insulin resistance through NF-κB pathway. IL-1β belongs to the IL-1 superfamily and is produced mainly by monocytes and macrophages and regulated by inflammasome activity [155]. The levels of IL-1β are increased during hyperglycemia [156], and elevation of IL-1β has been shown to increase the risk of T2D [157]. IL-1β binds to interleukin-1 receptor type I (IL-1R1) and triggers intracellular signaling cascades. IL-1R1 activates JAK protein kinases, then stimulates the translocation of NF-κB to the nucleus from a complex with IκB, thus promoting inflammatory gene expression [158]. IL-1β impairs insulin signaling in peripheral tissues and reduces insulin sensitivity and secretion in β-cells [159]. Gao et al. observed that macrophage-conditioned (MC) medium significantly reduces protein abundance of insulin signaling molecules in human adipocytes and blocks the actions of IL-1β, which can reverse the effects of MC medium on insulin signaling [155]. Additionally, IL-1β depletion completely changes the inhibitory effect of MC medium on insulin signaling molecules like IRS-1 and PI3K, which indicates that IL-1β is a key factor in mediating macrophage-induced insulin resistance in adipocytes [155].

Moreover, monocytes and tissue-resident macrophages express high levels of PPAR-γ [160]. PPAR-γ is a member of the nuclear receptor superfamily and is involved in the expression of the inflammatory response, cell differentiation, lipid, and glucose metabolism genes [161]. PPAR-γ natural ligands include various lipid and prostaglandin (PGs), and PGs could suppress PPAR-γ functions [162]. Under inflammation, the production of PGs increases to a considerable extent, which has a positive correlation with insulin resistance [163]. In contrast, PPAR-γ synthetic agonists significantly reduce insulin resistance and are widely used to treat diabetes [164,165]. PPAR-γ suppresses the NF-κB transcription activity and inhibits inflammation by interacting with p65 to induce ubiquitination and degradation. PPAR-γ also upregulates the IRS protein, which improves insulin resistance induced by obesity [166,167]. Macrophages with PPAR-γ knockout lead to decreased systematic glucose tolerance, increased insulin resistance, and increased levels of inflammatory factors expression in the muscles and liver [168].

4.3. JAK/STAT Pathway

IL-6 plays a crucial role in regulating metabolism and immunity. It is also elevated in obese patients compared to lean controls, which is detrimental to metabolic balance [169]. IL-6 works by binding to IL-6 receptor α chain and GP130 signaling chain complex in classical membrane-bound pathway, then initiating the JAK2/STAT3-dependent transcriptional activation of target genes, including SOCS-3 [170]. SOCS-3 is a negative regulator of IL-6 signaling and could impair insulin signal transduction at IRS protein level. IL-6-induced SOCS-3 leads to proteasomal degradation of IRS-1 [171]. Studies of IL-6 functions on insulin sensitivity have shown conflicting results. A very-low-calorie diet and weight loss decrease IL-6 levels significantly in adipose tissue and serum and improve insulin sensitivity compared to the control [172]. Acute IL-6 infusion of mice leads to insulin resistance without obesity [173]. However, IL-6 deficient mice develop insulin resistance and mature-onset obesity [174]. Another study showed that 4-month-old IL-6 deficient mice have glucose intolerance and increased fat pad weight [175]. Additional investigation is required to speculate on the effect of IL-6 on insulin sensitivity.

4.4. Other Pathways

Cytokines derived from macrophages, including TNF-α, IL-6, and IL-1β, could influence lipolysis. TNF-α affects lipid metabolism by inducing lipolysis, inhibiting FFAs uptake and lipoprotein lipase activity [176]. Starnes et al. administered TNF-α to patients and found that FFAs metabolism increased >60% [177], and TNF-α-deficient obese mice have lower levels of FFAs [140]. IL-6 enhances lipolysis and fatty acid oxidation both in mice and humans [178]. Wolsk et al. found that the unidirectional release of muscle fatty acids during IL-6 acute infusion leads to an increase in systemic fatty acids, which indicates that IL-6 may be a direct regulator of fat metabolism in skeletal muscle [179]. Moreover, IL-1β indirectly stimulates lipolysis by reducing the production and activity of proteins that inhibit lipolysis and increase the release of FFAs and glycerin [180]. Increased levels of lipid metabolites, including FFAs, ceramides, and diacylglycerol (DAG), may cause dysfunction and insulin resistance [181]. High levels of FFAs are considered markers of insulin resistance and T2D [182,183]. Elevated FFAs inhibit pyruvate dehydrogenase, increase serine phosphorylation of IRS-1, impair insulin-stimulated glucose uptake, and decrease glucose oxidation [184]. Several studies have found a correlation between the accumulation of DAG and impaired insulin function [185,186]. DAGs activate the PKCθ and PKCδ subtypes of protein kinase C (PKC) [187], and PKC prevents insulin-stimulated tyrosine phosphorylation of IRS-1 and directly interferes with the insulin signaling pathway [186]. PKC-θ knockout mice are protected against fat-induced insulin signaling defects and systemic insulin resistance [188]. Ceramides are implicated as antagonists of insulin action, and plasma ceramides are at high levels in obese or diabetic individuals [189]. Ceramide is mainly involved in the development of insulin resistance from two aspects: ceramide signal stimulates the binding of PKCζ and AKT, making AKT unable to bind phosphatidylinositol (3,4,5)-triphosphate (PIP3), thereby inhibiting insulin signaling [190]; on the other hand, ceramide activates protein phosphatase 2A (PP2A) and phosphorylates it, thereby impairing AKT [191]. Ceramides decrease the plasma content during pioglitazone treatment, and inhibition of ceramide synthesis or stimulation of ceramide degradation improves insulin signaling, indicating indispensable participation of ceramides in the development of obesity and insulin resistance [189].

Furthermore, galectin-3 (gal-3) is a member of the galectin family that induces insulin resistance [192,193]. Gal-3 binds directly to the insulin receptor and inhibits downstream signaling [192]. The amount of gal-3 in the blood is higher in the obese state than in the lean state [192]. Treatment of adipocytes, hepatocytes, and myocytes with gal-3 in vitro induces insulin resistance [192]. Administration of gal-3 in vivo can also cause glucose intolerance and insulin resistance in mice, and gal-3 knockout mice have higher insulin sensitivity and glucose tolerance [192]. The above results suggested that gal-3 may be a critical molecule in insulin resistance.

In addition to cytokines secreted from or related to macrophages, macrophage autophagy is crucial for the regulation of systemic insulin sensitivity [194]. In macrophages, autophagy controls inflammation by regulating mitochondria turnover and ROS generation [194]. During inflammation and obesity, autophagy is downregulated in macrophages, and macrophage-specific autophagy knockout mice have impaired insulin sensitivity in liver and adipose tissues when fed an HFD, inhibiting ROS in macrophages with antioxidants can restore insulin sensitivity of adipocytes [195]. (Figures 2 and 3)

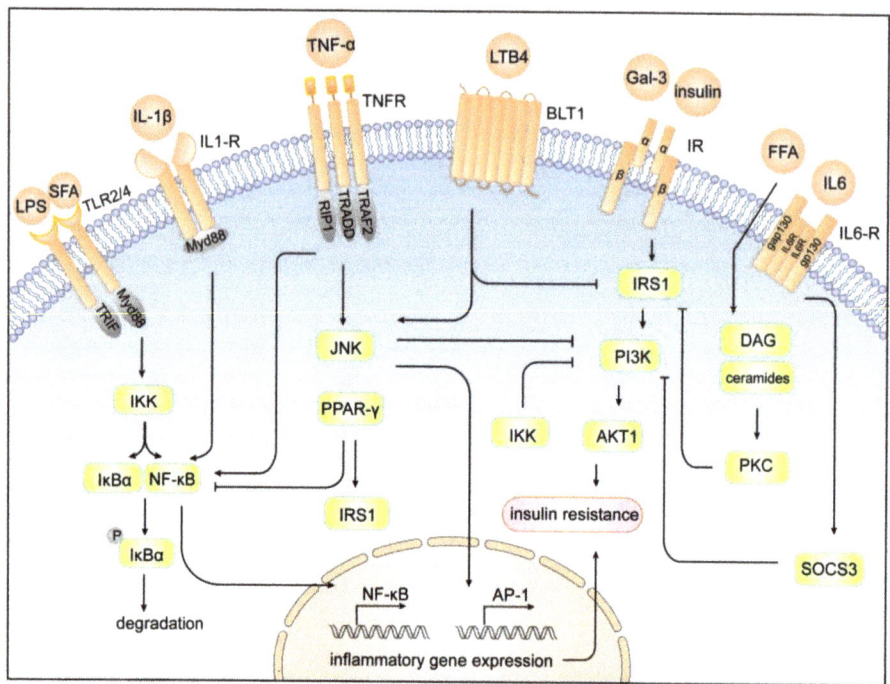

Figure 2. Cytokines regulate insulin sensitivity in insulin target cells. Activation of the insulin receptor leads to tyrosine phosphorylation of IRS-1 and initiates insulin signal transduction. Activation of TLR2/4 and TNFR results in the promotion of NF-κB and JNK signaling pathways. The serine kinases IKK and JNK-1 could reduce the signaling of IRS-1 and impair downstream insulin signaling. Moreover, the activation of IKK causes phosphorylation and degradation of IκB; thus, NF-κB could translocate into the nucleus. JNK promotes the formation of the AP-1 transcription factor, which in turn transactivates inflammatory gene expression by NF-κB and AP-1, further contributing to insulin resistance. PPAR-γ suppresses the NF-κB transcription activity and upregulates IRS protein, which favors the improvement insulin sensitivity. LTB4 promotes JNK activation through BLT-1 and leads to subsequent IRS-1 serine phosphorylation, ultimately promoting cellular insulin resistance. Gal-3 directly inhibits the insulin receptor and impairs all the major steps in the insulin signaling pathway. Additionally, IL6 induces SOCS-3 and leads to proteasomal degradation of IRS-1 through binding to the IL-6 receptor. IL-1β stimulates the translocation of NF-κB to the nucleus through IL-1R1, promoting inflammatory gene expression. Also, lipid metabolites, including FFAs, ceramides, and DAG, activate the PKC to impair IRS-1, which directly interfere with insulin signaling.

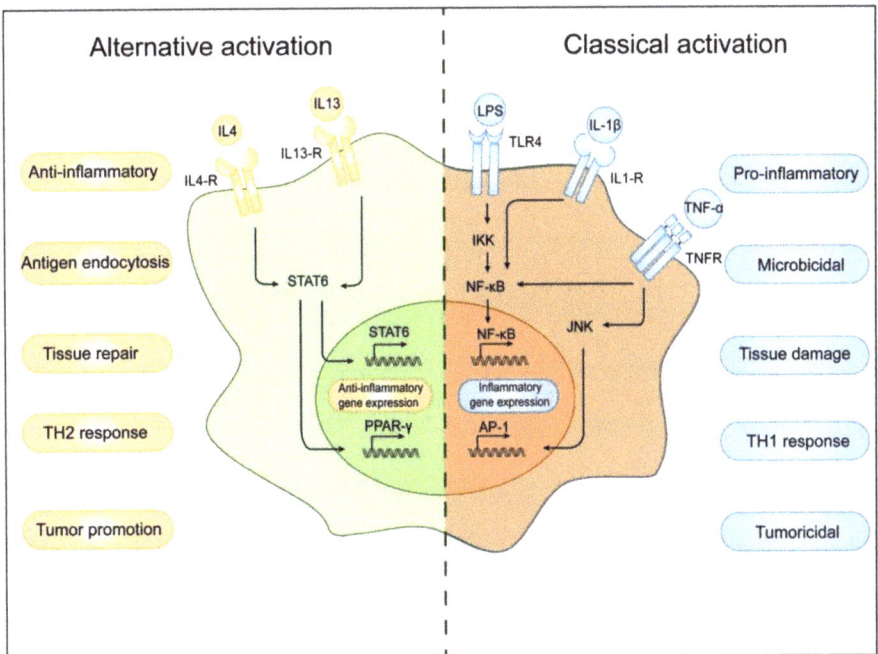

Figure 3. Cytokine stimulation leads to classical activation and alternative activation of macrophages. IL4 and IL13 activate macrophages to M2 polarization state through STAT6 and stimulate anti-inflammatory gene expression. M2 macrophages participate in Th2 response, anti-inflammatory, antigen endocytosis, and tumor promotion. On the other hand, when stimulated by LPS, IL-1β, and TNF-α, macrophages activate the inflammatory signaling cascades mediated by JNK and NF-κB, which stimulate M1 polarization of macrophages and inflammatory gene expression. M1 macrophages are involved in Th1 response, proinflammatory process, tissue damage, and so on.

5. Other Immune Cells and Insulin Resistance

In addition to macrophages, immune cells residing in adipose tissue and intestines, including cells of innate and adaptive immune systems, are also involved in chronic inflammation caused by obesity. In the process of obesity, immune cells, including Innate lymphoid type 1 cells (ILC1s), Innate lymphoid type 2 cells (ILC2s), eosinophils, mast cells, dendritic cells (DCs), neutrophils, T cells, and B cells, influence the polarization and recruitment of macrophages and play important roles in chronic inflammation and insulin resistance.

ILC2s and eosinophils participate in maintaining metabolic homeostasis states partially by maintaining the M2 polarization state of macrophages. ILC2s are a family of innate immune cells that mirror T cells [196]. They secrete Th2-associated cytokines, including IL-5 and IL-13, which promote the accumulation of M2 macrophages and eosinophils [197]. The deletion of ILC2s causes a significant decrease in VAT M2 macrophages and eosinophils and increases obesity and insulin resistance fed HFD [198]. Moreover, eosinophils have also been implicated in metabolic homeostasis and the maintenance of M2 macrophages [199]. Eosinophils content in adipose tissue is reduced in HFD-induced obesity and restored to lean levels when switching to a low-fat diet [200]. Eosinophils could produce IL-4 and IL-13, which promote differentiation of macrophages into the M2 state [198]. Impaired eosinophil accumulation in adipose tissue results in increased insulin resistance in obesity [198], and the absence of eosinophils leads to systemic insulin resistance [200].

Mast cells are first-line responders to invading pathogens by rapid degranulation ability [201], producing a wide range of inflammatory mediators, including histamines, prostaglandins, and proinflammatory cytokines (IFN-γ, TNF-α, IL-1β, IL-6), which trigger T-cell and M1 macrophage activation [202,203]. Liu et al. found that mast cells increased in obese adipose tissue, and mast cell deficiency can increase insulin sensitivity [204]. Additionally, some studies showed that DCs are involved in tissue recruitment and activation of macrophages; DC-deficient mice have a decreased number of ATMs and Kupffer cells, as well as improved glucose intolerance [205]. The transfer of bone-marrow-derived DCs to lean mice increases ATMs and Kupffer cells infiltration [205]. During obesity, neutrophils have high neutrophil elastase, neutrophil alkaline phosphatase, myeloperoxidase, IL-6, IL-1β, IL-12, IL-8, and TNF-α, and low expression of IL-10, which favors activation of M1 macrophages and development of chronic inflammation [206–210]. Neutrophil elastase impairs insulin signaling by promoting IRS-1 degradation, and elastase knockout in HFD mice improves glucose tolerance and increases insulin sensitivity [208]. Moreover, recent studies also found that ILC1s in the adipose tissue participate in developing inflammation and insulin resistance. HFD-induced obesity increases the number of ILC1s and induces them to produce IFN-γ and TNFα in the visceral adipose tissue (VAT), then ILC1s-derived IFN-γ and TNFα accelerate M1 macrophages accumulation and promote insulin resistance [211].

T cells, B cells, and macrophages are all in CLSs surrounding necrotic adipocytes [212]. Accumulation of macrophages and T cells within CLSs can predict the severity of obesity and insulin resistance [212]. T cells can be classified into CD4$^+$ and CD8$^+$ T cells by their phenotypic expression of the surface coreceptors. Increased recruitment and differentiation of CD8$^+$ T cells have been found in both animal and human obese WAT [213]. T cell receptor beta chain-deficient mice improve obesity-induced hyperglycemia and insulin resistance by suppressing macrophage infiltration and reducing inflammatory cytokine expression [214]. The number of Th1 cells increases and produces more IFN-γ in obesity, which promotes M1 polarization of ATMs [215,216]. Adoptive transfer of Th1 cells into HFD lymphocyte-free mice results in increased inflammation, impaired glucose tolerance, and macrophage infiltration [214]. Moreover, Treg cells secrete IL10 in a lean state, preserving an anti-inflammatory environment and M2 macrophage polarization [217]. Treg cells in VAT decrease dramatically during obesity in HFD feeding mice [218]. Treg cell deficiency in adipose tissue increases the production of proinflammatory cytokines, M1 macrophage polarization, and insulin resistance [217]. In contrast with CD4$^+$ T cells, CD8$^+$ T cells are mainly considered cytotoxic. CD8$^+$ T cells secrete perforins, granzymes, and cytokines that regulate the development and activation of macrophages [173]. Increased infiltration of CD8$^+$ T cells in WAT was found in obese mice, which induces adipose tissue inflammation and attracts macrophage recruitment [219]. Depletion of CD8$^+$ T cells could lower macrophage infiltration and adipose tissue inflammation and improve insulin resistance [219].

The impaired adaptive response of B cells leads to inflammation in obese people [220]. B cells secrete more IL-6 and NF-κB and less IL-10 in obese humans compared to lean individuals, which favors the recruitment of M1 macrophages [221]. Winer et al. demonstrated that B cells accumulate in VAT occurs early in HFD-fed mice and promote activation of T cells and M1 macrophages through the production of specific IgG antibodies, eventually inducing insulin resistance [222]. Obese B cell knockout mice have decreased systemic inflammation and improved insulin sensitivity and glucose tolerance compared to obese control mice [223] (Figure 4).

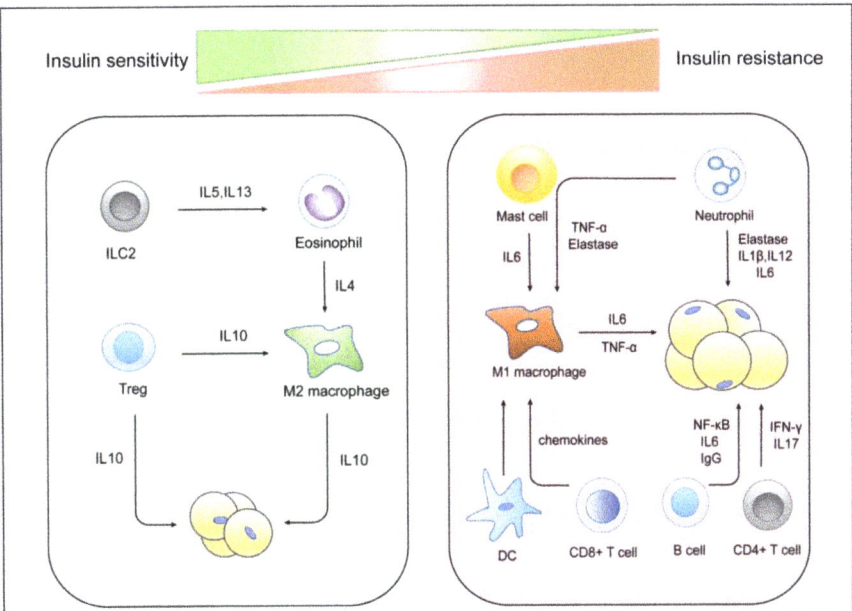

Figure 4. Role of the immune system in regulating polarization of macrophage and insulin resistance. In an insulin-sensitive state, ILC2 cells produce IL-5 and IL-13 to assist in the maturation and recruitment of eosinophils. Eosinophils and Treg cells promote the activation of M2 macrophages in the adipose tissue via IL-4 and IL-13 secretion. M2 macrophages and Treg cells secrete anti-inflammatory factors such as IL-10 to maintain insulin sensitivity in lean adipose tissue. In the obese state, recruitment of monocytes and differentiation into M1 macrophages are induced significantly. Mast cells produce IL-6 to trigger T-cell and M1 macrophage activation. Neutrophils contribute to M1 polarization of macrophages and impaired insulin signaling via the production of elastase, IL-6, and IL-1β. CD4+ and CD8+ T cells stimulate M1 macrophage polarization by secreting IFN-γ, IL17, and chemokines. B cells release NF-κB, IL6, and IgG that further contribute to M1 macrophage polarization and insulin resistance.

6. Macrophage-Related T2D Therapeutic Targets

Antidiabetic drugs act on adipose tissue and muscle to enhance insulin sensitivity and target the liver to inhibit glucose production, or stimulate β-cells to release insulin, thereby slowing the development of insulin resistance. However, they are not able to completely prevent or reverse the development of T2D, urgently necessitating new antidiabetic drugs [224]. Current studies used macrophage-derived factors or surface markers, including TNF-α, IL-1β, IL-6, miRNAs, and folate receptor (FR), as the therapeutic targets for diabetes, which have potential to be developed as pharmacological targets for the treatment of T2D [225,226].

TNF-α is identified as a potential target to treat insulin resistance in obesity; it is a classic proinflammatory cytokine and induces M1 polarization of macrophages. Treatment with shRNA to downregulate TNF-α contributes to improving IRS-1 phosphorylation and insulin response, which improves insulin sensitivity [227]. Burska et al. concluded that TNF-α inhibitor treatment improves insulin sensitivity in rheumatoid arthritis (RA) patients [228]. The topical addition of anti-TNF-α neutralizing antibodies could shift the macrophages towards M2 phenotype and accelerate wound healing [229]. Wang et al. reported a glucose-sensitive TNFα-antibody-delivery system for controlling local long-term inflammation and improving osteogenesis in T2D [230]. The clinical trials of anti-TNF-α antibodies Ro 45-2081 and CDP571 did not show any improvement in glucose homeostasis and insulin sensitivity [231,232]. Relevant studies are needed to prove the effectiveness of TNF-α target. In addition, when IKK/NF-κB pathway is inhibited by pharmacological inhibitors of IKK2 salicylates and aspirin, the animal models show improved obesity-induced insulin resistance and reduced TNF-α production [173].

IL-1β is elevated in obesity and induces insulin resistance by inhibiting the insulin signaling pathway [225,233]. IL-1β antibody treatment improves insulin resistance, glycemic control, and β-cell functions in mice with HFD-induced obesity [225]. IL-1R antagonist Anakinra also improves the glycemia β-cell functions and reduces systemic inflammation in patients with T2D; thus, it is approved for treating patients with RA (ClinicalTrials.gov identifier: NCT00303394) [234]. Human mAbs canakinumab and Xoma 052 are used to neutralize IL-1β specifically and support that blockade of IL-1β restores the regeneration of β-cells [235]. Canakinumab is tested in high-risk patients with T2D (ClinicalTrials.gov identifier: NCT01327846) and shows modest improvement in HbA1c, glycemia, and insulinemia [158]. Additional results of ongoing clinical trials are needed to clarify the function of IL-1β target.

IL-6 is another proinflammatory cytokine that participates in the development of T2D. Human monoclonal antibody Tocilizumab could inhibit IL-6 signaling selectively, and treatment with Tocilizumab causes a significant reduction of HOMA-IR and insulin resistance in non-diabetic patients with RA [236]. These studies suggest that inhibiting IL6 may improve insulin resistance and T2D. Further, IL-10 is an anti-inflammatory factor, which induces M2 activation of macrophages and improves obesity-induced insulin resistance [119]. Recombinant IL-10 has been proved safe in clinical trials to treat autoimmune diseases, neurodegenerative disorders, and so on [237]. Thus IL-10 may also be a promising target for treating T2D.

Macrophages could secrete miRNAs encapsulated in extracellular vesicles to exert anti-inflammatory or proinflammatory effects, and miRNAs may also contribute to the development of insulin resistance by regulating macrophage polarization. Since miRNAs are endogenous regulators whose levels are often deregulated in T2D, the therapeutic goal is to restore miRNAs to normal levels [226]. Presently, there are two main therapeutic methods: miRNA mimics to restore the miRNAs downregulated in diabetes, miRNA mimics that are synthetic RNA duplexes, liposomes, and adeno-associated virus preparations designed to package miRNAs [238,239]; the other method is to inhibit miRNAs that express significantly higher than normal, locked nucleic acid anti-miRNAs and morpholinos that are efficient inhibitors of miRNA decrease the plasma cholesterol with very low toxicity in mice [240,241]. Due to the instability of miRNA mimics and the difficulty in specific targeting, miRNA therapy needs to be developed further to treat T2D.

Moreover, therapeutic drugs with folate conjugates could selectively impair FR active macrophages [242]. FR is a marker of macrophage activation. While nonactivated resident macrophages do not express FR, other cells, including granulocytes, lymphocytes, or erythrocyte-enriched populations, show poor folate-conjugate binding. Furthermore, folate-FITC binding to active macrophages is FR-specific, which makes the folate receptor an optimal target for active macrophages involved in insulin resistance [243].

7. Conclusions

Accumulating evidence showed that macrophages play central roles in chronic inflammation and insulin resistance induced by obesity. Macrophages participate in inflammatory pathways including JNK, IKK/NF-κB, and JAK/STAT through secreting inflammatory factors, such as TNF-α, IL-6, IL-1β, and LTB4, thereby inducing chronic inflammation of adipose tissue, liver, and muscle, further leading to insulin resistance. Other immune cells, including ILC2s, eosinophils, mast cells, DCs, neutrophils, T cells, and B cells, affect the polarization state of macrophages, which in turn participate in the induction of insulin resistance and T2D. In recent years, there have been many discoveries in the field of immune metabolism, and direct or indirect targeting of macrophage-secreted factors or macrophage-related markers can improve insulin resistance and reduce the development of

T2D by mechanisms including enhancing insulin sensitivity, reducing oxidative stress, and reducing inflammation et al. Current research hotspots include targeted therapy of TNF-α, IL-1β, IL-6, and miRNAs. Although many problems remain unsolved, macrophages may be considered as promising targets for the treatment of T2D.

Author Contributions: H.L., Y.M., S.H., X.T., Y.Z., X.Z., L.W. and W.Z. listed have made a substantial, direct, and intellectual contribution to the work, and approved it for publication. All authors have read and agreed to the published version of the manuscript.

Funding: This work was supported by the CAMS Innovation Fund for Medical Sciences (CIFMS) (2021-I2M-1-026, 2022-I2M-JB-012,2022-I2M-2-002).

Conflicts of Interest: The authors declare no conflict of interest.

References

1. Chooi, Y.C.; Ding, C.; Magkos, F. The epidemiology of obesity. *Metabolism* **2019**, *92*, 6–10. [CrossRef]
2. Bhurosy, T.; Jeewon, R. Overweight and obesity epidemic in developing countries: A problem with diet, physical activity, or socioeconomic status? *Sci. World J.* **2014**, *2014*, 964236. [CrossRef]
3. Pulgaron, E.R.; Delamater, A.M. Obesity and type 2 diabetes in children: Epidemiology and treatment. *Curr. Diabetes Rep.* **2014**, *14*, 508. [CrossRef] [PubMed]
4. Zubrzycki, A.; Cierpka-Kmiec, K.; Kmiec, Z.; Wronska, A. The role of low-calorie diets and intermittent fasting in the treatment of obesity and type-2 diabetes. *J. Physiol. Pharmacol.* **2018**, *69*, 663–683.
5. Singh, G.M.; Danaei, G.; Farzadfar, F.; Stevens, G.A.; Woodward, M.; Wormser, D.; Kaptoge, S.; Whitlock, G.; Qiao, Q.; Lewington, S.; et al. The age-specific quantitative effects of metabolic risk factors on cardiovascular diseases and diabetes: A pooled analysis. *PLoS ONE* **2013**, *8*, e65174. [CrossRef] [PubMed]
6. Patell, R.; Dosi, R.; Joshi, H.; Sheth, S.; Shah, P.; Jasdanwala, S. Non-Alcoholic Fatty Liver Disease (NAFLD) in Obesity. *J. Clin. Diagn. Res.* **2014**, *8*, 62–66. [PubMed]
7. Yki-Järvinen, H. Non-alcoholic fatty liver disease as a cause and a consequence of metabolic syndrome. *Lancet Diabetes Endocrinol.* **2014**, *2*, 901–910. [CrossRef]
8. Lu, F.B.; Hu, E.D.; Xu, L.M.; Chen, L.; Wu, J.L.; Li, H.; Chen, D.Z.; Chen, Y.P. The relationship between obesity and the severity of non-alcoholic fatty liver disease: Systematic review and meta-analysis. *Expert Rev. Gastroenterol. Hepatol.* **2018**, *12*, 491–502. [CrossRef] [PubMed]
9. Lovren, F.; Teoh, H.; Verma, S. Obesity and atherosclerosis: Mechanistic insights. *Can. J. Cardiol.* **2015**, *31*, 177–183. [CrossRef]
10. Reardon, C.A.; Lingaraju, A.; Schoenfelt, K.Q.; Zhou, G.; Cui, C.; Jacobs-El, H.; Babenko, I.; Hoofnagle, A.; Czyz, D.; Shuman, H.; et al. Obesity and Insulin Resistance Promote Atherosclerosis through an IFNgamma-Regulated Macrophage Protein Network. *Cell Rep.* **2018**, *23*, 3021–3030. [CrossRef]
11. El-Khani, U.; Ahmed, A.; Hakky, S.; Nehme, J.; Cousins, J.; Chahal, H.; Purkayastha, S. The impact of obesity surgery on musculoskeletal disease. *Obes. Surg.* **2014**, *24*, 2175–2192. [CrossRef]
12. Salaun, H.; Thariat, J.; Vignot, M.; Merrouche, Y.; Vignot, S. Obesity and cancer. *Bull. Cancer* **2017**, *104*, 30–41. [CrossRef]
13. Lennon, H.; Sperrin, M.; Badrick, E.; Renehan, A.G. The Obesity Paradox in Cancer: A Review. *Curr. Oncol. Rep.* **2016**, *18*, 56. [CrossRef]
14. Himbert, C.; Delphan, M.; Scherer, D.; Bowers, L.W.; Hursting, S.; Ulrich, C.M. Signals from the Adipose Microenvironment and the Obesity-Cancer Link-A Systematic Review. *Cancer Prev. Res.* **2017**, *10*, 494–506. [CrossRef]
15. Barazzoni, R.; Gortan Cappellari, G.; Ragni, M.; Nisoli, E. Insulin resistance in obesity: An overview of fundamental alterations. *Eat. Weight Disord.* **2018**, *23*, 149–157. [CrossRef]
16. Alberti, K.G.; Eckel, R.H.; Grundy, S.M.; Zimmet, P.Z.; Cleeman, J.I.; Donato, K.A.; Fruchart, J.C.; James, W.P.; Loria, C.M.; Smith, S.C. Harmonizing the metabolic syndrome: A joint interim statement of the International Diabetes Federation Task Force on Epidemiology and Prevention; National Heart, Lung, and Blood Institute; American Heart Association; World Heart Federation; International Atherosclerosis Society; and International Association for the Study of Obesity. *Circulation* **2009**, *120*, 1640–1645.
17. Lackey, D.E.; Olefsky, J.M. Regulation of metabolism by the innate immune system. *Nat. Rev. Endocrinol.* **2016**, *12*, 15–28. [CrossRef]
18. Rafaqat, S.; Rafaqat, S.; Rafaqat, S. Pathophysiological aspects of insulin resistance in Atrial Fibrillation: Novel therapeutic approaches. *Int. J. Arrhythm.* **2022**, *23*, 6. [CrossRef]
19. Weisberg, S.P.; McCann, D.; Desai, M.; Rosenbaum, M.; Leibel, R.L.; Ferrante, A.W., Jr. Obesity is associated with macrophage accumulation in adipose tissue. *J. Clin. Investig.* **2003**, *112*, 1796–1808. [CrossRef]
20. Defronzo, R.A. Banting Lecture. From the triumvirate to the ominous octet: A new paradigm for the treatment of type 2 diabetes mellitus. *Diabetes* **2009**, *58*, 773–795. [CrossRef]
21. DeFronzo, R.A. Pathogenesis of type 2 diabetes mellitus. *Med. Clin. North Am.* **2004**, *88*, 787–835. [CrossRef] [PubMed]
22. Abdul-Ghani, M.A.; DeFronzo, R.A. Pathogenesis of insulin resistance in skeletal muscle. *J. Biomed. Biotechnol.* **2010**, *2010*, 476279. [CrossRef] [PubMed]

23. Sinha, R.; Dufour, S.; Petersen, K.F.; LeBon, V.; Enoksson, S.; Ma, Y.Z.; Savoye, M.; Rothman, D.L.; Shulman, G.I.; Caprio, S. Assessment of skeletal muscle triglyceride content by (1)H nuclear magnetic resonance spectroscopy in lean and obese adolescents: Relationships to insulin sensitivity, total body fat, and central adiposity. *Diabetes* **2002**, *51*, 1022–1027. [CrossRef] [PubMed]
24. Roden, M.; Bernroider, E. Hepatic glucose metabolism in humans—Its role in health and disease. *Best Pract. Res. Clin. Endocrinol. Metab.* **2003**, *17*, 365–383. [CrossRef]
25. Araujo, E.P.; De Souza, C.T.; Ueno, M.; Cintra, D.E.; Bertolo, M.B.; Carvalheira, J.B.; Saad, M.J.; Velloso, L.A. Infliximab restores glucose homeostasis in an animal model of diet-induced obesity and diabetes. *Endocrinology* **2007**, *148*, 5991–5997. [CrossRef]
26. Wu, M.; Wang, X.; Duan, Q.; Lu, T. Arachidonic acid can significantly prevent early insulin resistance induced by a high-fat diet. *Ann. Nutr. Metab.* **2007**, *51*, 270–276. [CrossRef]
27. DeFronzo, R.A.; Banerji, M.A.; Bray, G.A.; Buchanan, T.A.; Clement, S.; Henry, R.R.; Kitabchi, A.E.; Mudaliar, S.; Musi, N.; Ratner, R.; et al. Determinants of glucose tolerance in impaired glucose tolerance at baseline in the Actos Now for Prevention of Diabetes (ACT NOW) study. *Diabetologia* **2010**, *53*, 435–445. [CrossRef]
28. Osborn, O.; Olefsky, J.M. The cellular and signaling networks linking the immune system and metabolism in disease. *Nat. Med.* **2012**, *18*, 363–374. [CrossRef]
29. Wu, H.; Ballantyne, C.M. Skeletal muscle inflammation and insulin resistance in obesity. *J. Clin. Investig.* **2017**, *127*, 43–54. [CrossRef]
30. Esser, N.; Legrand-Poels, S.; Piette, J.; Scheen, A.J.; Paquot, N. Inflammation as a link between obesity, metabolic syndrome and type 2 diabetes. *Diabetes Res. Clin. Pract.* **2014**, *105*, 141–150. [CrossRef]
31. Asghar, A.; Sheikh, N. Role of immune cells in obesity induced low grade inflammation and insulin resistance. *Cell. Immunol.* **2017**, *315*, 18–26. [CrossRef]
32. Gentek, R.; Molawi, K.; Sieweke, M.H. Tissue macrophage identity and self-renewal. *Immunol. Rev.* **2014**, *262*, 56–73. [CrossRef]
33. Unanue, E.R. Antigen-presenting function of the macrophage. *Annu. Rev. Immunol.* **1984**, *2*, 395–428. [CrossRef]
34. Martinez, F.O.; Gordon, S. The M1 and M2 paradigm of macrophage activation: Time for reassessment. *F1000Prime Rep.* **2014**, *6*, 13. [CrossRef]
35. Vogel, D.Y.; Glim, J.E.; Stavenuiter, A.W.; Breur, M.; Heijnen, P.; Amor, S.; Dijkstra, C.D.; Beelen, R.H. Human macrophage polarization in vitro: Maturation and activation methods compared. *Immunobiology* **2014**, *219*, 695–703. [CrossRef]
36. Funes, S.C.; Rios, M.; Escobar-Vera, J.; Kalergis, A.M. Implications of macrophage polarization in autoimmunity. *Immunology* **2018**, *154*, 186–195. [CrossRef]
37. Mantovani, A.; Sica, A.; Sozzani, S.; Allavena, P.; Vecchi, A.; Locati, M. The chemokine system in diverse forms of macrophage activation and polarization. *Trends Immunol.* **2004**, *25*, 677–686. [CrossRef]
38. Mantovani, A.; Sica, A.; Locati, M. Macrophage polarization comes of age. *Immunity* **2005**, *23*, 344–346. [CrossRef]
39. Shaul, M.E.; Bennett, G.; Strissel, K.J.; Greenberg, A.S.; Obin, M.S. Dynamic, M2-like remodeling phenotypes of CD11c+ adipose tissue macrophages during high-fat diet–induced obesity in mice. *Diabetes* **2010**, *59*, 1171–1181. [CrossRef]
40. Verreck, F.A.W.; de Boer, T.; Langenberg, D.M.L.; Hoeve, M.A.; Kramer, M.; Vaisberg, E.; Kastelein, R.; Kolk, A.; de Waal-Malefyt, R.; Ottenhoff, T.H. Human IL-23-producing type 1 macrophages promote but IL-10-producing type 2 macrophages subvert immunity to (myco)bacteria. *Proc. Natl. Acad. Sci. USA* **2004**, *101*, 4560–4565. [CrossRef]
41. Gordon, S.; Taylor, P.R. Monocyte and macrophage heterogeneity. *Nat. Rev. Immunol.* **2005**, *5*, 953–964. [CrossRef]
42. Mosser, D.M. The many faces of macrophage activation. *J. Leukoc. Biol.* **2003**, *73*, 209–212. [CrossRef]
43. Mantovani, A.; Sozzani, S.; Locati, M.; Allavena, P.; Sica, A. Macrophage polarization: Tumor-associated macrophages as a paradigm for polarized M2 mononuclear phagocytes. *Trends Immunol.* **2002**, *23*, 549–555. [CrossRef]
44. Martinez, F.O.; Helming, L.; Gordon, S. Alternative activation of macrophages: An immunologic functional perspective. *Annu. Rev. Immunol.* **2009**, *27*, 451–483. [CrossRef] [PubMed]
45. Thorp, E.; Subramanian, M.; Tabas, I. The role of macrophages and dendritic cells in the clearance of apoptotic cells in advanced atherosclerosis. *Eur. J. Immunol.* **2011**, *41*, 2515–2518. [CrossRef]
46. Avila-Ponce de León, U.; Vázquez-Jiménez, A.; Matadamas-Guzman, M.; Pelayo, R.; Resendis-Antonio, O. Transcriptional and microenvironmental landscape of macrophage transition in cancer: A boolean analysis. *Front Immunol.* **2021**, *12*, 642842. [CrossRef]
47. Wang, L.X.; Zhang, S.X.; Wu, H.J.; Rong, X.L.; Guo, J. M2b macrophage polarization and its roles in diseases. *J. Leukoc. Biol.* **2019**, *106*, 345–358. [CrossRef]
48. Galvan-Pena, S.; O'Neill, L.A. Metabolic reprograming in macrophage polarization. *Front. Immunol.* **2014**, *5*, 420.
49. Jaitin, D.A.; Adlung, L.; Thaiss, C.A.; Weiner, A.; Li, B.; Descamps, H.; Lundgren, P.; Bleriot, C.; Liu, Z.; Deczkowska, A.; et al. Lipid-Associated Macrophages Control Metabolic Homeostasis in a Trem2-Dependent Manner. *Cell* **2019**, *178*, 686–698.e14. [CrossRef] [PubMed]
50. Cochain, C.; Vafadarnejad, E.; Arampatzi, P.; Pelisek, J.; Winkels, H.; Ley, K.; Wolf, D.; Saliba, A.E.; Zernecke, A. Single-Cell RNA-Seq Reveals the Transcriptional Landscape and Heterogeneity of Aortic Macrophages in Murine Atherosclerosis. *Circ. Res.* **2018**, *122*, 1661–1674. [CrossRef] [PubMed]
51. Rai, V.; Rao, V.H.; Shao, Z.; Agrawal, D.K. Dendritic Cells Expressing Triggering Receptor Expressed on Myeloid Cells-1 Correlate with Plaque Stability in Symptomatic and Asymptomatic Patients with Carotid Stenosis. *PLoS ONE* **2016**, *11*, e0154802. [CrossRef]

52. Saccani, A.; Schioppa, T.; Porta, C.; Biswas, S.K.; Nebuloni, M.; Vago, L.; Bottazzi, B.; Colombo, M.P.; Mantovani, A.; Sica, A. p50 Nuclear Factor- B Overexpression in Tumor-Associated Macrophages Inhibits M1 Inflammatory Responses and Antitumor Resistance. *Cancer Res.* **2006**, *66*, 11432–11440. [CrossRef]
53. Sica, A.; Mantovani, A. Macrophage plasticity and polarization: In vivo veritas. *J. Clin. Investig.* **2012**, *122*, 787–795. [CrossRef]
54. Escribese, M.M.; Casas, M.; Corbí, A.L. Influence of low oxygen tensions on macrophage polarization. *Immunobiology* **2012**, *217*, 1233–1240. [CrossRef]
55. Italiani, P.; Boraschi, D. From Monocytes to M1/M2 Macrophages: Phenotypical vs. Functional Differentiation. *Front. Immunol.* **2014**, *5*, 514. [CrossRef]
56. Murray, P.J.; Wynn, T.A. Protective and pathogenic functions of macrophage subsets. *Nat. Rev. Immunol.* **2011**, *11*, 723–737. [CrossRef]
57. Raes, G.; Van den Bergh, R.; De Baetselier, P.; Ghassabeh, G.H.; Scotton, C.; Locati, M.; Mantovani, A.; Sozzani, S. Arginase-1 and Ym1 are markers for murine, but not human, alternatively activated myeloid cells. *J. Immunol.* **2005**, *174*, 6561. [CrossRef]
58. Beattie, L.; Sawtell, A.; Mann, J.; Frame, T.C.M.; Teal, B.; de Labastida Rivera, F.; Brown, N.; Walwyn-Brown, K.; Moore, J.; MacDonald, S.; et al. Bone marrow-derived and resident liver macrophages display unique transcriptomic signatures but similar biological functions. *J. Hepatol.* **2016**, *65*, 758–768. [CrossRef]
59. Scott, C.L.; Zheng, F.; De Baetselier, P.; Martens, L.; Saeys, Y.; De Prijck, S.; Lippens, S.; Abels, C.; Schoonooghe, S.; Raes, G.; et al. Bone marrow-derived monocytes give rise to self-renewing and fully differentiated Kupffer cells. *Nat. Commun.* **2016**, *7*, 10321. [CrossRef]
60. Ramachandran, P.; Dobie, R.; Wilson-Kanamori, J.R.; Dora, E.F.; Henderson, B.E.P.; Luu, N.T.; Portman, J.R.; Matchett, K.P.; Brice, M.; Marwick, J.A.; et al. Resolving the fibrotic niche of human liver cirrhosis at single-cell level. *Nature* **2019**, *575*, 512–518. [CrossRef]
61. Charo, I.F. Macrophage polarization and insulin resistance: PPARgamma in control. *Cell Metab.* **2007**, *6*, 96–98. [CrossRef]
62. Lumeng, C.N.; Bodzin, J.L.; Saltiel, A.R. Obesity induces a phenotypic switch in adipose tissue macrophage polarization. *J. Clin. Investig.* **2007**, *117*, 175–184. [CrossRef]
63. Patsouris, D.; Li, P.-P.; Thapar, D.; Chapman, J.; Olefsky, J.M.; Neels, J.G. Ablation of CD11c-Positive Cells Normalizes Insulin Sensitivity in Obese Insulin Resistant Animals. *Cell Metab.* **2008**, *8*, 301–309. [CrossRef]
64. Subramanian, V.; Ferrante, A.W., Jr. Obesity, inflammation, and macrophages. *Nestle Nutr. Workshop Ser. Pediatr. Program.* **2009**, *63*, 151–159.
65. Li, C.; Xu, M.M.; Wang, K.; Adler, A.J.; Vella, A.T.; Zhou, B. Macrophage polarization and meta-inflammation. *Transl. Res.* **2018**, *191*, 29–44. [CrossRef]
66. Hotamisligil, G.S.; Shargill, N.S.; Spiegelman, B.M. Adipose expression of tumor necrosis factor-alpha: Direct role in obesity-linked insulin resistance. *Science* **1993**, *259*, 87–91. [CrossRef]
67. Gregor, M.F.; Hotamisligil, G.S. Inflammatory mechanisms in obesity. *Annu. Rev. Immunol.* **2011**, *29*, 415–445. [CrossRef] [PubMed]
68. Hassnain Waqas, S.F.; Noble, A.; Hoang, A.C.; Ampem, G.; Popp, M.; Strauss, S.; Guille, M.; Röszer, T. Adipose tissue macrophages develop from bone marrow-independent progenitors in Xenopus laevis and mouse. *J. Leukoc. Biol.* **2017**, *102*, 845–855. [CrossRef]
69. Schulz, C.; Gomez Perdiguero, E.; Chorro, L.; Szabo-Rogers, H.; Cagnard, N.; Kierdorf, K.; Prinz, M.; Wu, B.; Jacobsen, S.E.; Pollard, J.W.; et al. A lineage of myeloid cells independent of Myb and hematopoietic stem cells. *Science* **2012**, *336*, 86–90. [CrossRef] [PubMed]
70. Geissmann, F.; Jung, S.; Littman, D.R. Blood monocytes consist of two principal subsets with distinct migratory properties. *Immunity* **2003**, *19*, 71–82. [CrossRef]
71. Cho, C.H.; Koh, Y.J.; Han, J.; Sung, H.K.; Jong Lee, H.; Morisada, T.; Schwendener, R.A.; Brekken, R.A.; Kang, G.; Oike, Y.; et al. Angiogenic role of LYVE-1-positive macrophages in adipose tissue. *Circ. Res.* **2007**, *100*, e47–e57. [CrossRef]
72. Wang, Q.A.; Tao, C.; Gupta, R.K.; Scherer, P.E. Tracking adipogenesis during white adipose tissue development, expansion and regeneration. *Nat. Med.* **2013**, *19*, 1338–1344. [CrossRef]
73. Hill, D.A.; Lim, H.W.; Kim, Y.H.; Ho, W.Y.; Foong, Y.H.; Nelson, V.L.; Nguyen, H.; Chegireddy, K.; Kim, J.; Habertheuer, A.; et al. Distinct macrophage populations direct inflammatory versus physiological changes in adipose tissue. *Proc. Natl. Acad. Sci. USA* **2018**, *115*, E5096–E5105. [CrossRef]
74. Chakarov, S.; Lim, H.Y.; Tan, L.; Lim, S.Y.; See, P.; Lum, J.; Zhang, X.M.; Foo, S.; Nakamizo, S.; Duan, K.; et al. Two distinct interstitial macrophage populations coexist across tissues in specific subtissular niches. *Science* **2019**, *363*, eaau0964. [CrossRef]
75. Fujisaka, S. The role of adipose tissue M1/M2 macrophages in type 2 diabetes mellitus. *Diabetol. Int.* **2021**, *12*, 74–79. [CrossRef]
76. Wu, D.; Molofsky, A.B.; Liang, H.E.; Ricardo-Gonzalez, R.R.; Jouihan, H.A.; Bando, J.K.; Chawla, A.; Locksley, R.M. Eosinophils sustain adipose alternatively activated macrophages associated with glucose homeostasis. *Science* **2011**, *332*, 243–247. [CrossRef]
77. Odegaard, J.I.; Ricardo-Gonzalez, R.R.; Goforth, M.H.; Morel, C.R.; Subramanian, V.; Mukundan, L.; Red Eagle, A.; Vats, D.; Brombacher, F.; Ferrante, A.W., Jr.; et al. Macrophage-specific PPARγ controls alternative activation and improves insulin resistance. *Nature* **2007**, *447*, 1116–1120. [CrossRef]
78. Liang, W.; Qi, Y.; Yi, H.; Mao, C.; Meng, Q.; Wang, H.; Zheng, C. The Roles of Adipose Tissue Macrophages in Human Disease. *Front. Immunol.* **2022**, *13*, 908749. [CrossRef]

79. Nguyen, K.D.; Qiu, Y.; Cui, X.; Goh, Y.P.; Mwangi, J.; David, T.; Mukundan, L.; Brombacher, F.; Locksley, R.M.; Chawla, A. Alternatively activated macrophages produce catecholamines to sustain adaptive thermogenesis. *Nature* **2011**, *480*, 104–108. [CrossRef]
80. Zhang, Y.; Yang, P.; Cui, R.; Zhang, M.; Li, H.; Qian, C.; Sheng, C.; Qu, S.; Bu, L. Eosinophils Reduce Chronic Inflammation in Adipose Tissue by Secreting Th2 Cytokines and Promoting M2 Macrophages Polarization. *Int. J. Endocrinol.* **2015**, *2015*, 565760. [CrossRef]
81. Fischer, K.; Ruiz, H.H.; Jhun, K.; Finan, B.; Oberlin, D.J.; van der Heide, V.; Kalinovich, A.V.; Petrovic, N.; Wolf, Y.; Clemmensen, C.; et al. Alternatively activated macrophages do not synthesize catecholamines or contribute to adipose tissue adaptive thermogenesis. *Nat. Med.* **2017**, *23*, 623–630. [CrossRef]
82. Camell, C.D.; Sander, J.; Spadaro, O.; Lee, A.; Nguyen, K.Y.; Wing, A.; Goldberg, E.L.; Youm, Y.H.; Brown, C.W.; Elsworth, J.; et al. Inflammasome-driven catecholamine catabolism in macrophages blunts lipolysis during ageing. *Nature* **2017**, *550*, 119–123. [CrossRef] [PubMed]
83. Czech, M.P. Macrophages dispose of catecholamines in adipose tissue. *Nat. Med.* **2017**, *23*, 1255–1257. [CrossRef] [PubMed]
84. Wellen, K.E.; Hotamisligil, G.S. Obesity-induced inflammatory changes in adipose tissue. *J. Clin. Investig.* **2003**, *112*, 1785–1788. [CrossRef] [PubMed]
85. Alkhouri, N.; Gornicka, A.; Berk, M.P.; Thapaliya, S.; Dixon, L.J.; Kashyap, S.; Schauer, P.R.; Feldstein, A.E. Adipocyte apoptosis, a link between obesity, insulin resistance, and hepatic steatosis. *J. Biol. Chem.* **2010**, *285*, 3428–3438. [CrossRef]
86. Zheng, C.; Yang, Q.; Cao, J.; Xie, N.; Liu, K.; Shou, P.; Qian, F.; Wang, Y.; Shi, Y. Local proliferation initiates macrophage accumulation in adipose tissue during obesity. *Cell Death Dis.* **2016**, *7*, e2167. [CrossRef]
87. Lumeng, C.N.; DelProposto, J.B.; Westcott, D.J.; Saltiel, A.R. Phenotypic switching of adipose tissue macrophages with obesity is generated by spatiotemporal differences in macrophage subtypes. *Diabetes* **2008**, *57*, 3239–3246. [CrossRef]
88. Poret, J.M.; Souza-Smith, F.; Marcell, S.J.; Gaudet, D.A.; Tzeng, T.H.; Braymer, H.D.; Harrison-Bernard, L.M.; Primeaux, S.D. High fat diet consumption differentially affects adipose tissue inflammation and adipocyte size in obesity-prone and obesity-resistant rats. *Int. J. Obes.* **2018**, *42*, 535–541. [CrossRef]
89. Ramkhelawon, B.; Hennessy, E.J.; Ménager, M.; Ray, T.D.; Sheedy, F.J.; Hutchison, S.; Wanschel, A.; Oldebeken, S.; Geoffrion, M.; Spiro, W.; et al. Netrin-1 promotes adipose tissue macrophage retention and insulin resistance in obesity. *Nat. Med.* **2014**, *20*, 377–384. [CrossRef]
90. Murano, I.; Barbatelli, G.; Parisani, V.; Latini, C.; Muzzonigro, G.; Castellucci, M.; Cinti, S. Dead adipocytes, detected as crown-like structures, are prevalent in visceral fat depots of genetically obese mice. *J. Lipid Res.* **2008**, *49*, 1562–1568. [CrossRef]
91. Gao, B. Basic liver immunology. *Cell. Mol. Immunol.* **2016**, *13*, 265–266. [CrossRef] [PubMed]
92. Kubes, P.; Jenne, C. Immune Responses in the Liver. *Annu. Rev. Immunol.* **2018**, *36*, 247–277. [CrossRef] [PubMed]
93. Xu, M.; Wang, H.; Wang, J.; Burhan, D.; Shang, R.; Wang, P.; Zhou, Y.; Li, R.; Liang, B.; Evert, K.; et al. mTORC2 signaling is necessary for timely liver regeneration after partial hepatectomy. *Am. J. Pathol.* **2020**, *190*, 817–829. [CrossRef] [PubMed]
94. Dong, X.L.J.; Xu, Y.; Cao, H. Role of macrophages in experimental liver injury and repair in mice. *Exp. Ther. Med.* **2019**, *17*, 3835–3847. [CrossRef]
95. Jager, J.; Aparicio-Vergara, M.; Aouadi, M. Liver innate immune cells and insulin resistance: The multiple facets of Kupffer cells. *J. Intern. Med.* **2016**, *280*, 209–220. [CrossRef]
96. Krenkel, O.; Tacke, F. Liver macrophages in tissue homeostasis and disease. *Nat. Rev. Immunol.* **2017**, *17*, 306–321. [CrossRef]
97. Obstfeld, A.E.; Sugaru, E.; Thearle, M.; Francisco, A.M.; Gayet, C.; Ginsberg, H.N.; Ables, E.V.; Ferrante, A.W., Jr. C-C chemokine receptor 2 (CCR2) regulates the hepatic recruitment of myeloid cells that promote obesity-induced hepatic steatosis. *Diabetes* **2010**, *59*, 916–925. [CrossRef]
98. Ju, C.; Tacke, F. Hepatic macrophages in homeostasis and liver diseases: From pathogenesis to novel therapeutic strategies. *Cell. Mol. Immunol.* **2016**, *13*, 316–327. [CrossRef]
99. Morinaga, H.; Mayoral, R.; Heinrichsdorff, J.; Osborn, O.; Franck, N.; Hah, N.; Walenta, E.; Bandyopadhyay, G.; Pessentheiner, A.R.; Chi, T.J.; et al. Characterization of distinct subpopulations of hepatic macrophages in HFD/obese mice. *Diabetes* **2015**, *64*, 1120–1130. [CrossRef]
100. Ying, W.; Mahata, S.; Bandyopadhyay, G.K.; Zhou, Z.; Wollam, J.; Vu, J.; Mayoral, R.; Chi, N.W.; Webster, N.; Corti, A.; et al. Catestatin Inhibits Obesity-Induced Macrophage Infiltration and Inflammation in the Liver and Suppresses Hepatic Glucose Production, Leading to Improved Insulin Sensitivity. *Diabetes* **2018**, *67*, 841–848. [CrossRef]
101. Davies, L.C.; Jenkins, S.J.; Allen, J.E.; Taylor, P.R. Tissue-resident macrophages. *Nat. Immunol.* **2013**, *14*, 986–995. [CrossRef]
102. Meshkani, R.; Adeli, K. Hepatic insulin resistance, metabolic syndrome and cardiovascular disease. *Clin. Biochem.* **2009**, *42*, 1331–1346. [CrossRef] [PubMed]
103. Yki-Jarvinen, H. Fat in the liver and insulin resistance. *Ann. Med.* **2005**, *37*, 347–356. [CrossRef]
104. Lanthier, N.; Molendi-Coste, O.; Horsmans, Y.; van Rooijen, N.; Cani, P.D.; Leclercq, I.A. Kupffer cell activation is a causal factor for hepatic insulin resistance. *Am. J. Physiol. Gastrointest. Liver Physiol.* **2010**, *298*, G107–G116. [CrossRef]
105. Neyrinck, A.M.; Cani, P.D.; Dewulf, E.M.; De Backer, F.; Bindels, L.B.; Delzenne, N.M. Critical role of Kupffer cells in the management of diet-induced diabetes and obesity. *Biochem. Biophys. Res. Commun.* **2009**, *385*, 351–356. [CrossRef]
106. Lopez, B.G.; Tsai, M.S.; Baratta, J.L.; Longmuir, K.J.; Robertson, R.T. Characterization of Kupffer cells in livers of developing mice. *Comp. Hepatol.* **2011**, *10*, 2. [CrossRef]

107. Neyrinck, A.M.; Gomez, C.; Delzenne, N.M. Precision-cut liver slices in culture as a tool to assess the physiological involvement of Kupffer cells in hepatic metabolism. *Comp. Hepatol.* **2004**, *3* (Suppl. 1), S45. [CrossRef]
108. Wunderlich, F.T.; Strohle, P.; Konner, A.C.; Gruber, S.; Tovar, S.; Bronneke, H.S.; Juntti-Berggren, L.; Li, L.S.; van Rooijen, N.; Libert, C.; et al. Interleukin-6 signaling in liver-parenchymal cells suppresses hepatic inflammation and improves systemic insulin action. *Cell Metab.* **2010**, *12*, 237–249. [CrossRef]
109. Van Herpen, N.A.; Schrauwen-Hinderling, V.B. Lipid accumulation in non-adipose tissue and lipotoxicity. *Physiol. Behav.* **2008**, *94*, 231–241. [CrossRef]
110. Lauterbach, M.A.; Wunderlich, F.T. Macrophage function in obesity-induced inflammation and insulin resistance. *Pflug. Arch.* **2017**, *469*, 385–396. [CrossRef] [PubMed]
111. Haines, M.S.; Dichtel, L.E.; Santoso, K.; Torriani, M.; Miller, K.K.; Bredella, M.A. Association between muscle mass and insulin sensitivity independent of detrimental adipose depots in young adults with overweight/obesity. *Int. J. Obes.* **2020**, *44*, 1851–1858. [CrossRef]
112. Son, J.W.; Lee, S.S.; Kim, S.R.; Yoo, S.J.; Cha, B.Y.; Son, H.Y.; Cho, N.H. Low muscle mass and risk of type 2 diabetes in middle-aged and older adults: Findings from the KoGES. *Diabetologia* **2017**, *60*, 865–872. [CrossRef] [PubMed]
113. DeFronzo, R.A.; Tripathy, D. Skeletal muscle insulin resistance is the primary defect in type 2 diabetes. *Diabetes Care* **2009**, *32* (Suppl. 2), S157–S163. [CrossRef] [PubMed]
114. Pillon, N.J.; Bilan, P.J.; Fink, L.N.; Klip, A. Cross-talk between skeletal muscle and immune cells: Muscle-derived mediators and metabolic implications. *Am. J. Physiol. Endocrinol. Metab.* **2013**, *304*, E453–E465. [CrossRef]
115. Khan, I.M.; Perrard, X.Y.; Brunner, G.; Lui, H.; Sparks, L.M.; Smith, S.R.; Wang, X.; Shi, Z.Z.; Lewis, D.E.; Wu, H.; et al. Intermuscular and perimuscular fat expansion in obesity correlates with skeletal muscle T cell and macrophage infiltration and insulin resistance. *Int. J. Obes.* **2015**, *39*, 1607–1618. [CrossRef]
116. Chen, L.; Chen, R.; Wang, H.; Liang, F. Mechanisms Linking Inflammation to Insulin Resistance. *Int. J. Endocrinol.* **2015**, *2015*, 508409. [CrossRef]
117. Varma, V.; Yao-Borengasser, A.; Rasouli, N.; Nolen, G.T.; Phanavanh, B.; Starks, T.; Gurley, C.; Simpson, P.; McGehee, R.E., Jr.; Kern, P.A.; et al. Muscle inflammatory response and insulin resistance: Synergistic interaction between macrophages and fatty acids leads to impaired insulin action. *Am. J. Physiol. Endocrinol. Metab.* **2009**, *296*, E1300–E1310. [CrossRef]
118. Patsouris, D.; Cao, J.J.; Vial, G.; Bravard, A.; Lefai, E.; Durand, A.; Durand, C.; Chauvin, M.A.; Laugerette, F.; Debard, C.; et al. Insulin resistance is associated with MCP1-mediated macrophage accumulation in skeletal muscle in mice and humans. *PLoS ONE* **2014**, *9*, e110653. [CrossRef]
119. Hong, E.G.; Ko, H.J.; Cho, Y.R.; Kim, H.J.; Ma, Z.; Yu, T.Y.; Friedline, R.H.; Kurt-Jones, E.; Finberg, R.; Fischer, M.A.; et al. Interleukin-10 prevents diet-induced insulin resistance by attenuating macrophage and cytokine response in skeletal muscle. *Diabetes* **2009**, *58*, 2525–2535. [CrossRef]
120. Rachek, L.I. Free Fatty Acids and Skeletal Muscle Insulin Resistance. Glucose Homeostatis and the Pathogenesis of Diabetes Mellitus. *Prog. Mol. Biol. Transl. Sci.* **2014**, *121*, 267–292.
121. Boren, J.; Taskinen, M.R.; Olofsson, S.O.; Levin, M. Ectopic lipid storage and insulin resistance: A harmful relationship. *J. Intern. Med.* **2013**, *274*, 25–40. [CrossRef] [PubMed]
122. Banaei-Bouchareb, L.; Gouon-Evans, V.; Samara-Boustani, D.; Castellotti, M.C.; Czernichow, P.; Pollard, J.W.; Polak, M. Insulin cell mass is altered in Csf1op/Csf1op macrophage-deficient mice. *J. Leukoc. Biol.* **2004**, *76*, 359–367. [CrossRef] [PubMed]
123. Maedler, K.; Schumann, D.M.; Sauter, N.; Ellingsgaard, H.; Bosco, D.; Baertschiger, R.; Iwakura, Y.; Oberholzer, J.; Wollheim, C.B.; Gauthier, B.R.; et al. Low concentration of interleukin-1beta induces FLICE-inhibitory protein-mediated beta-cell proliferation in human pancreatic islets. *Diabetes* **2006**, *55*, 2713–2722. [CrossRef] [PubMed]
124. Ehses, J.A.; Perren, A.; Eppler, E.; Ribaux, P.; Pospisilik, J.A.; Maor-Cahn, R.; Gueripel, X.; Ellingsgaard, H.; Schneider, M.K.; Biollaz, G.; et al. Increased number of islet-associated macrophages in type 2 diabetes. *Diabetes* **2007**, *56*, 2356–2370. [CrossRef]
125. Kamata, K.; Mizukami, H.; Inaba, W.; Tsuboi, K.; Tateishi, Y.; Yoshida, T.; Yagihashi, S. Islet amyloid with macrophage migration correlates with augmented beta-cell deficits in type 2 diabetic patients. *Amyloid* **2014**, *21*, 191–201. [CrossRef]
126. Eguchi, K.; Manabe, I.; Oishi-Tanaka, Y.; Ohsugi, M.; Kono, N.; Ogata, F.; Yagi, N.; Ohto, U.; Kimoto, M.; Miyake, K.; et al. Saturated fatty acid and TLR signaling link beta cell dysfunction and islet inflammation. *Cell Metab.* **2012**, *15*, 518–533. [CrossRef]
127. Han, Z.; Boyle, D.L.; Chang, L.; Bennett, B.; Karin, M.; Yang, L.; Manning, A.M.; Firestein, G.S. c-Jun N-terminal kinase is required for metalloproteinase expression and joint destruction in inflammatory arthritis. *J. Clin. Investig.* **2001**, *108*, 73–81. [CrossRef]
128. Zhao, J.; Wang, L.; Dong, X.; Hu, X.; Zhou, L.; Liu, Q.; Song, B.; Wu, Q.; Li, L. The c-Jun N-terminal kinase (JNK) pathway is activated in human interstitial cystitis (IC) and rat protamine sulfate induced cystitis. *Sci. Rep.* **2016**, *6*, 19870. [CrossRef]
129. Chen, Y.R.; Tan, T.H. The c-Jun N-terminal kinase pathway and apoptotic signaling (review). *Int. J. Oncol.* **2000**, *16*, 651–662. [CrossRef]
130. Mitchell, S.; Vargas, J.; Hoffmann, A. Signaling via the NFkappaB system. *Wiley Interdiscip. Rev. Syst. Biol. Med.* **2016**, *8*, 227–241. [CrossRef]
131. Rios, R.; Silva, H.; Carneiro, N.V.Q.; Pires, A.O.; Carneiro, T.C.B.; Costa, R.D.S.; Marques, C.R.; Machado, M.; Velozo, E.; Silva, T.; et al. Solanum paniculatum L. decreases levels of inflammatory cytokines by reducing NFKB, TBET and GATA3 gene expression in vitro. *J. Ethnopharmacol.* **2017**, *209*, 32–40. [CrossRef]
132. Yang, R.; Tonnessen, T.I. DAMPs and sterile inflammation in drug hepatotoxicity. *Hepatol. Int.* **2019**, *13*, 42–50. [CrossRef]

133. Franklin, T.C.; Xu, C.; Duman, R.S. Depression and sterile inflammation: Essential role of danger associated molecular patterns. *Brain Behav. Immun.* **2018**, *72*, 2–13. [CrossRef]
134. Patel, S. Danger-Associated Molecular Patterns (DAMPs): The Derivatives and Triggers of Inflammation. *Curr. Allerg. Asthma Rep.* **2018**, *18*, 63. [CrossRef]
135. Tang, D.; Kang, R.; Coyne, C.B.; Zeh, H.J.; Lotze, M.T. PAMPs and DAMPs: Signal 0s that spur autophagy and immunity. *Immunol. Rev.* **2012**, *249*, 158–175. [CrossRef]
136. Zindel, J.; Kubes, P. DAMPs, PAMPs, and LAMPs in Immunity and Sterile Inflammation. *Annu. Rev. Pathol.* **2020**, *15*, 493–518. [CrossRef]
137. Akash, M.S.H.; Rehman, K.; Liaqat, A. Tumor Necrosis Factor-Alpha: Role in Development of Insulin Resistance and Pathogenesis of Type 2 Diabetes Mellitus. *J. Cell Biochem.* **2018**, *119*, 105–110. [CrossRef]
138. Xu, H.; Barnes, G.T.; Yang, Q.; Tan, G.; Yang, D.; Chou, C.J.; Sole, J.; Nichols, A.; Ross, J.S.; Tartaglia, L.A.; et al. Chronic inflammation in fat plays a crucial role in the development of obesity-related insulin resistance. *J. Clin. Investig.* **2003**, *112*, 1821–1830. [CrossRef]
139. De Taeye, B.M.; Novitskaya, T.; McGuinness, O.P.; Gleaves, L.; Medda, M.; Covington, J.W.; Vaughan, D.E. Macrophage TNF-alpha contributes to insulin resistance and hepatic steatosis in diet-induced obesity. *Am. J. Physiol. Endocrinol. Metab.* **2007**, *293*, E713–E725. [CrossRef]
140. Uysal, K.T.; Wiesbrock, S.M.; Marino, M.W.; Hotamisligil, G.S. Protection from obesity-induced insulin resistance in mice lacking TNF-alpha function. *Nature* **1997**, *389*, 610–614. [CrossRef]
141. Tang, F.; Tang, G.; Xiang, J.; Dai, Q.; Rosner, M.R.; Lin, A. The absence of NF-kappaB-mediated inhibition of c-Jun N-terminal kinase activation contributes to tumor necrosis factor alpha-induced apoptosis. *Mol. Cell. Biol.* **2002**, *22*, 8571–8579. [CrossRef]
142. Bandyopadhyay, G.K.; Yu, J.G.; Ofrecio, J.; Olefsky, J.M. Increased p85/55/50 expression and decreased phosphotidylinositol 3-kinase activity in insulin-resistant human skeletal muscle. *Diabetes* **2005**, *54*, 2351–2359. [CrossRef]
143. Cai, D.; Yuan, M.; Frantz, D.F.; Melendez, P.A.; Hansen, L.; Lee, J.; Shoelson, S.E. Local and systemic insulin resistance resulting from hepatic activation of IKK-beta and NF-kappaB. *Nat. Med.* **2005**, *11*, 183–190. [CrossRef]
144. Sabio, G.; Davis, R.J. cJun NH2-terminal kinase 1 (JNK1): Roles in metabolic regulation of insulin resistance. *Trends Biochem. Sci.* **2010**, *35*, 490–496. [CrossRef]
145. Rui, L.; Aguirre, V.; Kim, J.K.; Shulman, G.I.; Lee, A.; Corbould, A.; Dunaif, A.; White, M.F. Insulin/IGF-1 and TNF-alpha stimulate phosphorylation of IRS-1 at inhibitory Ser307 via distinct pathways. *J. Clin. Investig.* **2001**, *107*, 181–189. [CrossRef]
146. Hotamisligil, G.S.; Murray, D.L.; Choy, L.N.; Spiegelman, B.M. Tumor necrosis factor alpha inhibits signaling from the insulin receptor. *Proc. Natl. Acad. Sci. USA* **1994**, *91*, 4854–4858. [CrossRef]
147. Tanti, J.F.; Gremeaux, T.; van Obberghen, E.; Le Marchand-Brustel, Y. Serine/threonine phosphorylation of insulin receptor substrate 1 modulates insulin receptor signaling. *J. Biol. Chem.* **1994**, *269*, 6051–6057. [CrossRef]
148. Li, P.; Oh, D.Y.; Bandyopadhyay, G.; Lagakos, W.S.; Talukdar, S.; Osborn, O.; Johnson, A.; Chung, H.; Maris, M.; Ofrecio, J.M.; et al. LTB4 promotes insulin resistance in obese mice by acting on macrophages, hepatocytes and myocytes. *Nat. Med.* **2015**, *21*, 239–247. [CrossRef]
149. Higham, A.; Cadden, P.; Southworth, T.; Rossall, M.; Kolsum, U.; Lea, S.; Knowles, R.; Singh, D. Leukotriene B4 levels in sputum from asthma patients. *ERJ Open Res.* **2016**, *2*, 00088–2015. [CrossRef]
150. Brandt, S.L.; Serezani, C.H. Too much of a good thing: How modulating LTB4 actions restore host defense in homeostasis or disease. *Semin. Immunol.* **2017**, *33*, 37–43. [CrossRef]
151. Liu, T.; Zhang, L.; Joo, D.; Sun, S.C. NF-kappaB signaling in inflammation. *Signal Transduct. Target. Ther.* **2017**, *2*, 17023. [CrossRef] [PubMed]
152. Lawrence, T. The nuclear factor NF-kappaB pathway in inflammation. *Cold Spring Harb. Perspect. Biol.* **2009**, *1*, a001651. [CrossRef] [PubMed]
153. Yuan, M.; Konstantopoulos, N.; Lee, J.; Hansen, L.; Li, Z.W.; Karin, M.; Shoelson, S.E. Reversal of obesity- and diet-induced insulin resistance with salicylates or targeted disruption of Ikkbeta. *Science* **2001**, *293*, 1673–1677. [CrossRef] [PubMed]
154. Chiang, S.H.; Bazuine, M.; Lumeng, C.N.; Geletka, L.M.; Mowers, J.; White, N.M.; Ma, J.T.; Zhou, J.; Qi, N.; Westcott, D.; et al. The protein kinase IKKepsilon regulates energy balance in obese mice. *Cell* **2009**, *138*, 961–975. [CrossRef]
155. Gao, D.; Madi, M.; Ding, C.; Fok, M.; Steele, T.; Ford, C.; Hunter, L.; Bing, C. Interleukin-1beta mediates macrophage-induced impairment of insulin signaling in human primary adipocytes. *Am. J. Physiol. Endocrinol. Metab.* **2014**, *307*, E289–E304. [CrossRef]
156. Koenen, T.B.; Stienstra, R.; van Tits, L.J.; de Graaf, J.; Stalenhoef, A.F.; Joosten, L.A.; Tack, C.J.; Netea, M.G. Hyperglycemia activates caspase-1 and TXNIP-mediated IL-1beta transcription in human adipose tissue. *Diabetes* **2011**, *60*, 517–524. [CrossRef]
157. Spranger, J.; Kroke, A.; Mohlig, M.; Hoffmann, K.; Bergmann, M.M.; Ristow, M.; Boeing, H.; Pfeiffer, A.F. Inflammatory cytokines and the risk to develop type 2 diabetes: Results of the prospective population-based European Prospective Investigation into Cancer and Nutrition (EPIC)-Potsdam Study. *Diabetes* **2003**, *52*, 812–817. [CrossRef]
158. Peiro, C.; Lorenzo, O.; Carraro, R.; Sanchez-Ferrer, C.F. IL-1beta Inhibition in Cardiovascular Complications Associated to Diabetes Mellitus. *Front. Pharmacol.* **2017**, *8*, 363. [CrossRef]
159. Boni-Schnetzler, M.; Donath, M.Y. How biologics targeting the IL-1 system are being considered for the treatment of type 2 diabetes. *Br. J. Clin. Pharmacol.* **2013**, *76*, 263–268. [CrossRef]

160. Chawla, A.; Barak, Y.; Nagy, L.; Liao, D.; Tontonoz, P.; Evans, R.M. PPAR-gamma dependent and independent effects on macrophage-gene expression in lipid metabolism and inflammation. *Nat. Med.* **2001**, *7*, 48–52. [CrossRef]
161. Olefsky, J.; Saltiel, A. PPARγ and the Treatment of Insulin Resistance. *Trends Endocrinol. Metab.* **2000**, *11*, 362–368. [CrossRef]
162. Grygiel-Gorniak, B. Peroxisome proliferator-activated receptors and their ligands: Nutritional and clinical implications—A review. *Nutr. J.* **2014**, *13*, 17. [CrossRef]
163. Henkel, J.; Neuschafer-Rube, F.; Pathe-Neuschafer-Rube, A.; Puschel, G.P. Aggravation by prostaglandin E2 of interleukin-6-dependent insulin resistance in hepatocytes. *Hepatology* **2009**, *50*, 781–790. [CrossRef]
164. Gross, B.; Staels, B. PPAR agonists: Multimodal drugs for the treatment of type-2 diabetes. *Best Pract. Res. Clin. Endocrinol. Metab.* **2007**, *21*, 687–710. [CrossRef]
165. Sugii, S.; Olson, P.; Sears, D.D.; Saberi, M.; Atkins, A.R.; Barish, G.D.; Hong, S.H.; Castro, G.L.; Yin, Y.Q.; Nelson, M.C.; et al. PPARgamma activation in adipocytes is sufficient for systemic insulin sensitization. *Proc. Natl. Acad. Sci. USA* **2009**, *106*, 22504–22509. [CrossRef]
166. Leonardini, A.; Laviola, L.; Perrini, S.; Natalicchio, A.; Giorgino, F. Cross-Talk between PPARgamma and Insulin Signaling and Modulation of Insulin Sensitivity. *PPAR Res.* **2009**, *2009*, 818945. [CrossRef]
167. Feng, X.; Weng, D.; Zhou, F.; Owen, Y.D.; Qin, H.; Zhao, J.; Wen, Y.; Huang, Y.; Chen, J.; Fu, H.; et al. Activation of PPARgamma by a Natural Flavonoid Modulator, Apigenin Ameliorates Obesity-Related Inflammation Via Regulation of Macrophage Polarization. *eBioMedicine* **2016**, *9*, 61–76. [CrossRef]
168. Hevener, A.L.; Olefsky, J.M.; Reichart, D.; Nguyen, M.T.; Bandyopadyhay, G.; Leung, H.Y.; Watt, M.J.; Benner, C.; Febbraio, M.A.; Nguyen, A.K.; et al. Macrophage PPAR gamma is required for normal skeletal muscle and hepatic insulin sensitivity and full antidiabetic effects of thiazolidinediones. *J. Clin. Investig.* **2007**, *117*, 1658–1669. [CrossRef]
169. Nonogaki, K.; Fuller, G.M.; Fuentes, N.L.; Moser, A.H.; Staprans, I.; Grunfeld, C.; Feingold, K.R. Interleukin-6 stimulates hepatic triglyceride secretion in rats. *Endocrinology* **1995**, *136*, 2143–2149. [CrossRef]
170. Heinrich, P.C.; Behrmann, I.; Muller-Newen, G.; Schaper, F.; Graeve, L. Interleukin-6-type cytokine signalling through the gp130/Jak/STAT pathway. *Biochem. J.* **1998**, *334 Pt 2*, 297–314. [CrossRef]
171. Ueki, K.; Kondo, T.; Kahn, C.R. Suppressor of cytokine signaling 1 (SOCS-1) and SOCS-3 cause insulin resistance through inhibition of tyrosine phosphorylation of insulin receptor substrate proteins by discrete mechanisms. *Mol. Cell. Biol.* **2004**, *24*, 5434–5446. [CrossRef]
172. Bastard, J.P.; Jardel, C.; Bruckert, E.; Blondy, P.; Capeau, J.; Laville, M.; Vidal, H.; Hainque, B. Elevated levels of interleukin 6 are reduced in serum and subcutaneous adipose tissue of obese women after weight loss. *J. Clin. Endocrinol. Metab.* **2000**, *85*, 3338–3342.
173. Lee, B.C.; Lee, J. Cellular and molecular players in adipose tissue inflammation in the development of obesity-induced insulin resistance. *Biochim. Biophys. Acta* **2014**, *1842*, 446–462. [CrossRef]
174. Wallenius, V.; Wallenius, K.; Ahren, B.; Rudling, M.; Carlsten, H.; Dickson, S.L.; Ohlsson, C.; Jansson, J.O. Interleukin-6-deficient mice develop mature-onset obesity. *Nat. Med.* **2002**, *8*, 75–79. [CrossRef]
175. Kurauti, M.A.; Costa-Junior, J.M.; Ferreira, S.M.; Santos, G.J.; Sponton, C.H.G.; Carneiro, E.M.; Telles, G.D.; Chacon-Mikahil, M.; Cavaglieri, C.R.; Rezende, L.F.; et al. Interleukin-6 increases the expression and activity of insulin-degrading enzyme. *Sci. Rep.* **2017**, *7*, 46750. [CrossRef]
176. Chen, X.; Xun, K.; Chen, L.; Wang, Y. TNF-alpha, a potent lipid metabolism regulator. *Cell Biochem. Funct.* **2009**, *27*, 407–416. [CrossRef]
177. Starnes, H.F., Jr.; Warren, R.S.; Jeevanandam, M.; Gabrilove, J.L.; Larchian, W.; Oettgen, H.F.; Brennan, M.F. Tumor necrosis factor and the acute metabolic response to tissue injury in man. *J. Clin. Investig.* **1988**, *82*, 1321–1325. [CrossRef]
178. Wedell-Neergaard, A.S.; Lang Lehrskov, L.; Christensen, R.H.; Legaard, G.E.; Dorph, E.; Larsen, M.K.; Launbo, N.; Fagerlind, S.R.; Seide, S.K.; Nymand, S.; et al. Exercise-Induced Changes in Visceral Adipose Tissue Mass Are Regulated by IL-6 Signaling: A Randomized Controlled Trial. *Cell Metab.* **2019**, *29*, 844–855.e3. [CrossRef]
179. Wolsk, E.; Mygind, H.; Grondahl, T.S.; Pedersen, B.K.; van Hall, G. IL-6 selectively stimulates fat metabolism in human skeletal muscle. *Am. J. Physiol. Endocrinol. Metab.* **2010**, *299*, E832–E840. [CrossRef]
180. Speaker, K.J.; Fleshner, M. Interleukin-1 beta: A potential link between stress and the development of visceral obesity. *BMC Physiol.* **2012**, *12*, 8. [CrossRef]
181. Schaffer, J.E. Lipotoxicity: When tissues overeat. *Curr. Opin. Lipidol.* **2003**, *14*, 281–287. [CrossRef] [PubMed]
182. Ma, X.L.; Meng, L.; Li, L.L.; Ma, L.N.; Mao, X.M. Plasma Free Fatty Acids Metabolic Profile Among Uyghurs and Kazaks With or Without Type 2 Diabetes Based on GC-MS. *Exp. Clin. Endocrinol. Diabetes* **2018**, *126*, 604–611. [CrossRef] [PubMed]
183. Makarova, E.; Makrecka-Kuka, M.; Vilks, K.; Volska, K.; Sevostjanovs, E.; Grinberga, S.; Zarkova-Malkova, O.; Dambrova, M.; Liepinsh, E. Decreases in Circulating Concentrations of Long-Chain Acylcarnitines and Free Fatty Acids During the Glucose Tolerance Test Represent Tissue-Specific Insulin Sensitivity. *Front. Endocrinol.* **2019**, *10*, 870. [CrossRef] [PubMed]
184. Samuel, V.T.; Shulman, G.I. Mechanisms for insulin resistance: Common threads and missing links. *Cell* **2012**, *148*, 852–871. [CrossRef]
185. Jornayvaz, F.R.; Birkenfeld, A.L.; Jurczak, M.J.; Kanda, S.; Guigni, B.A.; Jiang, D.C.; Zhang, D.; Lee, H.Y.; Samuel, V.T.; Shulman, G.I. Hepatic insulin resistance in mice with hepatic overexpression of diacylglycerol acyltransferase 2. *Proc. Natl. Acad. Sci. USA* **2011**, *108*, 5748–5752. [CrossRef]

186. Metcalfe, L.K.; Smith, G.C.; Turner, N. Defining lipid mediators of insulin resistance—Controversies and challenges. *J. Mol. Endocrinol.* **2018**, *62*, R65–R82. [CrossRef]
187. Szendroedi, J.; Yoshimura, T.; Phielix, E.; Koliaki, C.; Marcucci, M.; Zhang, D.; Jelenik, T.; Müller, J.; Herder, C.; Nowotny, P.; et al. Role of diacylglycerol activation of PKCtheta in lipid-induced muscle insulin resistance in humans. *Proc. Natl. Acad. Sci. USA* **2014**, *111*, 9597–9602. [CrossRef]
188. Kim, J.K.; Fillmore, J.J.; Sunshine, M.J.; Albrecht, B.; Higashimori, T.; Kim, D.W.; Liu, Z.X.; Soos, T.J.; Cline, G.W.; O'Brien, W.R.; et al. PKC-θ knockout mice are protected from fat-induced insulin resistance. *J. Clin. Investig.* **2004**, *114*, 823–827. [CrossRef]
189. Sokolowska, E.; Blachnio-Zabielska, A. The Role of Ceramides in Insulin Resistance. *Front. Endocrinol.* **2019**, *10*, 577. [CrossRef]
190. Fox, T.E.; Houck, K.L.; O'Neill, S.M.; Nagarajan, M.; Stover, T.C.; Pomianowski, P.T.; Unal, O.; Yun, J.K.; Naides, S.J.; Kester, M. Ceramide recruits and activates protein kinase C ζ (PKCζ) within structured membrane microdomains. *J. Biol. Chem.* **2007**, *282*, 12450–12457. [CrossRef]
191. Chavez, J.A.; Knotts, T.A.; Wang, L.P.; Li, G.; Dobrowsky, R.T.; Florant, G.L.; Summers, S.A. A role for ceramide, but not diacylglycerol, in the antagonism of insulin signal transduction by saturated fatty acids. *J. Biol. Chem.* **2003**, *278*, 10297–10303. [CrossRef]
192. Li, P.; Liu, S.; Lu, M.; Bandyopadhyay, G.; Oh, D.; Imamura, T.; Johnson, A.; Sears, D.; Shen, Z.; Cui, B.; et al. Hematopoietic-Derived Galectin-3 Causes Cellular and Systemic Insulin Resistance. *Cell* **2016**, *167*, 973–984.e12. [CrossRef]
193. Dong, R.; Zhang, M.; Hu, Q.; Zheng, S.; Soh, A.; Zheng, Y.; Yuan, H. Galectin-3 as a novel biomarker for disease diagnosis and a target for therapy (Review). *Int. J. Mol. Med.* **2018**, *41*, 599–614. [CrossRef]
194. Nakahira, K.; Haspel, J.A.; Rathinam, V.A.; Lee, S.J.; Dolinay, T.; Lam, H.C.; Englert, J.A.; Rabinovitch, M.; Cernadas, M.; Kim, H.P.; et al. Autophagy proteins regulate innate immune responses by inhibiting the release of mitochondrial DNA mediated by the NALP3 inflammasome. *Nat. Immunol.* **2011**, *12*, 222–230. [CrossRef]
195. Kang, Y.H.; Cho, M.H.; Kim, J.Y.; Kwon, M.S.; Peak, J.J.; Kang, S.W.; Yoon, S.Y.; Song, Y. Impaired macrophage autophagy induces systemic insulin resistance in obesity. *Oncotarget* **2016**, *7*, 35577–35591. [CrossRef]
196. Bonamichi, B.; Lee, J. Unusual Suspects in the Development of Obesity-Induced Inflammation and Insulin Resistance: NK cells, iNKT cells, and ILCs. *Diabetes Metab. J.* **2017**, *41*, 229–250. [CrossRef]
197. Jonckheere, A.C.; Bullens, D.M.A.; Seys, S.F. Innate lymphoid cells in asthma: Pathophysiological insights from murine models to human asthma phenotypes. *Curr. Opin. Allergy. Clin. Immunol.* **2019**, *19*, 53–60. [CrossRef]
198. Molofsky, A.B.; Nussbaum, J.C.; Liang, H.E.; Van Dyken, S.J.; Cheng, L.E.; Mohapatra, A.; Chawla, A.; Locksley, R.M. Innate lymphoid type 2 cells sustain visceral adipose tissue eosinophils and alternatively activated macrophages. *J. Exp. Med.* **2013**, *210*, 535–549. [CrossRef]
199. Liu, W.; Zeng, Q.; Chen, Y.; Luo, R.Z. Role of Leptin/Osteopontin Axis in the Function of Eosinophils in Allergic Rhinitis with Obesity. *Mediat. Inflamm.* **2018**, *2018*, 9138904. [CrossRef]
200. Bolus, W.R.; Kennedy, A.J.; Hasty, A.H. Obesity-induced reduction of adipose eosinophils is reversed with low-calorie dietary intervention. *Physiol. Rep.* **2018**, *6*, e13919. [CrossRef] [PubMed]
201. Zelechowska, P.; Agier, J.; Kozlowska, E.; Brzezinska-Blaszczyk, E. Mast cells participate in chronic low-grade inflammation within adipose tissue. *Obes. Rev.* **2018**, *19*, 686–697. [CrossRef] [PubMed]
202. Milling, S. Adipokines and the control of mast cell functions: From obesity to inflammation? *Immunology* **2019**, *158*, 1–2. [CrossRef] [PubMed]
203. Xu, J.M.; Shi, G.P. Emerging role of mast cells and macrophages in cardiovascular and metabolic diseases. *Endocr. Rev.* **2012**, *33*, 71–108. [CrossRef] [PubMed]
204. Liu, J.; Divoux, A.; Sun, J.; Zhang, J.; Clement, K.; Glickman, J.N.; Sukhova, G.K.; Wolters, P.J.; Du, J.; Gorgun, C.Z.; et al. Genetic deficiency and pharmacological stabilization of mast cells reduce diet-induced obesity and diabetes in mice. *Nat. Med.* **2009**, *15*, 940–945. [CrossRef]
205. Stefanovic-Racic, M.; Yang, X.; Turner, M.S.; Mantell, B.S.; Stolz, D.B.; Sumpter, T.L.; Sipula, I.J.; Dedousis, N.; Scott, D.K.; Morel, P.A.; et al. Dendritic cells promote macrophage infiltration and comprise a substantial proportion of obesity-associated increases in CD11c+ cells in adipose tissue and liver. *Diabetes* **2012**, *61*, 2330–2339. [CrossRef]
206. Xu, X.; Su, S.; Wang, X.; Barnes, V.; De Miguel, C.; Ownby, D.; Pollock, J.; Snieder, H.; Chen, W.; Wang, X. Obesity is associated with more activated neutrophils in African American male youth. *Int. J. Obes.* **2015**, *39*, 26–32. [CrossRef]
207. Medeiros, N.I.; Mattos, R.T.; Menezes, C.A.; Fares, R.C.G.; Talvani, A.; Dutra, W.O.; Rios-Santos, F.; Correa-Oliveira, R.; Gomes, J. IL-10 and TGF-beta unbalanced levels in neutrophils contribute to increase inflammatory cytokine expression in childhood obesity. *Eur. J. Nutr.* **2018**, *57*, 2421–2430. [CrossRef]
208. Talukdar, S.; Oh, D.Y.; Bandyopadhyay, G.; Li, D.; Xu, J.; McNelis, J.; Lu, M.; Li, P.; Yan, Q.; Zhu, Y.; et al. Neutrophils mediate insulin resistance in mice fed a high-fat diet through secreted elastase. *Nat. Med.* **2012**, *18*, 1407–1412. [CrossRef]
209. Pan, Y.; Choi, J.H.; Shi, H.; Zhang, L.; Su, S.; Wang, X. Discovery and Validation of a Novel Neutrophil Activation Marker Associated with Obesity. *Sci. Rep.* **2019**, *9*, 3433. [CrossRef]
210. Uribe-Querol, E.; Rosales, C. Neutrophils Actively Contribute to Obesity-Associated Inflammation and Pathological Complications. *Cells* **2022**, *11*, 1883. [CrossRef]
211. Chen, H.; Sun, L.; Feng, L.; Yin, Y.; Zhang, W. Role of Innate lymphoid Cells in Obesity and Insulin Resistance. *Front. Endocrinol.* **2022**, *13*, 855197. [CrossRef]

212. McDonnell, M.E.; Ganley-Leal, L.M.; Mehta, A.; Bigornia, S.J.; Mott, M.; Rehman, Q.; Farb, M.G.; Hess, D.T.; Joseph, L.; Gokce, N.; et al. B lymphocytes in human subcutaneous adipose crown-like structures. *Obesity* **2012**, *20*, 1372–1378. [CrossRef]
213. Acosta, J.R.; Douagi, I.; Andersson, D.P.; Backdahl, J.; Ryden, M.; Arner, P.; Laurencikiene, J. Increased fat cell size: A major phenotype of subcutaneous white adipose tissue in non-obese individuals with type 2 diabetes. *Diabetologia* **2016**, *59*, 560–570. [CrossRef]
214. Khan, I.M.; Dai Perrard, X.Y.; Perrard, J.L.; Mansoori, A.; Smith, C.W.; Wu, H.; Ballantyne, C.M. Attenuated adipose tissue and skeletal muscle inflammation in obese mice with combined CD4+ and CD8+ T cell deficiency. *Atherosclerosis* **2014**, *233*, 419–428. [CrossRef]
215. Pacifico, L.; Di Renzo, L.; Anania, C.; Osborn, J.F.; Ippoliti, F.; Schiavo, E.; Chiesa, C. Increased T-helper interferon-gamma-secreting cells in obese children. *Eur. J. Endocrinol.* **2006**, *154*, 691–697. [CrossRef]
216. Rocha, V.Z.; Folco, E.J.; Sukhova, G.; Shimizu, K.; Gotsman, I.; Vernon, A.H.; Libby, P. Interferon-gamma, a Th1 cytokine, regulates fat inflammation: A role for adaptive immunity in obesity. *Circ. Res.* **2008**, *103*, 467–476. [CrossRef]
217. Feuerer, M.; Herrero, L.; Cipolletta, D.; Naaz, A.; Wong, J.; Nayer, A.; Lee, J.; Goldfine, A.B.; Benoist, C.; Shoelson, S.; et al. Lean, but not obese, fat is enriched for a unique population of regulatory T cells that affect metabolic parameters. *Nat. Med.* **2009**, *15*, 930–939. [CrossRef]
218. Winer, S.; Chan, Y.; Paltser, G.; Truong, D.; Tsui, H.; Bahrami, J.; Dorfman, R.; Wang, Y.; Zielenski, J.; Mastronardi, F.; et al. Normalization of obesity-associated insulin resistance through immunotherapy. *Nat. Med.* **2009**, *15*, 921–929. [CrossRef]
219. Nishimura, S.; Manabe, I.; Nagasaki, M.; Eto, K.; Yamashita, H.; Ohsugi, M.; Hara, K.; Ueki, K.; Sugiura, S.; Yoshimura, K.; et al. CD8+ effector T cells contribute to macrophage recruitment and adipose tissue inflammation in obesity. *Nat. Med.* **2009**, *15*, 914–920. [CrossRef]
220. Zhai, X.; Qian, G.; Wang, Y.; Chen, X.; Lu, J.; Zhang, Y.; Huang, Q.; Wang, Q. Elevated B Cell Activation is Associated with Type 2 Diabetes Development in Obese Subjects. *Cell. Physiol. Biochem.* **2016**, *38*, 1257–1266. [CrossRef]
221. Jiang, C.; Ting, A.T.; Seed, B. PPAR-γ agonists inhibit production of monocyte inflammatory cytokines. *Nature* **1998**, *391*, 82–86. [CrossRef]
222. Winer, D.A.; Winer, S.; Shen, L.; Wadia, P.P.; Yantha, J.; Paltser, G.; Tsui, H.; Wu, P.; Davidson, M.G.; Alonso, M.N.; et al. B cells promote insulin resistance through modulation of T cells and production of pathogenic IgG antibodies. *Nat. Med.* **2011**, *17*, 610–617. [CrossRef]
223. DeFuria, J.; Belkina, A.C.; Jagannathan-Bogdan, M.; Snyder-Cappione, J.; Carr, J.D.; Nersesova, Y.R.; Markham, D.; Strissel, K.J.; Watkins, A.A.; Zhu, M.; et al. B cells promote inflammation in obesity and type 2 diabetes through regulation of T-cell function and an inflammatory cytokine profile. *Proc. Natl. Acad. Sci. USA* **2013**, *110*, 5133–5138. [CrossRef] [PubMed]
224. Carpino, P.A.; Goodwin, B. Diabetes area participation analysis: A review of companies and targets described in the 2008–2010 patent literature. *Expert Opin. Ther. Pat.* **2010**, *20*, 1627–1651. [CrossRef]
225. Osborn, O.; Brownell, S.E.; Sanchez-Alavez, M.; Salomon, D.; Gram, H.; Bartfai, T. Treatment with an Interleukin 1 beta antibody improves glycemic control in diet-induced obesity. *Cytokine* **2008**, *44*, 141–148. [CrossRef]
226. Mao, Y.; Mohan, R.; Zhang, S.; Tang, X. MicroRNAs as pharmacological targets in diabetes. *Pharmacol. Res.* **2013**, *75*, 37–47. [CrossRef] [PubMed]
227. Alipourfard, I.; Datukishvili, N.; Mikeladze, D. TNF-alpha Downregulation Modifies Insulin Receptor Substrate 1 (IRS-1) in Metabolic Signaling of Diabetic Insulin-Resistant Hepatocytes. *Mediat. Inflamm.* **2019**, *2019*, 3560819. [CrossRef] [PubMed]
228. Burska, A.N.; Sakthiswary, R.; Sattar, N. Effects of Tumour Necrosis Factor Antagonists on Insulin Sensitivity/Resistance in Rheumatoid Arthritis: A Systematic Review and Meta-Analysis. *PLoS ONE* **2015**, *10*, e0128889. [CrossRef] [PubMed]
229. Taylor, P.C.; Feldmann, M. Anti-TNF biologic agents: Still the therapy of choice for rheumatoid arthritis. *Nat. Rev. Rheumatol.* **2009**, *5*, 578–582. [CrossRef]
230. Wang, Q.; Li, H.; Xiao, Y.; Li, S.; Li, B.; Zhao, X.; Ye, L.; Guo, B.; Chen, X.; Ding, Y.; et al. Locally controlled delivery of TNFalpha antibody from a novel glucose-sensitive scaffold enhances alveolar bone healing in diabetic conditions. *J. Control. Release* **2015**, *206*, 232–242. [CrossRef] [PubMed]
231. Paquot, N.; Castillo, M.J.; Lefebvre, P.J.; Scheen, A.J. No increased insulin sensitivity after a single intravenous administration of a recombinant human tumor necrosis factor receptor: Fc fusion protein in obese insulin-resistant patients. *J. Clin. Endocrinol. Metab.* **2000**, *85*, 1316–1319. [PubMed]
232. Ofei, F.; Hurel, S.; Newkirk, J.; Sopwith, M.; Taylor, R. Effects of an engineered human anti-TNF-alpha antibody (CDP571) on insulin sensitivity and glycemic control in patients with NIDDM. *Diabetes* **1996**, *45*, 881–885. [CrossRef] [PubMed]
233. Jager, J.; Gremeaux, T.; Cormont, M.; Le Marchand-Brustel, Y.; Tanti, J.F. Interleukin-1beta-induced insulin resistance in adipocytes through down-regulation of insulin receptor substrate-1 expression. *Endocrinology* **2007**, *148*, 241–251. [CrossRef]
234. Larsen, C.M.; Faulenbach, M.; Vaag, A.; Volund, A.; Ehses, J.A.; Seifert, B.; Mandrup-Poulsen, T.; Donath, M.Y. Interleukin-1-receptor antagonist in type 2 diabetes mellitus. *N. Engl. J. Med.* **2007**, *356*, 1517–1526. [CrossRef]
235. Dinarello, C.A. A clinical perspective of IL-1beta as the gatekeeper of inflammation. *Eur. J. Immunol.* **2011**, *41*, 1203–1217. [CrossRef]
236. Schultz, O.; Oberhauser, F.; Saech, J.; Rubbert-Roth, A.; Hahn, M.; Krone, W.; Laudes, M. Effects of inhibition of interleukin-6 signalling on insulin sensitivity and lipoprotein (a) levels in human subjects with rheumatoid diseases. *PLoS ONE* **2010**, *5*, e14328. [CrossRef]

237. Dagdeviren, S.; Jung, D.Y.; Friedline, R.H.; Noh, H.L.; Kim, J.H.; Patel, P.R.; Tsitsilianos, N.; Inashima, K.; Tran, D.A.; Hu, X.; et al. IL-10 prevents aging-associated inflammation and insulin resistance in skeletal muscle. *FASEB J.* **2017**, *31*, 701–710. [CrossRef]
238. De Fougerolles, A.; Vornlocher, H.P.; Maraganore, J.; Lieberman, J. Interfering with disease: A progress report on siRNA-based therapeutics. *Nat. Rev. Drug Discov.* **2007**, *6*, 443–453. [CrossRef]
239. Xie, J.; Ameres, S.L.; Friedline, R.; Hung, J.H.; Zhang, Y.; Xie, Q.; Zhong, L.; Su, Q.; He, R.; Li, M.; et al. Long-term, efficient inhibition of microRNA function in mice using rAAV vectors. *Nat. Methods* **2012**, *9*, 403–409. [CrossRef]
240. Vester, B.; Wengel, J. LNA (locked nucleic acid): High-affinity targeting of complementary RNA and DNA. *Biochemistry* **2004**, *43*, 13233–13241. [CrossRef]
241. Elmen, J.; Lindow, M.; Schutz, S.; Lawrence, M.; Petri, A.; Obad, S.; Lindholm, M.; Hedtjärn, M.; Hansen, H.F.; Berger, U.; et al. LNA-mediated microRNA silencing in non-human primates. *Nature* **2008**, *452*, 896–899. [CrossRef] [PubMed]
242. Paulos, C.M.; Varghese, B.; Widmer, W.R.; Breur, G.J.; Vlashi, E.; Low, P.S. Folate-targeted immunotherapy effectively treats established adjuvant and collagen-induced arthritis. *Arthritis Res. Ther.* **2006**, *8*, R77. [CrossRef] [PubMed]
243. Xia, W.; Hilgenbrink, A.R.; Matteson, E.L.; Lockwood, M.B.; Cheng, J.X.; Low, P.S. A functional folate receptor is induced during macrophage activation and can be used to target drugs to activated macrophages. *Blood* **2009**, *113*, 438–446. [CrossRef] [PubMed]

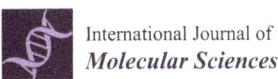

Article

Idiopathic Plasmacytic Lymphadenopathy Forms an Independent Subtype of Idiopathic Multicentric Castleman Disease

Asami Nishikori [1], Midori Filiz Nishimura [1,2,*], Yoshito Nishimura [3,4], Fumio Otsuka [3], Kanna Maehama [1], Kumiko Ohsawa [5], Shuji Momose [5], Naoya Nakamura [6] and Yasuharu Sato [1,*]

1. Department of Molecular Hematopathology, Okayama University Graduate School of Health Sciences, Okayama 700-8558, Japan
2. Department of Pathology, Okayama University Hospital, Okayama 700-8558, Japan
3. Department of General Medicine, Okayama University Graduate School of Medicine, Dentistry, and Pharmaceutical Sciences, Okayama 700-8558, Japan
4. Department of Medicine, John A. Burns School of Medicine, University of Hawai'i, Honolulu, HI 96813, USA
5. Department of Pathology, Saitama Medical Center, Saitama Medical University, Saitama 350-8550, Japan
6. Department of Pathology, Tokai University School of Medicine, Kanagawa 259-1193, Japan
* Correspondence: p2hq21br@s.okayama-u.ac.jp (M.F.N.); satou-y@okayama-u.ac.jp (Y.S.); Tel.: +81-86-235-7150 (Y.S.)

Abstract: Idiopathic multicentric Castleman disease (iMCD) is a type of Castleman disease that is not related to KSHV/HHV8 infection. Currently, iMCD is classified into iMCD-TAFRO (thrombocytopenia, anasarca, fever, reticulin fibrosis, and organomegaly) and iMCD-NOS (not otherwise specified). The former has been established as a relatively homogeneous disease unit that has been recently re-defined, while the latter is considered to be a heterogeneous disease that could be further divided into several subtypes. In 1980, Mori et al. proposed the concept of idiopathic plasmacytic lymphadenopathy (IPL), a disease presenting with polyclonal hypergammaglobulinemia and a sheet-like proliferation of mature plasma cells in the lymph nodes. Some researchers consider IPL to be a part of iMCD-NOS, although it has not been clearly defined to date. This is the first paper to analyze iMCD-NOS clinicopathologically, to examine whether IPL forms a uniform disease unit in iMCD. Histologically, the IPL group showed prominent plasmacytosis and the hyperplasia of germinal centers, while the non-IPL group showed prominent vascularity. Clinically, the IPL group showed significant thrombocytosis and elevated serum IgG levels compared to the non-IPL group ($p = 0.007$, $p < 0.001$, respectively). Pleural effusion and ascites were less common in the IPL group ($p < 0.001$). The IPL group was more likely to have an indolent clinical course and a good response to the anti-IL-6 receptor antibody, while the non-IPL counterpart frequently required more aggressive medical interventions. Thus, the IPL group is a clinicopathologically uniform entity that forms an independent subtype of iMCD.

Keywords: Castleman disease; idiopathic multicentric Castleman disease; idiopathic plasmacytic lymphadenopathy; plasma cell morphology

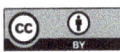

1. Introduction

Castleman disease (CD) is a rare lymphoproliferative disorder described by Castleman et al. in 1956 [1]. CD is clinically classified into unicentric and multicentric types. Unicentric CD (UCD) is characterized by a localized lymphadenopathy with or without minimal systemic symptoms, and the resection of the affected lymph node is often curative [2]. In contrast, multicentric CD (MCD) shows a generalized lymphadenopathy with systemic inflammatory symptoms, such as generalized weakness and fever [3]. The infection status of Kaposi sarcoma-associated herpesvirus/Human herpesvirus type 8 (KSHV/HHV8) defines the etiology of MCD [4]. Idiopathic MCD (iMCD) is defined as a group of KSHV/HHV8-negative MCD without POEMS syndrome (polyneuropathy, organomegaly, endocrinopathy, M-proteins, and skin changes) [5]. Clinically, iMCD is classified into iMCD-TAFRO (thrombocytopenia, anasarca, fever, reticulin fibrosis, and organomegaly) [6–8] and iMCD-NOS (not otherwise specified). Histologically, there are two main pathological variants in iMCD: plasma cell (PC) and hypervascular (HyperV) types [5,9,10]. The mixed type shows the features of both the PC and HyperV variants, but no clear pathological definition [11,12]. Commonly, iMCD-TAFRO is histologically associated with the HyperV type, and iMCD-NOS frequently has PC morphology [5]. As the name suggests, iMCD-NOS is a heterogenous entity. Previous studies have suggested that iMCD-NOS could include atypical and undiagnosed autoimmune diseases [13]. Moreover, it could potentially be further classified into several subtypes with research efforts, including clinicopathological analyses and genomic sequencing [14,15]. One potential candidate that is to be separated from the current iMCD-NOS is idiopathic plasmacytic lymphadenopathy (IPL). IPL was initially proposed in 1980 by Mori et al., characterized by polyclonal hypergammaglobulinemia and a sheet-like proliferation of mature plasma cells in the lymph nodes, as well as the exclusion of known diseases associated with hypergammaglobulinemias such as infections, collagen diseases, hyperthyroidism, allergic diseases, hepatitis, liver cirrhosis, and lymphoma [16]. In the clinical course, IPL was indolent, and all the cases achieved the remission of disease activity [13,16]. The concept of IPL was proposed before the establishment of MCD, and IPL was later considered as a part of iMCD-NOS, given the clinicopathological similarity [11,16]. However, there has been no study to validate whether or not IPL has distinct clinicopathologic features compared to other iMCD-NOS. In this study, we perform a comprehensive clinicopathological analysis of iMCD-NOS, with a focus on IPL or others (non-IPL) to examine if IPL needs to be defined as an independent iMCD subtype.

2. Results

2.1. Clinical Findings

The main clinical findings are summarized in Table 1. See Supplementary Table S1 for details of each case.

Table 1. Clinicopathological findings of iMCD-NOS.

	IPL (n = 34)	Non-IPL (n = 8)	p-Value
Age (median ± SD)	54.8 ± 12.2	57.9 ± 16.9	0.471
Sex (M/F)	21/13	3/5	
WBC ($\times 10^3/\mu L$)	7.7 ± 2.5 †	14.1 ± 9.1 ‡	0.200
CRP (mg/dL)	6.5 ± 3.5 †	13.2 ± 8.4 ‡	0.391
Hb (g/dL)	10.1 ± 2.1 †	9.3 ± 1.6	0.080
Plt ($\times 10^4/\mu L$)	36.9 ± 15.2 †	23.8 ± 10.9 ‡	0.007 *
Serum IgG (mg/dL)	5140.3 ± 1453.1	2502.0 ± 752.3	<0.001 **
Serum IL-6 (pg/mL)	27.3 ± 16.8 †	107.2 ± 94.2 ‡	0.149
Pleural effusions or/and ascites (%)	1 (2.9)	5 (62.5)	<0.001 **
Disease-specific autoantibody (%)	6/26 (23.1)	3/6 (50.0)	0.420

Significant p-values are in bold. Significance was calculated using the Mann–Whitney U test. Fisher's exact analysis or chi-square test were used for the statistical analysis of nominal scales. * $p < 0.05$, ** $p < 0.001$. iMCD-NOS, idiopathic multicentric Castleman disease not otherwise specified; SD, standard deviation; IPL, idiopathic plasmacytic lymphadenopathy; WBC, white blood cells; CRP, C-reactive protein; Hb, hemoglobin; Plt, platelet; Ig, immunoglobulin; IL-6, interleukin 6. Normal ranges: WBC, 3.9–9.8 × $10^3/\mu L$; CRP, 0.0–0.3 mg/dL; Hb, 13.5–17.6 g/dL (male), 11.3–15.2 g/dL (female); Plt, 13.0–36.9 × $10^4/\mu L$; serum IgG, 870–1700 mg/dL; serum IL-6, 0.0–4.0 pg/mL. † WBC, CRP, Hb, Plt, and IL-6 levels were available for 21, 33, 31, 31, and 11 patients with IPL, respectively. ‡ WBC, CRP, Plt, and IL-6 levels were available for 7, 7, 7, and 5 patients with non-IPL, respectively.

Of the 42 included cases, 34 (81.0%) and 8 (19.0%) were classified as the IPL group and the non-IPL group, respectively. In the IPL group, there were 21 males and 13 females, aged 34–76 years, with a median age of 54.8. In the non-IPL group, three were males and five were females, aged 32–89 years, with a median age of 57.9. There was no significant difference in age between the two groups ($p = 0.471$). Regarding laboratory findings, there were no significant differences in the white blood cells (WBC) nor the C-reactive protein (CRP) between the two groups ($p = 0.200$, $p = 0.391$, respectively). While hemoglobin (Hb) was considerably lower in the non-IPL group compared to the IPL group, there was no significant difference ($p = 0.080$). By contrast, platelet count (Plt) and serum immunoglobulin G (IgG) were significantly higher in the IPL group ($p = 0.007$, $p < 0.001$, respectively). All cases had elevated serum interleukin-6 (IL-6), but there was no significant difference between the two groups ($p = 0.149$). In total, 6/26 (23.1%) in the IPL group and 3/6 (50.0%) in the non-IPL group had disease-specific autoantibodies ($p = 0.420$). In the IPL group, the following specific autoantibodies were detected: myeloperoxidase-anti-neutrophil cytoplasmic antibodies (MPO-ANCA) (3/6, 50.0%), proteinase-3-anti-neutrophil cytoplasmic antibodies (PR3-ANCA) (2/6, 33.3%), anti-double-strand DNA antibody (ds-DNA) (2/6, 33.3%), anti-single-strand DNA antibody (ss-DNA) (1/6, 16.7%), anti-ribonucleoprotein antibody (RNP) (1/6, 16.7%), anti-cardiolipin antibody (1/6, 16.7%), and anti-mitochondrial M2 antibody (AMA2) (1/6, 16.7%). In contrast, the following specific autoantibodies were detected in the non-IPL group: anti-SS-A antibodies (SS-A) (2/3, 66.7%), anti-cardiolipin antibody (2/3, 66.7%), anti-platelet-associated IgG (PA-IgG) (2/3, 66.7%), ds-DNA (1/3, 33.3%), AMA2 (1/3, 33.3%), MPO-ANCA (1/3, 33.3%), and anti-SS-B antibodies (SS-B) (1/3, 33.3%). Regarding imaging, 5/8 (62.5%) in the non-IPL group had pleural effusions or/and ascites, while this was only noted in 1/34 (2.9%) in the IPL group ($p < 0.001$).

2.2. Pathological Findings

The pathological findings of the two groups are summarized in Table 2.

Table 2. Pathological findings of iMCD-NOS.

	IPL ($n = 34$)	Non-IPL ($n = 8$)	p-Value
Vascularity			
Median	0.7	2.0	0.003 *
Grade 0 (%)	17 (50.0)	1 (12.5)	
Grade 1 (%)	11 (32.4)	2 (25.0)	
Grade 2 (%)	4 (11.8)	1 (12.5)	
Grade 3 (%)	2 (5.9)	4 (50.0)	
Plasmacytosis			
Median	2.9	2.1	0.001 *
Grade 0 (%)	0 (0.0)	0 (0.0)	
Grade 1 (%)	0 (0.0)	1 (12.5)	
Grade 2 (%)	3 (8.8)	5 (62.5)	
Grade 3 (%)	31 (91.2)	2 (25.0)	
Regressed GCs			
Median	0.9	1.4	0.255
Grade 0 (%)	8 (23.5)	2 (25.0)	
Grade 1 (%)	20 (58.8)	3 (37.5)	
Grade 2 (%)	6 (17.6)	1 (12.5)	
Grade 3 (%)	0 (0.0)	2 (25.0)	
Hyperplastic GCs			
Median	2.4	0.9	0.003 *
Grade 0 (%)	1 (2.9)	5 (62.5)	
Grade 1 (%)	6 (17.6)	0 (0.0)	
Grade 2 (%)	7 (20.6)	2 (25.0)	
Grade 3 (%)	20 (58.8)	1 (12.5)	

Significant p-values are in bold. Significance was calculated using the Mann–Whitney U test. * $p < 0.05$. GCs, germinal centers.

In the IPL group, various levels of vascularity were noted with a median score of 0.70, including 17/34 with grade 0 (50.0%), 11/34 with grade 1 (32.4%), 4/34 with grade 2 (11.8%), and 2/34 with grade 3 (5.9%). The median level of plasmacytosis was 2.9, including

3/34 with grade 2 (8.8%) and 31/34 with grade 3 (91.2%). The median score of regressed GCs was 0.90, including 8/34 with grade 0 (23.5%), 20/34 with grade 1 (58.8%), and 6/34 with grade 2 (17.6%). Regarding hyperplastic GCs, the median score was 2.4, including 1/34 with grade 0 (2.9%), 6/34 with grade 1 (17.6%), 7/34 with grade 2 (20.6%), and 20/34 with grade 3 (58.8%). The typical histological findings of the IPL group are shown in Figure 1.

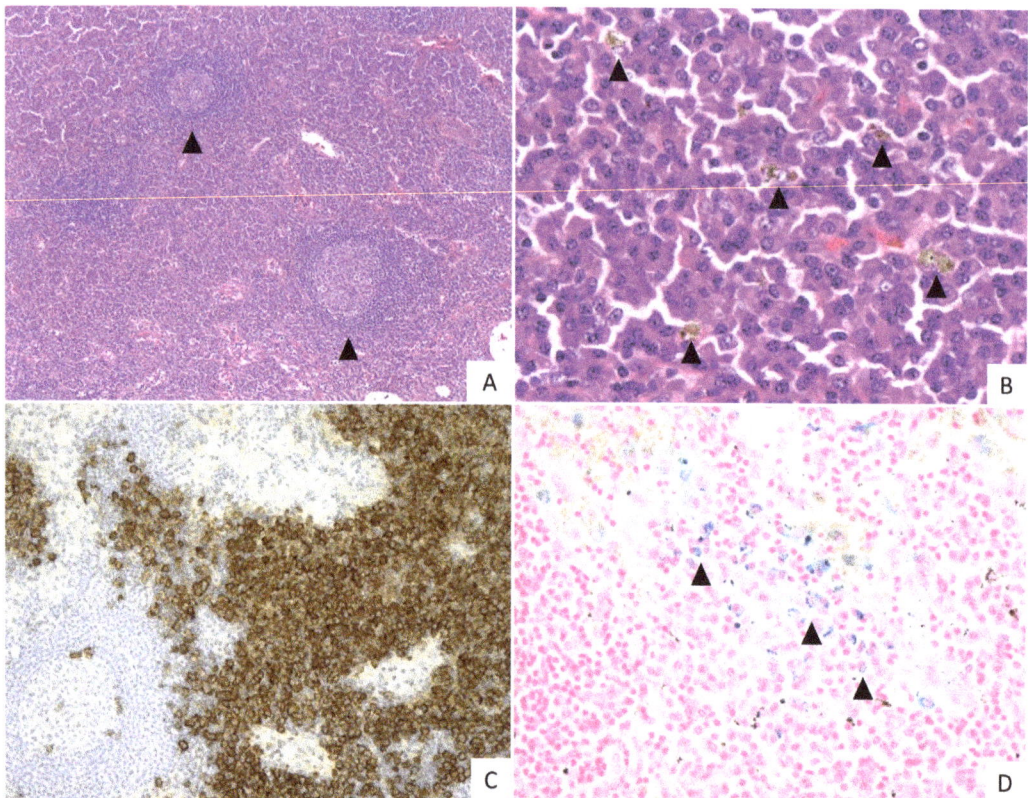

Figure 1. Histopathological features of the IPL group. (**A**) Interfollicular areas are expanded and germinal centers (GCs) appear hyperplastic (arrowheads) (H&E, 10×). (**B**) The sheet-like proliferation of mature plasma cells in the interfollicular areas and hemosiderin deposition are observed (arrow heads) (H&E,40×). (**C**) Numerous plasma cells are observed in the interfollicular areas (CD138, 20×). (**D**) Hemosiderin deposition is observed (arrowheads) (Berlin blue staining, 40×). This case was scored: vascularity grade 0, plasmacytosis grade 3, regressed GC grade 2, and hyperplastic GC grade 2.

Among the non-IPL group, the median level of vascularity was 2.0, including 1/8 with grade 0 (12.5%), 2/8 with grade 1 (25.0%), 1/8 with grade 2 (12.5%), and 4/8 with grade 3 (50.0%), respectively. In addition, the median score of the plasmacytosis was 2.1, including 1/8 with grade 1 (12.5%), 5/8 with grade 2 (62.5%), and 2/8 with grade 3 (25.0%), respectively. The median score of the regressed GCs was 1.4, including 2/8 with grade 0 (25.0%), 3/8 with grade 1 (37.5%), 1/8 with grade 2 (12.5%) and 2/8 with grade 3 (25.0%). The hyperplastic GCs showed a median score of 0.90, including 5/8 with grade 0 (62.5%), 2/8 with grade 2 (25.0%), and 1/8 with grade 3 (12.5%). The histological features of the non-IPL group are shown in Figure 2.

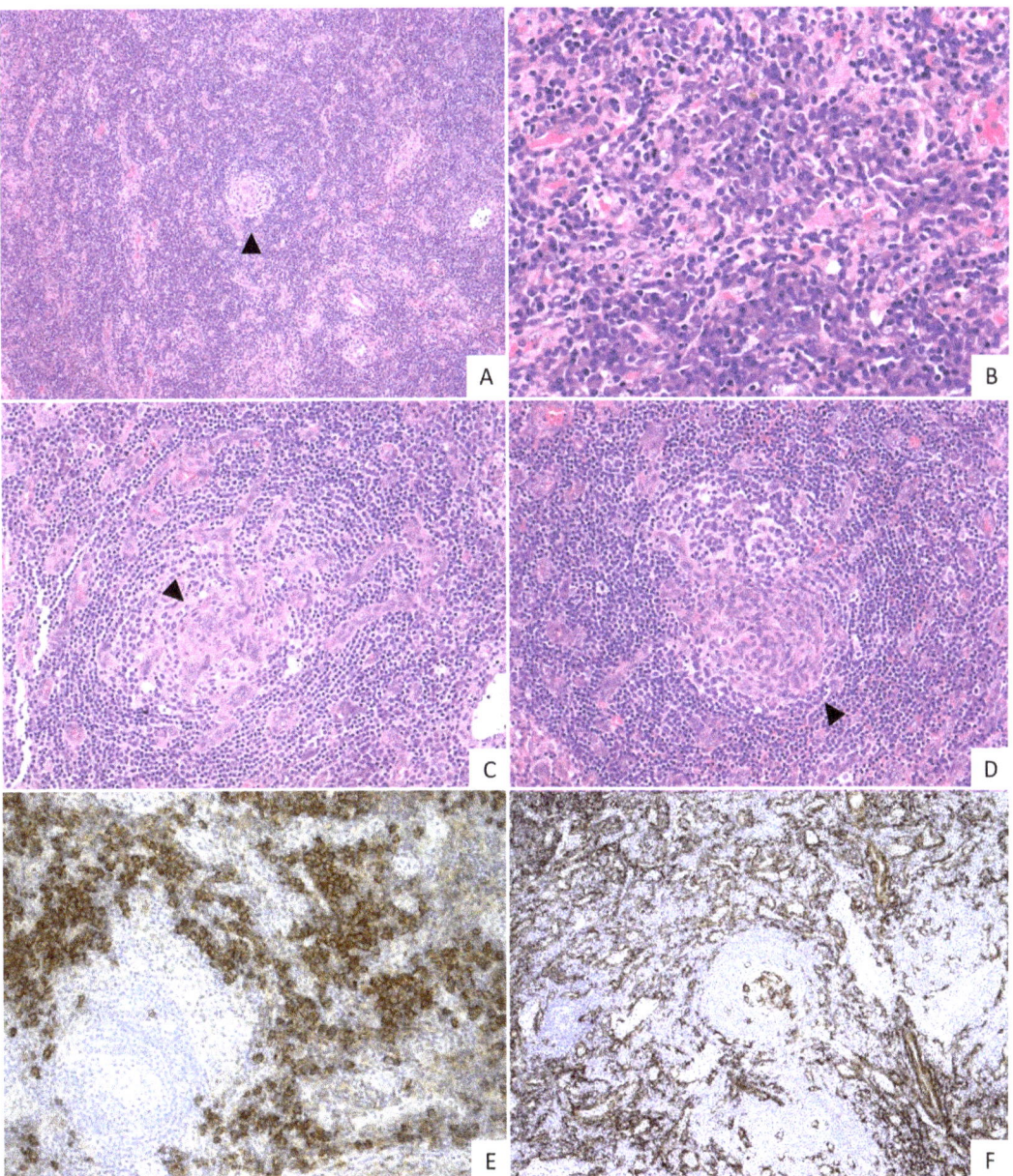

Figure 2. Histopathological features of the non-IPL group. (**A**) Extended interfollicular areas and severe vascularization are observed. Germinal center (GC) is atrophic (arrowhead) (H&E, 10×). (**B**) Mature plasma cells are observed within prominent vascularization (H&E, 40×). (**C,D**) Marked hypervascularization penetrating the GC is observed. The blood vessels show a branching pattern ((**C**), arrowhead) and whirl-like pattern ((**D**), arrowhead) (H&E, 20×). (**E**) Numerous plasma cells are observed in the interfollicular areas (CD138, 20×). (**F**) Vascular in the GC and interfollicular areas were α-SMA-positive (α-SMA, 10×). This case was scored vascularity grade 3, plasmacytosis grade 2, regressed GC grade 3 and hyperplastic GC grade 0.

The IPL group had less significant vascularity, more frequent hyperplastic GCs, and severe plasmacytosis compared to the non-IPL group ($p = 0.003$, $p = 0.003$, $p = 0.001$, respectively). While the non-IPL group was more likely to have extensive regressed GCs, there was no significant difference between the two groups ($p = 0.255$). In addition, branching and/or whirl-like patterns of the vessels (Figure 2C–E) were observed in the GCs of the cases with prominent vascularization. Such findings were seen in 1/34 cases of the IPL group (2.9%) and 2/8 cases of the non-IPL group (25.0%).

2.3. Treatment and Clinical Course

Outpatient follow-up data were available for 23/34 cases in the IPL group and for 5/8 cases in the non-IPL group, with a median follow-up period of 65.5 months (Table 3).

Table 3. Treatment and clinical courses of iMCD-NOS.

Subtype	Case No.	Age/Sex	1st Treatment	2nd Treatment	3rd Treatment	Outcome	Follow-Up Period (Month)
IPL	1	35/F	PSL 20 mg	rituximab	tocilizumab	Improved	122
	2	62/M	PSL 30 mg	tocilizumab		Improved	93
	3	55/F	tocilizumab			Improved	57
	4	37/M	follow-up			- †	4
	5	39/M	tocilizumab			Improved	39
	6	49/F	tocilizumab			Improved	38
	7	59/M	PSL 50 mg			no response	39
	8	64/M	PSL 30 mg	tocilizumab		Improved	130
	9	70/M	PSL 30 mg	tocilizumab		Improved	32
	10	54/F	follow-up			no change	161
	11	65/M	PSL 25 mg	PSL 6 mg		Improved ‡	37
	12	62/F	PSL 10 mg	PSL 5 mg		Improved	175
	13	55/F	tocilizumab			Improved	13
	14	74/F	tocilizumab			Improved	10
	15	52/F	tocilizumab			Improved ‡	202
	16	70/M	follow-up			no change	198
	17	43/M	PSL 15 mg	tocilizumab		Improved	131
	18	41/M	PSL 5 mg			no response	126
	19	49/M	PSL 30 mg			Improved	90
	20	48/F	PSL 15 mg	tocilizumab		Improved	77
	21	76/M	PSL 40 mg	PSL 10 mg		Improved	6
	22	67/M	PSL 20 mg	tocilizumab		Improved	4
	23	72/M	tocilizumab			Improved	4
non-IPL	1	52/F	PSL 50 mg + tocilizumab	rituximab		PR	96
	2	89/M	PSL 60 mg			Repeatedly worsened during tapering	10
	3	73/F	PSL 35 mg			Improved	74
	4	49/F	follow-up			progression	41
	5	49/F	mPSL 500 mg	PSL 40 mg		no response	143

Treatment information was available for 23 cases of the IPL group and 5 cases of the non-IPL group. PR, partial remission; mPSL, methylprednisolone; PSL, prednisolone. "Outcome" represents the clinical condition of the patient at the last visit. "Partial remission" represents improvement in some laboratory data or subjective symptoms. "Complete remission" represents improvement in all laboratory data, objective symptoms, and radiographic findings. "No response" represents all clinical findings and subjective symptoms unchanged. "No change" represents no worsening nor improving of the disease during follow-up. "Progression" represents a worsening of laboratory findings, subjective symptoms, or radiographic findings. † Case 4: Lost to follow-up. ‡ Cases 11 and 15 achieved PR, but expired from non-iMCD disease (lung cancer) and post-surgical bleeding, respectively.

For the first-line treatment, corticosteroids were used in 13/23 (56.5%) cases in the IPL group and 4/5 (80%) cases in the non-IPL group. One patient in the non-IPL group

(Case 1) received corticosteroid and tocilizumab. Among those treated with corticosteroids, corticosteroids were successfully tapered in 3/13 (23.1%) patients in the IPL group and 1/4 (25.0%) patients in the non-IPL group. One case in the IPL group (Case 11) expired during the follow-up period with corticosteroid monotherapy, likely due to lung cancer.

Overall, 14/23 (60.9%) patients in the IPL group and 1/5 (20.0%) patients in the non-IPL group received tocilizumab during the follow-up period. Those in the IPL group who received tocilizumab achieved an improvement in disease activity. One patient in the IPL group treated with tocilizumab expired due to post-surgical bleeding that was unrelated to IPL (Case 15). In contrast, the non-IPL case treated with tocilizumab had a progressive disease and required rituximab as a second-line therapy to achieve a partial remission of disease activity.

3. Discussion

iMCD is a rare lymphoproliferative disorder that is characterized by multiple lymphadenopathies with unknown etiology [17]. In particular, iMCD-NOS is a heterogenous entity, likely including undefined disease [11,18–21]. The present results show that IPL is likely to be a separate subtype of iMCD, along with iMCD-TAFRO and iMCD-NOS, given its unique clinicopathological characteristics.

Our results show that the IPL group had distinct clinicopathological features compared to the non-IPL iMCD-NOS cases. Pathologically, the IPL group had less significant vascularity, as well as more prominent plasmacytosis and hyperplastic GCs than the non-IPL group. By contrast, the non-IPL group showed marked hypervascularization both in GCs and in interfollicular areas. Clinically, the IPL group had higher platelet counts and serum IgG levels, and fewer signs of fluid retention in third space such as pleural effusions and/or ascites, than the non-IPL group.

In 2008, before the current iMCD criteria were proposed, Kojima et al. reported that iMCD had at least two clinical subtypes, IPL and non-IPL, with the latter showing more thrombocytopenia, fluid retention, positive autoantibodies, and relatively aggressive clinical symptoms [13]. They also suggested that non-IPL may be associated with autoimmune diseases. In addition, Frizzera et al. reported multiple lesions of CD, which led to the term MCD being established [3,22]. Some of their MCD cases included those with clinical and laboratory findings characteristic of systemic lupus erythematosus (SLE), Sjögren's syndrome, or both [3]. Currently, such cases may be considered ill-defined autoimmune diseases [23–25]. Moreover, SLE cases with MCD-like histology [24,26] and iMCD cases with various autoantibodies [23] have been reported. Although no significant differences were observed for disease-specific autoantibodies in the present results, this may be due to a lack of power to detect the difference, given the small number of non-IPL cases. Combined with the context and the present results, it may be crucial to closely follow-up with non-IPL patients on an outpatient basis to find clinical signs of autoimmune diseases.

The two groups also had different clinical courses and treatment responses. There were a few patients who were treated with tocilizumab (an anti-IL-6 receptor monoclonal antibody approved in Japan for the treatment of iMCD [27]), and all patients with IPL who received tocilizumab achieved a remission of disease activity. In contrast, the non-IPL case that had a poor response to tocilizumab also required rituximab. Despite the second-line non-IL-6 therapy, the patient still had progressive disease during the follow-up period. The results concur with previous studies suggesting that IPL may have an indolent clinical course compared to the non-IPL group, with a superior response to anti-IL-6 agents. In recent studies, the PI3K/Akt/mTOR pathway, JAK/STAT3 pathway, and type I IFN have focused on the treatment targets in iMCD cases refractory to IL-6-targeted therapy [28–31]. While non-IPL iMCD-NOS cases could be heterogenous, as discussed, efforts to identify a primary etiology (for example, possible autoimmune disease) by molecular analysis and targeted therapies for the cellular signals may need to be considered.

In conclusion, the present results suggest that IPL is clinicopathologically a uniform disease entity, and may be an independent subtype of iMCD. Future studies are warranted to identify diagnostics, treatment, and follow-up plans that are specific to IPL. Given the heterogeneity of the non-IPL cases, clinicians are urged to identify a primary etiology of such cases, including atypical autoimmune diseases. These cases may benefit from molecular analysis to clarify underlying pathology.

4. Materials and Methods

4.1. Patients

Forty-two Japanese patients with lymph node involvement of iMCD-NOS were included in this study. All cases were selected from pathology consultation files at the Department of Pathology, Okayama University. All patients had systemic or multiple lymphadenopathies, and the detailed sites are summarized in Supplementary Table S1. All iMCD-NOS patients met the consensus diagnostic criteria for iMCD [5]. All cases were serologically or immunohistochemically negative for KSHV/HHV8.

4.2. Histological Evaluation

All lymph node specimens were fixed in 10% formalin and embedded in paraffin. Paraffin-embedded tissue blocks were sliced into 3 μm thin sections and stained with hematoxylin and eosin (H&E), immunohistochemical staining and Berlin blue staining.

Immunohistochemical staining was performed using an automated BOND-III instrument (Leica Biosystems, Wetzlar, Germany) with the primary antibody of HHV-8 (13B10, 1:40; LifeSpan Biosciences, Seattle, WA, USA), CD138 (MI15, 1:200; DAKO, Carpinteria, CA, USA) and α-SMA (1A4, 1:50; DAKO, Carpinteria, CA, USA). In situ hybridization was also performed for the κ and λ light chains (Leica Biosystems, Wetzlar, Germany).

The pathological findings of all cases were reviewed with H&E stained by the authors (Y.S., M.F.N. and A.N.). The following histopathological features were graded on a scale of 0 to 3: vascularity, plasmacytosis, regressed germinal centers (GCs), and hyperplastic GCs, based on previous reports [5,28].

4.3. Classification of iMCD-NOS

According to a previous report [13], we defined IPL as a case meeting all the following four criteria: (1) prominent polyclonal hypergammaglobulinemia (γ-globulin > 4.0 g/dL or serum IgG level >3500 mg/dL), (2) multicentric lymphadenopathy, (3) an absence of definite autoimmune disease, and (4) normal germinal centers and a sheet-like infiltration of polyclonal plasma cells in the lymph node lesion. Cases that did not meet the criteria were defined as non-IPL.

4.4. Statistical Analysis

Statistical analyses were conducted using SPSS for Windows version 23.0 (SPSS, Chicago, IL, USA). Statistical significance was set at $p < 0.05$.

Supplementary Materials: The following supporting information can be downloaded at: https://www.mdpi.com/article/10.3390/ijms231810301/s1.

Author Contributions: Conceptualization, A.N., M.F.N. and Y.S.; methodology, A.N.; formal analysis, A.N.; investigation, A.N., F.O., K.M., K.O., S.M. and N.N.; data curation, A.N.; writing—original draft preparation, A.N.; writing—review and editing, Y.N.; supervision, M.F.N. and Y.S. All authors have read and agreed to the published version of the manuscript.

Funding: This work was supported by JST, the establishment of university fellowships towards the creation of science technology innovation, Grant Number JPMJFS2128, and a Grant-in-Aid for Scientific Research (C) (JSPS KAKENHI Grant Number JP 20K07407), from the Japan Society for the Promotion of Science.

Institutional Review Board Statement: The study was conducted in accordance with the Declaration of Helsinki, and approved by the Institutional Review Board of Okayama University (approval number: 2007-033).

Informed Consent Statement: Comprehensive informed consent was obtained from all patients through an opt-out methodology.

Data Availability Statement: Not applicable.

Conflicts of Interest: The authors declare no conflict of interest.

References

1. Castleman, B.; Iverson, L.; Menendez, V.P. Localized mediastinal lymphnode hyperplasia resembling thymoma. *Cancer* **1956**, *9*, 822–830. [CrossRef]
2. Nishimura, M.F.; Nishimura, Y.; Nishikori, A.; Maekawa, Y.; Maehama, K.; Yoshino, T.; Sato, Y. Clinical and Pathological Characteristics of Hyaline-Vascular Type Unicentric Castleman Disease: A 20-Year Retrospective Analysis. *Diagnostics* **2021**, *11*, 2008. [CrossRef] [PubMed]
3. Frizzera, G.; Banks, P.M.; Massarelli, G.; Rosai, J. A systemic lymphoproliferative disorder with morphologic features of Castleman's disease. Pathological findings in 15 patients. *Am. J. Surg. Pathol.* **1983**, *7*, 211–231. [CrossRef]
4. Soulier, J.; Grollet, L.; Oksenhendler, E.; Cacoub, P.; Cazals-Hatem, D.; Babinet, P.; d'Agay, M.F.; Clauvel, J.P.; Raphael, M.; Degos, L.; et al. Kaposi's sarcoma-associated herpesvirus-like DNA sequences in multicentric Castleman's disease. *Blood* **1995**, *86*, 1276–1280. [CrossRef]
5. Fajgenbaum, D.C.; Uldrick, T.S.; Bagg, A.; Frank, D.; Wu, D.; Srkalovic, G.; Simpson, D.; Liu, A.Y.; Menke, D.; Chandrakasan, S.; et al. International, evidence-based consensus diagnostic criteria for HHV-8-negative/idiopathic multicentric Castleman disease. *Blood* **2017**, *129*, 1646–1657. [CrossRef] [PubMed]
6. Iwaki, N.; Fajgenbaum, D.C.; Nabel, C.S.; Gion, Y.; Kondo, E.; Kawano, M.; Masunari, T.; Yoshida, I.; Moro, H.; Nikkuni, K.; et al. Clinicopathologic analysis of TAFRO syndrome demonstrates a distinct subtype of HHV-8-negative multicentric Castleman disease. *Am. J. Hematol.* **2016**, *91*, 220–226. [CrossRef]
7. Nishimura, Y.; Fajgenbaum, D.C.; Pierson, S.K.; Iwaki, N.; Nishikori, A.; Kawano, M.; Nakamura, N.; Izutsu, K.; Takeuchi, K.; Nishimura, M.F.; et al. Validated international definition of the thrombocytopenia, anasarca, fever, reticulin fibrosis, renal insufficiency, and organomegaly clinical subtype (TAFRO) of idiopathic multicentric Castleman disease. *Am. J. Hematol.* **2021**, *96*, 1241–1252. [CrossRef] [PubMed]
8. Nishimura, Y.; Nishimura, M.F.; Sato, Y. International definition of iMCD-TAFRO: Future perspectives. *J. Clin. Exp. Hematop.* **2022**, *62*, 73–78. [CrossRef] [PubMed]
9. Keller, A.R.; Hochholzer, L.; Castleman, B. Hyaline-vascular and plasma-cell types of giant lymph node hyperplasia of the mediastinum and other locations. *Cancer* **1972**, *29*, 670–683. [CrossRef]
10. Frizzera, G. Castleman's disease and related disorders. *Semin. Diagn. Pathol.* **1988**, *5*, 346–364.
11. Wang, H.W.; Pittaluga, S.; Jaffe, E.S. Multicentric Castleman disease: Where are we now? *Semin Diagn. Pathol.* **2016**, *33*, 294–306. [CrossRef]
12. Frizzera, G.; Peterson, B.A.; Bayrd, E.D.; Goldman, A. A systemic lymphoproliferative disorder with morphologic features of Castleman's disease: Clinical findings and clinicopathologic correlations in 15 patients. *J. Clin. Oncol.* **1985**, *3*, 1202–1216. [CrossRef]
13. Kojima, M.; Nakamura, N.; Tsukamoto, N.; Otuski, Y.; Shimizu, K.; Itoh, H.; Kobayashi, S.; Kobayashi, H.; Murase, T.; Masawa, N.; et al. Clinical implications of idiopathic multicentric castleman disease among Japanese: A report of 28 cases. *Int. J. Surg. Pathol.* **2008**, *16*, 391–398. [CrossRef]
14. Pierson, S.K.; Shenoy, S.; Oromendia, A.B.; Gorzewski, A.M.; Langan Pai, R.A.; Nabel, C.S.; Ruth, J.R.; Parente, S.A.T.; Arenas, D.J.; Guilfoyle, M.; et al. Discovery and validation of a novel subgroup and therapeutic target in idiopathic multicentric Castleman disease. *Blood Adv.* **2021**, *5*, 3445–3456. [CrossRef]
15. Endo, Y.; Koga, T.; Ubara, Y.; Sumiyoshi, R.; Furukawa, K.; Kawakami, A. Mediterranean fever gene variants modify clinical phenotypes of idiopathic multi-centric Castleman disease. *Clin. Exp. Immunol.* **2021**, *206*, 91–98. [CrossRef] [PubMed]
16. Mori, S.; Mohri, N. Clinicopathological analysis of systemic nodal plasmacytosis with severe polyclonal hyperimmunoglobulinemia. *Proc. Jpn. Soc. Pathol.* **1978**, *67*, 252–253.
17. Han, E.J.; O, J.H.; Jung, S.E.; Park, G.; Choi, B.O.; Jeon, Y.W.; Min, G.J.; Cho, S.G. FDG PET/CT Findings of Castleman Disease Assessed by Histologic Subtypes and Compared with Laboratory Findings. *Diagnostics* **2020**, *10*, 998. [CrossRef] [PubMed]
18. Nishimura, M.F.; Nishimura, Y.; Nishikori, A.; Yoshino, T.; Sato, Y. Historical and pathological overview of Castleman disease. *J. Clin. Exp. Hematop.* **2022**, *62*, 60–72. [CrossRef] [PubMed]
19. Han, Y.; Igawa, T.; Ogino, K.; Nishikori, A.; Gion, Y.; Yoshino, T.; Sato, Y. Hemosiderin deposition in lymph nodes of patients with plasma cell-type Castleman disease. *J. Clin. Exp. Hematop.* **2020**, *60*, 1–6. [CrossRef]
20. Nishikori, A.; Nishimura, M.F.; Nishimura, Y.; Notohara, K.; Satou, A.; Moriyama, M.; Nakamura, S.; Sato, Y. Investigation of IgG4-positive cells in idiopathic multicentric Castleman disease and validation of the 2020 exclusion criteria for IgG4-related disease. *Pathol. Int.* **2022**, *72*, 43–52. [CrossRef] [PubMed]
21. Nishimura, M.F.; Igawa, T.; Gion, Y.; Tomita, S.; Inoue, D.; Izumozaki, A.; Ubara, Y.; Nishimura, Y.; Yoshino, T.; Sato, Y. Pulmonary Manifestations of Plasma Cell Type Idiopathic Multicentric Castleman Disease: A Clinicopathological Study in Comparison with IgG4-Related Disease. *J. Pers. Med.* **2020**, *10*, 269. [CrossRef]

22. Takeuchi, K. Idiopathic plasmacytic lymphadenopathy: A conceptual history along with a translation of the original Japanese article published in 1980. *J. Clin. Exp. Hematop.* **2022**, *62*, 79–84. [CrossRef] [PubMed]
23. Nishimura, Y.; Nishikori, A.; Sawada, H.; Czech, T.; Otsuka, Y.; Nishimura, M.F.; Mizuno, H.; Sawa, N.; Momose, S.; Ohsawa, K.; et al. Idiopathic multicentric Castleman disease with positive antiphospholipid antibody: Atypical and undiagnosed autoimmune disease? *J. Clin. Exp. Hematop.* **2022**, *62*, 99–105. [CrossRef]
24. Kojima, M.; Nakamura, S.; Itoh, H.; Yoshida, K.; Asano, S.; Yamane, N.; Komatsumoto, S.; Ban, S.; Joshita, T.; Suchi, T. Systemic lupus erythematosus (SLE) lymphadenopathy presenting with histopathologic features of Castleman' disease: A clinicopathologic study of five cases. *Pathol. Res. Pract.* **1997**, *193*, 565–571. [CrossRef]
25. Kojima, M.; Nakamura, N.; Tsukamoto, N.; Yokohama, A.; Itoh, H.; Kobayashi, S.; Kashimura, M.; Masawa, N.; Nakamura, S. Multicentric Castleman's disease representing effusion at initial clinical presentation: Clinicopathological study of seven cases. *Lupus* **2011**, *20*, 44–50. [CrossRef] [PubMed]
26. Kojima, M.; Motoori, T.; Asano, S.; Nakamura, S. Histological diversity of reactive and atypical proliferative lymph node lesions in systemic lupus erythematosus patients. *Pathol. Res. Pract.* **2007**, *203*, 423–431. [CrossRef]
27. Narazaki, M.; Kishimoto, T. The Two-Faced Cytokine IL-6 in Host Defense and Diseases. *Int. J. Mol. Sci.* **2018**, *19*, 3528. [CrossRef] [PubMed]
28. Fajgenbaum, D.C.; Langan, R.A.; Japp, A.S.; Partridge, H.L.; Pierson, S.K.; Singh, A.; Arenas, D.J.; Ruth, J.R.; Nabel, C.S.; Stone, K.; et al. Identifying and targeting pathogenic PI3K/AKT/mTOR signaling in IL-6-blockade-refractory idiopathic multicentric Castleman disease. *J. Clin. Investig.* **2019**, *129*, 4451–4463. [CrossRef]
29. Sumiyoshi, R.; Koga, T.; Kawakami, A. Candidate biomarkers for idiopathic multicentric Castleman disease. *J. Clin. Exp. Hematop.* **2022**, *62*, 85–90. [CrossRef] [PubMed]
30. Arenas, D.J.; Floess, K.; Kobrin, D.; Pai, R.L.; Srkalovic, M.B.; Tamakloe, M.A.; Rasheed, R.; Ziglar, J.; Khor, J.; Parente, S.A.T.; et al. Increased mTOR activation in idiopathic multicentric Castleman disease. *Blood* **2020**, *135*, 1673–1684. [CrossRef] [PubMed]
31. Pai, R.L.; Japp, A.S.; Gonzalez, M.; Rasheed, R.F.; Okumura, M.; Arenas, D.; Pierson, S.K.; Powers, V.; Layman, A.A.K.; Kao, C.; et al. Type I IFN response associated with mTOR activation in the TAFRO subtype of idiopathic multicentric Castleman disease. *JCI Insight* **2020**, *5*, e135031. [CrossRef] [PubMed]

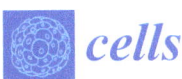

Article

Quartz Crystal Microbalance Measurement of Histidine-Rich Glycoprotein and Stanniocalcin-2 Binding to Each Other and to Inflammatory Cells

Tor Persson Skare [1], Hiroshi Kaito [1,†], Claudia Durall [2], Teodor Aastrup [2] and Lena Claesson-Welsh [1,*]

1. Science for Life and Beijer Laboratories, Department of Immunology, Genetics and Pathology, Uppsala University, Dag Hammarskjöldsv 20, 751 85 Uppsala, Sweden
2. Attana AB, Greta Arwidssons Väg 21, 114 19 Stockholm, Sweden
* Correspondence: lena.welsh@igp.uu.se
† Present affiliation: Department of Nephrology, Hyogo Prefectural Kobe Children's Hospital, Kobe 650-0047, Japan.

Abstract: The plasma protein histidine-rich glycoprotein (HRG) is implicated in the polarization of macrophages to an M1 antitumoral phenotype. The broadly expressed secreted protein stanniocalcin 2 (STC2), also implicated in tumor inflammation, is an HRG interaction partner. With the aim to biochemically characterize the HRG and STC2 complex, binding of recombinant HRG and STC2 preparations to each other and to cells was explored using the quartz crystal microbalance (QCM) methodology. The functionality of recombinant proteins was tested in a phagocytosis assay, where HRG increased phagocytosis by monocytic U937 cells while STC2 suppressed HRG-induced phagocytosis. The binding of HRG to STC2, measured using QCM, showed an affinity between the proteins in the nanomolar range, and both HRG and STC2 bound individually and in combination to vitamin D3-treated, differentiated U937 monocytes. HRG, but not STC2, also bound to formaldehyde-fixed U937 cells irrespective of their differentiation stage in part through the interaction with heparan sulfate. These data show that HRG and STC2 bind to each other as well as to U937 monocytes with high affinity, supporting the relevance of these interactions in monocyte/macrophage polarity.

Keywords: histidine-rich glycoprotein; stanniocalcin-2; protein complex; inflammatory cells; quartz crystal microbalance

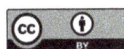

1. Introduction

Histidine-rich glycoprotein (HRG) is a 75 kDa abundant plasma protein produced by hepatocytes and implicated in cancer immune responsiveness [1]. HRG is organized as a multi-domain structure of two N-terminal cystatin-like domains, followed by a histidine–proline-rich (His/Pro-rich) domain containing 12 pentapeptide repeats of Gly-His-His-Pro-His. The His/Pro repeats, which are highly conserved among mammalian species [2], are flanked by two Pro-rich regions and a C-terminal domain [3]. The cystatin domains have been implicated in HRG's antibacterial effects [4] and in IgG and complement C1q binding [5]. The His/Pro-rich domain binds heparan sulfate in a Zn^{2+} dependent manner [6]. This domain is also critical for the anti-angiogenic properties of HRG [7]. The structure of HRG's NH_2-terminal domain has been solved, indicating a redox-regulated release of the NH2-terminal domain from the His/Pro-rich domain [8]. HRG has also been classified as an intrinsically unstructured protein, unable to attain an ordered or fixed conformation [9].

HRG's multi-domain organization allows for interactions with a range of proteins, both intracellular such as tropomyosin, extracellular such as stanniocalcin 2 (STC2), and proteins participating in the coagulation cascade, including plasminogen, plasmin and fibrinogen [10,11]. Consequently, HRG is involved in diverse processes including defense against bacterial infections, regulation of coagulation and fibrinolysis, inflammation and angiogenesis. Thus, HRG exerts antibacterial effects and may serve as a clinical biomarker for sepsis [12]. Moreover, HRG accelerates both coagulation and fibrinolysis in a $Hrg^{-/-}$ mouse model [13]. Rare familiar cases of HRG deficiency support the role of HRG in the regulation of coagulation [14]. Certain HRG effects are dependent on changes in gene regulation in monocytes/macrophages, promoting a phenotypic switch towards anti-tumor immunity and dampened tumor growth and metastasis [1]. While HRG administration to tumor-bearing wildtype mice results in suppressed tumor growth and metastasis, tumor growth is accelerated in $Hrg^{-/-}$ mice, and tumor macrophages are predominantly of an M2 phenotype in these Hrg-deficient mice [1,7,15].

We previously investigated the immunomodulatory role of HRG on inflammatory cells and found that HRG appears in complex with STC2 and that HRG modulates STC2-mediated gene regulation on U937 monocytic cells [16]. STC2 is a glycosylated homodimeric protein expressed in the placenta, endothelial cells, fibroblasts and cardiomyocytes [17]. In mouse glioma, tumor-infiltrating leukocytes express STC2 [16]. Like HRG, STC2 is involved in inflammatory processes and in Ca^{2+} and PO_4 homeostasis [18,19]. $Stc2^{-/-}$ mice show decreased overall growth, suggesting an important role for STC2 in muscle and bone development [20].

To explore the biochemical properties of HRG, STC2 and the complex of the two, purified proteins were analyzed using a novel quartz crystal microbalance (QCM) technique. Through the QCM analyses, the affinity and kinetics of the HRG-STC2 interaction as well as the binding of HRG and STC2 to the U937 monocyte cell surface were tested [21]. U937 is a human histiocytic lymphoma cell line, which differentiates towards a macrophage phenotype after treatment with vitamin D3 (vitD3) [22]. The functionality of the HRG and STC2 recombinant protein preparations were assessed by the induction of phagocytosis by differentiated U937 monocytes. While HRG administration stimulated phagocytosis, STC2 abrogated this HRG-dependent effect. In the QCM system, vitD3 differentiated live U937 cells, but not undifferentiated cells, bound both HRG and STC2, with an affinity in the micromolar range. HRG, but not STC2, also bound to fixed U937 cells, possibly representing HRG interactions with heparan sulfate exposed through the fixation. Thus, digestion with heparinase revealed high affinity binding sites for HRG on the differentiated, fixed U937 cells. Combined, these findings confirm the specificity of the HRG-STC2 interaction and show high affinity binding sites on the monocytic cell surface.

2. Materials and Methods

2.1. Differentiation of U937 Cells

The human histiocytic lymphoma cell line U937 [23] (American Type Culture Collection, ATCC 1593, RRID:CVCL_0007) was a kind gift from Professor Kenneth Nilsson, Uppsala University. The cells were cultured in an RPMI 1640 medium supplemented with 10% fetal bovine serum (FBS) and 1% penicillin/streptomycin (cat. no. 61870036; Life Technologies, Grand Island, NY, USA). For monocyte differentiation, U937 cells were incubated in 10 nM 1α,25-Dihydroxyvitamin D3 (vitD3; cat. no. 17936, Merck Life Science, Darmstadt, Germany) for 15 h, centrifuged (1500 rpm, 5 min), and resuspended in fresh medium. Differentiation was determined by real-time reverse transcriptase-PCR (qPCR) to detect CD14 transcripts. The mRNA was extracted from cells using the RNAeasy mini kit (Qiagen, Germantown, MD, USA) and RNA was reverse transcribed with iScript adv (cat. no. 1725038, Bio-Rad, Hercules, CA, USA). Gene expression was determined using TaqMan universal master mix (cat. no. 4304437, Life Technologies, Grand Island, NY, USA) in the CFX96 Real-Time PCR Detection System (Bio-Rad, Hercules, CA, USA) with TaqMan primers against human CD14 (cat. no. Hs 00169122, Life Technologies, Grand Island, NY, USA) and human GAPDH (cat no. 4352934, Applied Biosystems, Waltham, MA, USA). Cycle threshold values were calculated with CFX Maestro v. 1.1 software (Bio-Rad, Hercules, CA, USA).

2.2. Purified Proteins and Phagocytosis Assay

The U937 cells were seeded at 10^4 cells per well in 8-well chamber slides (cat. no. 80826, ibidi, Fitchburg, WI, USA). At the start of the experiment, cells were incubated with 10 nM vitD3, recombinant, in-house purified HRG (mouse) at 1 µg/mL (13.3 nM) [24], and STC2 (mouse) (cat. no. STC2-16118 M, Creative Biomart, Shirley, NY, USA) or inactive HRG protein at equivalent molar concentrations together with sterile green E. coli bioparticles (cat. no. 4616, Essen Bioscience, Ann Arbor, MI, USA) at 33 µg/mL. Following 20 h incubation at 37 °C in 5% CO_2, cells were imaged at 10× with a Zeiss LSM 700 Microscope with AxioCam HRm and Zen Black software (Zeiss, Oberkochen, Germany). Quantification was completed by counting of fluorescent cells in relation to all cells per image, using ImageJ (NIH).

2.3. Co-Immunoprecipitation and Immunoblotting

Equimolar concentrations of active or inactive HRG and STC2 were incubated on ice for 30 min followed by incubation with an anti-STC2 antibody (cat. no. hpa045372; Merck Life Science, Darmstadt, Germany) for 1 h. Protein G Sepharose (cat. no. 71708300 AM, GE Healthcare, Chicago, IL, USA) was added and incubated at 4 °C for 1 h. Following centrifugation and washes, samples were heated at 97 °C for 3 min for dissociation. Samples were separated by SDS-PAGE, transferred to a PVDF membrane (Millipore, Burlington, MA, USA), blocked in blocking buffer (5% milk in Tris-buffered saline and 0.1% Tween20) for 1 h and incubated with primary anti-human HRG antibody raised in rabbit (#0119) [7] overnight at 4 °C. Membranes were washed and incubated with HRP-conjugated secondary anti-rabbit antibody (Life Technologies, Grand Island, NY, USA) in blocking buffer for 1 h at room temperature. The development was performed with ECL prime (GE Healthcare, Chicago, IL, USA) and the luminescence signals detected using ChemiDoc MP (Bio-Rad; Hercules, CA, USA). Next, membranes were re-incubated with the STC2 antibody (cat. no. hpa045372, Merck Life Science, Darmstadt, Germany) overnight at 4 °C and developed again as described above.

2.4. Binding of HRG to STC2

Low noise block (LNB) chips were pre-wet with HEPES-buffered Steinberg's solution (HBS-T) and inserted into an Attana Cell^{TM}200 instrument. When the signal was stabilized (<0.2 Hz/min), STC2 or HRG protein (50 µg/mL) were immobilized on the surface with a flow rate of 10 µL/min at 22 °C using the amine coupling kit. Different concentrations of HRG (3.12, 6.25 and 12.5 µg/mL (each in triplicate)) and STC2 (7.5, 15 and 30 µg/mL) were injected after blank injections (phosphate-buffered saline; PBS) followed by regeneration injections at pH 1 for 30 s. PBS was used as the running buffer for the blank injections and to dilute HRG. Glycine (10 mM, pH 1) was used as the regeneration buffer. The biochemical assay was carried out at a flow rate of 10 µL/min, at 22 °C and with a 500 s dissociation time. The data were prepared by subtracting the blank injections from the HRG injections using the Attana evaluation software (version 3.5.0.7, Attana AB Stockholm, Stockholm, Sweden). The curve fitting was performed with Tracedrawer (Ridgeview Instruments AB, Uppsala, Sweden), using the 1:1 global interaction model. The number of independent experiments (mostly 3) performed are given in the figure legends.

2.5. Binding of HRG and STC2 to U937 Cells Treated or Not with Heparinase and Fixative

LNB-CC chips were pre-wet with HBS-T and then inserted into an Attana Cell^{TM} 200 (Attana AB, Stockholm, Sweden). When the signal was stabilized (<0.2 Hz), lectin (50 µg/mL) was coupled by amine coupling. Cells were then seeded at a density of 2×10^5 cells per chip and left to settle for 45 min at room temperature. After seeding, the cells were washed with PBS, stained with Hoechst 33342 solution for 15 min, and washed three times, followed by imaging using a fluorescence microscope (Nikon Eclipse 80i, Minato City, Tokyo, Japan). Next, the chips were inserted in the instrument (Attana Cell^{TM} 200, Stockholm, Sweden) and left to equilibrate (<0.2 Hz/min) under flow (RPMI 1640 medium, 20 µL/min at 37 °C). STC2, HRG or a mix of the two (10 µg/mL) were injected manually over the cells and the responses were recorded for 30 min. Between injections, chip surfaces were regenerated using Glycine (10 mM pH 1) for 50 s for experiments involving fixed cells.

When indicated, cells were treated with heparinase using a mixture of heparinase-I, -II, and -III (IBEX Pharmaceuticals, Montreal, QC, Canada), which was added to the cultures to a final concentration of 3.4 mU/mL for each enzyme for 1 h at 37 °C before seeding the cells on the activated chips. The fixation of cells was performed just after seeding by removing the PBS and adding 50 µL of a 3.7% formaldehyde solution. Subsequently, the chips were incubated at 4 °C for 10 min followed by washing with PBS three times. The data were prepared by subtracting the blank injections from the analyte injections using the Attana evaluation software (version 3.5.0.7, Attana AB Stockholm, Stockholm, Sweden). The signal output is given in frequency (Hz) and is directly related to changes in mass on the sensor surface. The negative changes of resonance frequency are depicted. The curve fitting was performed with Tracedrawer (Ridgeview Instruments, Uppsala, Sweden), using the 1:1 or 1:2 binding models (only one component reported) and global interaction model. At least two independent experiments were performed with 3 technical repeats within each experiment.

3. Results

3.1. HRG Increases Phagocytosis by U937 Monocytes

First, the bioactivity of purified, recombinant STC2 and HRG preparations were determined. To ensure that the recombinant proteins could form a complex, as previously shown by co-immunoprecipitation from co-expressing cells [16], antibodies against STC2 were used for pull-down from a mixture of the two proteins, followed by immunoblotting (Figure 1A; see Supplemental Figure S1 for uncropped blots). In parallel, a preparation of HRG serendipitously denatured during purification, and was used as a negative control ("inactive HRG"). Active HRG was efficiently co-immunoprecipitated with STC2 while the inactive HRG was only inefficiently pulled down by STC2 (Figure 1B). Still, the inactive HRG was detected by the polyclonal anti-HRG antibody upon immunoblotting, ensuring that this preparation indeed consisted of HRG. The inactive HRG-preparation was used as a negative control in subsequent experiments.

3.2. HRG and STC2 Interact with Nanomolar Affinity

HRG and STC2 are both secreted proteins, and therefore, it is not immediately obvious how they exert their modulatory effects on inflammatory cells. To investigate the interactions of the individual proteins and the complex with each other and with cells, we employed QCM technology [25], which allowed for real-time and label-free evaluation of the protein interactions in both a cell-free and cellular environment.

First, STC2 was immobilized on the QCM chip surface (Figure 2A). Next, the binding of increasing concentrations of HRG to the STC2-coated chip was analyzed using a kinetic 1:1 global interaction model, which showed an association rate constant (K_{a1}) of 2.6×10^4 $M^{-1} \cdot s^{-1}$ and dissociation rate constant (K_{d1}) of 1.4×10^{-3} s^{-1}, resulting in an estimated binding affinity of 55 nM between HRG and STC2 (Figure 2B). In contrast, the inactive HRG failed to bind to the immobilized STC2 (Figure 2C). Moreover, when HRG was immobilized on the grid, STC2 was not retained (Figure 2D). This result indicates that the interaction between HRG and STC2 may be dependent on HRG's conformation or that a binding pocket in HRG, involved in the retention of STC2, was compromised when HRG was immobilized onto the chip. HRG is classified as an intrinsically unstructured protein [9], i.e., a protein that lacks a fixed three-dimensional structure, and it may therefore be structurally less stable and, in particular, not retain a more complex binding epitope upon immobilization.

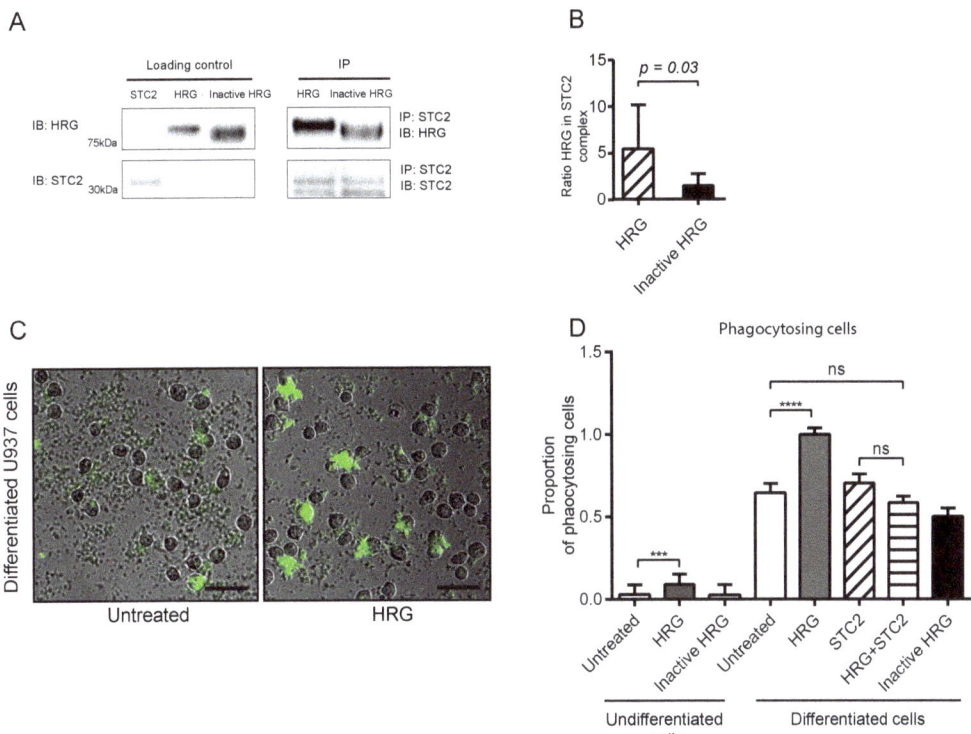

Figure 1. Recombinant HRG binds STC2 and modulates phagocytosis of bioparticles. (**A**) Co-immunoprecipitation of HRG but not inactive HRG with STC2. Recombinant proteins (2 μg each) were separated on SDS-PAGE as individual preparations (loading control) or after mixing and immunoprecipitation (IP) using antibodies against STC2, followed by immunoblotting (IB) as indicated. (**B**) Ratio of HRG (active or inactive) band intensities in the STC2 immunoprecipitate normalized to corresponding active and inactive HRG loading controls. Statistical analysis; Student's t-test. (**C**) Representative microscope images of U937 monocytes without (left) or with treatment with active HRG (right) in the phagocytosis assay. Green cells have engulfed pH-sensitive fluorescent bioparticles. Scale bar; 50 μm. (**D**) Quantification of phagocytosis efficiency in the different treatment conditions. The proportion of positive (green) phagocytic U937 cells to all cells per field of vision is shown in relation to the positive cells/total cells in the vitD3 differentiated HRG-treated condition (set to 1). Statistical analysis; Tukey's multiple comparisons test (**D**). *** $p < 0.001$; **** $p < 0.0001$.

3.3. Live U937 Cells Bind HRG after vitD3 Differentiation

Next, we assessed binding of HRG, STC2 and the complex to live U937 cells, vitD3-differentiated or not (Figure 3A). First, we confirmed the ability of U937 cells to differentiate to monocytes on the chip surface in response to vitD3. Relative CD14 expression increased >1000-fold after vitD3 treatment, ensuring that the cells indeed had differentiated to monocytes in response to vitD3 (Figure 3B). This is in agreement with previously reported effects of HRG treatment on CD14 expression in vitD3-induced U937 cells [15]. Binding of both HRG and STC2 to the undifferentiated U937 cells was low and binding increased markedly when cells were induced to differentiate by vitD3 treatment (Figure 3C–F). The association rate constants of HRG and STC2 binding tested individually (Figure 3C–F) or in combination (Figure 3G,H) increased slightly with differentiation, in keeping with the increased expression of a specific binding protein(s) expressed on the U937 surface in response to the vitD3 treatment. When a mixture of HRG and STC2 was tested on the differentiated U937 cells, the binding affinity remained in the µM range, similar to that recorded for the individual proteins (Figure 3G,H).

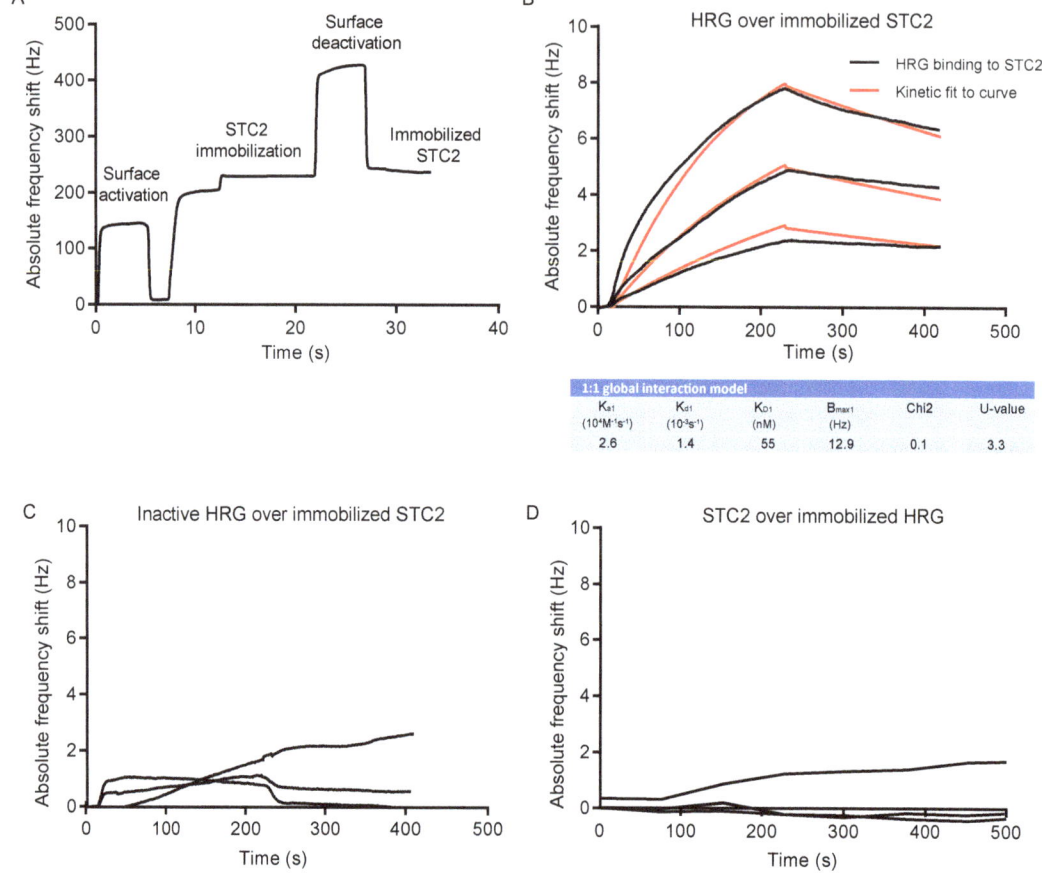

Figure 2. Affinity determination of HRG's binding to STC2 using QCM. (**A**) The immobilization of STC2 on the QCM LNB sensor surface. (**B**) Sensorgram and kinetic analysis showing chip-immobilized STC2 and binding of HRG at three different concentrations: 50, 100 and 200 nM. Black lines: experimental curves. Red lines: fitted curves. For representative sensorgram shown, three injections per concentration, two independent experiments. (**C**) Sensorgram showing chip-immobilized STC2 and lack of binding of inactive HRG tested at three different concentrations: 50, 100 and 200 nM. For representative sensorgram shown, three injections per concentration, two independent experiments. (**D**) Sensorgram showing chip-immobilized HRG and lack of binding of STC2, tested at three different concentrations: 200 nM, 450 nM and 900 nM. For representative sensorgram shown, two injections per concentration, three independent experiments.

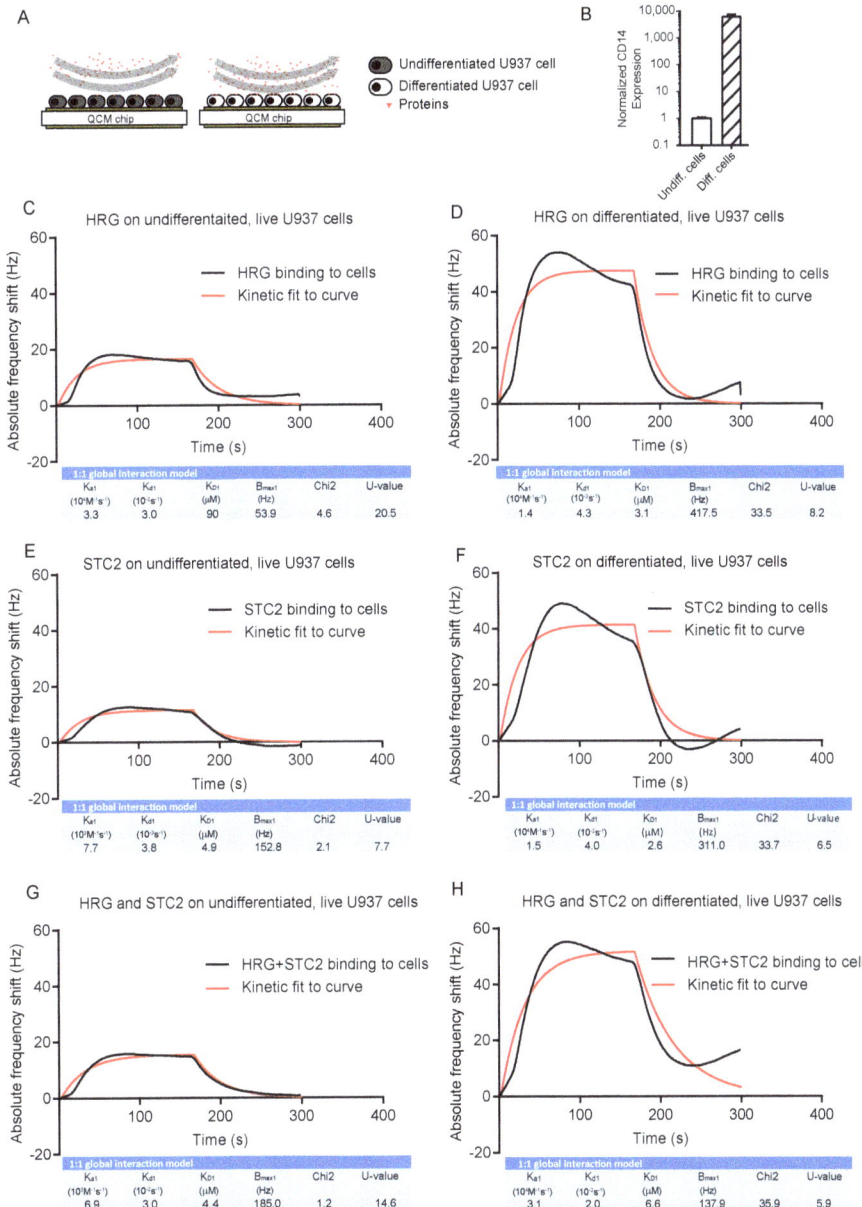

Figure 3. Binding of HRG and STC2 individually and together to live U937 cells. (**A**) Schematic outline of the experimental setup. Undifferentiated or vitD3 differentiated U937 cells, immobilized on QCM LNB chips with HRG, STC2 or a mix of the two, injected over chip surfaces. (**B**) Real-time qPCR data of CD14 expression normalized to GAPDH on undifferentiated and vitD3 differentiated U937 cells seeded on the QCM chip. Three independent analyses. (**C**–**F**) Representative sensorgram showing frequency response from injections over undifferentiated (**C**,**E**,**G**) and vitD3 differentiated (**D**,**F**,**H**) live U937 cells. Black lines: experimental curves. Red lines: fitted curves of the 1:1 interaction model. For representative sensorgrams shown, three injections per concentration, two independent experiments.

We conclude that both HRG and STC2 bound to U937 monocytes with affinities in the µM range and with an estimated 1:1 interaction mode both for the individual proteins and the mixture.

3.4. Binding of HRG to Fixed U937 Cells Is Independent of vitD3-Induced Differentiation

Due to the potential challenge in separating interaction properties from interaction-induced changes in the live U937 monocytes immobilized on the QCM chip surface, cells were then fixed, and the binding of HRG and STC2 was determined. As expected, inactive HRG, used as a negative control, displayed no interaction with U937 cells, differentiated or not, even at high concentrations (100 µg/mL) (Figure 4A). In addition, STC2 failed to bind both to undifferentiated and differentiated cells in a specific manner, with the response dropping down to baseline immediately after the end of injection (Figure 4B). In contrast, bioactive HRG interacted with the fixed cells with an affinity around 3.5 nM to undifferentiated cells and 166 nM to differentiated cells (Figure 4C,D) with a 1:1 interaction mode. In combination, these data show very different properties for STC2 and HRG interactions with fixed cells, as fixation exposed binding sites for HRG on undifferentiated cells were recorded while not observed with live cells. However, we cannot categorically exclude that the binding sites exposed upon fixation, at least in part, could represent intracellular ligands for HRG [3], either proteinase K-resistant or -sensitive.

Instead, we hypothesized that these binding sites for HRG on undifferentiated, fixed cells may involve heparan sulfate epitopes [6]. To investigate this possibility further, cells were treated with heparinase before HRG binding. The treatment with heparinase changed the dissociation curve to a 1:2 interaction mode [26]. The affinities for the two categories of HRG binding to heparinase-treated undifferentiated cells were 88 nM and 0.84 µM, respectively (Figure 4E). Heparinase-digestion of differentiated U937 cells on the other hand revelated affinities for HRG of 0.03 nM and 0.4 µM, respectively (Figure 4F). We suggest that this non-heparan sulfate-dependent, high-affinity binding of HRG to fixed, differentiated cells may represent binding to a molecular entity responsible for transducing the biological effects of HRG, such as increased phagocytosis.

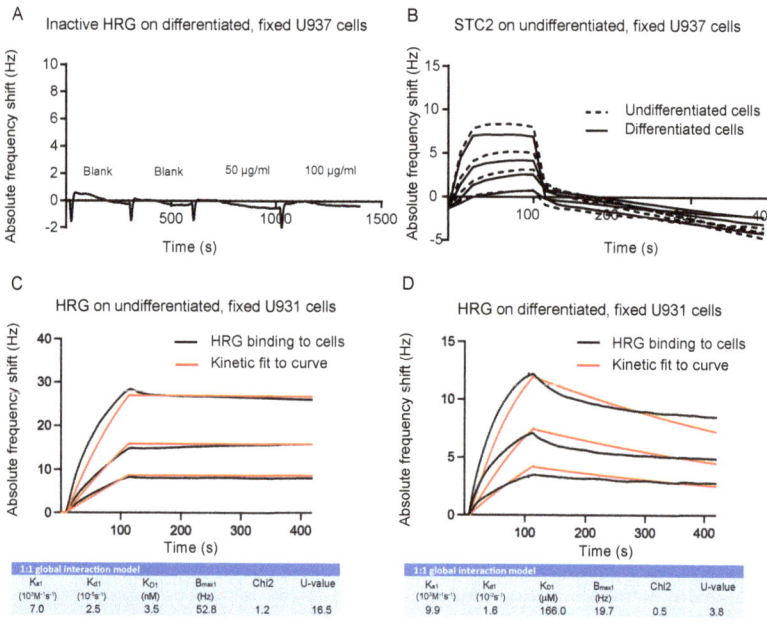

Figure 4. *Cont.*

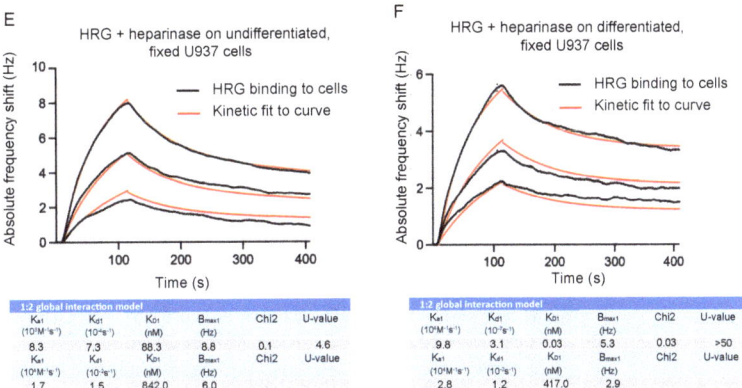

1:2 global interaction model					
K_{a1} ($10^4 M^{-1}s^{-1}$)	K_{d1} ($10^{-4} s^{-1}$)	K_{D1} (nM)	B_{max1} (Hz)	Chi2	U-value
8.3	7.3	88.3	8.8	0.1	4.6
K_{a1} ($10^4 M^{-1}s^{-1}$)	K_{d1} ($10^{-3} s^{-1}$)	K_{D1} (nM)	B_{max1} (Hz)	Chi2	U-value
1.7	1.5	842.0	6.0		

1:2 global interaction model					
K_{a1} ($10^4 M^{-1}s^{-1}$)	K_{d1} ($10^{-7} s^{-1}$)	K_{D1} (nM)	B_{max1} (Hz)	Chi2	U-value
9.8	3.1	0.03	5.3	0.03	>50
K_{a1} ($10^4 M^{-1}s^{-1}$)	K_{d1} ($10^{-3} s^{-1}$)	K_{D1} (nM)	B_{max1} (Hz)	Chi2	U-value
2.8	1.2	417.0	2.9		

Figure 4. Affinity of HRG for binding to fixed U937 cells. (**A**) Sensorgram showing frequency response to inactive HRG over vitD3 differentiated, fixed U937 cells. (**B**) Sensorgram showing frequency response to four concentrations (125 nM, 250 nM, 500 nM, 1 µM) of STC2 over fixed, undifferentiated (dashed lines) and vitD3 differentiated (straight lines) U937 cells. The mean of two injections is shown. (**C,D**) Sensorgram and kinetic analysis show the binding of HRG at three concentrations (25, 50 and 100 nM) to undifferentiated (**C**) or vitD3 differentiated (**D**), fixed U937 cells. Black lines: experimental curves. Red lines: fitted curves of the 1:1 interaction model. For representative sensorgrams shown, three injections per concentration, three independent experiments. (**E,F**) Sensorgram and kinetic analysis showing frequency response to three concentrations of HRG (25, 50 and 100 nM) to fixed, undifferentiated (**E**) or vitD3 differentiated (**F**) U937 cells after treatment with heparinase. Black lines: experimental curves. Red lines: fitted curves of 1:2 interaction model. For representative sensorgrams shown, three injections per concentration, three independent experiments.

4. Discussion

This study aimed to understand the binding properties of the soluble plasma proteins HRG and STC2, motivated by their induction of gene regulatory programs that steer the phenotype of the monocyte/macrophage towards pro- or anti-inflammatory activities. We have previously shown that HRG, either administered as a recombinant protein, overexpressed by tumor cells, or delivered through adenovirus-mediated gene therapy, polarizes monocytes/macrophages to an anti-tumor immune profile, allowing for the recruitment of cytotoxic T cells to the tumor [1,16,24]. The effect of HRG is accompanied by tumor vessel normalization and suppressed tumor growth [1,27]. In a screen to identify HRG binding partners on the surface of monocytes mediating HRG's gene regulatory effects, STC2 was identified and shown to have broad effects on inflammatory gene regulation [16]. Here, we asked whether HRG and STC2 bind to a common cell surface molecule ("receptor") to steer monocyte gene regulation in a concerted action, based on the characteristics of binding to U937 monocytic cells.

To explore the binding properties of HRG and STC2, we employed a QCM biosensor methodology using unmodified, label-free proteins. This is important as modifications such as fluorescent peptide linkers or fusion partners, e.g., green fluorescent protein, can affect the folding of the modified protein and cause unnatural protein interactions. Moreover, radioactive labelling of proteins to determine protein interactions can harm the protein through the harsh methods used to introduce the label. In QCM, a thin quartz crystal disk is sandwiched between two electrodes. Changes in mass, e.g., upon binding of HRG to the surface of immobilized cells, results in a mechanical deformation of the disk, which mediates a frequency change in the quartz crystal that is proportional to the change in mass, which allows for calculations of affinity [28,29]. The technology also allows for real-time tracking of the kinetics of the interaction. However, the application of live cells, in particular the issues with non-adherent cells undergoing a differentiation process, are not trivial for

QCM analyses. The cells need to remain on the grid, unaffected by the flow of the medium and pursue the differentiation program. By measuring CD14 expression, we could show that the U937 cells on the grid indeed could be induced by vitD3 to differentiate towards the monocyte lineage. However, as live cells may react to the binding component, in this case, HRG and STC2, kinetic measurements may represent both interaction properties and interaction-induced cell surface modifications. We, therefore, analyzed the binding of HRG and STC2 also to fixed cells. The utilization of fixed cells allowed for repeated measurements and different concentrations of analyte on the same cell surfaces. This increases reproducibility and leads to more robust data. However, fixation may interfere with protein–protein interactions and affect binding. The formaldehyde fixation utilized here is a preferred fixative for preserved immunoreactivity [30]. Unexpectedly, upon fixation of the cells, STC2 failed to bind to cells irrespective of the differentiation stage, while HRG bound to fixed cells both with and without vitD3 treatment (Figure 4). We therefore suggest that STC2 and HRG bind to distinct molecular entities on the U937 cells, and that the STC2 interactive surface was denatured upon fixation, however, definite proof for this assumption requires identification of the binding surfaces for HRG and STC2.

The binding of HRG to undifferentiated, fixed U937 cells may be due to fixation-induced exposure of heparan sulfate. HRG is known to bind with heparan sulfate in a Zn^{2+}-dependent manner, and this interaction is required for the anti-angiogenic effects of HRG [6]. We addressed the role of heparan sulfate by incubating cells with heparinase. Although incomplete, as revealed by the remaining binding of HRG to undifferentiated U937 cells, the digestion resulted in a change of the interaction mode from a 1:1 model with linear dissociation curves to a 1:2 model. This change supports the hypothesis that HRG binds to two classes of binding epitopes with different affinities—a lower affinity heparan sulfate-dependent binding and a higher affinity binding epitope that we hypothesize may represent the signal transducing cell surface expressed receptor mediating the gene regulatory effects of HRG. Further studies include determining whether the interaction between STC2 and HRG is Zn^{2+}-dependent, to identify, in each protein, the minimal binding stretch for their interaction and ultimately, to identify the cell surface expressed binding proteins/receptors for HRG and STC2.

5. Conclusions

The main findings from this study are (1) HRG and STC2 promote distinct U937 differentiation programs as STC2 suppressed the HRG-induced increase in phagocytosis. Moreover, (2) HRG and STC2 bind to each other with nanomolar affinity, and the interaction is stable, as evidenced by the relatively slow dissociation rate. Both proteins also (3) bind to differentiated, live U937 cells with μM affinities, i.e., to cells that, in response to vitD3, have initiated a gene regulatory program similar to that accompanying monocyte differentiation marked by the expression of CD14 [31]. It is possible that the binding of both HRG and STC2 to live cells is, in part, heparan sulfate-dependent and that differentiation is required to induce expression of a particular category of heparan sulfated proteoglycans. Finally, (4) while STC2 fails to bind to fixed U937 cells, the high-affinity binding of HRG to heparinase-treated fixed cells may represent the interaction with a specific cell surface receptor mediating the biological effects of HRG. These results indicate that STC2 and HRG interact with distinct rather than shared cell surface binding epitopes.

Supplementary Materials: The following supporting information can be downloaded at: https://www.mdpi.com/article/10.3390/cells11172684/s1, Figure S1: Uncropped blots corresponding to Figure 1A. Uncropped immunoblots for HRG (top panel), STC2 (short exposure; middle panel) and STC2 (long exposure, lower panel) were used to compose Figure 1A. Box 1, Box 2, Box 3 and Box 4 in the three blots correspond to parts in the composite in Figure 1A as follows: Box 1; upper left part of the composite, box 2; upper right, box 3; lower left, and box 4; lower right part of the composite, respectively. Migration positions for HRG, STC2 and IgG heavy and light chains are indicated.

Author Contributions: Conceptualization: T.P.S., H.K. and L.C.-W.; Investigation: T.P.S. and C.D.; Methodology development: C.D. and T.A.; Evaluation: All authors.; Statistics: T.P.S., C.D. and T.A.; Writing original draft: T.P.S. and L.C.-W.; Editing: All authors. All authors have read and agreed to the published version of the manuscript.

Funding: This study was supported by the following grants to L.C.-W.: Swedish Cancer Society (19 0119 Pj 01 H), the Swedish Research Council (2020-01349), the Knut and Alice Wallenberg foundation (project grant KAW 2020.0057) and Wallenberg Scholar grant (2015.0275).

Institutional Review Board Statement: Not applicable.

Data Availability Statement: Data supporting the results shown in this paper can be obtained from the lead authors (T.A. and L.C.W.) upon reasonable request.

Conflicts of Interest: T.P.S., H.K. and L.C.W. declare no financial interest. C.D. is an employee and T.A. is the founder and CEO of Attana Ab.

References

1. Rolny, C.; Mazzone, M.; Tugues, S.; Laoui, D.; Johansson, I.; Coulon, C.; Squadrito, M.L.; Segura, I.; Li, X.; Knevels, E.; et al. HRG inhibits tumor growth and metastasis by inducing macrophage polarization and vessel normalization through downregulation of PlGF. *Cancer Cell* **2011**, *19*, 31–44. [CrossRef] [PubMed]
2. Wakabayashi, S. Chapter Nine—New Insights into the Functions of Histidine-Rich Glycoprotein. In *International Review of Cell and Molecular Biology*; Jeon, K.W., Ed.; Academic Press: Cambridge, MA, USA, 2013; pp. 467–493.
3. Poon, I.K.H.; Patel, K.K.; Davis, D.S.; Parish, C.R.; Hulett, M.D. Histidine-rich glycoprotein: The Swiss Army knife of mammalian plasma. *Blood* **2011**, *117*, 2093–2101. [CrossRef] [PubMed]
4. Shannon, O.; Rydengård, V.; Schmidtchen, A.; Mörgelin, M.; Alm, P.; Sørensen, O.E.; Björck, L. Histidine-rich glycoprotein promotes bacterial entrapment in clots and decreases mortality in a mouse model of sepsis. *Blood* **2010**, *116*, 2365–2372. [CrossRef]
5. Gorgani, N.N.; Parish, C.; Easterbrook Smith, S.B.; Altin, J.G. Histidine-Rich Glycoprotein Binds to Human IgG and C1q and Inhibits the Formation of Insoluble Immune Complexes. *Biochemistry* **1997**, *36*, 6653–6662. [CrossRef] [PubMed]
6. Vanwildemeersch, M.; Olsson, A.-K.; Gottfridsson, E.; Claesson-Welsh, L.; Lindahl, U.; Spillmann, D. The anti-angiogenic His/Pro-rich fragment of histidine-rich glycoprotein binds to endothelial cell heparan sulfate in a Zn^{2+}-dependent manner. *J. Biol. Chem.* **2006**, *281*, 10298–10304. [CrossRef] [PubMed]
7. Olsson, A.-K.; Larsson, H.; Dixelius, J.; Johansson, I.; Lee, C.; Oellig, C.; Björk, I.; Claesson-Welsh, L. A fragment of histidine-rich glycoprotein is a potent inhibitor of tumor vascularization. *Cancer Res.* **2004**, *64*, 599–605. [CrossRef]
8. Kassaar, O.; McMahon, S.A.; Thompson, R.; Botting, C.H.; Naismith, J.H.; Stewart, A.J. Crystal structure of histidine-rich glycoprotein N2 domain reveals redox activity at an interdomain disulfide bridge: Implications for angiogenic regulation. *Blood* **2014**, *123*, 1948–1955. [CrossRef]
9. Tompa, P. Intrinsically unstructured proteins. *Trends Biochem. Sci.* **2002**, *27*, 527–533. [CrossRef]
10. Blank, M.; Shoenfeld, Y. Histidine-rich glycoprotein modulation of immune/autoimmune, vascular, and coagulation systems. *Clin. Rev. Allergy Immunol.* **2008**, *34*, 307–312. [CrossRef]
11. Roche, F.; Sipilä, K.; Honjo, S.; Johansson, S.; Tugues, S.; Heino, J.; Claesson-Welsh, L. Histidine-rich glycoprotein blocks collagen-binding integrins and adhesion of endothelial cells through low-affinity interaction with alpha2 integrin. *Matrix Biol.* **2015**, *48*, 89–99. [CrossRef]
12. Kuroda, K.; Ishii, K.; Mihara, Y.; Kawanoue, N.; Wake, H.; Mori, S.; Yoshida, M.; Nishibori, M.; Morimatsu, H. Histidine-rich glycoprotein as a prognostic biomarker for sepsis. *Sci. Rep.* **2021**, *11*, 10223. [CrossRef] [PubMed]
13. Tsuchida-Straeten, N.; Ensslen, S.; Schäfer, C.; Wöltje, M.; Denecke, B.; Moser, M.; Gräber, S.; Wakabayashi, S.; Koide, T.; Jahnen-Dechent, W. Enhanced blood coagulation and fibrinolysis in mice lacking histidine-rich glycoprotein (HRG). *J. Thromb. Haemost.* **2005**, *3*, 865–872. [CrossRef]
14. Lee, C.; Bongcam-Rudloff, E.; Sollner, C.; Jahnen-Dechent, W.; Claesson-Welsh, L. Type 3 cystatins; fetuins, kininogen and histidine-rich glycoprotein. *Front. Biosci.* **2009**, *14*, 2911–2922. [CrossRef] [PubMed]
15. Tugues, S.; Honjo, S.; König, C.; Noguer, O.; Hedlund, M.; Botling, J.; Deschoemaeker, S.; Wenes, M.; Rolny, C.; Jahnen-Dechent, W.; et al. Genetic deficiency in plasma protein HRG enhances tumor growth and metastasis by exacerbating immune escape and vessel abnormalization. *Cancer Res.* **2012**, *72*, 1953–1963. [CrossRef] [PubMed]
16. Roche, F.P.; Pietilä, I.; Kaito, H.; Sjöström, E.O.; Sobotzki, N.; Noguer, O.; Skare, T.P.; Essand, M.; Wollscheid, B.; Welsh, M.; et al. Leukocyte Differentiation by Histidine-Rich Glycoprotein/Stanniocalcin-2 Complex Regulates Murine Glioma Growth through Modulation of Antitumor Immunity. *Mol. Cancer Ther.* **2018**, *17*, 1961–1972. [CrossRef]
17. Uhlén, M.; Fagerberg, L.; Hallström, B.M.; Lindskog, C.; Oksvold, P.; Mardinoglu, A.; Sivertsson, Å.; Kampf, C.; Sjöstedt, E.; Asplund, A.; et al. Proteomics. Tissue-based map of the human proteome. *Science* **2015**, *347*, 1260419. [CrossRef]
18. Joshi, A.D. New Insights Into Physiological and Pathophysiological Functions of Stanniocalcin 2. *Front. Endocrinol.* **2020**, *11*, 172. [CrossRef]
19. Yeung, B.H.; Law, A.Y.; Wong, C.K. Evolution and roles of stanniocalcin. *Mol. Cell Endocrinol.* **2012**, *349*, 272–280. [CrossRef]

20. Chang, A.C.; Hook, J.; Lemckert, F.A.; McDonald, M.; Nguyen, M.-A.T.; Hardeman, E.C.; Little, D.G.; Gunning, P.W.; Reddel, R. The murine stanniocalcin 2 gene is a negative regulator of postnatal growth. *Endocrinology* **2008**, *149*, 2403–2410. [CrossRef]
21. Gianneli, M.; Polo, E.; Lopez, H.; Castagnola, V.; Aastrup, T.; Dawson, K.A. Label-free in-flow detection of receptor recognition motifs on the biomolecular corona of nanoparticles. *Nanoscale* **2018**, *10*, 5474–5481. [CrossRef]
22. Olsson, I.; Gullberg, U.; Ivhed, I.; Nilsson, K. Induction of differentiation of the human histiocytic lymphoma cell line U-937 by 1 alpha,25-dihydroxycholecalciferol. *Cancer Res.* **1983**, *43*, 5862–5867. [PubMed]
23. Sundström, C.; Nilsson, K. Establishment and characterization of a human histiocytic lymphoma cell line (U-937). *Int. J. Cancer* **1976**, *17*, 565–577. [CrossRef] [PubMed]
24. Tugues, S.; Roche, F.; Noguer, O.; Orlova, A.; Bhoi, S.; Padhan, N.; Åkerud, P.; Honjo, S.; Selvaraju, R.K.; Mazzone, M.; et al. Histidine-rich glycoprotein uptake and turnover is mediated by mononuclear phagocytes. *PLoS ONE* **2014**, *9*, e107483.
25. Peiris, D.; Aastrup, T.; Altun, S.; Käck, C.; Gianneli, M.; Proverbio, D.; Jørgensen, L.M. Label-Free Cell-Based Assay for Characterization of Biomolecules and Receptors. In *Epitope Mapping Protocols*; Rockberg, J., Nilvebrant, J., Eds.; Springer: New York, NY, USA, 2018; pp. 53–63.
26. Forssén, P.; Multia, E.; Samuelsson, J.; Andersson, M.; Aastrup, T.; Altun, S.; Wallinder, D.; Wallbing, L.; Liangsupree, T.; Riekkola, M.-L.; et al. Reliable Strategy for Analysis of Complex Biosensor Data. *Anal. Chem.* **2018**, *90*, 5366–5374. [CrossRef] [PubMed]
27. Theek, B.; Baues, M.; Gremse, F.; Pola, R.; Pechar, M.; Negwer, I.; Koynov, K.; Weber, B.; Barz, M.; Jahnen-Dechent, W.; et al. Histidine-rich glycoprotein-induced vascular normalization improves EPR-mediated drug targeting to and into tumors. *J. Control. Release* **2018**, *282*, 25–34. [CrossRef]
28. Marx, K.A. Quartz Crystal Microbalance: A Useful Tool for Studying Thin Polymer Films and Complex Biomolecular Systems at the Solution−Surface Interface. *Biomacromolecules* **2003**, *4*, 1099–1120. [CrossRef]
29. Pei, Z.; Saint-Guirons, J.; Käck, C.; Ingemarsson, B.; Aastrup, T. Real-time analysis of the carbohydrates on cell surfaces using a QCM biosensor: A lectin-based approach. *Biosens. Bioelectron.* **2012**, *35*, 200–205. [CrossRef]
30. Paavilainen, L.; Edvinsson, Å.; Asplund, A.; Hober, S.; Kampf, C.; Pontén, F.; Wester, K. The impact of tissue fixatives on morphology and antibody-based protein profiling in tissues and cells. *J. Histochem. Cytochem.* **2010**, *58*, 237–246. [CrossRef]
31. Zamani, F.; Shahneh, F.Z.; Aghebati-Maleki, L.; Baradaran, B. Induction of CD14 Expression and Differentiation to Monocytes or Mature Macrophages in Promyelocytic Cell Lines: New Approach. *Adv. Pharm. Bull.* **2013**, *3*, 329–332.

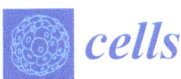

Review

The Interaction of Human Papillomavirus Infection and Prostaglandin E$_2$ Signaling in Carcinogenesis: A Focus on Cervical Cancer Therapeutics

Janice García-Quiroz [1], Bismarck Vázquez-Almazán [1], Rocío García-Becerra [2], Lorenza Díaz [1] and Euclides Avila [1,*]

[1] Departamento de Biología de la Reproducción Dr. Carlos Gual Castro, Instituto Nacional de Ciencias Médicas y Nutrición Salvador Zubirán, Av. Vasco de Quiroga No. 15, Col. Belisario Domínguez Sección XVI, Tlalpan, Mexico City 14080, Mexico

[2] Departamento de Biología Molecular y Biotecnología, Instituto de Investigaciones Biomédicas, Universidad Nacional Autónoma de México, Av. Universidad 3000, Coyoacán, Mexico City 04510, Mexico

* Correspondence: euclides.avilac@incmnsz.mx

Abstract: Chronic infection by high-risk human papillomaviruses (HPV) and chronic inflammation are factors associated with the onset and progression of several neoplasias, including cervical cancer. Oncogenic proteins E5, E6, and E7 from HPV are the main drivers of cervical carcinogenesis. In the present article, we review the general mechanisms of HPV-driven cervical carcinogenesis, as well as the involvement of cyclooxygenase-2 (COX-2)/prostaglandin E$_2$ (PGE$_2$) and downstream effectors in this pathology. We also review the evidence on the crosstalk between chronic HPV infection and PGE$_2$ signaling, leading to immune response weakening and cervical cancer development. Finally, the last section updates the current therapeutic and preventive options targeting PGE$_2$-derived inflammation and HPV infection in cervical cancer. These treatments include nonsteroidal anti-inflammatory drugs, prophylactic and therapeutical vaccines, immunomodulators, antivirals, and nanotechnology. Inflammatory signaling pathways are closely related to the carcinogenic nature of the virus, highlighting inflammation as a co-factor for HPV-dependent carcinogenesis. Therefore, blocking inflammatory signaling pathways, modulating immune response against HPV, and targeting the virus represent excellent options for anti-tumoral therapies in cervical cancer.

Keywords: cervical cancer; human papillomavirus; chronic inflammation; oncogenic proteins; cyclooxygenase-2; prostaglandin E$_2$; cervical cancer treatment

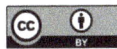

1. Introduction

Cancer encompasses a group of complex diseases characterized by uncontrolled growth, evasion of anti-growth signaling, resistance to cell death, and colonization of distant niches by malignant cells. Cancer develops by a progressive multistep process from normal diploid cells, which are spontaneously or carcinogen-transformed to cancer cells. These initial cancer cells without a distinctive phenotype progressively evolve towards a malignant phenotype by the driving force of DNA alterations or genetic instability [1]. Several factors are involved in the origin of cancer including chemical carcinogenesis, radiation, air pollution, nutritional factors, and viral infection, among others. In this regard, infections by a virus such as Epstein–Barr, human herpesvirus 8, hepatitis B and C viruses, human T-lymphotropic virus type 1 and Merkel cell polyomavirus are linked to Hodgkin lymphoma and Burkitt lymphoma, Kaposi's sarcoma, liver cancer, adult T-cell leukemia/lymphoma, and Merkel cell carcinoma, respectively [2]. Among causative viruses of cancer, human papillomaviruses (HPVs) are associated mainly with cervical cancer but also with neoplasias of the vulva, vagina, penis, anus, and oropharynx [2].

On the other hand, prostaglandin E$_2$ (PGE$_2$) is a lipid mediator of inflammation, which is one of the hallmarks of cancer [3]. Chronic inflammation promotes tumor development by enhancing survival, proliferation, and spreading of transformed cells while promoting tumor angiogenesis and evasion of tumor immune surveillance [3]. PGE$_2$ bioavailability and signaling are highly regulated processes, and disruption of this regulatory axis is related to various human cancers, including cervical cancer [4]. This review is focused on the molecular mechanisms of carcinogenesis driven by HPVs and the participation of PGE$_2$ signaling in cancer progression. Crosstalk between HPV infection and PGE$_2$ is also addressed in this review. Finally, therapeutic options in cervical cancer based on HPV and PGE$_2$ signaling are presented.

2. Cervical Cancer and Human Papillomavirus

Cervical cancer is by far the most clinically relevant HPV-related disease. In 2020, more than 600,000 women were diagnosed with cervical cancer worldwide, and about 342,000 women died. Accordingly, cervical cancer is the fourth most prevalent cancer among women globally, ranking after breast, colorectal, and lung cancer [5]. Although cervical cancer is still a disease with high mortality rates in developing countries, in high-income countries this type of cancer is one of the most preventable neoplasias, due to cytological screening of the cervix and prophylactic vaccination against HPV.

2.1. The Human Papillomavirus Life Cycle

HPVs are DNA viruses that probably represent the most prevalent sexually transmitted infection in both women and men worldwide. Based on their DNA sequence, more than 200 types of HPVs have been described; however, only a few HPV types are associated with health problems. HPVs are considered cutaneous or mucosal types according to their ability to infect epithelial cells of the skin or the inner lining of tissues. The last group of HPVs is important for cancer biology because they infect the lining of the mouth, respiratory tract, and anogenital epithelium. At least 20 HPVs are associated with lesions of the anogenital tract, which are further categorized as low-risk HPV (LR-HPVs types 6, 11, 42, 43 and 44, which cause benign warts) and high-risk HPVs (HR-HPVs types 16, 18, 31, 33, 34, 35, 39, 45, 51, 52, 56, 58, 59, 66, 68 and 70), which are associated with premalignant squamous lesions that are precursors of cancer [6]. HR-HPVs are detected in about 99% of cervical malignant lesions, HPV16 and HPV18 being responsible for at least 70% of all of them. Infection with an HR-HPV is necessary but not sufficient to cause cervical cancer because most HPV infections are efficiently cleared by the immune system without clinical disease.

HPVs are small non-enveloped double-stranded circular DNA viruses, in which only one of the DNA strands is transcribed. HPV DNA comprises approximately 8 kb organized into three functional regions: the early region encoding the non-structural proteins E1, E2, E4, E5, E6, and E7 that regulate viral gene expression and some of them, such as E1 and E2, also participate in DNA replication; the late region that encodes the structural proteins L1 and L2, needed for the viral capsid, and a long control region (LCR) that contains the regulatory sequences required for replication and transcription, namely, the origin of viral replication and the early promoter [7].

Although HPV replication requires E1 and E2 proteins, the participation of host proteins in this process are also required. HPVs infect only human epithelial cells, mainly keratinocytes. Cells located in the basal layer of the mucosa are the only cell type with the ability to divide and proliferate. This reservoir of basal cells is replenished by symmetric cell division of basal cells. However, asymmetric division of these cells generates two cells, one of them is used to renovate the basal cell population while the other one leaves the lower layer. Basal cells selected for terminal differentiation exit the cell cycle and stop DNA replication after they move out from the basal layer to the suprabasal layers. During this upward journey, cells acquire specialized properties and die when they arrive at the skin surface [8].

The HPV life cycle is closely linked with this renewal process occurring in the stratified squamous epithelium of the cervix. Because HPV infection is sexually transmitted, the viruses present in the anogenital region of HPV-infected men (mainly in the corona sulcus, glans, foreskin, and scrotum) are introduced in the inner female genital tract during sexual intercourse. HPVs gain access to the deepest layer via microabrasions or via hair follicles, finally reaching the single layer of epithelial cells located in the squamocolumnar junction between the endocervix and ectocervix. There, basal cells are infected by HPVs through the interaction of L1 capsid protein with heparan sulfate-containing proteoglycans which are thought to be the main HPV receptor [9]. In addition, keratinocyte-secreted laminin 5 [10] and cell adhesion α-6-integrin [11] also function as cellular co-receptors for HPVs. After specific binding on the keratinocyte cell surface, viral particles are slowly internalized by an actin cytoskeleton-dependent endocytic mechanism [12]. Inside basal cells, HPV capsid is disassembled, the viral genome is coated with L2 protein, packed inside transport vesicles, and delivered into the nucleus, whose envelope breaks down in early mitosis [13]. Like other DNA viruses, after mitosis and subsequent reformation of the nuclear membrane, the HPV genome-L2 protein complex harbored into the transport vesicles interact with promyelocytic leukemia nuclear bodies (also known as promyelocytic oncogenic domains), where transcription and replication take place [14,15].

In the initial phase of HPV replication, the viral genome in the form of episomes is maintained at a low copy number in infected basal cells [16]. HPV DNA replication requires the cooperation between the host DNA replication machinery and viral early proteins E1 and E2. HPV DNA replication starts with the binding of transcription factor E2 to specific sites located on LCR DNA, which results in the recruitment of E1 DNA helicase to the viral origin of replication, allowing the assembly of the DNA replication complex [17]. Initial infection with HPV is characterized by a low copy number of HPVs genomes (50–100 viral DNA copies per cell). An HPV persistent infection requires the production of a constant number of viral DNA in the nuclei of undifferentiated host cells during the cell cycle.

When HPV-infected basal cells move towards the epithelium surface, high levels of the HPV genome are synthesized, leading to the generation of progeny virions, which are sloughed from infected epithelia in the form of virion-laden squames. However, the HPV genome is often integrated into the host DNA in premalignant and malignant lesions of the cervix. HPV DNA integration represents a dead-end for the viral life cycle because infectious particles are no longer produced [6].

How does HPV maintain active DNA replication in arrested cell-cycle cells? HPVs have evolved successful strategies to actively replicate in infected growth-arrested host cells that are efficiently evading apoptotic signals. Among them, early proteins E5, E6, and E7 combined function are critical drivers of persistent viral infection and cellular transformation [18].

2.2. Mechanisms Underlying HPV-Driven Carcinogenesis

Unlike HPV E6 and E7 oncoproteins, little is known of the role of the E5 in the malignant transformation of the cervical epithelium. E5 is a multifunctional small hydrophobic polypeptide that is encoded by LR- and HR-HPVs and participates in key carcinogenesis points. Table 1 summarizes the role of high-risk HPV E5 on transformation, tumorigenesis, apoptosis, and immune modulation in cervical cancer. As noted, E5 oncoprotein contributes to cellular transformation driven by HPVs during the early stages of cervical carcinogenesis [19]. HPV DNA integration into the host's genome correlates with the loss of E2, E5, and increased expression of E6 and E7 oncoproteins [19].

Table 1. Summary of cancer-related processes triggered by high-risk HPV E5.

Process	References
HPV16 E5 triggers malignant transformation of murine keratinocytes	[20]
HPV16 E5 leads to cell growth in low serum and anchorage-independent growth of murine fibroblasts	[21]
HPV16 E5 stimulates the transforming activity of the epidermal growth factor receptor and lengthens receptor action by delaying its degradation	[22,23]
HPV16 E5 gene cooperates with E7 to stimulate cell proliferation and increases viral gene expression	[24]
HPV16 E5 enhances endothelin-1-induced keratinocyte growth	[25]
HPV16 E5 inhibits endocytic trafficking	[26]
HPV16 E5 impairs apoptosis in the early stages of viral infection in human keratinocytes	[27]
HPV16 E5 protects human foreskin keratinocytes from UV radiation-induced apoptosis	[28]
HPV16 E5 down-regulates surface HLA class I allowing persistent infection by avoiding host immune clearance	[29]
EGFR cooperates with HPV16 E5 to induce hyperplasia in mice	[30]
HPV16 E5 up-regulates COX-2 by a mechanism dependent on NF-kB and AP1	[31]
HPV16 E5 increases PTGER4 receptor for PGE$_2$ in cervical cancer cells	[32]
HPV16 E5 represses the expression of stress pathway genes -XBP-1 and COX-2 in genital keratinocytes	[33]
HPV16 E5 synergizes EGFR signaling to enhance cell cycle progression and down-regulation of p27	[34]
HPV16 E5 inhibits apoptosis by proteasome-dependent degradation of Bax in human cervical cancer cells	[35]
Expression of HPV16 E5 produces enlarged nuclei and polyploidy in human keratinocytes	[36]
HPV16 E5 modulates the expression of host microRNAs miR-146a, miR-203, and miR-324-5p, and their target genes	[37]
HPV16 E5 induces switching from FGFR2b to FGFR2c and epithelial–mesenchymal transition	[38]
HPV18 E5 supports cell cycle progression and impairs epithelial differentiation by modulating EGFR signaling	[39]
HPV16 E5 increases MET, a growth factor receptor critical for tumor progression in human keratinocytes	[40]
HPV18 E5 cooperates with E6 and E7 in promoting cell invasion and in modulating the cellular redox state	[41]

Both HR-HPV E6 and E7 are small proteins that cooperate together to keep HPV DNA replication and prevent apoptosis while inducing genome instability and immortalization of HPV-infected cells [7].

Transforming properties of HR-HPV E6 are closely linked to P53 activity, a tumor suppressor gene mutated in nearly half of human cancers [42]. P53 suppresses tumor development mainly by blocking the cellular proliferation of cells carrying damaged DNA and by induction of apoptosis in cancer cells. When DNA is damaged in proliferating cells, DNA repair is an essential process that prevents carcinogenesis. The lack of efficient DNA repair triggered by P53 and the suppression of apoptosis in HPV-infected cells are largely the main mechanisms of cellular transformation mediated by E6, resulting in damaged DNA accumulation and genomic instability [43].

Normal cells maintain very low levels of P53 protein through proteasomal degradation mainly by the action of E3 ligase murine double minute 2 (MDM2) [44] (Figure 1a). However, in response to genotoxic stress, several stimuli converge in the inhibition of MDM2, resulting in P53 accumulation in the nucleus. Activated P53, by both acetylation and phosphorylation, homotetramerizes and acts as a transcription factor that regulates genes involved in cell death, DNA repair, and cell cycle arrest, among others (Figure 1b). Hence, activation of the P53 pathway induces cell-cycle arrest at the G1 phase to provide an opportunity for cells to repair damaged DNA; however, when extensive DNA damage is detected, P53 activates apoptosis. HPV-infected cells cannot activate these anti-stress cellular processes because P53 protein levels are always insufficient (Figure 1c). HPV E6 binds to ubiquitin ligase E6-associated protein (E6AP), and this complex recruits P53, stimulating its ubiquitinylation and further degradation in the proteasome [45]. The P53 proteasomal degradation is not the only mechanism by which E6 abrogates P53 function. It was described that E6 reduces P53 transcriptional activity by targeting the coactivator CBP/p300 [46]. Thus, the presence of E6 on promoter regions switches CBP/p300 complex from an activating mode to a repressing state, leading to inhibition of P53-dependent transactivation [47]. Interestingly, in cells infected with types 5 and 8 HPV E6, the P53- and p300-dependent gene Ataxia Telangiectasia and Rad3-related (ATR), encoding for a phosphatidylinositol 3-kinase critical for the repair of UV-damaged DNA, is downregulated [48].

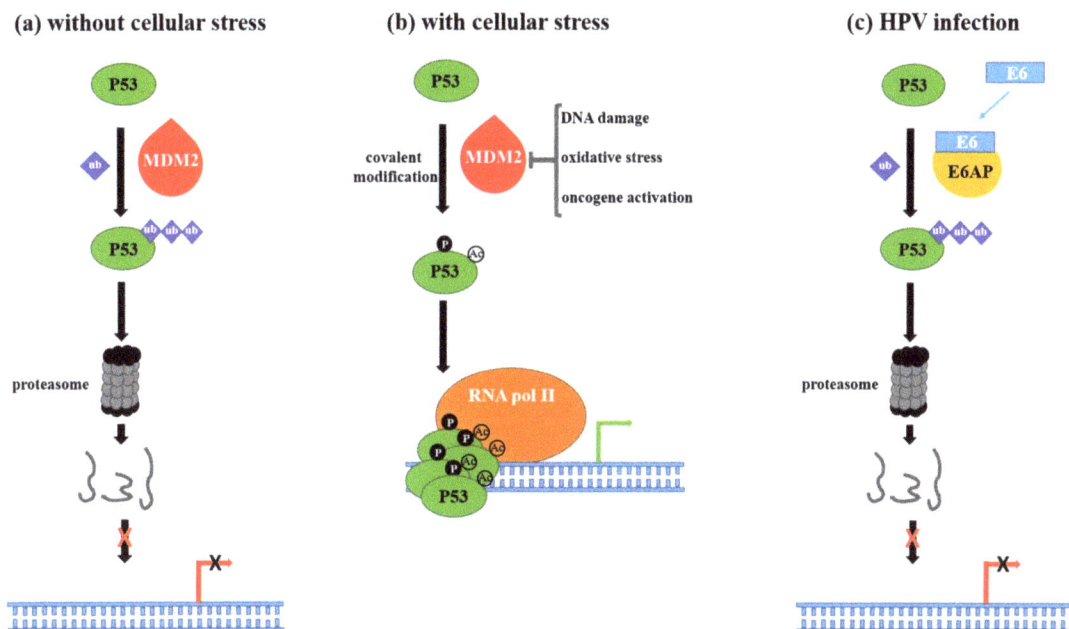

Figure 1. Role of P53 on normal cell physiology and during high-risk HPV infection. (**a**) In the absence of stressors, the coordinated action of MDM2 and proteasome maintain very low P53 bioavailability. (**b**) Stressor factors such as nutrient deprivation, genotoxic damage, and abnormal expression of oncogenes inhibit MDM2 activity while other cellular factors stabilize P53 by post-translational modification such as phosphorylation and acetylation. Acting as a homotetramer, P53 activates genes favoring DNA repair, apoptosis, and cell cycle arrest, among other processes involved in tumor development prevention. (**c**) Epithelial cells infected with HPV produce high levels of E6 oncogene, which binds E6AP. The complex E6AP-E6 targets P53 for degradation in the proteasome. Using this mechanism, E6 suppresses the protective response initiated by P53 against HPV infection. ub, ubiquitin; P, phosphorylation; Ac, acetylation.

Given the potential association of types 5 and 8 HPVs with non-melanoma skin cancer [49], it seems that E6 enhances the carcinogenic potential of UV radiation by downregulation of both P300 and ATR and the concomitant accumulation of thymine dimers increasing DNA mutation rates.

HPV E6 is also required to extend the life span indefinitely in infected keratinocytes. Immortalization properties of E6 are achieved by a range of cellular proteins. Both abrogation of the retinoblastoma protein (pRB) pathway and overexpression of telomerase reverse transcriptase (TERT) are the drivers for the immortalization of normal keratinocytes [50]. It was described in cervical cells that the TERT promoter is activated by E6 from oncogenic HPVs [51], contributing in this way to the increase in TERT's activity, needed for cervical carcinogenesis [52,53]. Another critical oncogene involved in the malignant transformation of the cervical epithelium is E7. This oncoprotein is an essential regulator of host transcription leading to cell cycle deregulation and immune evasion. E7 effects on host gene expression patterns are mediated by its interaction with several components of transcription and chromatin remodeling complexes, which are summarized in Table 2. Through these interactions, E7 exerts a broad impact on the host gene expression programs. Of particular importance is the interaction between E7 with members of the pRB family. pRB tumor suppressor is considered a key regulator of cellular processes such as cell cycle progression and apoptosis [54]. E7 targets pRB for proteasomal degradation [55], releasing the transcription factor E2F, which in turn activates genes needed for cell cycle progression into S-phase [56].

Table 2. Some interaction partners of high-risk HPV E7 oncoprotein.

Protein Name (Symbol, Common Name)	Consequence of Interaction with E7	Reference
Cyclin-dependent kinase inhibitor 1B (CDKN1B, p27)	A cyclin-dependent kinase inhibitor. Inactivation of p27 by E7 promotes cell cycle S phase entry	[57]
Cyclin E1 (CCNE1, cyclin E)	A modulator of the cell cycle that functions as a regulatory subunit of CDK2. Enhanced kinase activity mediated by E7 interaction favors cell cycle G1/S transition	[58]
Cyclin-dependent kinase inhibitor 1A (CDKN1A, p21)	Another cyclin-dependent kinase inhibitor. E7 interaction with p21 promotes pRB phosphorylation by activated CDK2-cyclin A, enabling cell cycle progression	[59]
TATA-box binding protein (TBP, TFIID)	A critical factor in transcription initiation. Interaction between E7 and TBP participates in the transformation of epithelial cells	[60]
Proteasome 26S subunit, ATPase 4 (PSMC4, S4 subunit of the 26S proteasome)	An ATPase essential for protein turnover by the 26S proteasome. Upon interaction with E7, this protein might participate in pRB degradation by 26S proteasome favoring in this way the cell cycle progression	[61]
Retinoblastoma (pRB) RB transcriptional corepressor like 1 (RBL1, p107) RB transcriptional corepressor like 2 (RBL2, p130)	Hypophosphorylated pRB, p107, and p130 tumor suppressors inhibit E2F-mediated transcription initiation. Interaction of these proteins with E7 alleviates transcriptional inhibition promoting premature entry into the S-phase of the cell cycle	[62]
Fork head box M1 (FOXM1, fork head domain transcription factor MPP2)	A transcription factor involved in cell proliferation regulation. E7 enhances the transactivation and transformation properties of matrix metallopeptidase (MMP)-2	[63]
POU class 5 homeobox 1 (POU5F1, OCT4)	OCT4 is a transcription factor essential for stem cell pluripotency and embryonic development. E7 expression in differentiated cells stimulates OCT4 activity	[64]
Interferon regulatory factor 1 (IRF1, IRF-1)	A tumor suppressor gene with transcriptional regulation activity involved in immune responses. E7 direct inactivation of IRF1 promotes immune evasion of HPV in cancer	[65]
E1A binding protein P300 (EP300, Transcriptional coactivator P300)	A general transcriptional coactivator. By binding to P300, E7 impaired transcriptional regulation	[66]
Lysine acetyltransferase 2B (KAT2B, PCAF)	Another general transcriptional coactivator. E7 interaction reduces acetyltransferase activity impairing transcriptional regulation	[67]
Cyclin A2 (CCNA2, cyclin A)	A critical cell cycle regulator whose function activates cyclin-dependent kinase 2 (CDK2). E7 promotes cell cycle transition through G1/S and G2/M by activation of CDK2/cyclin A	[68]

Table 2. Cont.

Protein Name (Symbol, Common Name)	Consequence of Interaction with E7	Reference
E2F transcription factor 6 (E2F6, transcription factor E2F6)	E2F6 is a transcription factor that negatively regulates transcription. Interaction between E2F6 and E7 abrogates inhibitory action of E2F6, which extends the S-phase	[69]
Rho GTPase activating protein 35 (ARHGAP35, p190RhoGAP)	A GTPase activating protein for RhoA. Binding of E7 alters actin cytoskeleton dynamics and cell migration	[70]

This mechanism and those summarized in Table 2 are responsible for the immortalization of HPV-infected cells and the induction of tumorigenesis.

Thus, early proteins E5, E6, and E7 encoded by HPVs play a pivotal role in the HPV life cycle and are required for the malignant transformation of the cervical epithelium by increasing host genomic instability and by blocking pivotal cell cycle checkpoints [18]. Other HPV proteins have a small contribution to cervical transformation. For instance, HPV16 E4 collapse the epithelial cell intermediate filament network in human keratinocytes by specific interaction with cytokeratins [71]. The cumulative sum of cellular alterations driven by HPV products leads to the onset of precancerous squamous lesions in the cervical tissue known as low-grade squamous intraepithelial lesions [LSIL, or cervical intraepithelial neoplasia grade I (CIN-I)], which can progress to high-grade squamous intraepithelial lesions [HSIL, a histological stage that encompasses the former entities CIN-2, CIN-3, moderate and severe dysplasia] and finally invasive squamous cell carcinoma [72]. Although the oncogenic role of HPV is well established, only a small number of HPV-infected women develop cervical cancer. Other cancer risk factors that promote persistent chronic HPV infection are cigarette smoking [73] and alcohol consumption [74]. Another cofactor for cancer development is chronic inflammation caused by HPV [75]. Chronic inflammation is considered a hallmark of human cancer, and proinflammatory factors are involved in cancer development [76].

3. Role of the Axis Cyclooxygenases/PGE$_2$ and Its Receptors in Normal Physiology and Cancer

PGE$_2$ exerts diverse physiologic and pathologic effects [77,78], regulating cellular processes in the immune [79], renal [80], cardiovascular [81], gastrointestinal [82,83], respiratory [84], and reproductive systems [85,86]. Additionally, PGE$_2$ evokes important actions in bone metabolism [87], hematopoiesis [88], and is a crucial mediator of inflammation, fever, and pain [89–92].

3.1. PGE$_2$ Biosynthesis and Metabolism

The prostaglandins (PGs) D2, E2, F2α, and I2 are eicosanoids that belong to the prostanoid family, which also includes thromboxanes (TXs) and prostacyclins. The basic chemical structure of prostanoids is a prostanoic acid with a cyclopentane ring and two carbon chains. The precursor molecule for these lipid mediators is arachidonic acid (AA), an essential polyunsaturated fatty acid that is stored in membrane phospholipids and released by the action of phospholipase A2 (PLA$_2$) (Figure 2) [93–95]. Several signals activate PLA$_2$, including phosphorylation by mitogen-activated protein kinase and an increase in intracellular calcium [96].

AA is afterward bis-dioxygenated by cyclooxygenase (COX) enzymes COX-1 and COX-2 (officially named prostaglandin endoperoxide synthases 1 and 2, respectively) to generate hydroperoxy endoperoxide PGG$_2$, which is then reduced to the intermediate prostaglandin H2 (PGH$_2$). COX-1 is constitutively expressed in most tissues and is responsible for the production of 'housekeeping' PGs that control a wide range of physiological effects, including maintaining homeostasis and gastrointestinal protection. On the other hand, COX-2 isoform expression is inducible at sites of inflammation and vascular trauma by a range of pro-inflammatory stimuli such as cytokines, growth factors, and ulcerogenic stimuli but particularly during infection and inflammation [97]. However, the COX-2 constitutive expression was also reported in selected organs in the absence of inflammation in the kidneys, gastrointestinal tract, and brain [98]. COX-2 expression is regulated mainly at the transcriptional level by inflammatory agents, cytokines, and growth factors [93].

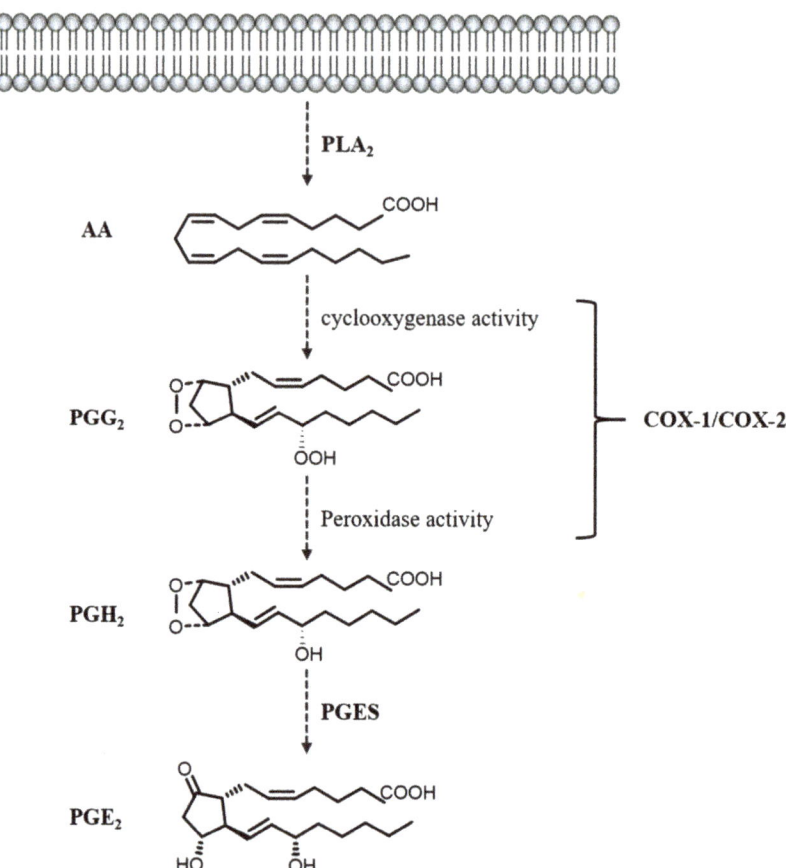

Figure 2. PGE_2 biosynthesis. Arachidonic acid (AA) is released from membrane phospholipids by cytoplasmic phospholipase A2 (PLA_2). The cyclooxygenase (COX) enzymes COX-1 and COX-2 convert AA to prostaglandin G2 (PGG_2) and then prostaglandin H2 (PGH_2). Subsequently, the enzyme PGE_2 synthase (PGES) converts PGH_2 to prostaglandin E2 (PGE_2).

Several specific isomerases and oxidoreductases convert PGH_2 to the different types of PGs, such as PGE_2, PGD_2, PGI_2, $PGF_{2\alpha}$, and TXA_2 [93–95]. Biosynthesis of these metabolites depends on the tissue type and stimulus; specifically, PGE_2, which is the most widely produced prostanoid in the body, is synthesized by PGE_2 synthases (PGES) in a broad range of cell types [99]. After its synthesis, PGE_2 is transported into the extracellular microenvironment by multidrug resistance-associated protein 4 [100,101]. PGE_2 is metabolized mainly by nicotinamide adenine dinucleotide (NAD+)-dependent 15-hydroxyprostaglandin dehydrogenase to generate 15-keto-prostaglandin E_2, which has significantly lower biological activity [102].

3.2. PGE$_2$ Receptors

PGE$_2$ performs its biological functions via interaction with four prostaglandin E receptor subtypes (PTGER1-4, also known as EP1-4) [103,104]. These receptors share around 30% sequence identity and belong to the G-protein-coupled, rhodopsin-type receptor superfamily [104]. PTGER1, PTGER2, PTGER3, and PTGER4 are located on human chromosomes 19, 14, 1, and 5, respectively [105–107]. The human PTGERs genes encode proteins of 402, 358, 390, and 488 amino acids with molecular masses of 42, 53, 43, and 53 kDa, respectively. PGE$_2$ binds PTGER1, PTGER2, PTGER3, and PTGER4 with Kd values of 21, 40, 3, and 11 nM, respectively [104]. All of them exhibit differences in tissue distribution, signal transduction, and expression regulation [104,108]. PGE$_2$ also has an affinity for other prostanoid receptors, such as the PGD$_2$ DP1 receptor, and the PGF$_{2\alpha}$ FP receptor [109].

Upon being activated by PGE$_2$, PTGER1 couples with G proteins and the Gαq subunit promotes the activation of phospholipase C (PLC), which hydrolyzes phosphatidylinositol 4,5-bisphosphate (PIP2) to diacylglycerol (DAG) and inositol 1,4,5-trisphosphate (IP3), leading to intracellular calcium mobilization and activation of protein kinase C (PKC) (Figure 3). Additionally, PKC activation induces desensitization of PTGER1, being PKC an important feedback regulator of the signal transduction of PTGER1 [110]. The PTGER1 activation also increases intracellular calcium mainly due to extracellular calcium influx through a pathway independent of PLC activation [110]. Both PTGER2 and PTGER4 are coupled to Gαs proteins to activate the adenylate cyclase (AC) enzyme increasing intracellular cyclic adenosine monophosphate (cAMP) levels (Figure 3) [103,104,111].

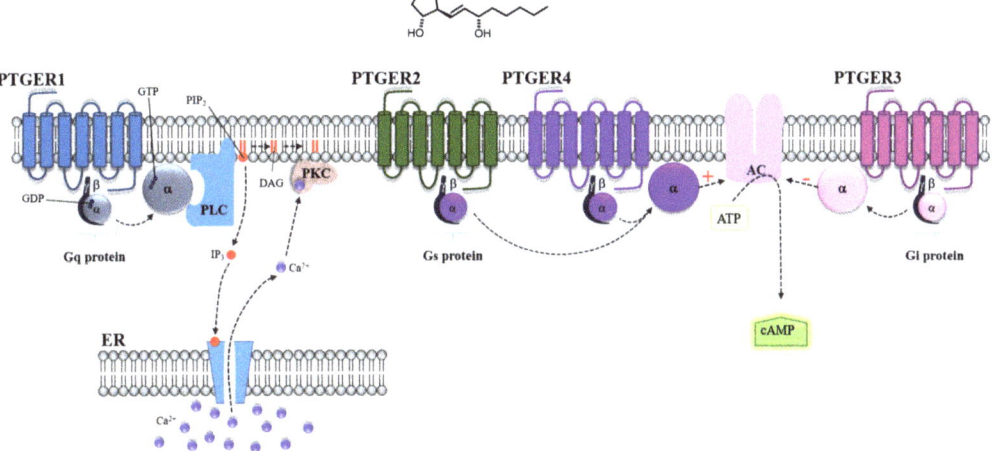

Figure 3. PGE$_2$ activates four receptors, PTGER1-4. Prostaglandin E$_2$ (PGE$_2$) binds to G protein-coupled receptors identified as PTGER1-4. The binding of PGE$_2$ to PTGER1 causes the exchange of guanosine diphosphate (GDP) for guanosine triphosphate (GTP) in the Gαq subunit allowing its dissociation from the βγ complex. The α subunit moves to phospholipase C (PLC) and activates it. This enzyme catalyzes the cleavage of the membrane phospholipid phosphatidylinositol 4,5-bisphosphate (PIP$_2$) to produce two intracellular second messenger diacylglycerol (DAG) and inositol 1,4,5-trisphosphate (IP3). IP3 binds to specific calcium (Ca^{2+}) channels releasing Ca^{2+} into the cytosol. Both IP3 and DAG contribute to activating protein kinase C (PKC). Regarding PTGER2 and PTGER4, the activation of adenylate cyclase (AC) by Gαs causes an increase in the intracellular cyclic adenosine monophosphate (cAMP) concentration formed from adenosine triphosphate (ATP). In contrast, the binding of PGE$_2$ to PTGER3 causes inhibition of the activity of AC, resulting in diminished production of cAMP through the Gαi subunit. The activation of PTGER receptors regulates many cellular processes.

Even though fewer intracellular cAMP formation has been reported in cells expressing PTGER4 than in those expressing PTGER2 [112], the desensitization and internalization of PGE_2-PTGER4 are faster than PGE_2-PTGER2 [113].

PTGER2 and PTGER4 activate multiple signaling pathways; PTGER2, besides causing AMP production and protein kinase A (PKA) activation, increases the epidermal growth factor receptor (EGFR) and Src through its association with β-arrestin1, this leading to the subsequent activation of H-Ras/extracellular signal-regulated kinases (ERK), and phosphatidylinositol 3 kinase (PI3K)/protein kinase B (AKT) [114]. PTGER4 also activates PI3K, causing ERK phosphorylation [115]. PTGER2 is implicated in beneficial and adverse roles in the central nervous system, female reproduction, vascular hypertension, tumorigenesis, and peripheral diseases [116,117]. PTGER4 activation is associated with ductus arteriosus closure and inflammation-associated bone resorption [117].

PTGER3 activation induces its coupling to Gαi proteins, which inhibit AC decreasing intracellular cAMP concentration [103,104,111] (Figure 3). However, the splicing variants of the PTGER3 are coupled to different signaling pathways that act to both increase or decrease cAMP levels [104]. PTGER3 plays a crucial role in several biological events, such as fever, gastric mucosal protection, pain hypersensitivity, kidney function, and anti-allergic response [117]. Interestingly, PTGER3 expression is associated as a prognostic marker for cervical cancer [118].

3.3. Role of the COXs/PGE$_2$/PTGERs Axis in Human Cancer

The axis COX-2/PGE_2/PTGERs is involved in cancer progression through multiple pathways that regulate fundamental oncogenic process as cell proliferation, metastasis, angiogenesis, immune evasion, and cell death (Table 3).

Malignancies linked to HPV infection as cervical cancer, present high levels of COX-1/COX-2 and elevated synthesis of PGE_2 [119,120]. In this regard, the incubation of HeLa cells with seminal plasma, which contains high levels of PGE_2, up-regulated COX-2 expression and mRNAs of PTGER1, PTGER2, and PTGER4 [121]. Interestingly, seminal plasma alters vascular function by enhanced expression of angiogenic chemokines, such as interleukin (IL)-8, and growth-regulated oncogene alpha by mechanisms dependent on EGFR/ERK/COX and nuclear factor-kappa B (NF-κB) [122]. PTGER2 expression increases while PTGER3 expression decreases during cervical neoplasia development [118,123], suggesting these receptors might be considered as positive and negative prognostic markers of cervical cancer lesions, respectively. PTGER2 expression is a prognostic factor for the overall survival in the subgroup of negative PTGER3, and high galectin-3 expressed cervical cancer patients [124]. PTGER3 signaling promotes the migration of cervical cancer cells through the modulation of the urokinase-type plasminogen activator receptor [125]. Hence, the COX-2/PGE_2/PTGERs axis plays an important role in the inflammatory environment seen in cervical cancer development.

Table 3. Participation of COX-2/PGE_2/PTGERs axis in human cancer.

Cancer Type	COX-2/PGE2/PTGER1-4	Tumorigenic Role	Factors and Associated Genes	References
Colorectal	COX-2/PGE_2/PTGER2	Angiogenesis	VEGF and Ang-2	[126,127]
Colon	COX-2/PGE_2/PTGER2	Tumor microenvironment	CXCL1, IL6, WNT (2, 2B, 5A), MMP12	[128]
Gastric	COX-2/PGE_2/PTGER4	Tumor microenvironment, metastasis	ADAM metalloproteases, EGFR ligands	[129]
	PTGER2/PTGER4	Cell growth inhibition		[130]

Table 3. Cont.

Cancer Type	COX-2/PGE2/PTGER1-4	Tumorigenic Role	Factors and Associated Genes	References
Cervical	PTGER2	Prognostic marker of disease		[123]
	COX-2/PGE$_2$/PTGER3	Metastasis	uPAR	[125]
	COX-2/PGE$_2$/PTGER4	Carcinogenesis		[32]
Lung	COX-2	Tumor microenvironment and inflammation	Cancer promoting cytokines	[131]
	COX-2/PGE$_2$/PTGER4	Cell migration		[132]
	COX-2/PGE$_2$/PTGER1	Cell proliferation and migration	ERK phosphorylation, β1 integrin activation	[133,134]
	COX-2/PGE$_2$/PTGER3	Cell migration	MMP 2-9 VEGF, TGFβ, p-Smad 2-3	[135]
Breast	COX-2	Metastasis	MMP1	[136]
		Chemoresistance	MFGE8, KLK5, and KLK7	[137]
	PTGER3	Prognostic factor for progression-free survival		[138]
	COX-2/PGE$_2$/PTGER2/PTGER4	Angiogenesis, cell proliferation and stemness	MMP 2-9	[139,140]
	Nuclear PTGER1	Good prognosis marker		[141]
Bladder	COX-2	Stemness	Oct3/4, CD44v6	[142]
Vulva	COX-2/PGE$_2$/PTGER4	Negative prognostic factor		[143]
Bone	COX-2	Cell migration		[144]
		Cell growth and progression, poor survival		[145]
Liver	COX-2	Activation of AKT and mTOR oncogenic pathways	AKT, TET1, MTOR, LTBP1, ADCY5 and PRKCZ	[146]
Prostate	COX-2/PGE$_2$/PTGER4	Cell proliferation and migration	RANKL, RUNX2, MMP 2-9	[147]
Oral squamous carcinoma	COX-2/PGE$_2$	Cell growth inhibition		[148]

4. Crosstalk between HPV Infection and PGE$_2$/PTGERs Signaling on Cancer Progression

A long-lasting infection can cause chronic inflammation, while inflammation by itself is responsible for causing as much as 25% of human cancers [149,150]. HPV may induce cancer through several mechanisms involving its viral oncoproteins, mainly E5, E6, and E7. These mechanisms produce a pro-tumorigenic environment that eventually can cause increased proliferation, inhibition of the host immune response, inactivation of tumor suppressor genes, mutations/immortalization, and malignant transformation, which are all considered hallmarks of cancer [151]. Notably, HPV carcinogenic mechanisms crosstalk with inflammatory pathways, favoring the tumorigenic process. Carcinogenic pathways of both the virus and inflammation intermingle at different points, involving distinct PGE$_2$ receptors and viral oncoproteins that activate specific signaling pathways, as described in detail as follows and in Figure 4.

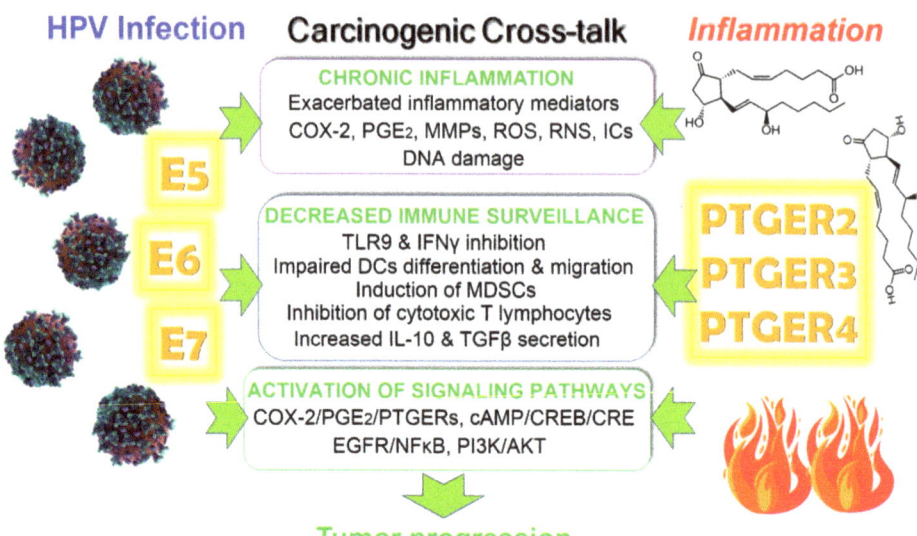

Figure 4. Crosstalk between HPV infection and PGE$_2$ signaling on cancer progression. Cervical neoplasia may be promoted by HPV infection or chronic inflammation, processes that greatly interact to fuel tumorigenesis. HPV viral oncoproteins E5, E6 and E7 produce chronic inflammation by up-regulating COX-2 expression and consequently prostaglandin E2 (PGE$_2$) production. HPV may also induce other inflammatory mediators such as reactive oxygen and nitrogen species (ROS, RNS), and PGE$_2$ receptors (PTGER) expression. Likewise, PTGER activation results in increased expression/release of inflammatory cytokines (ICs) and metalloproteinases, as well as COX-2 activity/expression. Notably, ROS and RNS may cause DNA damage, facilitating HPV–DNA integration. Another important oncogenic mechanism in cervical HPV-dependent neoplasia is immune response evasion. Viral oncoproteins can drive dendritic cells (DCs) and lymphocytes towards a protolerogenic phenotype, inhibiting the expression of Toll-like receptor 9 (TLR9), down-regulating ICs such as interferon-gamma (IFNγ) while up-regulating immunosuppressive cytokines, including interleukin-10 (IL-10) and transforming growth factor beta (TGFβ), allowing HPV to survive. Furthermore, increased inflammatory mediators were associated with the induction of immunosuppressive myeloid-derived suppressor cells (MDSCs). Finally, known signaling pathways involved in the crosstalk between HPV infection and inflammation include PI3K/AKT, the epidermal growth factor receptor (EGFR)/nuclear factor-kappa B (NF-κB), COX-2/PGE$_2$/PTGERs, and the cyclic AMP (cAMP)/cAMP-response element binding protein (CREB)/cAMP-responsive element (CRE).

4.1. Chronic Inflammation

The knowledge that chronic inflammation can predispose an individual to develop cancer is now well established. A variety of factors can cause chronic inflammation, including bacterial infections, oxidative stress, chemical insults, and viral agents. In the case of HPV infection of neoplastic cervical epithelial cells, the viral oncoproteins E6 and E7 produce chronic inflammation by up-regulating COX-2 expression, and therefore PGE$_2$ production [152]. The inductive effects of E6 and E7 were shown to be mediated by enhanced binding of activator protein-1 to the cAMP-responsive element (CRE) of the COX-2 promoter. E5 also up-regulates COX-2 expression but does so through EGFR/NF-κB signaling [31]. Moreover, the HPV E5 oncoprotein is known to induce the expression of the PTGER4 subtype in a cAMP-response element binding protein (CREB)/CRE-dependent pathway, potentiating in this way the proinflammatory activity of HPV [32]. Notably, HPV infection-dependent inflammation may generate reactive oxygen species (ROS) and nitrogen species (RNS), which can contribute to cancer initiation and progression by inducing

DNA damage. Indeed, it was proposed that ROS and RNS generated by infection-related inflammatory processes have the potential to create DNA strand breaks, facilitating HPV–DNA integration, and contributing in this manner to carcinogenesis [153,154]. Therefore, inflammation and oxidative stress are widely interconnected, being free radicals an active component of both HPV infection and inflammation processes [149].

On the other hand, in the case of inflammation-induced carcinogenesis, known proinflammatory mediators involved in this process include matrix metallopeptidases (MMPs), cytokines such as tumor necrosis factor-alpha (TNFα), diverse interleukins, and COX-2. In particular, proinflammatory cytokines' constant release activates signaling pathways that result in the formation of ROS and RNS [154]. Particularly in the setting of gynecological tumors, the COX-2-PGE$_2$-PTGERs signaling is the central inflammatory pathway involved in carcinogenesis [155]. In this regard, PTGER2/PTGER4 PGE$_2$ receptors are of clinical relevance in various tumors because of their involvement in stimulating COX-2 activity and/or expression and, consequently, PGE$_2$ production [119], converging in this manner with the effects of E6 and E7 oncoproteins. Due to PGE$_2$ being a recognized inflammatory prostaglandin, its role in maintaining chronic inflammation and creating an oncogenic environment is at sight. Indeed, inflammation is considered a cofactor in HPV-associated carcinogenesis [153]. PTGER2/PTGER4 mediate their effects on target cells via activating AC, increasing cAMP intracellular levels, which in turn activate the PKA pathway [121,155,156]. However, the PI3K/AKT signaling pathway was also linked to the PTGER2/PTGER4-triggered COX-2 transcriptional induction after PGE$_2$ stimulation of cancer cells [157].

4.2. Immune Response Evasion

In cervical cancer, immune evasion is of the greatest importance for HPV to persist and cause malignant transformation. Viral oncoproteins and inflammation can both cause a local protolerogenic immune response, converging in the modulation of the activity of antigen-presenting cells (APCs), such as DCs, which can polarize the immune response. A tolerogenic immune response may help tumor cells and viral agents escape the immune system, allowing them to survive and grow [158]. In this regard, E6 and E7 oncogenes integrated into the host DNA of their target cells produce transcription products that inhibit TLR9 expression in DCs, causing their impaired differentiation, and consequently, down-regulation of immune surveillance. These HPV16 oncoproteins induce NF-κB to translocate into the nucleus, down-regulating TLR9 expression [159]. TLR9 down-regulation by HPV E7 oncoprotein was also demonstrated in HPV16-positive keratinocytes and cervical cell lines, through a mechanism that combines epigenetic and transcriptional events [160,161]. TLRs are expressed on both immune and nonimmune cells and are important for host defense activation because they can sense pathogen-derived products. Specifically, TLR9 is involved in sensing double-stranded DNA, such as that from HPVs. Furthermore, HPV can inhibit interferon (IFN) synthesis and its antiviral duties through E6 and E7 oncoproteins [162,163].

Notably, E6 was also described to inhibit the migration of DCs by increasing PGE$_2$ in cervical lesions, which is another interconnecting point between HPV infection and PGE$_2$ signaling [164]. In addition, E5 and E7 may block the activation of T lymphocytes, thus, helping infected cells expressing these oncoproteins to escape cytotoxic T-lymphocytes attack [165].

On the other hand, infected cancer cells per se also contribute to polarizing the tumor immune milieu, as it was found that supernatants from HPV-transformed cell cultures contained IL-10 and transforming growth factor (TGFβ), both immunosuppressive cytokines, while the analysis of HPV-positive cervical cancer biopsies showed a predominant immunosuppressive expression profile [158].

In a similar manner, in the case of inflammation, although counterintuitive to the proinflammatory activity of PGE$_2$, this prostaglandin is known to promote immune tolerance through PTGER2 and PTGER3 receptors by inducing secretion of IL-10 in DCs [166].

Of note, upon PTGER2 and PTGER3 activation, the transcription factor CREB is phosphorylated. This suggests that both PTGER2 and PTGER3 induce cAMP mobilization, even though PTGER3 is typically associated with cAMP inhibition, as depicted in Figure 3. In addition, PTGER2 and PTGER4 are known to down-regulate the anti-tumor activity of PTGER-expressing natural killer cells, which are a type of cytotoxic T-lymphocytes (CTLs), by inhibiting their ability to kill tumor cells, cytokine synthesis, and chemotactic activity; thus, contributing to the pro-tumorigenic environment [167,168]. High PGE_2 levels and other inflammatory mediators were also associated with stimulation of COX-2 expression in monocytes, contributing to the induction and persistence of immunosuppressive myeloid-derived suppressor cells (MDSC), which highlights the central role of COX-2/PGE_2 signaling in tumor progression [169]. Indeed, MDSCs comprise a population of immature myeloid cells involved in suppressing antitumor immunity while stimulating cancer cell proliferation and tumor metastasis [170]. In particular, PGE_2, via PTGER2 and PTGER4 expressed on MDSCs, inhibits the development of CTLs, impairing T cell functions [171]. As mentioned earlier, PGE_2 is able to induce the rapid accumulation of cAMP, a process coupled with PTGER2/PTGER4 receptors [121]. This is very relevant to explaining the immunomodulatory effects of PGE_2, given the well-known immunosuppressive effects of cAMP [172].

Considering this all together, it is clear that the COX-2-PGE_2-PTGERs axis and cAMP/CREB signaling improve the oncogenic ability of HPV by promoting chronic inflammation in cervical cancer. In addition, the immunodepression caused by both HPV infection and inflammatory response is an additional pro-tumorigenic factor in cervical cancer progression. Thus, inflammation and immune modulation remain the main targets for therapies in cervical cancer.

5. Therapeutic Targeting of the COX/PGE_2 Axis in Cancer

COX enzymes are the primary target of non-steroidal anti-inflammatory drugs (NSAIDs), which are widely used to relieve pain, fever, and other inflammatory processes. These drugs are classified according to their selectivity into non-selective NSAIDS and COX-2-selective NSAIDs [97].

5.1. The Non-Selective NSAIDS as Antineoplastic Agents in Cervical Cancer

The non-selective NSAIDs inhibit both COX-1 and COX-2 enzymes, and it was demonstrated that their long-term use may decrease the risk of colorectal, esophageal, breast, lung, prostate, liver, skin, and cervical cancers [173], which is in accordance with the previously discussed oncogenic role of inflammation. Regarding cervical cancer, few studies have reported this relationship, and most of them include the use of aspirin, whose long-term use is associated with decreased risk of cervical cancer [174]. Indeed, aspirin inhibits cervical cancer cell proliferation and colony formation in a time- and concentration-dependent manner, induces apoptosis, alters cell cycle distribution, and inhibits EGFR downstream cell survival signaling pathways [175–177]. The combined treatment of aspirin with radiation decreases cervical cancer cell proliferation to a greater extent than each condition alone and induces apoptosis by bcl-2 repression and caspase-3 induction [176]. Ibuprofen inhibits the growth and induces apoptotic cell death in cervical cancer cells while having no significant cytotoxicity on non-cancerous cells [175,178]. Meclofenolic acid exhibits great toxicity in cervical cancer both in vitro and in vivo, showing a significant reduction in tumor growth and increased survival of tumor-bearing mice. Other non-selective NSAIDs such as sulindac and indomethacin also inhibit cervical cancer cell proliferation and colony formation in a time and concentration-dependent manner; while nimesulide shows partial cytotoxicity [176,179].

5.2. COX-2 Selective NSAIDs as Antineoplastic Agents in Cervical Cancer

In addition to its typical therapeutical effects, some selective COX-2 inhibitors have chemopreventive and chemotherapeutic effects [180]. The mechanism of action of celecoxib to induce apoptosis could be independent of COX-2 inhibition, and rather the apoptosis may be due to the activation of caspase-8 and -9 with Bid cleavage and the loss of mitochondrial membrane potential, using as a possible target NF-κβ [181]. In a pilot study, it was determined that treating cervical cancer patients with celecoxib (400 mg twice daily/10 days) decreased the expression of COX-2, Ki-67, PGE_2, and microvessel density in tumor biopsies [182]. Additionally, in a phase II randomized, double-blind placebo-controlled trial of celecoxib in patients with moderate and severe cervical dysplasia, the most of patients who received celecoxib had a good clinical response compared to the placebo group [183]. In another clinical trial carried out in patients with CIN-3 lesions and elevated serum vascular endothelial growth factor (VEGF) levels, the treatment with celecoxib showed greater regression than in the placebo group and decreased expression of COX-2 in cervical biopsies from treated patients was observed [184]. Moreover, the combinatorial effect of celecoxib with chemo- and radiotherapy have resulted in increased neoplastic cell sensitivity in different kinds of tumors [185,186], including patients with locally advanced cervical cancer in which the combination was associated with toxicity [187,188].

5.3. Corticosteroids in Cervical Cancer

Corticosteroids may inhibit the inflammatory process through modulating the transcription of anti-inflammatory and pro-inflammatory genes, including the down-regulation of COX-2 in monocytes and epithelial cells, so they are used to treat several inflammatory and immune diseases [189]. Taking into account the benefits of corticosteroids as anti-inflammatory agents in addition to their antiemetic effects, the synthetic corticosteroid dexamethasone was used as co-medication with radiotherapy in lymphoma and solid tumors [190]. Moreover, the corticosteroids protect cardiomyocytes from apoptosis induced by the cytotoxic doxorubicin, an antineoplastic drug known for its side effect of inducing cardiomyopathy [191]. While corticosteroids generally support therapy of lymphoid tumor cells, some studies describe interference of cancer therapy in cell lines of solid tumors. In this regard, dexamethasone inhibits cisplatin and 5-fluorouracil-induced apoptosis and promotes the growth of the majority of cells from solid tumors, but not of lymphoid cells [192]. Additionally, dexamethasone inhibits radiation-induced apoptosis in cervical carcinoma cell lines, which depends upon increased HPV E6 and E7; in contrast, the glucocorticoid had no effect on apoptosis of cells that either lack HPV or in which HPV E6 and E7 transcription is repressed by dexamethasone [193]. Part of the mechanism involved in dexamethasone-mediated proliferation and survival of cancer cells from solid tumors involves glucocorticoid receptor-mediated activation or suppression of target genes, modulation of the P53-dependent miR-145 expression in HPV-positive cervical cancer cells, and activation of HPV through the responsiveness of the upstream regulatory region (URR) of the virus [194,195]. The URR is responsible for the transcriptional regulation of the HPV major early promoter, which controls the expression of early genes of the virus, and interestingly, the URR of HPV18 is inducible by dexamethasone [195].

6. Targeting the Human Papillomavirus in Cancer

Epidemiological studies have shown the presence of HPV in up to 99% of cervical cancers and in a high percentage of other genital tract cancers [196]. Indeed, HPV is considered the main causative agent of genital tract cancers; offering a unique opportunity for infection prevention and treatment, which was addressed by the introduction of both prophylactic and therapeutic vaccines, among other treatments.

6.1. Preventing HPV Transmission Using Prophylactic Vaccines

Prophylactic vaccines are prepared using purified virus-like particles (VLPs) self-assembled by the major capsid protein L1, generating the recombinant proteins L1-VLPs, which are morphologically and immunologically similar to HPV virions, but that do not contain a viral genome. The L1-VLPs promote the generation of neutralizing antibodies directed against viral capsid proteins, blocking the adherence and internalization of HPV in the basal cells of the epithelium [197]. Several prophylactic vaccines were introduced into the market, including the bivalent, tetravalent, and nonavalent vaccines, named accordingly to the number of HPVs that can neutralize [196]. The bivalent vaccine is composed of the recombinant protein LI-VLPs of HPV16 and 18, the tetravalent contains LI-VLPs of HPV6, 11, 16, and 18, and the nonavalent is formed by LI-VLPs of HPV31, 33, 45, 52, 58, 6, 11, 16 and 18 [198]. Although prophylactic vaccines are effective in preventing HPV infection, they are not effective in eradicating it because they act by inducing neutralizing antibodies against L1 viral capsid protein, which is lost when HPV integrates into the host genome [196]. The problem that these vaccines have no therapeutic efficacy, the high demand for an efficient way to clear an established HPV infection, as well as the interest in the regression of precancerous and cancerous lesions have prompted the design of therapeutic vaccines [198].

6.2. Therapeutic Vaccines Targeting HPV Oncoproteins

Vaccines made against HPV oncoproteins may induce an immune response able to kill cervical cancer cells, representing a good therapeutic strategy and a promising treatment alternative to clear HR-HPV infections and associated malignancies. Among the proteins encoded by HPV, E6 and E7 are the main targets for the development of potential therapeutic vaccines due to: (1) their constitutive expression in infected cells, (2) both are functionally important for the development of tumor cells, and (3) they are readily recognized by the adaptive immune system as tumor antigens [196,198]. Other targets include E1, E2, and E5; however, their effectiveness is restricted because they are lost when the viral genome is integrated. Regarding HPV-therapeutic vaccines, several strategies were applied in their development, including the use of vectors (attenuated bacterial and viral)-based, nucleic acid-based, peptide/protein-based, and cellular-based vaccines [198].

6.2.1. HPV-Therapeutic Vaccines Designed with Bacterial Vectors

Bacterial vector vaccines utilize attenuated bacteria to transport genes of interest into the cell. The bacterial vectors include *Lactobacillus casei, Listeria monocytogenes, Lactobacillus lactis, Lactobacillus plantarum*, and *Salmonella* species.

A recombinant *Lactobacillus casei* modified HPV16 antigen E7 vaccine completed the phase I/IIa clinical trial in patients diagnosed with CIN-3 positive to HPV16; interestingly, nine of these patients experienced disease regression to CIN-2, while five patients remarkably regressed to LSIL [198]. Another immunotherapeutic bacterial vector is *Listeria monocytogenes* (Lm), which is internalized via phagocytosis by APCs, where they can follow two routes. In the first, most bacteria are killed, providing a source of antigens for major histocompatibility complex (MHC) class II for activation of CD4+ helper T-cell. In the second, Lm being inside of phagolysosome, secretes the listeriolysin O (LLO), a pore-forming toxin that destroys the phagosomal membrane allowing it to escape and enter the cytosol, where it can be degraded by the proteasome and loaded onto MHC class I molecules for presentation to cytotoxic T cells [199]. The natural mechanism of infection of Lm was used to develop the HPV therapeutic vaccine, Lm-LLO-E7 (ADXS11-001 or AXAL), engineering by fusing HPV16 antigen E7 with a non-hemolytic fragment of LLO. The recombinant Lm secrets the tumor-associated antigens HPV16 E7 as fusion proteins with Lm antigens allowing both MHC class I and class II antigen presentation [196]. In a first study, mice xenografted with a cancer cell line expressing HPV antigen E6 and E7 were vaccinated with recombinant Lm expressing E7 alone or E7 as a fusion protein with LLO. Remarkably, in the last case, complete regression of 75% of tumors was achieved [200]. Afterward, numerous preclinical studies demonstrated Lm-LLO-E7 ability to induce regression of HPV-transformed tumors, leading to its advancement into multiple clinical trials [200]. The safety of Lm-LLO-E7 was evaluated in fifteen patients with metastatic, refractory, or recurrent invasive carcinoma of the cervix (ICC); the study showed that a live-attenuated Lm is safe to be administrated to late-stage ICC patients and a reduction in total tumor size was observed in four patients [201]. After the promising safe results of this clinical trial, multiple clinical trials followed, among them NCT02853604, an active phase III study of ADXS11-001 administered following chemo-radiation as adjuvant treatment for high-risk locally advanced cervical cancer, designed to compare the disease-free survival (study completion on October 2024, https://www.clinicaltrials.gov/ct2/results?cond=cervical+cancer&term=ADXS11-001+&cntry=&state=&city=&dist; accessed on 1 August 2022). The GTL001 vaccine was designed to induce a T-cell immune response to HPV16 and HPV18 and prevent the development of high-grade lesions in infected women who still have normal cervical cytology or minor abnormalities [202]. This vaccine was engineered by fusing HPV16 and HPV18 antigen E7 proteins with the catalytically inactive AC from *Bordetella pertussis* [203]. *Bordetella pertussis* secrets the AC-E7 protein fusion, which binds to the $\alpha M\beta 2$ integrin receptor on the cell membrane of DCs and delivers its N-terminal catalytic AC domain into the cytoplasm, whose characteristic is used as the vector for antigen delivery into APC and subsequent antigen presentation [204].

6.2.2. HPV-Therapeutic Vaccines Designed with Viral Vectors

Viral vectors are able to infect a variety of cell types and efficiently express encoded antigens, which makes them attractive candidates for the development of therapeutic HPV vaccines. Among the potential vectors evaluated in the development of therapeutic vaccines are vaccinia virus, adenovirus, adeno-associated virus and alphavirus [205].

Vaccinia virus is used to deliver E6 and E7 antigens for therapeutic HPV vaccination. Among the therapeutic vaccinia based-vaccine developed to treat genital cancers is the tissue-antigen HPV vaccine (TA-HPV), which expresses modified forms of E6 and E7 fusion proteins from HPV16 and HPV18, whose safety, immunogenicity, and efficacy were confirmed in patients with clinical early and late-stage of cervical cancer as well as vulval intraepithelial neoplasia and vaginal intraepithelial neoplasia [206–208]. The clinical benefits of this vaccine were enhanced by combining it with other therapeutic vaccines [209,210], local treatments such as surgery (NCT00002916), or immunomodulators (NCT00788164). Other vaccinia-based vaccine expresses LLO fused to HPV16 E7, which induces a strong immune response and causes the regression of established HPV16 immortalized tumors in C57BL/6 mice [211]. Modified Vaccinia Ankara (MVA) virus serves as a powerful vector system for developing vaccines against cancer, such as cervical cancer [212]. At this point, a recombinant vaccine expressing the MVA virus and the bovine papilloma virus E2 (MVA-E2) was created [213]. The orthotopic injection of MVA-E2 in murine models arrested tumor growth or promoted tumor regression [213,214]. Similarly, in clinical studies, direct injection of MVA-E2 virus particles in precancerous lesions of the cervix, anus, vulva, urethra, and uterus promoted their regression or complete elimination [215–217]. Additionally, the treated patients exhibited viral load reduction or even total clearance, and induction of long-lasting immune cytotoxic response correlating with no lesion recurrence [217]. Another recombinant MVA virus-based vaccine is MVA–HPV–IL2 (TG4001/R3484), which is engineered to express HPV16 E6, E7, and IL-2. The immunization of CIN-2/3 patients with this vaccine exhibited HPV16 clearance after 6 months of vaccination, and at 12 months, seven out of eight patients had no signs of CIN-2/3 relapse or HPV16 infection [218]. Likewise, the vaccination of mice with a replication-deficient adenovirus vector expressing calreticulin-HPV16 E7 fusion protein induced a stronger E7-specific immune response, inhibited tumor growth in pre-vaccinated mice xenografted with E7-expressing TC-1 cells, generating long-term memory against E7 and in established tumors resulted in complete tumor regression in all animals [219].

6.2.3. Nucleic Acid-Based Vaccines against HPV

Nucleic acid vaccines are a method of immunization where DNA or mRNA sequences are delivered into the body to generate proteins, mimicking pathogens' antigens to stimulate immune response [220]. VGX-3100 is a DNA-based vaccine consisting of two DNA plasmids containing codon-optimized sequences corresponding to the E6 and E7 genes of

HPV16 and HPV18, whose safety, tolerability, efficacy, immunogenicity, and durability of response, were assessed in patients with HPV-related pre-cancerous conditions. VGX-3100 can drive the induction of robust immune responses to antigens from HR-HPV serotypes and could contribute to HPV16 and HPV18 elimination with complete histopathological regression of the dysplastic infectious process [221–223]. Other DNA-based vaccines targeting multiple HPV types are GX188E and pBI-1, which have completed phase I clinical trials exhibiting positive results regarding tolerance, CIN regression, and HPV clearance [224]. Regarding GX188E, it was demonstrated that electroporation-enhanced immunization with this vaccine, preferentially targeting HPV antigens to DCs, elicits a significant E6/E7-specific IFNγ producing a T-cell response in all evaluated CIN-3 patients [225,226]. Although different types of therapeutic vaccines exist, the best results have been achieved with MVA-E2, VGX-3100, GX-188E, and pBI-11. Particularly, MVA-E2 and VGX-3100 have reached phase III trials; however, their licenses are not yet authorized for marketing [224]. Other DNA-based vaccines candidates have also demonstrated a good safety and efficacy profile, including pNGVL4a-Sig/E7(detox)/HSP70 and pNGVL4a-CRT/E7(detox) [198].

6.2.4. Peptide/Protein-Based Vaccines against HPV

Peptide-based vaccines have the potential to induce cellular immune responses mainly by the induction of cytotoxic T cells, with the capacity to recognize non-auto immunogenic cancer antigens eliminating malignant cells [227]. The peptide-based vaccine HPV-16-SLP consists of nine HPV16 E6 and four HPV16 E7 synthetic long peptides (SLP), whose immunogenicity and efficacy were investigated in HPV16-induced high-grade vulvar, vaginal, CIN, and pre-malignant disorders of the uterine cervix. Several clinical trials determined that the clinical responses to HPV-16-SLP correlated with the strength of HPV 16-specific T-cell immunity [228–232]. A clinical trial carried out in patients with HPV16 dependent vulval intraepithelial neoplasia (VIN) grade 3 exhibited increased clinical response according to the time elapsed after the last vaccination, and approximately 50% of them ended displaying a complete response, which correlated with kinetics and phenotype of induced T-cell responses [228,229]. Another peptide-based vaccine is PepCan, which consists of four synthetic peptides covering the HPV16 E6 protein and Candida skin test reagents as an adjuvant, whose safety and biological response was demonstrated in a clinical trial carried out in patients with CIN-2/3 lesions. This study demonstrated that the vaccine is safe while inducing a detectable immune response to E6 in 65% of the patients [233]. TA-CIN is a fusion protein vaccine that incorporates HPV-16 L2, E6, and E7, for the treatment of HPV16-associated genital disease. Vaccination of healthy volunteers with TA-CIN administrated without adjuvants reported no serious adverse events [234] and induction of L2-specific serum antibodies that neutralized several papillomavirus species [235]. The combination of TA-CIN with adjuvants elicited protective humoral and cell-mediated immunity to a greater extent than TA-CIN alone [236]. To date, a current pilot clinical trial is assessing the safety and feasibility of intramuscular administration of the TA-CIN vaccine as adjuvant therapy for patients with a history of HPV16-associated cervical cancer (NCT02405221).

These vaccines typically have increased stability during storage and transport as compared to DNA vaccines; however, they induce lower immunogenicity and poor stability in vivo, which remain their major drawbacks [227]. Additionally, other vaccines are currently under investigation, including DC-based vaccines, tumor cell-based vaccines, and T cell-based vaccines [205].

7. Immunomodulators

Imiquimod, an imidazoquinoline amine, is an immunomodulator approved for the treatment of external anogenital warts, small superficial basal cell carcinoma, and other malignancies [237,238]. Imiquimod activates innate and adaptive immune responses through activation of the TLR7, leading to inflammatory cell infiltration within the application area and apoptosis of diseased tissue [238]. The low patient compliance and high recurrence rate are significant problems for the treatment of genital warts by imiquimod; therefore, the combined use of this drug with therapeutic vaccines was proposed. Regarding this, a phase I clinical trial is currently studying the pNGVL4a-Sig/E7 (detox)/HSP70 DNA and TA-HPB vaccines side effects, the best dose scheme and clinical outcome when given with or without imiquimod in CIN-3 patients. The final data collection date for the primary outcome measure is expected in July 2023 (NCT00788164). In another phase I clinical trial, topic imiquimod was combined with GTL001 vaccine in patients infected with HPV16 or HPV18 with normal cytology, showing an acceptable safety profile and good antigen-specific cellular immune response [202]. In addition, a similar clinical trial determined that topical imiquimod with GTL001 vaccination induced antigen-specific CD8+ T cell responses leading to tumor regression in a murine model [203]. Co-administration of imiquimod with TA-CIN in VIN patients was investigated in a phase II clinical trial, showing significant infiltration of CD4+ and CD8+ T-cells in lesion responders at week 20 of treatment while complete lesion regression in 63% of patients was found at week 52 [239].

8. Chemical Antivirals

HPV DNA replication is an attractive target for HPV antivirals because its inhibition would result in fewer genomes available for viral protein synthesis and integration, a critical step in the development of HPV-dependent cancers [240]. Several studies and clinical trials have identified and demonstrated the robust anti-HPV potential of certain acyclic nucleoside phosphonates, antivirals targeting proteins encoded by HPV, and other host proteins utilized by HPV as targets of antiviral therapy [198].

8.1. Acyclic Nucleoside Phosphonates

Among the acyclic nucleoside phosphonates, cidofovir and adefovir are acyclic analogs of the corresponding monophosphates of deoxycytidine and deoxyadenosine. The active dephosphorylated forms of these antivirals are deoxynucleoside triphosphate analogs, potent inhibitors of viral DNA polymerases, reducing viral DNA synthesis [241]. Cidofovir has broad-spectrum antiviral against cytomegalovirus, herpes viruses, poxviruses, and papilloma viruses [241]. In HPV16 transformed keratinocytes lacking a viral DNA polymerase, cidofovir suppressed cell proliferation in a dose-dependent manner, induced DNA fragmentation, reduced P21 levels, and inhibited cell cycle progression in S-phase [242]. In cervical carcinoma and head and neck squamous cell carcinoma cell lines, cidofovir reduced E6 and E7 expression, induced P21, P53, and pRB accumulation, promoted the cell cycle arrest, reduced cyclin A, induced antiproliferative activity, triggered programmed cell death and radio-sensitized HPV-positive cells [243,244]. Cidofovir exhibited antiproliferative effects in HPV-positive and negative tumor cells, through its incorporation into DNA, causing its damage [245]. In vivo studies demonstrated significant tumor reduction with cidofovir in nude mice xenografted with HPV-positive cervical cancer cells [246]. Clinical trials have evaluated topical cidofovir in the treatment of patients with CIN and VIN, where the 60.8% and 46.1% of patients, respectively, were free of malignancy [247]. The antitumoral effect of cidofovir was also evaluated in combination with chemotherapy and radiotherapy, among others. In a phase I clinical trial carried out in patients with stage IB-IVA cervical cancer, it was determined that cidofovir (5 mg/kg/week) combined with chemo-radiotherapy appeared well tolerable and yielded significant tumor regressions [248]. On the other hand, some pro-drugs of adefovir and tenofovir showed significantly more antiproliferative activity against SiHa (HPV16), HeLa (HPV18), and C33A (HPV negative) cervical cancer cells, in comparison to their parent compounds [241].

8.2. Other Antivirals Targeting HPV Proteins Interaction

HPV-E1 and -E2 proteins are excellent targets for developing antivirals; on one side, HPV-E1 is an ATPase and helicase required for viral DNA replication, while on the other hand, E2 is required for transcription activation and repression. E2 recruits E1 at the beginning of replication, forming a ternary complex with viral DNA and the inhibition of this interaction blocks viral DNA replicating activity [17]. The indandiones are capable to inhibit E1–E2 protein interaction, acting by binding to the E2 N-terminal transactivation domain, the same protein region that interacts with E1. These antivirals display potent activity against E2 proteins of HPV6 and HPV11 [249]. Other compounds that inhibit HPV protein interaction are biphenylsulfonacetic acid and its derivatives, which are competitive inhibitors of the ATPase activity of HPV6 E1 helicase, inhibiting ATP hydrolysis by an allosteric mechanism involving tyrosine 486 [250].

9. Therapeutic Strategy against Cervical Cancer Using Nanoparticles and Gene Therapy

Nanotechnology is the approach to manufacturing nanoparticles, nanotubes, nanosheets, and nanorods, with a size from 1 to 100 nm in at least one dimension [251]. The development of nanotechnology drew attention to be used in medicine, with the idea of inserting nanorobots into patients to treat several diseases, including cancer [252]. The application of nanotechnology in cancer is named nano-oncology, which includes both diagnosis and therapeutic, employing nanomaterials that increase drug absorption, delivery, specificity, efficacy, and decreased side effects [252]. In cervical cancer, nanotechnology is being explored to enhance early diagnosis and improve treatment and vaccine efficacy; while HPV vaccines are usually delivered by intramuscular injection, nanotechnology offers a new approach for delivering vaccines by microneedles patch that efficiently delivers the vaccines into the epidermis and dermis region, which contain many Langerhans and DCs [251]. The microneedle array contains the vaccine antigen in the form of solution or suspension encapsulated in nanoparticles that induces a robust immune response [253]. Regarding this, in preclinical studies, the HPV vaccine Gardasil was intradermally delivered by Nanopatch, which comprises 10,000 micro projections/cm^2 each 250 μm long, enhancing the antigenicity of the vaccine [254]. Additionally, in different preclinical studies, the efficacy of nanoparticles loaded with siRNA against E6 and/or E7 HPV oncoproteins was evaluated [255,256]. One of them assessed the efficacy of chitosan/HPV16 E7 siRNA nanoparticles, which were efficiently delivered into CaSki cervical cells and were observed to induce apoptosis [255]. Moreover, nanoparticles co-loaded with paclitaxel and E7 siRNA were developed with the aim to be simultaneously delivered to preclinical models of cervical cancer showing synergistic anti-tumor effect [257].

10. Conclusions

Standard treatments for advanced cervical cancer include surgery, radiotherapy, and chemotherapy, some of which are invasive and others have adverse side effects. In HPV-related malignancies such as cervical cancer, the COX-2–PGE_2–PTGERs inflammatory signaling pathway, together with the cAMP/CREB/CRE cascade, are closely intermingled with the carcinogenic nature of the virus, highlighting inflammation as a co-factor for HPV-dependent carcinogenesis. Furthermore, the attenuation of the immune response caused by both the virus and inflammatory mediators represents an additional pro-tumorigenic process involved with cervical cancer development. Therefore, inflammation and immune modulation remain the main targets for anti-tumoral therapies in cervical cancer. In this regard, accessible therapeutic options for cervical cancer treatment and prevention have been developed in the last years. For instance, anti-inflammatory drugs constitute an excellent therapeutic strategy in cervical cancer patients. Indeed, it was suggested that some of these drugs may be re-purposed as antineoplastic agents, such as aspirin and celecoxib. On the other hand, HPV infection is considered the leading causative agent of genital tract cancers, representing an attractive therapeutic target for preventing and treating cervical cancer. Prophylactic vaccines against HPV made with recombinant DNA technology have been very effective in preventing persistent HPV infection and lesions that lead to cervical cancer. Highly immunogenic prophylactic vaccines induce a strong humoral immune response with the production of HPV-neutralizing antibodies that inhibit viral infection. The development of therapeutic vaccines for cervical cancer is based on activating cellular immunity against cancer cells instead of neutralizing antibodies. Among the different therapeutic vaccines developed against cervical cancer, the best results were achieved with MVA-E2, VGX-3100, GX-188E, and pBI-11. Particularly, MVA-E2 and VGX-3100 have reached the phase III trial; however, they have not been licensed for use yet. Additionally, the clinical benefits of HPV-therapeutic vaccines were enhanced by combining them with each other and local treatments or immunomodulators such as Imiquimod. The potency of therapeutic vaccines has been increased in preclinical studies employing nanotechnology, such as in the case of Nanopatch, which delivers a Gardasil prophylactic vaccine intradermally using microneedles. Finally, another way to target HPV is through antivirals, resulting in fewer genomes available for viral protein synthesis and integration, a critical step in the development of HPV-dependent cancers.

Author Contributions: J.G.-Q. wrote the section dedicated to the therapeutic and preventive options targeting inflammation derived by both prostaglandin E_2 and HPV infection in cervical cancer, made the concluding section, gave feedback on all other sections and had oversight of the overall article. B.V.-A. wrote the section on the role of the cyclooxygenases, prostaglandin E_2 synthesis and PTGER receptors in human cancer with a focus on cervical malignancies and made Table 3. R.G.-B. wrote the section dedicated to the role of the cyclooxygenases, prostaglandin E_2 synthesis and PTGER receptors in normal human physiology and drew Figures 2 and 3. L.D. wrote the section on the crosstalk between prostaglandin E_2 signaling and HPV infection on cervical cancer progression and drew Figure 4. E.A. conceived the outline of the review, wrote the synopsis, wrote the abstract, wrote the introductory section dedicated to the HPV infection, drew Figure 1 and made Tables 1 and 2; gave feedback on all other sections and had oversight of the overall article. All authors read and gave feedback on all sections, and approved the final version of the review. All authors have read and agreed to the published version of the manuscript.

Funding: This work was partially supported by Instituto Nacional de Ciencias Médicas y Nutrición Salvador Zubirán, grant number BRE-2848 (E.A.).

Institutional Review Board Statement: Not applicable.

Informed Consent Statement: Not applicable.

Data Availability Statement: Not applicable.

Acknowledgments: This review is part of the academic work of B. V. A. who is a student from Doctorado en Ciencias Biológicas, Universidad Nacional Autónoma de México (UNAM) and is receiving a fellowship from Consejo Nacional de Ciencia y Tecnología (CONACyT, México).

Conflicts of Interest: The authors declare no conflict of interest.

Abbreviations

AA	Arachidonic acid
AC	Adenylate cyclase
AKT	Protein kinase B
APC	Antigen-presenting cells
ATR	Ataxia Telangiectasia and Rad3-related
cAMP	Cyclic adenosine monophosphate
CIN	Cervical intraepithelial neoplasia
COX	Cyclooxygenase
CRE	cAMP-responsive element
CREB	cAMP-response element binding protein
CTL	Cytotoxic T-lymphocytes
DAG	Diacylglycerol
DC	Dendritic cells
EGFR	Epidermal growth factor receptor
ERK	Extracellular signal-regulated kinase
HPV	Human papillomavirus
HSIL	High-grade squamous intraepithelial lesion
IC	Inflammatory cytokines
ICC	Invasive carcinoma of the cervix

IFNγ	Interferon-gamma
IL	Interleukin
IP3	Inositol 1,4,5-trisphosphate
LCR	Long control region
LLO	Listeriolysin O
Lm	Listeria monocytogenes
LSIL	Low-grade squamous intraepithelial lesion
MDSCs	Myeloid-derived suppressor cells
MHC	Major histocompatibility complex
MMP	Matrix metallopeptidase
mTOR	Mammalian target of rapamycin
MVA	Modified Vaccinia Ankara
NF-κB	Nuclear factor-kappa B
NSAIDS	Non-steroidal anti-inflammatory drugs
PGE$_2$	Prostaglandin E$_2$
PGES	Prostaglandin E$_2$ synthase
PI3K	Phosphatidylinositol 3-kinase
PIP2	Phosphatidylinositol 4,5-bisphosphate
PKA	Protein kinase A
PKC	Protein kinase C
PLA$_2$	Phospholipase A2
PLC	Phospholipase C
PTGER	Prostaglandin E$_2$ receptor
pRB	Retinoblastoma protein
RNS	Reactive nitrogen species
ROS	Reactive oxygen species
SLP	Synthetic long peptides
TERT	Telomerase reverse transcriptase
TGFβ	Transforming growth factor-beta
TLR	Toll-like receptor
TNFα	Tumor necrosis factor-alpha
TX	Thromboxane
URR	Upstream regulatory region
VEGF	Vascular endothelial growth factor
VIN	Vulval intraepithelial neoplasia
VLPs	Virus-like particles

References

1. Duesberg, P.; Li, R. Multistep carcinogenesis: A chain reaction of aneuploidizations. *Cell Cycle* **2003**, *2*, 202–210. [CrossRef] [PubMed]
2. Chen, C.J.; Hsu, W.L.; Yang, H.I.; Lee, M.H.; Chen, H.C.; Chien, Y.C.; You, S.L. Epidemiology of virus infection and human cancer. *Recent Results Cancer Res.* **2014**, *193*, 11–32. [CrossRef] [PubMed]
3. Colotta, F.; Allavena, P.; Sica, A.; Garlanda, C.; Mantovani, A. Cancer-related inflammation, the seventh hallmark of cancer: Links to genetic instability. *Carcinogenesis* **2009**, *30*, 1073–1081. [CrossRef] [PubMed]
4. Finetti, F.; Travelli, C.; Ercoli, J.; Colombo, G.; Buoso, E.; Trabalzini, L. Prostaglandin E2 and Cancer: Insight into Tumor Progression and Immunity. *Biology* **2020**, *9*, 434. [CrossRef] [PubMed]
5. Arbyn, M.; Weiderpass, E.; Bruni, L.; de Sanjose, S.; Saraiya, M.; Ferlay, J.; Bray, F. Estimates of incidence and mortality of cervical cancer in 2018: A worldwide analysis. *Lancet Glob. Health* **2020**, *8*, e191–e203. [CrossRef]
6. Schiffman, M.; Castle, P.E.; Jeronimo, J.; Rodriguez, A.C.; Wacholder, S. Human papillomavirus and cervical cancer. *Lancet* **2007**, *370*, 890–907. [CrossRef]
7. Graham, S.V. Human papillomavirus: Gene expression, regulation and prospects for novel diagnostic methods and antiviral therapies. *Future Microbiol.* **2010**, *5*, 1493–1506. [CrossRef]
8. Graham, S.V. Keratinocyte Differentiation-Dependent Human Papillomavirus Gene Regulation. *Viruses* **2017**, *9*, 245. [CrossRef]
9. Shafti-Keramat, S.; Handisurya, A.; Kriehuber, E.; Meneguzzi, G.; Slupetzky, K.; Kirnbauer, R. Different heparan sulfate proteoglycans serve as cellular receptors for human papillomaviruses. *J. Virol.* **2003**, *77*, 13125–13135. [CrossRef]

10. Culp, T.D.; Budgeon, L.R.; Marinkovich, M.P.; Meneguzzi, G.; Christensen, N.D. Keratinocyte-secreted laminin 5 can function as a transient receptor for human papillomaviruses by binding virions and transferring them to adjacent cells. *J. Virol.* **2006**, *80*, 8940–8950. [CrossRef]
11. Yoon, C.S.; Kim, K.D.; Park, S.N.; Cheong, S.W. Alpha(6) Integrin is the main receptor of human papillomavirus type 16 VLP. *Biochem. Biophys. Res. Commun.* **2001**, *283*, 668–673. [CrossRef]
12. Schelhaas, M.; Shah, B.; Holzer, M.; Blattmann, P.; Kuhling, L.; Day, P.M.; Schiller, J.T.; Helenius, A. Entry of human papillomavirus type 16 by actin-dependent, clathrin- and lipid raft-independent endocytosis. *PLoS Pathog.* **2012**, *8*, e1002657. [CrossRef]
13. Popa, A.; Zhang, W.; Harrison, M.S.; Goodner, K.; Kazakov, T.; Goodwin, E.C.; Lipovsky, A.; Burd, C.G.; DiMaio, D. Direct binding of retromer to human papillomavirus type 16 minor capsid protein L2 mediates endosome exit during viral infection. *PLoS Pathog.* **2015**, *11*, e1004699. [CrossRef]
14. Day, P.M.; Baker, C.C.; Lowy, D.R.; Schiller, J.T. Establishment of papillomavirus infection is enhanced by promyelocytic leukemia protein (PML) expression. *Proc. Natl. Acad. Sci. USA* **2004**, *101*, 14252–14257. [CrossRef]
15. Guion, L.G.; Sapp, M. The Role of Promyelocytic Leukemia Nuclear Bodies During HPV Infection. *Front. Cell. Infect. Microbiol.* **2020**, *10*, 35. [CrossRef]
16. Doorbar, J.; Quint, W.; Banks, L.; Bravo, I.G.; Stoler, M.; Broker, T.R.; Stanley, M.A. The biology and life-cycle of human papillomaviruses. *Vaccine* **2012**, *30* (Suppl. S5), F55–F70. [CrossRef]
17. Sanders, C.M.; Stenlund, A. Recruitment and loading of the E1 initiator protein: An ATP-dependent process catalysed by a transcription factor. *EMBO J.* **1998**, *17*, 7044–7055. [CrossRef]
18. Valle, G.F.; Banks, L. The human papillomavirus (HPV)-6 and HPV-16 E5 proteins co-operate with HPV-16 E7 in the transformation of primary rodent cells. *J. Gen. Virol.* **1995**, *76 Pt 5*, 1239–1245. [CrossRef]
19. Venuti, A.; Paolini, F.; Nasir, L.; Corteggio, A.; Roperto, S.; Campo, M.S.; Borzacchiello, G. Papillomavirus E5: The smallest oncoprotein with many functions. *Mol. Cancer* **2011**, *10*, 140. [CrossRef]
20. Leptak, C.; Ramon y Cajal, S.; Kulke, R.; Horwitz, B.H.; Riese, D.J., 2nd; Dotto, G.P.; DiMaio, D. Tumorigenic transformation of murine keratinocytes by the E5 genes of bovine papillomavirus type 1 and human papillomavirus type 16. *J. Virol.* **1991**, *65*, 7078–7083. [CrossRef]
21. Leechanachai, P.; Banks, L.; Moreau, F.; Matlashewski, G. The E5 gene from human papillomavirus type 16 is an oncogene which enhances growth factor-mediated signal transduction to the nucleus. *Oncogene* **1992**, *7*, 19–25. [PubMed]
22. Pim, D.; Collins, M.; Banks, L. Human papillomavirus type 16 E5 gene stimulates the transforming activity of the epidermal growth factor receptor. *Oncogene* **1992**, *7*, 27–32. [PubMed]
23. Straight, S.W.; Herman, B.; McCance, D.J. The E5 oncoprotein of human papillomavirus type 16 inhibits the acidification of endosomes in human keratinocytes. *J. Virol.* **1995**, *69*, 3185–3192. [CrossRef] [PubMed]
24. Bouvard, V.; Matlashewski, G.; Gu, Z.M.; Storey, A.; Banks, L. The human papillomavirus type 16 E5 gene cooperates with the E7 gene to stimulate proliferation of primary cells and increases viral gene expression. *Virology* **1994**, *203*, 73–80. [CrossRef]
25. Venuti, A.; Salani, D.; Poggiali, F.; Manni, V.; Bagnato, A. The E5 oncoprotein of human papillomavirus type 16 enhances endothelin-1-induced keratinocyte growth. *Virology* **1998**, *248*, 1–5. [CrossRef]
26. Thomsen, P.; van Deurs, B.; Norrild, B.; Kayser, L. The HPV16 E5 oncogene inhibits endocytic trafficking. *Oncogene* **2000**, *19*, 6023–6032. [CrossRef]
27. Kabsch, K.; Alonso, A. The human papillomavirus type 16 E5 protein impairs TRAIL- and FasL-mediated apoptosis in HaCaT cells by different mechanisms. *J. Virol.* **2002**, *76*, 12162–12172. [CrossRef]
28. Zhang, B.; Spandau, D.F.; Roman, A. E5 protein of human papillomavirus type 16 protects human foreskin keratinocytes from UV B-irradiation-induced apoptosis. *J. Virol.* **2002**, *76*, 220–231. [CrossRef]
29. Ashrafi, G.H.; Haghshenas, M.R.; Marchetti, B.; O'Brien, P.M.; Campo, M.S. E5 protein of human papillomavirus type 16 selectively downregulates surface HLA class I. *Int. J. Cancer* **2005**, *113*, 276–283. [CrossRef]
30. Genther Williams, S.M.; Disbrow, G.L.; Schlegel, R.; Lee, D.; Threadgill, D.W.; Lambert, P.F. Requirement of epidermal growth factor receptor for hyperplasia induced by E5, a high-risk human papillomavirus oncogene. *Cancer Res.* **2005**, *65*, 6534–6542. [CrossRef]
31. Kim, S.H.; Oh, J.M.; No, J.H.; Bang, Y.J.; Juhnn, Y.S.; Song, Y.S. Involvement of NF-kappaB and AP-1 in COX-2 upregulation by human papillomavirus 16 E5 oncoprotein. *Carcinogenesis* **2009**, *30*, 753–757. [CrossRef]
32. Oh, J.M.; Kim, S.H.; Lee, Y.I.; Seo, M.; Kim, S.Y.; Song, Y.S.; Kim, W.H.; Juhnn, Y.S. Human papillomavirus E5 protein induces expression of the EP4 subtype of prostaglandin E2 receptor in cyclic AMP response element-dependent pathways in cervical cancer cells. *Carcinogenesis* **2009**, *30*, 141–149. [CrossRef]
33. Sudarshan, S.R.; Schlegel, R.; Liu, X. The HPV-16 E5 protein represses expression of stress pathway genes XBP-1 and COX-2 in genital keratinocytes. *Biochem. Biophys. Res. Commun.* **2010**, *399*, 617–622. [CrossRef]
34. Pedroza-Saavedra, A.; Lam, E.W.; Esquivel-Guadarrama, F.; Gutierrez-Xicotencatl, L. The human papillomavirus type 16 E5 oncoprotein synergizes with EGF-receptor signaling to enhance cell cycle progression and the down-regulation of p27(Kip1). *Virology* **2010**, *400*, 44–52. [CrossRef]
35. Oh, J.M.; Kim, S.H.; Cho, E.A.; Song, Y.S.; Kim, W.H.; Juhnn, Y.S. Human papillomavirus type 16 E5 protein inhibits hydrogen-peroxide-induced apoptosis by stimulating ubiquitin-proteasome-mediated degradation of Bax in human cervical cancer cells. *Carcinogenesis* **2010**, *31*, 402–410. [CrossRef]

36. Hu, L.; Potapova, T.A.; Li, S.; Rankin, S.; Gorbsky, G.J.; Angeletti, P.C.; Ceresa, B.P. Expression of HPV16 E5 produces enlarged nuclei and polyploidy through endoreplication. *Virology* **2010**, *405*, 342–351. [CrossRef]
37. Greco, D.; Kivi, N.; Qian, K.; Leivonen, S.K.; Auvinen, P.; Auvinen, E. Human papillomavirus 16 E5 modulates the expression of host microRNAs. *PLoS ONE* **2011**, *6*, e21646. [CrossRef]
38. Ranieri, D.; Belleudi, F.; Magenta, A.; Torrisi, M.R. HPV16 E5 expression induces switching from FGFR2b to FGFR2c and epithelial-mesenchymal transition. *Int. J. Cancer* **2015**, *137*, 61–72. [CrossRef]
39. Wasson, C.W.; Morgan, E.L.; Muller, M.; Ross, R.L.; Hartley, M.; Roberts, S.; Macdonald, A. Human papillomavirus type 18 E5 oncogene supports cell cycle progression and impairs epithelial differentiation by modulating growth factor receptor signalling during the virus life cycle. *Oncotarget* **2017**, *8*, 103581–103600. [CrossRef]
40. Scott, M.L.; Coleman, D.T.; Kelly, K.C.; Carroll, J.L.; Woodby, B.; Songock, W.K.; Cardelli, J.A.; Bodily, J.M. Human papillomavirus type 16 E5-mediated upregulation of Met in human keratinocytes. *Virology* **2018**, *519*, 1–11. [CrossRef]
41. Hochmann, J.; Parietti, F.; Martinez, J.; Lopez, A.C.; Carreno, M.; Quijano, C.; Boccardo, E.; Sichero, L.; Moller, M.N.; Mirazo, S.; et al. Human papillomavirus type 18 E5 oncoprotein cooperates with E6 and E7 in promoting cell viability and invasion and in modulating the cellular redox state. *Mem. Inst. Oswaldo Cruz* **2020**, *115*, e190405. [CrossRef] [PubMed]
42. Hollstein, M.; Sidransky, D.; Vogelstein, B.; Harris, C.C. p53 mutations in human cancers. *Science* **1991**, *253*, 49–53. [CrossRef] [PubMed]
43. Aubrey, B.J.; Kelly, G.L.; Janic, A.; Herold, M.J.; Strasser, A. How does p53 induce apoptosis and how does this relate to p53-mediated tumour suppression? *Cell Death Differ.* **2018**, *25*, 104–113. [CrossRef] [PubMed]
44. Haupt, Y.; Maya, R.; Kazaz, A.; Oren, M. Mdm2 promotes the rapid degradation of p53. *Nature* **1997**, *387*, 296–299. [CrossRef]
45. Scheffner, M.; Takahashi, T.; Huibregtse, J.M.; Minna, J.D.; Howley, P.M. Interaction of the human papillomavirus type 16 E6 oncoprotein with wild-type and mutant human p53 proteins. *J. Virol.* **1992**, *66*, 5100–5105. [CrossRef]
46. Zimmermann, H.; Degenkolbe, R.; Bernard, H.U.; O'Connor, M.J. The human papillomavirus type 16 E6 oncoprotein can down-regulate p53 activity by targeting the transcriptional coactivator CBP/p300. *J. Virol.* **1999**, *73*, 6209–6219. [CrossRef]
47. Thomas, M.C.; Chiang, C.M. E6 oncoprotein represses p53-dependent gene activation via inhibition of protein acetylation independently of inducing p53 degradation. *Mol. Cell* **2005**, *17*, 251–264. [CrossRef]
48. Wallace, N.A.; Robinson, K.; Howie, H.L.; Galloway, D.A. HPV 5 and 8 E6 abrogate ATR activity resulting in increased persistence of UVB induced DNA damage. *PLoS Pathog.* **2012**, *8*, e1002807. [CrossRef]
49. Hasche, D.; Vinzon, S.E.; Rosl, F. Cutaneous Papillomaviruses and Non-melanoma Skin Cancer: Causal Agents or Innocent Bystanders? *Front. Microbiol.* **2018**, *9*, 874. [CrossRef]
50. Kiyono, T.; Foster, S.A.; Koop, J.I.; McDougall, J.K.; Galloway, D.A.; Klingelhutz, A.J. Both Rb/p16INK4a inactivation and telomerase activity are required to immortalize human epithelial cells. *Nature* **1998**, *396*, 84–88. [CrossRef]
51. Van Doorslaer, K.; Burk, R.D. Association between hTERT activation by HPV E6 proteins and oncogenic risk. *Virology* **2012**, *433*, 216–219. [CrossRef] [PubMed]
52. Oh, S.T.; Kyo, S.; Laimins, L.A. Telomerase activation by human papillomavirus type 16 E6 protein: Induction of human telomerase reverse transcriptase expression through Myc and GC-rich Sp1 binding sites. *J. Virol.* **2001**, *75*, 5559–5566. [CrossRef] [PubMed]
53. Nakano, K.; Watney, E.; McDougall, J.K. Telomerase activity and expression of telomerase RNA component and telomerase catalytic subunit gene in cervical cancer. *Am. J. Pathol.* **1998**, *153*, 857–864. [CrossRef]
54. Weinberg, R.A. The retinoblastoma protein and cell cycle control. *Cell* **1995**, *81*, 323–330. [CrossRef]
55. Boyer, S.N.; Wazer, D.E.; Band, V. E7 protein of human papilloma virus-16 induces degradation of retinoblastoma protein through the ubiquitin-proteasome pathway. *Cancer Res.* **1996**, *56*, 4620–4624.
56. Shan, B.; Lee, W.H. Deregulated expression of E2F-1 induces S-phase entry and leads to apoptosis. *Mol. Cell. Biol.* **1994**, *14*, 8166–8173. [CrossRef]
57. Zerfass-Thome, K.; Zwerschke, W.; Mannhardt, B.; Tindle, R.; Botz, J.W.; Jansen-Durr, P. Inactivation of the cdk inhibitor p27KIP1 by the human papillomavirus type 16 E7 oncoprotein. *Oncogene* **1996**, *13*, 2323–2330.
58. McIntyre, M.C.; Ruesch, M.N.; Laimins, L.A. Human papillomavirus E7 oncoproteins bind a single form of cyclin E in a complex with cdk2 and p107. *Virology* **1996**, *215*, 73–82. [CrossRef]
59. Funk, J.O.; Waga, S.; Harry, J.B.; Espling, E.; Stillman, B.; Galloway, D.A. Inhibition of CDK activity and PCNA-dependent DNA replication by p21 is blocked by interaction with the HPV-16 E7 oncoprotein. *Genes Dev.* **1997**, *11*, 2090–2100. [CrossRef]
60. Massimi, P.; Pim, D.; Banks, L. Human papillomavirus type 16 E7 binds to the conserved carboxy-terminal region of the TATA box binding protein and this contributes to E7 transforming activity. *J. Gen. Virol.* **1997**, *78 Pt 10*, 2607–2613. [CrossRef]
61. Berezutskaya, E.; Bagchi, S. The human papillomavirus E7 oncoprotein functionally interacts with the S4 subunit of the 26 S proteasome. *J. Biol. Chem.* **1997**, *272*, 30135–30140. [CrossRef]
62. Lee, J.O.; Russo, A.A.; Pavletich, N.P. Structure of the retinoblastoma tumour-suppressor pocket domain bound to a peptide from HPV E7. *Nature* **1998**, *391*, 859–865. [CrossRef]
63. Luscher-Firzlaff, J.M.; Westendorf, J.M.; Zwicker, J.; Burkhardt, H.; Henriksson, M.; Muller, R.; Pirollet, F.; Luscher, B. Interaction of the fork head domain transcription factor MPP2 with the human papilloma virus 16 E7 protein: Enhancement of transformation and transactivation. *Oncogene* **1999**, *18*, 5620–5630. [CrossRef]

64. Brehm, A.; Ohbo, K.; Zwerschke, W.; Botquin, V.; Jansen-Durr, P.; Scholer, H.R. Synergism with germ line transcription factor Oct-4: Viral oncoproteins share the ability to mimic a stem cell-specific activity. *Mol. Cell. Biol.* **1999**, *19*, 2635–2643. [CrossRef]
65. Park, J.S.; Kim, E.J.; Kwon, H.J.; Hwang, E.S.; Namkoong, S.E.; Um, S.J. Inactivation of interferon regulatory factor-1 tumor suppressor protein by HPV E7 oncoprotein. Implication for the E7-mediated immune evasion mechanism in cervical carcinogenesis. *J. Biol. Chem.* **2000**, *275*, 6764–6769. [CrossRef]
66. Bernat, A.; Avvakumov, N.; Mymryk, J.S.; Banks, L. Interaction between the HPV E7 oncoprotein and the transcriptional coactivator p300. *Oncogene* **2003**, *22*, 7871–7881. [CrossRef]
67. Avvakumov, N.; Torchia, J.; Mymryk, J.S. Interaction of the HPV E7 proteins with the pCAF acetyltransferase. *Oncogene* **2003**, *22*, 3833–3841. [CrossRef]
68. He, W.; Staples, D.; Smith, C.; Fisher, C. Direct activation of cyclin-dependent kinase 2 by human papillomavirus E7. *J. Virol.* **2003**, *77*, 10566–10574. [CrossRef]
69. McLaughlin-Drubin, M.E.; Huh, K.W.; Munger, K. Human papillomavirus type 16 E7 oncoprotein associates with E2F6. *J. Virol.* **2008**, *82*, 8695–8705. [CrossRef]
70. Todorovic, B.; Nichols, A.C.; Chitilian, J.M.; Myers, M.P.; Shepherd, T.G.; Parsons, S.J.; Barrett, J.W.; Banks, L.; Mymryk, J.S. The human papillomavirus E7 proteins associate with p190RhoGAP and alter its function. *J. Virol.* **2014**, *88*, 3653–3663. [CrossRef]
71. Doorbar, J.; Ely, S.; Sterling, J.; McLean, C.; Crawford, L. Specific interaction between HPV-16 E1-E4 and cytokeratins results in collapse of the epithelial cell intermediate filament network. *Nature* **1991**, *352*, 824–827. [CrossRef]
72. Nayar, R.; Wilbur, D.C. The Bethesda System for Reporting Cervical Cytology: A Historical Perspective. *Acta Cytol.* **2017**, *61*, 359–372. [CrossRef]
73. Giuliano, A.R.; Sedjo, R.L.; Roe, D.J.; Harri, R.; Baldwi, S.; Papenfuss, M.R.; Abrahamsen, M.; Inserra, P. Clearance of oncogenic human papillomavirus (HPV) infection: Effect of smoking (United States). *Cancer Causes Control* **2002**, *13*, 839–846. [CrossRef]
74. Oh, H.Y.; Seo, S.S.; Kim, M.K.; Lee, D.O.; Chung, Y.K.; Lim, M.C.; Kim, J.Y.; Lee, C.W.; Park, S.Y. Synergistic effect of viral load and alcohol consumption on the risk of persistent high-risk human papillomavirus infection. *PLoS ONE* **2014**, *9*, e104374. [CrossRef]
75. Boccardo, E.; Lepique, A.P.; Villa, L.L. The role of inflammation in HPV carcinogenesis. *Carcinogenesis* **2010**, *31*, 1905–1912. [CrossRef]
76. Coussens, L.M.; Werb, Z. Inflammation and cancer. *Nature* **2002**, *420*, 860–867. [CrossRef]
77. Gerritsen, M.E. Physiological and pathophysiological roles of eicosanoids in the microcirculation. *Cardiovasc. Res.* **1996**, *32*, 720–732. [CrossRef]
78. Narumiya, S. Physiology and pathophysiology of prostanoid receptors. *Proc. Jpn. Academy. Ser. B Phys. Biol. Sci.* **2007**, *83*, 296–319. [CrossRef]
79. Diao, G.; Huang, J.; Zheng, X.; Sun, X.; Tian, M.; Han, J.; Guo, J. Prostaglandin E2 serves a dual role in regulating the migration of dendritic cells. *Int. J. Mol. Med.* **2021**, *47*, 207–218. [CrossRef]
80. Li, Y.; Wei, Y.; Zheng, F.; Guan, Y.; Zhang, X. Prostaglandin E2 in the Regulation of Water Transport in Renal Collecting Ducts. *Int. J. Mol. Sci.* **2017**, *18*, 2539. [CrossRef]
81. Bryson, T.D.; Harding, P. Prostaglandin E2 EP receptors in cardiovascular disease: An update. *Biochem. Pharmacol.* **2022**, *195*, 114858. [CrossRef] [PubMed]
82. Heeney, A.; Rogers, A.C.; Mohan, H.; Mc Dermott, F.; Baird, A.W.; Winter, D.C. Prostaglandin E2 receptors and their role in gastrointestinal motility—Potential therapeutic targets. *Prostaglandins Other Lipid Mediat.* **2021**, *152*, 106499. [CrossRef] [PubMed]
83. Dey, I.; Lejeune, M.; Chadee, K. Prostaglandin E2 receptor distribution and function in the gastrointestinal tract. *Br. J. Pharmacol.* **2006**, *149*, 611–623. [CrossRef] [PubMed]
84. Tilley, S.L.; Hartney, J.M.; Erikson, C.J.; Jania, C.; Nguyen, M.; Stock, J.; McNeish, J.; Valancius, C.; Panettieri, R.A., Jr.; Penn, R.B.; et al. Receptors and pathways mediating the effects of prostaglandin E2 on airway tone. *Am. J. Physiol. Lung Cell. Mol. Physiol.* **2003**, *284*, L599–L606. [CrossRef]
85. Robertson, R.P. Molecular regulation of prostaglandin synthesis Implications for endocrine systems. *Trends Endocrinol. Metab. TEM* **1995**, *6*, 293–297. [CrossRef]
86. Niringiyumukiza, J.D.; Cai, H.; Xiang, W. Prostaglandin E2 involvement in mammalian female fertility: Ovulation, fertilization, embryo development and early implantation. *Reprod. Biol. Endocrinol. RBE* **2018**, *16*, 43. [CrossRef]
87. Li, M.; Thompson, D.D.; Paralkar, V.M. Prostaglandin E(2) receptors in bone formation. *Int. Orthop.* **2007**, *31*, 767–772. [CrossRef]
88. Durand, E.M.; Zon, L.I. Newly emerging roles for prostaglandin E2 regulation of hematopoiesis and hematopoietic stem cell engraftment. *Curr. Opin. Hematol.* **2010**, *17*, 308–312. [CrossRef]
89. Kalinski, P. Regulation of immune responses by prostaglandin E2. *J. Immunol.* **2012**, *188*, 21–28. [CrossRef]
90. Kawahara, K.; Hohjoh, H.; Inazumi, T.; Tsuchiya, S.; Sugimoto, Y. Prostaglandin E2-induced inflammation: Relevance of prostaglandin E receptors. *Biochim. Biophys. Acta* **2015**, *1851*, 414–421. [CrossRef]
91. Kawabata, A. Prostaglandin E2 and pain—An update. *Biol. Pharm. Bull.* **2011**, *34*, 1170–1173. [CrossRef]
92. Coceani, F.; Akarsu, E.S. Prostaglandin E2 in the pathogenesis of fever. An update. *Ann. N. Y. Acad. Sci.* **1998**, *856*, 76–82. [CrossRef]
93. Smith, W.L.; Dewitt, D.L. Prostaglandin endoperoxide H synthases-1 and -2. *Adv. Immunol.* **1996**, *62*, 167–215. [CrossRef]
94. Sreeramkumar, V.; Fresno, M.; Cuesta, N. Prostaglandin E2 and T cells: Friends or foes? *Immunol. Cell Biol.* **2012**, *90*, 579–586. [CrossRef]

95. Samuelsson, B.; Goldyne, M.; Granstrom, E.; Hamberg, M.; Hammarstrom, S.; Malmsten, C. Prostaglandins and thromboxanes. *Annu. Rev. Biochem.* **1978**, *47*, 997–1029. [CrossRef]
96. Gijon, M.A.; Leslie, C.C. Regulation of arachidonic acid release and cytosolic phospholipase A2 activation. *J. Leukoc. Biol.* **1999**, *65*, 330–336. [CrossRef]
97. Hawkey, C.J. COX-1 and COX-2 inhibitors. *Best Pract. Res. Clin. Gastroenterol.* **2001**, *15*, 801–820. [CrossRef]
98. Kirkby, N.S.; Chan, M.V.; Zaiss, A.K.; Garcia-Vaz, E.; Jiao, J.; Berglund, L.M.; Verdu, E.F.; Ahmetaj-Shala, B.; Wallace, J.L.; Herschman, H.R.; et al. Systematic study of constitutive cyclooxygenase-2 expression: Role of NF-kappaB and NFAT transcriptional pathways. *Proc. Natl. Acad. Sci. USA* **2016**, *113*, 434–439. [CrossRef]
99. Smith, W.L.; Marnett, L.J.; DeWitt, D.L. Prostaglandin and thromboxane biosynthesis. *Pharmacol. Ther.* **1991**, *49*, 153–179. [CrossRef]
100. Ritter, C.A.; Jedlitschky, G.; Meyer zu Schwabedissen, H.; Grube, M.; Kock, K.; Kroemer, H.K. Cellular export of drugs and signaling molecules by the ATP-binding cassette transporters MRP4 (ABCC4) and MRP5 (ABCC5). *Drug Metab. Rev.* **2005**, *37*, 253–278. [CrossRef]
101. Kochel, T.J.; Reader, J.C.; Ma, X.; Kundu, N.; Fulton, A.M. Multiple drug resistance-associated protein (MRP4) exports prostaglandin E2 (PGE2) and contributes to metastasis in basal/triple negative breast cancer. *Oncotarget* **2017**, *8*, 6540–6554. [CrossRef]
102. Na, H.K.; Park, J.M.; Lee, H.G.; Lee, H.N.; Myung, S.J.; Surh, Y.J. 15-Hydroxyprostaglandin dehydrogenase as a novel molecular target for cancer chemoprevention and therapy. *Biochem. Pharmacol.* **2011**, *82*, 1352–1360. [CrossRef]
103. Narumiya, S.; Sugimoto, Y.; Ushikubi, F. Prostanoid receptors: Structures, properties, and functions. *Physiol. Rev.* **1999**, *79*, 1193–1226. [CrossRef]
104. Ushikubi, F.; Hirata, M.; Narumiya, S. Molecular biology of prostanoid receptors; an overview. *J. Lipid Mediat. Cell Signal.* **1995**, *12*, 343–359. [CrossRef]
105. Duncan, A.M.; Anderson, L.L.; Funk, C.D.; Abramovitz, M.; Adam, M. Chromosomal localization of the human prostanoid receptor gene family. *Genomics* **1995**, *25*, 740–742. [CrossRef]
106. Smock, S.L.; Pan, L.C.; Castleberry, T.A.; Lu, B.; Mather, R.J.; Owen, T.A. Cloning, structural characterization, and chromosomal localization of the gene encoding the human prostaglandin E(2) receptor EP2 subtype. *Gene* **1999**, *237*, 393–402. [CrossRef]
107. Foord, S.M.; Marks, B.; Stolz, M.; Bufflier, E.; Fraser, N.J.; Lee, M.G. The structure of the prostaglandin EP4 receptor gene and related pseudogenes. *Genomics* **1996**, *35*, 182–188. [CrossRef]
108. Sugimoto, Y.; Narumiya, S. Prostaglandin E receptors. *J. Biol. Chem.* **2007**, *282*, 11613–11617. [CrossRef]
109. Abramovitz, M.; Adam, M.; Boie, Y.; Carriere, M.; Denis, D.; Godbout, C.; Lamontagne, S.; Rochette, C.; Sawyer, N.; Tremblay, N.M.; et al. The utilization of recombinant prostanoid receptors to determine the affinities and selectivities of prostaglandins and related analogs. *Biochim. Biophys. Acta* **2000**, *1483*, 285–293. [CrossRef]
110. Katoh, H.; Watabe, A.; Sugimoto, Y.; Ichikawa, A.; Negishi, M. Characterization of the signal transduction of prostaglandin E receptor EP1 subtype in cDNA-transfected Chinese hamster ovary cells. *Biochim. Biophys. Acta* **1995**, *1244*, 41–48. [CrossRef]
111. O'Callaghan, G.; Houston, A. Prostaglandin E2 and the EP receptors in malignancy: Possible therapeutic targets? *Br. J. Pharmacol.* **2015**, *172*, 5239–5250. [CrossRef] [PubMed]
112. Fujino, H.; West, K.A.; Regan, J.W. Phosphorylation of glycogen synthase kinase-3 and stimulation of T-cell factor signaling following activation of EP2 and EP4 prostanoid receptors by prostaglandin E2. *J. Biol. Chem.* **2002**, *277*, 2614–2619. [CrossRef] [PubMed]
113. Nishigaki, N.; Negishi, M.; Ichikawa, A. Two Gs-coupled prostaglandin E receptor subtypes, EP2 and EP4, differ in desensitization and sensitivity to the metabolic inactivation of the agonist. *Mol. Pharmacol.* **1996**, *50*, 1031–1037. [PubMed]
114. Chun, K.S.; Lao, H.C.; Trempus, C.S.; Okada, M.; Langenbach, R. The prostaglandin receptor EP2 activates multiple signaling pathways and beta-arrestin1 complex formation during mouse skin papilloma development. *Carcinogenesis* **2009**, *30*, 1620–1627. [CrossRef] [PubMed]
115. Fujino, H.; Xu, W.; Regan, J.W. Prostaglandin E2 induced functional expression of early growth response factor-1 by EP4, but not EP2, prostanoid receptors via the phosphatidylinositol 3-kinase and extracellular signal-regulated kinases. *J. Biol. Chem.* **2003**, *278*, 12151–12156. [CrossRef] [PubMed]
116. Ganesh, T. Prostanoid receptor EP2 as a therapeutic target. *J. Med. Chem.* **2014**, *57*, 4454–4465. [CrossRef] [PubMed]
117. Murakami, M.; Kudo, I. Recent advances in molecular biology and physiology of the prostaglandin E2-biosynthetic pathway. *Prog. Lipid Res.* **2004**, *43*, 3–35. [CrossRef]
118. Hester, A.; Ritzer, M.; Kuhn, C.; Schmoeckel, E.; Mayr, D.; Kolben, T.; Dannecker, C.; Mahner, S.; Jeschke, U.; Kolben, T.M. The role of EP3-receptor expression in cervical dysplasia. *J. Cancer Res. Clin. Oncol.* **2019**, *145*, 313–319. [CrossRef]
119. Sales, K.J.; Katz, A.A.; Davis, M.; Hinz, S.; Soeters, R.P.; Hofmeyr, M.D.; Millar, R.P.; Jabbour, H.N. Cyclooxygenase-2 expression and prostaglandin E(2) synthesis are up-regulated in carcinomas of the cervix: A possible autocrine/paracrine regulation of neoplastic cell function via EP2/EP4 receptors. *J. Clin. Endocrinol. Metab.* **2001**, *86*, 2243–2249. [CrossRef]
120. Sales, K.J.; Katz, A.A.; Howard, B.; Soeters, R.P.; Millar, R.P.; Jabbour, H.N. Cyclooxygenase-1 is up-regulated in cervical carcinomas: Autocrine/paracrine regulation of cyclooxygenase-2, prostaglandin e receptors, and angiogenic factors by cyclooxygenase-1. *Cancer Res.* **2002**, *62*, 424–432.

121. Sales, K.J.; Katz, A.A.; Millar, R.P.; Jabbour, H.N. Seminal plasma activates cyclooxygenase-2 and prostaglandin E2 receptor expression and signalling in cervical adenocarcinoma cells. *Mol. Hum. Reprod.* **2002**, *8*, 1065–1070. [CrossRef]
122. Sales, K.J.; Sutherland, J.R.; Jabbour, H.N.; Katz, A.A. Seminal plasma induces angiogenic chemokine expression in cervical cancer cells and regulates vascular function. *Biochim. Biophys. Acta* **2012**, *1823*, 1789–1795. [CrossRef]
123. Schmoeckel, E.; Fraungruber, P.; Kuhn, C.; Jeschke, U.; Mahner, S.; Kolben, T.M.; Kolben, T.; Vilsmaier, T.; Hester, A.; Heidegger, H.H. The role of EP-2 receptor expression in cervical intraepithelial neoplasia. *Histochem. Cell Biol.* **2020**, *154*, 655–662. [CrossRef]
124. Dietlmeier, S.; Ye, Y.; Kuhn, C.; Vattai, A.; Vilsmaier, T.; Schroder, L.; Kost, B.P.; Gallwas, J.; Jeschke, U.; Mahner, S.; et al. The prostaglandin receptor EP2 determines prognosis in EP3-negative and galectin-3-high cervical cancer cases. *Sci. Rep.* **2020**, *10*, 1154. [CrossRef]
125. Ye, Y.; Peng, L.; Vattai, A.; Deuster, E.; Kuhn, C.; Dannecker, C.; Mahner, S.; Jeschke, U.; von Schonfeldt, V.; Heidegger, H.H. Prostaglandin E2 receptor 3 (EP3) signaling promotes migration of cervical cancer via urokinase-type plasminogen activator receptor (uPAR). *J. Cancer Res. Clin. Oncol.* **2020**, *146*, 2189–2203. [CrossRef]
126. Sonoshita, M.; Takaku, K.; Sasaki, N.; Sugimoto, Y.; Ushikubi, F.; Narumiya, S.; Oshima, M.; Taketo, M.M. Acceleration of intestinal polyposis through prostaglandin receptor EP2 in Apc(Delta 716) knockout mice. *Nat. Med.* **2001**, *7*, 1048–1051. [CrossRef]
127. Yoshida, S.; Amano, H.; Hayashi, I.; Kitasato, H.; Kamata, M.; Inukai, M.; Yoshimura, H.; Majima, M. COX-2/VEGF-dependent facilitation of tumor-associated angiogenesis and tumor growth in vivo. *Lab. Investig.* **2003**, *83*, 1385–1394. [CrossRef]
128. Ma, X.; Aoki, T.; Tsuruyama, T.; Narumiya, S. Definition of Prostaglandin E2-EP2 Signals in the Colon Tumor Microenvironment That Amplify Inflammation and Tumor Growth. *Cancer Res.* **2015**, *75*, 2822–2832. [CrossRef]
129. Oshima, H.; Popivanova, B.K.; Oguma, K.; Kong, D.; Ishikawa, T.O.; Oshima, M. Activation of epidermal growth factor receptor signaling by the prostaglandin E(2) receptor EP4 pathway during gastric tumorigenesis. *Cancer Sci.* **2011**, *102*, 713–719. [CrossRef]
130. Okuyama, T.; Ishihara, S.; Sato, H.; Rumi, M.A.; Kawashima, K.; Miyaoka, Y.; Suetsugu, H.; Kazumori, H.; Cava, C.F.; Kadowaki, Y.; et al. Activation of prostaglandin E2-receptor EP2 and EP4 pathways induces growth inhibition in human gastric carcinoma cell lines. *J. Lab. Clin. Med.* **2002**, *140*, 92–102. [CrossRef]
131. Grace, V.M.B.; Wilson, D.D.; Anushya, R.; Siddikuzzaman. Regulation of inflammation and COX-2 gene expression in benzo (a) pyrene induced lung carcinogenesis in mice by all trans retinoic acid (ATRA). *Life Sci.* **2021**, *285*, 119867. [CrossRef]
132. Kim, J.I.; Lakshmikanthan, V.; Frilot, N.; Daaka, Y. Prostaglandin E2 promotes lung cancer cell migration via EP4-betaArrestin1-c-Src signalsome. *Mol. Cancer Res.* **2010**, *8*, 569–577. [CrossRef]
133. Krysan, K.; Reckamp, K.L.; Dalwadi, H.; Sharma, S.; Rozengurt, E.; Dohadwala, M.; Dubinett, S.M. Prostaglandin E2 activates mitogen-activated protein kinase/Erk pathway signaling and cell proliferation in non-small cell lung cancer cells in an epidermal growth factor receptor-independent manner. *Cancer Res.* **2005**, *65*, 6275–6281. [CrossRef]
134. Bai, X.; Yang, Q.; Shu, W.; Wang, J.; Zhang, L.; Ma, J.; Xia, S.; Zhang, M.; Cheng, S.; Wang, Y.; et al. Prostaglandin E2 upregulates beta1 integrin expression via the E prostanoid 1 receptor/nuclear factor kappa-light-chain-enhancer of activated B cells pathway in non-small-cell lung cancer cells. *Mol. Med. Rep.* **2014**, *9*, 1729–1736. [CrossRef]
135. Li, L.; Lv, Y.; Yan, D. Inhibition of Ep3 attenuates migration and promotes apoptosis of non-small cell lung cancer cells via suppression of TGF-beta/Smad signaling. *Oncol. Lett.* **2018**, *16*, 5645–5654. [CrossRef]
136. Harati, R.; Mabondzo, A.; Tlili, A.; Khoder, G.; Mahfood, M.; Hamoudi, R. Combinatorial targeting of microRNA-26b and microRNA-101 exerts a synergistic inhibition on cyclooxygenase-2 in brain metastatic triple-negative breast cancer cells. *Breast Cancer Res. Treat.* **2021**, *187*, 695–713. [CrossRef]
137. Tian, J.; Wang, V.; Wang, N.; Khadang, B.; Boudreault, J.; Bakdounes, K.; Ali, S.; Lebrun, J.J. Identification of MFGE8 and KLK5/7 as mediators of breast tumorigenesis and resistance to COX-2 inhibition. *Breast Cancer Res.* **2021**, *23*, 23. [CrossRef]
138. Semmlinger, A.; von Schoenfeldt, V.; Wolf, V.; Meuter, A.; Kolben, T.M.; Kolben, T.; Zeder-Goess, C.; Weis, F.; Gallwas, J.; Wuerstlein, R.; et al. EP3 (prostaglandin E2 receptor 3) expression is a prognostic factor for progression-free and overall survival in sporadic breast cancer. *BMC Cancer* **2018**, *18*, 431. [CrossRef]
139. Cheuk, I.W.; Shin, V.Y.; Siu, M.T.; Tsang, J.Y.; Ho, J.C.; Chen, J.; Tse, G.M.; Wang, X.; Kwong, A. Association of EP2 receptor and SLC19A3 in regulating breast cancer metastasis. *Am. J. Cancer Res.* **2015**, *5*, 3389–3399.
140. Majumder, M.; Xin, X.; Liu, L.; Tutunea-Fatan, E.; Rodriguez-Torres, M.; Vincent, K.; Postovit, L.M.; Hess, D.; Lala, P.K. COX-2 Induces Breast Cancer Stem Cells via EP4/PI3K/AKT/NOTCH/WNT Axis. *Stem Cells* **2016**, *34*, 2290–2305. [CrossRef]
141. Thorat, M.A.; Morimiya, A.; Mehrotra, S.; Konger, R.; Badve, S.S. Prostanoid receptor EP1 expression in breast cancer. *Mod. Pathol.* **2008**, *21*, 15–21. [CrossRef] [PubMed]
142. Thanan, R.; Murata, M.; Ma, N.; Hammam, O.; Wishahi, M.; El Leithy, T.; Hiraku, Y.; Oikawa, S.; Kawanishi, S. Nuclear localization of COX-2 in relation to the expression of stemness markers in urinary bladder cancer. *Mediat. Inflamm.* **2012**, *2012*, 165879. [CrossRef] [PubMed]
143. Buchholz, A.; Vattai, A.; Furst, S.; Vilsmaier, T.; Kuhn, C.; Schmoeckel, E.; Mayr, D.; Dannecker, C.; Mahner, S.; Jeschke, U.; et al. EP4 as a Negative Prognostic Factor in Patients with Vulvar Cancer. *Cancers* **2021**, *13*, 1410. [CrossRef] [PubMed]
144. Lee, E.J.; Choi, E.M.; Kim, S.R.; Park, J.H.; Kim, H.; Ha, K.S.; Kim, Y.M.; Kim, S.S.; Choe, M.; Kim, J.I.; et al. Cyclooxygenase-2 promotes cell proliferation, migration and invasion in U2OS human osteosarcoma cells. *Exp. Mol. Med.* **2007**, *39*, 469–476. [CrossRef]

145. Urakawa, H.; Nishida, Y.; Naruse, T.; Nakashima, H.; Ishiguro, N. Cyclooxygenase-2 overexpression predicts poor survival in patients with high-grade extremity osteosarcoma: A pilot study. *Clin. Orthop. Relat. Res.* **2009**, *467*, 2932–2938. [CrossRef]
146. Chen, H.; Cai, W.; Chu, E.S.H.; Tang, J.; Wong, C.C.; Wong, S.H.; Sun, W.; Liang, Q.; Fang, J.; Sun, Z.; et al. Hepatic cyclooxygenase-2 overexpression induced spontaneous hepatocellular carcinoma formation in mice. *Oncogene* **2017**, *36*, 4415–4426. [CrossRef]
147. Xu, S.; Zhou, W.; Ge, J.; Zhang, Z. Prostaglandin E2 receptor EP4 is involved in the cell growth and invasion of prostate cancer via the cAMPPKA/PI3KAkt signaling pathway. *Mol. Med. Rep.* **2018**, *17*, 4702–4712. [CrossRef]
148. ElAttar, T.M.; Lin, H.S. Inhibition of human oral squamous carcinoma cell (SCC-25) proliferation by prostaglandin E2 and vitamin E succinate. *J. Oral Pathol. Med.* **1993**, *22*, 425–427. [CrossRef]
149. Kawanishi, S.; Ohnishi, S.; Ma, N.; Hiraku, Y.; Murata, M. Crosstalk between DNA Damage and Inflammation in the Multiple Steps of Carcinogenesis. *Int. J. Mol. Sci.* **2017**, *18*, 1808. [CrossRef]
150. Landskron, G.; De la Fuente, M.; Thuwajit, P.; Thuwajit, C.; Hermoso, M.A. Chronic inflammation and cytokines in the tumor microenvironment. *J. Immunol. Res.* **2014**, *2014*, 149185. [CrossRef]
151. Hanahan, D. Hallmarks of Cancer: New Dimensions. *Cancer Discov.* **2022**, *12*, 31–46. [CrossRef]
152. Subbaramaiah, K.; Dannenberg, A.J. Cyclooxygenase-2 transcription is regulated by human papillomavirus 16 E6 and E7 oncoproteins: Evidence of a corepressor/coactivator exchange. *Cancer Res.* **2007**, *67*, 3976–3985. [CrossRef]
153. Georgescu, S.R.; Mitran, C.I.; Mitran, M.I.; Caruntu, C.; Sarbu, M.I.; Matei, C.; Nicolae, I.; Tocut, S.M.; Popa, M.I.; Tampa, M. New Insights in the Pathogenesis of HPV Infection and the Associated Carcinogenic Processes: The Role of Chronic Inflammation and Oxidative Stress. *J. Immunol. Res.* **2018**, *2018*, 5315816. [CrossRef]
154. Williams, V.M.; Filippova, M.; Soto, U.; Duerksen-Hughes, P.J. HPV-DNA integration and carcinogenesis: Putative roles for inflammation and oxidative stress. *Future Virol.* **2011**, *6*, 45–57. [CrossRef]
155. Ye, Y.; Wang, X.; Jeschke, U.; von Schonfeldt, V. COX-2-PGE2-EPs in gynecological cancers. *Arch. Gynecol. Obstet.* **2020**, *301*, 1365–1375. [CrossRef]
156. Jabbour, H.N.; Milne, S.A.; Williams, A.R.; Anderson, R.A.; Boddy, S.C. Expression of COX-2 and PGE synthase and synthesis of PGE(2) in endometrial adenocarcinoma: A possible autocrine/paracrine regulation of neoplastic cell function via EP2/EP4 receptors. *Br. J. Cancer* **2001**, *85*, 1023–1031. [CrossRef]
157. Hsu, H.H.; Lin, Y.M.; Shen, C.Y.; Shibu, M.A.; Li, S.Y.; Chang, S.H.; Lin, C.C.; Chen, R.J.; Viswanadha, V.P.; Shih, H.N.; et al. Prostaglandin E2-Induced COX-2 Expressions via EP2 and EP4 Signaling Pathways in Human LoVo Colon Cancer Cells. *Int. J. Mol. Sci.* **2017**, *18*, 1132. [CrossRef]
158. Alcocer-Gonzalez, J.M.; Berumen, J.; Tamez-Guerra, R.; Bermudez-Morales, V.; Peralta-Zaragoza, O.; Hernandez-Pando, R.; Moreno, J.; Gariglio, P.; Madrid-Marina, V. In vivo expression of immunosuppressive cytokines in human papillomavirus-transformed cervical cancer cells. *Viral. Immunol.* **2006**, *19*, 481–491. [CrossRef]
159. Hirsch, I.; Caux, C.; Hasan, U.; Bendriss-Vermare, N.; Olive, D. Impaired Toll-like receptor 7 and 9 signaling: From chronic viral infections to cancer. *Trends Immunol.* **2010**, *31*, 391–397. [CrossRef]
160. Hasan, U.A.; Bates, E.; Takeshita, F.; Biliato, A.; Accardi, R.; Bouvard, V.; Mansour, M.; Vincent, I.; Gissmann, L.; Iftner, T.; et al. TLR9 expression and function is abolished by the cervical cancer-associated human papillomavirus type 16. *J. Immunol.* **2007**, *178*, 3186–3197. [CrossRef]
161. Hasan, U.A.; Zannetti, C.; Parroche, P.; Goutagny, N.; Malfroy, M.; Roblot, G.; Carreira, C.; Hussain, I.; Muller, M.; Taylor-Papadimitriou, J.; et al. The human papillomavirus type 16 E7 oncoprotein induces a transcriptional repressor complex on the Toll-like receptor 9 promoter. *J. Exp. Med.* **2013**, *210*, 1369–1387. [CrossRef]
162. Barnard, P.; Payne, E.; McMillan, N.A. The human papillomavirus E7 protein is able to inhibit the antiviral and anti-growth functions of interferon-alpha. *Virology* **2000**, *277*, 411–419. [CrossRef]
163. Beglin, M.; Melar-New, M.; Laimins, L. Human papillomaviruses and the interferon response. *J. Interf. Cytokine Res.* **2009**, *29*, 629–635. [CrossRef]
164. Huang, J.; Diao, G.; Zhang, Q.; Chen, Y.; Han, J.; Guo, J. E6regulated overproduction of prostaglandin E2 may inhibit migration of dendritic cells in human papillomavirus 16positive cervical lesions. *Int. J. Oncol.* **2020**, *56*, 921–931. [CrossRef]
165. Ferreira, A.R.; Ramalho, A.C.; Marques, M.; Ribeiro, D. The Interplay between Antiviral Signalling and Carcinogenesis in Human Papillomavirus Infections. *Cancers* **2020**, *12*, 646. [CrossRef]
166. Florez-Grau, G.; Cabezon, R.; Borgman, K.J.E.; Espana, C.; Lozano, J.J.; Garcia-Parajo, M.F.; Benitez-Ribas, D. Up-regulation of EP2 and EP3 receptors in human tolerogenic dendritic cells boosts the immunosuppressive activity of PGE2. *J. Leukoc. Biol.* **2017**, *102*, 881–895. [CrossRef]
167. Kundu, N.; Ma, X.; Holt, D.; Goloubeva, O.; Ostrand-Rosenberg, S.; Fulton, A.M. Antagonism of the prostaglandin E receptor EP4 inhibits metastasis and enhances NK function. *Breast Cancer Res. Treat.* **2009**, *117*, 235–242. [CrossRef]
168. Mao, Y.; Sarhan, D.; Steven, A.; Seliger, B.; Kiessling, R.; Lundqvist, A. Inhibition of tumor-derived prostaglandin-e2 blocks the induction of myeloid-derived suppressor cells and recovers natural killer cell activity. *Clin. Cancer Res.* **2014**, *20*, 4096–4106. [CrossRef]
169. Obermajer, N.; Muthuswamy, R.; Lesnock, J.; Edwards, R.P.; Kalinski, P. Positive feedback between PGE2 and COX2 redirects the differentiation of human dendritic cells toward stable myeloid-derived suppressor cells. *Blood* **2011**, *118*, 5498–5505. [CrossRef]
170. Wu, L.; Liu, H.; Guo, H.; Wu, Q.; Yu, S.; Qin, Y.; Wang, G.; Wu, Q.; Zhang, R.; Wang, L.; et al. Circulating and tumor-infiltrating myeloid-derived suppressor cells in cervical carcinoma patients. *Oncol. Lett.* **2018**, *15*, 9507–9515. [CrossRef]

171. Ching, M.M.; Reader, J.; Fulton, A.M. Eicosanoids in Cancer: Prostaglandin E2 Receptor 4 in Cancer Therapeutics and Immunotherapy. *Front. Pharmacol.* **2020**, *11*, 819. [CrossRef] [PubMed]
172. Mosenden, R.; Tasken, K. Cyclic AMP-mediated immune regulation–overview of mechanisms of action in T cells. *Cell Signal.* **2011**, *23*, 1009–1016. [CrossRef] [PubMed]
173. Alfonso, L.; Ai, G.; Spitale, R.C.; Bhat, G.J. Molecular targets of aspirin and cancer prevention. *Br. J. Cancer* **2014**, *111*, 61–67. [CrossRef] [PubMed]
174. Friel, G.; Liu, C.S.; Kolomeyevskaya, N.V.; Hampras, S.S.; Kruszka, B.; Schmitt, K.; Cannioto, R.A.; Lele, S.B.; Odunsi, K.O.; Moysich, K.B. Aspirin and Acetaminophen Use and the Risk of Cervical Cancer. *J. Low. Genit. Tract Dis.* **2015**, *19*, 189–193. [CrossRef]
175. Ahmadi, R.; Karimi Ghezeli, Z.; Gravand, F.; Naghshineh, M. The Effect of Aspirin and Ibuprofen on the Proliferation of Cervical Cancer Cells (HeLa) Compared to Non-Cancerous Cells (HEK 293) in Cell Culture Medium. *Qom Univ. Med. Sci. J.* **2018**, *12*, 16–24. [CrossRef]
176. Kim, K.Y.; Seol, J.Y.; Jeon, G.A.; Nam, M.J. The combined treatment of aspirin and radiation induces apoptosis by the regulation of bcl-2 and caspase-3 in human cervical cancer cell. *Cancer Lett.* **2003**, *189*, 157–166. [CrossRef]
177. Xiang, S.; Sun, Z.; He, Q.; Yan, F.; Wang, Y.; Zhang, J. Aspirin inhibits ErbB2 to induce apoptosis in cervical cancer cells. *Med. Oncol.* **2010**, *27*, 379–387. [CrossRef]
178. Sakonlaya, D.; Tapanadechopone, P.; Poomkokruk, A.; Charoenvilaisiri, S. Do NSAIDs inhibit growth of precancerous cervical cells in vitro? *J. Med. Assoc. Thai.* **2012**, *95* (Suppl. S1), S65–S73.
179. Soriano-Hernandez, A.D.; Madrigal-Perez, D.; Galvan-Salazar, H.R.; Martinez-Fierro, M.L.; Valdez-Velazquez, L.L.; Espinoza-Gomez, F.; Vazquez-Vuelvas, O.F.; Olmedo-Buenrostro, B.A.; Guzman-Esquivel, J.; Rodriguez-Sanchez, I.P.; et al. Anti-inflammatory drugs and uterine cervical cancer cells: Antineoplastic effect of meclofenamic acid. *Oncol. Lett.* **2015**, *10*, 2574–2578. [CrossRef]
180. Kolawole, O.R.; Kashfi, K. NSAIDs and Cancer Resolution: New Paradigms beyond Cyclooxygenase. *Int. J. Mol. Sci.* **2022**, *23*, 1432. [CrossRef]
181. Kim, S.H.; Song, S.H.; Kim, S.G.; Chun, K.S.; Lim, S.Y.; Na, H.K.; Kim, J.W.; Surh, Y.J.; Bang, Y.J.; Song, Y.S. Celecoxib induces apoptosis in cervical cancer cells independent of cyclooxygenase using NF-kappaB as a possible target. *J. Cancer Res. Clin. Oncol.* **2004**, *130*, 551–560. [CrossRef]
182. Ferrandina, G.; Ranelletti, F.O.; Legge, F.; Lauriola, L.; Salutari, V.; Gessi, M.; Testa, A.C.; Werner, U.; Navarra, P.; Tringali, G.; et al. Celecoxib modulates the expression of cyclooxygenase-2, ki67, apoptosis-related marker, and microvessel density in human cervical cancer: A pilot study. *Clin. Cancer Res.* **2003**, *9*, 4324–4331.
183. Farley, J.H.; Truong, V.; Goo, E.; Uyehara, C.; Belnap, C.; Larsen, W.I. A randomized double-blind placebo-controlled phase II trial of the cyclooxygenase-2 inhibitor Celecoxib in the treatment of cervical dysplasia. *Gynecol. Oncol.* **2006**, *103*, 425–430. [CrossRef]
184. Rader, J.S.; Sill, M.W.; Beumer, J.H.; Lankes, H.A.; Benbrook, D.M.; Garcia, F.; Trimble, C.; Tate Thigpen, J.; Lieberman, R.; Zuna, R.E.; et al. A stratified randomized double-blind phase II trial of celecoxib for treating patients with cervical intraepithelial neoplasia: The potential predictive value of VEGF serum levels: An NRG Oncology/Gynecologic Oncology Group study. *Gynecol. Oncol.* **2017**, *145*, 291–297. [CrossRef]
185. Nakata, E.; Mason, K.A.; Hunter, N.; Husain, A.; Raju, U.; Liao, Z.; Ang, K.K.; Milas, L. Potentiation of tumor response to radiation or chemoradiation by selective cyclooxygenase-2 enzyme inhibitors. *Int. J. Radiat. Oncol. Biol. Phys.* **2004**, *58*, 369–375. [CrossRef]
186. Raju, U.; Nakata, E.; Yang, P.; Newman, R.A.; Ang, K.K.; Milas, L. In vitro enhancement of tumor cell radiosensitivity by a selective inhibitor of cyclooxygenase-2 enzyme: Mechanistic considerations. *Int. J. Radiat. Oncol. Biol. Phys.* **2002**, *54*, 886–894. [CrossRef]
187. Herrera, F.G.; Chan, P.; Doll, C.; Milosevic, M.; Oza, A.; Syed, A.; Pintilie, M.; Levin, W.; Manchul, L.; Fyles, A. A prospective phase I-II trial of the cyclooxygenase-2 inhibitor celecoxib in patients with carcinoma of the cervix with biomarker assessment of the tumor microenvironment. *Int. J. Radiat. Oncol. Biol. Phys.* **2007**, *67*, 97–103. [CrossRef]
188. Gaffney, D.K.; Winter, K.; Dicker, A.P.; Miller, B.; Eifel, P.J.; Ryu, J.; Avizonis, V.; Fromm, M.; Greven, K. A Phase II study of acute toxicity for Celebrex (celecoxib) and chemoradiation in patients with locally advanced cervical cancer: Primary endpoint analysis of RTOG 0128. *Int. J. Radiat. Oncol. Biol. Phys.* **2007**, *67*, 104–109. [CrossRef]
189. Barnes, P.J. Anti-inflammatory actions of glucocorticoids: Molecular mechanisms. *Clin. Sci.* **1998**, *94*, 557–572. [CrossRef]
190. Grunberg, S.M. Antiemetic activity of corticosteroids in patients receiving cancer chemotherapy: Dosing, efficacy, and tolerability analysis. *Ann. Oncol.* **2007**, *18*, 233–240. [CrossRef]
191. Chen, Q.M.; Alexander, D.; Sun, H.; Xie, L.; Lin, Y.; Terrand, J.; Morrissy, S.; Purdom, S. Corticosteroids inhibit cell death induced by doxorubicin in cardiomyocytes: Induction of antiapoptosis, antioxidant, and detoxification genes. *Mol. Pharmacol.* **2005**, *67*, 1861–1873. [CrossRef]
192. Zhang, C.; Beckermann, B.; Kallifatidis, G.; Liu, Z.; Rittgen, W.; Edler, L.; Buchler, P.; Debatin, K.M.; Buchler, M.W.; Friess, H.; et al. Corticosteroids induce chemotherapy resistance in the majority of tumour cells from bone, brain, breast, cervix, melanoma and neuroblastoma. *Int. J. Oncol.* **2006**, *29*, 1295–1301. [CrossRef]
193. Kamradt, M.C.; Mohideen, N.; Krueger, E.; Walter, S.; Vaughan, A.T. Inhibition of radiation-induced apoptosis by dexamethasone in cervical carcinoma cell lines depends upon increased HPV E6/E7. *Br. J. Cancer* **2000**, *82*, 1709–1716. [CrossRef]

194. Shi, M.; Du, L.; Liu, D.; Qian, L.; Hu, M.; Yu, M.; Yang, Z.; Zhao, M.; Chen, C.; Guo, L.; et al. Glucocorticoid regulation of a novel HPV-E6-p53-miR-145 pathway modulates invasion and therapy resistance of cervical cancer cells. *J. Pathol.* **2012**, *228*, 148–157. [CrossRef]
195. Bromberg-White, J.L.; Meyers, C. Comparison of the basal and glucocorticoid-inducible activities of the upstream regulatory regions of HPV18 and HPV31 in multiple epithelial cell lines. *Virology* **2003**, *306*, 197–202. [CrossRef]
196. Crusz, S.M.; El-Shakankery, K.; Miller, R.E. Targeting HPV in gynaecological cancers—Current status, ongoing challenges and future directions. *Womens Health* **2020**, *16*, 1745506520961709. [CrossRef]
197. Hellner, K.; Munger, K. Human papillomaviruses as therapeutic targets in human cancer. *J. Clin. Oncol.* **2011**, *29*, 1785–1794. [CrossRef]
198. Liu, Y.; Li, H.; Pi, R.; Yang, Y.; Zhao, X.; Qi, X. Current strategies against persistent human papillomavirus infection (Review). *Int. J. Oncol.* **2019**, *55*, 570–584. [CrossRef]
199. Flickinger, J.C., Jr.; Rodeck, U.; Snook, A.E. Listeria monocytogenes as a Vector for Cancer Immunotherapy: Current Understanding and Progress. *Vaccines* **2018**, *6*, 48. [CrossRef]
200. Gunn, G.R.; Zubair, A.; Peters, C.; Pan, Z.K.; Wu, T.C.; Paterson, Y. Two Listeria monocytogenes vaccine vectors that express different molecular forms of human papilloma virus-16 (HPV-16) E7 induce qualitatively different T cell immunity that correlates with their ability to induce regression of established tumors immortalized by HPV-16. *J. Immunol.* **2001**, *167*, 6471–6479. [CrossRef] [PubMed]
201. Maciag, P.C.; Radulovic, S.; Rothman, J. The first clinical use of a live-attenuated Listeria monocytogenes vaccine: A Phase I safety study of Lm-LLO-E7 in patients with advanced carcinoma of the cervix. *Vaccine* **2009**, *27*, 3975–3983. [CrossRef] [PubMed]
202. Van Damme, P.; Bouillette-Marussig, M.; Hens, A.; De Coster, I.; Depuydt, C.; Goubier, A.; Van Tendeloo, V.; Cools, N.; Goossens, H.; Hercend, T.; et al. GTL001, A Therapeutic Vaccine for Women Infected with Human Papillomavirus 16 or 18 and Normal Cervical Cytology: Results of a Phase I Clinical Trial. *Clin. Cancer Res.* **2016**, *22*, 3238–3248. [CrossRef] [PubMed]
203. Esquerre, M.; Bouillette-Marussig, M.; Goubier, A.; Momot, M.; Gonindard, C.; Keller, H.; Navarro, A.; Bissery, M.C. GTL001, a bivalent therapeutic vaccine against human papillomavirus 16 and 18, induces antigen-specific CD8+ T cell responses leading to tumor regression. *PLoS ONE* **2017**, *12*, e0174038. [CrossRef]
204. Simsova, M.; Sebo, P.; Leclerc, C. The adenylate cyclase toxin from Bordetella pertussis–a novel promising vehicle for antigen delivery to dendritic cells. *Int. J. Med. Microbiol.* **2004**, *293*, 571–576. [CrossRef]
205. Yang, A.; Farmer, E.; Lin, J.; Wu, T.C.; Hung, C.F. The current state of therapeutic and T cell-based vaccines against human papillomaviruses. *Virus Res.* **2017**, *231*, 148–165. [CrossRef]
206. Boursnell, M.E.; Rutherford, E.; Hickling, J.K.; Rollinson, E.A.; Munro, A.J.; Rolley, N.; McLean, C.S.; Borysiewicz, L.K.; Vousden, K.; Inglis, S.C. Construction and characterisation of a recombinant vaccinia virus expressing human papillomavirus proteins for immunotherapy of cervical cancer. *Vaccine* **1996**, *14*, 1485–1494. [CrossRef]
207. Borysiewicz, L.K.; Fiander, A.; Nimako, M.; Man, S.; Wilkinson, G.W.; Westmoreland, D.; Evans, A.S.; Adams, M.; Stacey, S.N.; Boursnell, M.E.; et al. A recombinant vaccinia virus encoding human papillomavirus types 16 and 18, E6 and E7 proteins as immunotherapy for cervical cancer. *Lancet* **1996**, *347*, 1523–1527. [CrossRef]
208. Baldwin, P.J.; van der Burg, S.H.; Boswell, C.M.; Offringa, R.; Hickling, J.K.; Dobson, J.; Roberts, J.S.; Latimer, J.A.; Moseley, R.P.; Coleman, N.; et al. Vaccinia-expressed human papillomavirus 16 and 18 e6 and e7 as a therapeutic vaccination for vulval and vaginal intraepithelial neoplasia. *Clin. Cancer Res.* **2003**, *9*, 5205–5213.
209. Maldonado, L.; Teague, J.E.; Morrow, M.P.; Jotova, I.; Wu, T.C.; Wang, C.; Desmarais, C.; Boyer, J.D.; Tycko, B.; Robins, H.S.; et al. Intramuscular therapeutic vaccination targeting HPV16 induces T cell responses that localize in mucosal lesions. *Sci. Transl. Med.* **2014**, *6*, 221ra213. [CrossRef]
210. Peng, S.; Ferrall, L.; Gaillard, S.; Wang, C.; Chi, W.Y.; Huang, C.H.; Roden, R.B.S.; Wu, T.C.; Chang, Y.N.; Hung, C.F. Development of DNA Vaccine Targeting E6 and E7 Proteins of Human Papillomavirus 16 (HPV16) and HPV18 for Immunotherapy in Combination with Recombinant Vaccinia Boost and PD-1 Antibody. *mBio* **2021**, *12*, e03224-20. [CrossRef]
211. Lamikanra, A.; Pan, Z.K.; Isaacs, S.N.; Wu, T.C.; Paterson, Y. Regression of established human papillomavirus type 16 (HPV-16) immortalized tumors in vivo by vaccinia viruses expressing different forms of HPV-16 E7 correlates with enhanced CD8(+) T-cell responses that home to the tumor site. *J. Virol.* **2001**, *75*, 9654–9664. [CrossRef]
212. Volz, A.; Sutter, G. Modified Vaccinia Virus Ankara: History, Value in Basic Research, and Current Perspectives for Vaccine Development. *Adv. Virus Res.* **2017**, *97*, 187–243. [CrossRef]
213. Rosales, C.; Graham, V.V.; Rosas, G.A.; Merchant, H.; Rosales, R. A recombinant vaccinia virus containing the papilloma E2 protein promotes tumor regression by stimulating macrophage antibody-dependent cytotoxicity. *Cancer Immunol. Immunother.* **2000**, *49*, 347–360. [CrossRef]
214. Valdez Graham, V.; Sutter, G.; Jose, M.V.; Garcia-Carranca, A.; Erfle, V.; Moreno Mendoza, N.; Merchant, H.; Rosales, R. Human tumor growth is inhibited by a vaccinia virus carrying the E2 gene of bovine papillomavirus. *Cancer* **2000**, *88*, 1650–1662. [CrossRef]
215. Corona Gutierrez, C.M.; Tinoco, A.; Navarro, T.; Contreras, M.L.; Cortes, R.R.; Calzado, P.; Reyes, L.; Posternak, R.; Morosoli, G.; Verde, M.L.; et al. Therapeutic vaccination with MVA E2 can eliminate precancerous lesions (CIN 1, CIN 2, and CIN 3) associated with infection by oncogenic human papillomavirus. *Hum. Gene Ther.* **2004**, *15*, 421–431. [CrossRef]

216. Garcia-Hernandez, E.; Gonzalez-Sanchez, J.L.; Andrade-Manzano, A.; Contreras, M.L.; Padilla, S.; Guzman, C.C.; Jimenez, R.; Reyes, L.; Morosoli, G.; Verde, M.L.; et al. Regression of papilloma high-grade lesions (CIN 2 and CIN 3) is stimulated by therapeutic vaccination with MVA E2 recombinant vaccine. *Cancer Gene Ther.* **2006**, *13*, 592–597. [CrossRef]
217. Rosales, R.; Lopez-Contreras, M.; Rosales, C.; Magallanes-Molina, J.R.; Gonzalez-Vergara, R.; Arroyo-Cazarez, J.M.; Ricardez-Arenas, A.; Del Follo-Valencia, A.; Padilla-Arriaga, S.; Guerrero, M.V.; et al. Regression of human papillomavirus intraepithelial lesions is induced by MVA E2 therapeutic vaccine. *Hum. Gene Ther.* **2014**, *25*, 1035–1049. [CrossRef]
218. Brun, J.L.; Dalstein, V.; Leveque, J.; Mathevet, P.; Raulic, P.; Baldauf, J.J.; Scholl, S.; Huynh, B.; Douvier, S.; Riethmuller, D.; et al. Regression of high-grade cervical intraepithelial neoplasia with TG4001 targeted immunotherapy. *Am. J. Obstet. Gynecol.* **2011**, *204*, 169.e1–169.e8. [CrossRef]
219. Gomez-Gutierrez, J.G.; Elpek, K.G.; Montes de Oca-Luna, R.; Shirwan, H.; Sam Zhou, H.; McMasters, K.M. Vaccination with an adenoviral vector expressing calreticulin-human papillomavirus 16 E7 fusion protein eradicates E7 expressing established tumors in mice. *Cancer Immunol. Immunother.* **2007**, *56*, 997–1007. [CrossRef]
220. Ho, W.; Gao, M.; Li, F.; Li, Z.; Zhang, X.Q.; Xu, X. Next-Generation Vaccines: Nanoparticle-Mediated DNA and mRNA Delivery. *Adv. Healthc. Mater.* **2021**, *10*, e2001812. [CrossRef]
221. Bagarazzi, M.L.; Yan, J.; Morrow, M.P.; Shen, X.; Parker, R.L.; Lee, J.C.; Giffear, M.; Pankhong, P.; Khan, A.S.; Broderick, K.E.; et al. Immunotherapy against HPV16/18 generates potent TH1 and cytotoxic cellular immune responses. *Sci. Transl. Med.* **2012**, *4*, 155ra138. [CrossRef] [PubMed]
222. Morrow, M.P.; Kraynyak, K.A.; Sylvester, A.J.; Dallas, M.; Knoblock, D.; Boyer, J.D.; Yan, J.; Vang, R.; Khan, A.S.; Humeau, L.; et al. Clinical and Immunologic Biomarkers for Histologic Regression of High-Grade Cervical Dysplasia and Clearance of HPV16 and HPV18 after Immunotherapy. *Clin. Cancer Res.* **2018**, *24*, 276–294. [CrossRef] [PubMed]
223. Bhuyan, P.K.; Dallas, M.; Kraynyak, K.; Herring, T.; Morrow, M.; Boyer, J.; Duff, S.; Kim, J.; Weiner, D.B. Durability of response to VGX-3100 treatment of HPV16/18 positive cervical HSIL. *Hum. Vaccines Immunother.* **2021**, *17*, 1288–1293. [CrossRef] [PubMed]
224. Tang, J.; Li, M.; Zhao, C.; Shen, D.; Liu, L.; Zhang, X.; Wei, L. Therapeutic DNA Vaccines against HPV-Related Malignancies: Promising Leads from Clinical Trials. *Viruses* **2022**, *14*, 239. [CrossRef]
225. Kim, T.J.; Jin, H.T.; Hur, S.Y.; Yang, H.G.; Seo, Y.B.; Hong, S.R.; Lee, C.W.; Kim, S.; Woo, J.W.; Park, K.S.; et al. Clearance of persistent HPV infection and cervical lesion by therapeutic DNA vaccine in CIN3 patients. *Nat. Commun.* **2014**, *5*, 5317. [CrossRef]
226. Choi, Y.J.; Hur, S.Y.; Kim, T.J.; Hong, S.R.; Lee, J.K.; Cho, C.H.; Park, K.S.; Woo, J.W.; Sung, Y.C.; Suh, Y.S.; et al. A Phase II, Prospective, Randomized, Multicenter, Open-Label Study of GX-188E, an HPV DNA Vaccine, in Patients with Cervical Intraepithelial Neoplasia 3. *Clin. Cancer Res.* **2020**, *26*, 1616–1623. [CrossRef]
227. Celis, E.; Sette, A.; Grey, H.M. Epitope selection and development of peptide based vaccines to treat cancer. *Semin. Cancer Biol.* **1995**, *6*, 329–336. [CrossRef]
228. Kenter, G.G.; Welters, M.J.; Valentijn, A.R.; Lowik, M.J.; Berends-van der Meer, D.M.; Vloon, A.P.; Essahsah, F.; Fathers, L.M.; Offringa, R.; Drijfhout, J.W.; et al. Vaccination against HPV-16 oncoproteins for vulvar intraepithelial neoplasia. *N. Engl. J. Med.* **2009**, *361*, 1838–1847. [CrossRef]
229. Welters, M.J.; Kenter, G.G.; de Vos van Steenwijk, P.J.; Lowik, M.J.; Berends-van der Meer, D.M.; Essahsah, F.; Stynenbosch, L.F.; Vloon, A.P.; Ramwadhdoebe, T.H.; Piersma, S.J.; et al. Success or failure of vaccination for HPV16-positive vulvar lesions correlates with kinetics and phenotype of induced T-cell responses. *Proc. Natl. Acad. Sci. USA* **2010**, *107*, 11895–11899. [CrossRef]
230. van Poelgeest, M.I.; Welters, M.J.; van Esch, E.M.; Stynenbosch, L.F.; Kerpershoek, G.; van Persijn van Meerten, E.L.; van den Hende, M.; Lowik, M.J.; Berends-van der Meer, D.M.; Fathers, L.M.; et al. HPV16 synthetic long peptide (HPV16-SLP) vaccination therapy of patients with advanced or recurrent HPV16-induced gynecological carcinoma, a phase II trial. *J. Transl. Med.* **2013**, *11*, 88. [CrossRef]
231. de Vos van Steenwijk, P.J.; Ramwadhdoebe, T.H.; Lowik, M.J.; van der Minne, C.E.; Berends-van der Meer, D.M.; Fathers, L.M.; Valentijn, A.R.; Oostendorp, J.; Fleuren, G.J.; Hellebrekers, B.W.; et al. A placebo-controlled randomized HPV16 synthetic long-peptide vaccination study in women with high-grade cervical squamous intraepithelial lesions. *Cancer Immunol. Immunother.* **2012**, *61*, 1485–1492. [CrossRef]
232. de Vos van Steenwijk, P.J.; van Poelgeest, M.I.; Ramwadhdoebe, T.H.; Lowik, M.J.; Berends-van der Meer, D.M.; van der Minne, C.E.; Loof, N.M.; Stynenbosch, L.F.; Fathers, L.M.; Valentijn, A.R.; et al. The long-term immune response after HPV16 peptide vaccination in women with low-grade pre-malignant disorders of the uterine cervix: A placebo-controlled phase II study. *Cancer Immunol. Immunother.* **2014**, *63*, 147–160. [CrossRef]
233. Greenfield, W.W.; Stratton, S.L.; Myrick, R.S.; Vaughn, R.; Donnalley, L.M.; Coleman, H.N.; Mercado, M.; Moerman-Herzog, A.M.; Spencer, H.J.; Andrews-Collins, N.R.; et al. A phase I dose-escalation clinical trial of a peptide-based human papillomavirus therapeutic vaccine with Candida skin test reagent as a novel vaccine adjuvant for treating women with biopsy-proven cervical intraepithelial neoplasia 2/3. *Oncoimmunology* **2015**, *4*, e1031439. [CrossRef]
234. de Jong, A.; O'Neill, T.; Khan, A.Y.; Kwappenberg, K.M.; Chisholm, S.E.; Whittle, N.R.; Dobson, J.A.; Jack, L.C.; St Clair Roberts, J.A.; Offringa, R.; et al. Enhancement of human papillomavirus (HPV) type 16 E6 and E7-specific T-cell immunity in healthy volunteers through vaccination with TA-CIN, an HPV16 L2E7E6 fusion protein vaccine. *Vaccine* **2002**, *20*, 3456–3464. [CrossRef]

235. Gambhira, R.; Gravitt, P.E.; Bossis, I.; Stern, P.L.; Viscidi, R.P.; Roden, R.B. Vaccination of healthy volunteers with human papillomavirus type 16 L2E7E6 fusion protein induces serum antibody that neutralizes across papillomavirus species. *Cancer Res.* **2006**, *66*, 11120–11124. [CrossRef]
236. Karanam, B.; Gambhira, R.; Peng, S.; Jagu, S.; Kim, D.J.; Ketner, G.W.; Stern, P.L.; Adams, R.J.; Roden, R.B. Vaccination with HPV16 L2E6E7 fusion protein in GPI-0100 adjuvant elicits protective humoral and cell-mediated immunity. *Vaccine* **2009**, *27*, 1040–1049. [CrossRef]
237. Yuan, J.; Ni, G.; Wang, T.; Mounsey, K.; Cavezza, S.; Pan, X.; Liu, X. Genital warts treatment: Beyond imiquimod. *Hum. Vaccines Immunother.* **2018**, *14*, 1815–1819. [CrossRef]
238. Bilu, D.; Sauder, D.N. Imiquimod: Modes of action. *Br. J. Dermatol.* **2003**, *149* (Suppl. S66), 5–8. [CrossRef]
239. Daayana, S.; Elkord, E.; Winters, U.; Pawlita, M.; Roden, R.; Stern, P.L.; Kitchener, H.C. Phase II trial of imiquimod and HPV therapeutic vaccination in patients with vulval intraepithelial neoplasia. *Br. J. Cancer* **2010**, *102*, 1129–1136. [CrossRef]
240. Archambault, J.; Melendy, T. Targeting human papillomavirus genome replication for antiviral drug discovery. *Antivir. Ther.* **2013**, *18*, 271–283. [CrossRef]
241. Cundy, K.C. Clinical pharmacokinetics of the antiviral nucleotide analogues cidofovir and adefovir. *Clin. Pharmacokinet.* **1999**, *36*, 127–143. [CrossRef]
242. Johnson, J.A.; Gangemi, J.D. Selective inhibition of human papillomavirus-induced cell proliferation by (S)-1-[3-hydroxy-2-(phosphonylmethoxy)propyl]cytosine. *Antimicrob. Agents Chemother.* **1999**, *43*, 1198–1205. [CrossRef]
243. Abdulkarim, B.; Sabri, S.; Deutsch, E.; Chagraoui, H.; Maggiorella, L.; Thierry, J.; Eschwege, F.; Vainchenker, W.; Chouaib, S.; Bourhis, J. Antiviral agent Cidofovir restores p53 function and enhances the radiosensitivity in HPV-associated cancers. *Oncogene* **2002**, *21*, 2334–2346. [CrossRef]
244. Yang, J.; Dai, L.X.; Chen, M.; Li, B.; Ding, N.; Li, G.; Liu, Y.Q.; Li, M.Y.; Wang, B.N.; Shi, X.L.; et al. Inhibition of antiviral drug cidofovir on proliferation of human papillomavirus-infected cervical cancer cells. *Exp. Ther. Med.* **2016**, *12*, 2965–2973. [CrossRef]
245. Mertens, B.; Nogueira, T.; Stranska, R.; Naesens, L.; Andrei, G.; Snoeck, R. Cidofovir is active against human papillomavirus positive and negative head and neck and cervical tumor cells by causing DNA damage as one of its working mechanisms. *Oncotarget* **2016**, *7*, 47302–47318. [CrossRef]
246. Andrei, G.; Snoeck, R.; Piette, J.; Delvenne, P.; De Clercq, E. Inhibiting effects of cidofovir (HPMPC) on the growth of the human cervical carcinoma (SiHa) xenografts in athymic nude mice. *Oncol. Res.* **1998**, *10*, 533–539.
247. Van Pachterbeke, C.; Bucella, D.; Rozenberg, S.; Manigart, Y.; Gilles, C.; Larsimont, D.; Vanden Houte, K.; Reynders, M.; Snoeck, R.; Bossens, M. Topical treatment of CIN 2+ by cidofovir: Results of a phase II, double-blind, prospective, placebo-controlled study. *Gynecol. Oncol.* **2009**, *115*, 69–74. [CrossRef]
248. Deutsch, E.; Haie-Meder, C.; Bayar, M.A.; Mondini, M.; Laporte, M.; Mazeron, R.; Adam, J.; Varga, A.; Vassal, G.; Magne, N.; et al. Phase I trial evaluating the antiviral agent Cidofovir in combination with chemoradiation in cervical cancer patients. *Oncotarget* **2016**, *7*, 25549–25557. [CrossRef]
249. Wang, Y.; Coulombe, R.; Cameron, D.R.; Thauvette, L.; Massariol, M.J.; Amon, L.M.; Fink, D.; Titolo, S.; Welchner, E.; Yoakim, C.; et al. Crystal structure of the E2 transactivation domain of human papillomavirus type 11 bound to a protein interaction inhibitor. *J. Biol. Chem.* **2004**, *279*, 6976–6985. [CrossRef]
250. White, P.W.; Faucher, A.M.; Massariol, M.J.; Welchner, E.; Rancourt, J.; Cartier, M.; Archambault, J. Biphenylsulfonacetic acid inhibitors of the human papillomavirus type 6 E1 helicase inhibit ATP hydrolysis by an allosteric mechanism involving tyrosine 486. *Antimicrob. Agents Chemother.* **2005**, *49*, 4834–4842. [CrossRef]
251. Chen, J.; Gu, W.; Yang, L.; Chen, C.; Shao, R.; Xu, K.; Xu, Z.P. Nanotechnology in the management of cervical cancer. *Rev. Med. Virol.* **2015**, *25* (Suppl. S1), 72–83. [CrossRef] [PubMed]
252. Jain, K.K. Nanomedicine: Application of nanobiotechnology in medical practice. *Med. Princ. Pract.* **2008**, *17*, 89–101. [CrossRef] [PubMed]
253. Menon, I.; Bagwe, P.; Gomes, K.B.; Bajaj, L.; Gala, R.; Uddin, M.N.; D'Souza, M.J.; Zughaier, S.M. Microneedles: A New Generation Vaccine Delivery System. *Micromachines* **2021**, *12*, 435. [CrossRef] [PubMed]
254. Meyer, B.K.; Kendall, M.A.F.; Williams, D.M.; Bett, A.J.; Dubey, S.; Gentzel, R.C.; Casimiro, D.; Forster, A.; Corbett, H.; Crichton, M.; et al. Immune response and reactogenicity of an unadjuvated intradermally delivered human papillomavirus vaccine using a first generation Nanopatch in rhesus macaques: An exploratory, pre-clinical feasibility assessment. *Vaccine X* **2019**, *2*, 100030. [CrossRef] [PubMed]
255. Yang, J.; Li, S.; Guo, F.; Zhang, W.; Wang, Y.; Pan, Y. Induction of apoptosis by chitosan/HPV16 E7 siRNA complexes in cervical cancer cells. *Mol. Med. Rep.* **2013**, *7*, 998–1002. [CrossRef] [PubMed]
256. Saengkrit, N.; Sanitrum, P.; Woramongkolchai, N.; Saesoo, S.; Pimpha, N.; Chaleawlert-Umpon, S.; Tencomnao, T.; Puttipipatkhachorn, S. The PEI-introduced CS shell/PMMA core nanoparticle for silencing the expression of E6/E7 oncogenes in human cervical cells. *Carbohydr. Polym.* **2012**, *90*, 1323–1329. [CrossRef]
257. Xu, C.; Liu, W.; Hu, Y.; Li, W.; Di, W. Bioinspired tumor-homing nanoplatform for co-delivery of paclitaxel and siRNA-E7 to HPV-related cervical malignancies for synergistic therapy. *Theranostics* **2020**, *10*, 3325–3339. [CrossRef]

MDPI
St. Alban-Anlage 66
4052 Basel
Switzerland
www.mdpi.com

MDPI Books Editorial Office
E-mail: books@mdpi.com
www.mdpi.com/books

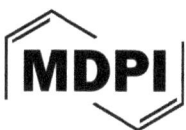

Disclaimer/Publisher's Note: The statements, opinions and data contained in all publications are solely those of the individual author(s) and contributor(s) and not of MDPI and/or the editor(s). MDPI and/or the editor(s) disclaim responsibility for any injury to people or property resulting from any ideas, methods, instructions or products referred to in the content.

www.ingramcontent.com/pod-product-compliance
Lightning Source LLC
LaVergne TN
LVHW070126100526
838202LV00016B/2239